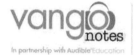
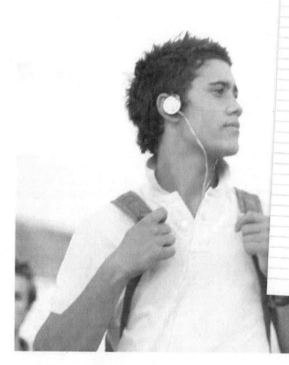

Prentice Hall Nursing Reviews & Rationales

Pathophysiology

Second Edition

Series Editor

Mary Ann Hogan, MSN, RN

Clinical Assistant Professor
University of Massachusetts–Amherst
Amherst, Massachusetts

Consulting Editors

Marcia Bower, CS, MSN, RN, CRNP

Assistant Professor
Holy Family University
Newton, Pennsylvania

Karen Hill, RN, MSN, PhD

Associate Professor
Southeastern Louisiana University
Hammond, Louisana

Kathleen S. Holm, RN, MSN, CNRN, FAAPM

Nursing Instructor
Reading Area Community College
Reading, Pennsylvania

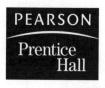

PEARSON
Prentice
Hall

Upper Saddle River, New Jersey 07458

Library of Congress Cataloging-in-Publication Data
Hogan, Mary Ann
Pathophysiology / Mary Ann Hogan
   p. ; cm. — (Prentice Hall nursing reviews & rationales)
   Rev. ed. of Pathophysiology / [edited by] Mary Ann
Hogan, Karen Hill
   Includes bibliographical references and index.
    ISBN-13: 978-0-13-178972-2
    ISBN-10: 0-13-178972-4
   1. Physiology, pathological—Outlines, syllabi, etc.
2. Nursing—Outlines, syllabi, etc.
    [DLNM: 1. Nursing Assessment—methods—Outlines.
2. Pathology—Outlines. WY 18.2 H714p 2008]
   RC113 .H625 2008
   616.07—dc21
                             2007104995

Notice: Care has been taken to confirm the accuracy of the information presented in this book. The authors, editors, and the publisher, however, cannot accept any responsibility for errors or omissions or for the consequences for application of the information in this book and make no warranty, express or implied, with respect to its contents.

The authors and the publisher have exerted every effort to ensure that drug selections and dosages set forth in this text are in accord with current recommendations and practice at time of publication. However, in view of ongoing research, changes in government regulations, and the constant flow of information relating to drug therapy and drug reactions, the reader is urged to check the package inserts of all drugs for any change in indications of dosage and for added warnings and precautions. This is particularly important when the recommended agent is a new and/or infrequently employed drug.

The authors and publisher disclaim all responsibility for any liability, loss, injury, or damage incurred as a consequence, directly or indirectly, of the use and application of any of the contents of this volume.

Publisher: Julie Levin Alexander
Assistant to Publisher: Regina Bruno
Editor-in-Chief: Maura Connor
Editorial Assistant: Marion Gottlieb
Developmental Editor: Danielle Doller
Managing Editor, Production: Patrick Walsh
Production Liaison: Anne Garcia
Production Editor: Jessica Balch, Pine Tree Composition
Manufacturing Manager: Ilene Sanford
Manufacturing Buyer: Pat Brown

Design Coordinator/Cover Designer: Mary Siener
Director of Marketing: Karen Allman
Senior Marketing Manager: Francisco Del Castillo
Marketing Coordinator: Michael Sirinides
Marketing Assistant: Anca David
Media Product Manager: John Jordan
New Media Project Manager: Stephen Hartner
Composition: Pine Tree Composition, Inc.
Printer/Binder: Courier Westford
Cover Printer: Phoenix Color Corp.

Pearson Prentice Hall™ is a trademark of Pearson Education, Inc.
Pearson® is a registered trademark of Pearson plc.
Prentice Hall® is a registered trademark of Pearson Education, Inc.

Pearson Education Ltd., *London*
Pearson Education Australia Pty. Limited, *Sydney*
Pearson Education Singapore, Pte. Ltd.
Pearson Education North Asia Ltd., *Hong Kong*
Pearson Education Canada, Ltd., *Toronto*

Pearson Educación de Mexico, S.A. de C.V.
Pearson Education—Japan, *Tokyo*
Pearson Education Malaysia, Pte. Ltd.
Pearson Education, Upper Saddle River, New Jersey

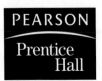

10 9 8 7 6 5 4 3 2
ISBN-13: 978-0-13-178972-2
ISBN-10:   0-13-178972-4
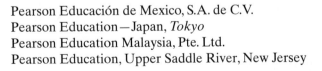

Contents

Welcome to the Prentice Hall Nursing Reviews & Rationales Series!

This series has been specifically designed to provide a clear and concentrated review of important nursing knowledge in the following content areas:

- Anatomy & Physiology
- Nursing Fundamentals
- Nutrition & Diet Therapy
- Fluids, Electrolytes, & Acid-Base Balance
- Medical-Surgical Nursing
- Pathophysiology
- Pharmacology
- Maternal-Newborn Nursing
- Child Health Nursing
- Mental Health Nursing
- Physical Assessment
- Community Health Nursing
- Leadership & Management

The books in this series are designed for use either by current nursing students as a study aid for nursing course work, for NCLEX-RN® licensing exam preparation, or by practicing nurses seeking a comprehensive yet concise review of a nursing specialty or subject area.

This series is truly unique. One of its most special features is that it has been developed and reviewed by a large team of nurse educators from across the United States and Canada to ensure that each chapter is edited by a nurse expert in the content area under study. The series editor, Mary Ann Hogan, designed the overall series in collaboration with a core Prentice Hall team to take full advantage of Prentice Hall's cutting-edge technology. The consulting editors for each book, also experts in that specialty area, then reviewed all chapters and test questions submitted for comprehensiveness and accuracy. Finally, Mary Ann Hogan reviewed the chapters in each book for consistency, accuracy, and applicability to the NCLEX-RN® Test Plan.

All books in the series are identical in their overall design for your convenience. As an added value, each book comes with a comprehensive support package, including a bonus **NCLEX-RN® Test Prep** CD-ROM and a tear-out **NursingNotes** card for clinical reference and quick review.

Study Tips

Use of this book should help simplify your review. To make the most of your valuable study time, also follow these simple but important suggestions:

1. Use a weekly calendar to schedule study sessions.
   - Outline the timeframes for all of your activities (home, school, appointments, etc.) on a weekly calendar.
   - Find the "holes" in your calendar, which are the times in which you can plan to study. Add study sessions to the calendar at times when you can expect to be mentally alert and follow it!
2. Create the optimal study environment.
   - Eliminate external sources of distraction, such as television, telephone, etc.
   - Eliminate internal sources of distraction, such as hunger, thirst, or dwelling on items or problems that cannot be worked on at the moment.
   - Take a break for 10 minutes or so after each hour of concentrated study both as a reward and an incentive to keep studying.
3. Use pre-reading strategies to increase comprehension of chapter material.
   - Skim read the headings in the chapter (because they identify chapter content).
   - Read the definitions of key terms, which will help you learn new words to comprehend chapter information.

- Review all graphic aids (figures, tables, boxes) because they are often used to explain important points in the chapter.
4. Read the chapter thoroughly but at a reasonable speed.
   - Comprehension and retention are actually enhanced by not reading too slowly.
   - Do take the time to reread any section that is unclear to you.
5. Summarize what you have learned.
   - Use questions supplied with this book and the *NCLEX-RN® Test Prep* CD-ROM to test your application of chapter content.
   - Review again any sections that correspond to questions you answered incorrectly or incompletely.

Test-Taking Strategies

We added new test-taking strategies to the rationales for every question in the series. These strategies will enable you to select the correct answer by breaking down the question, even if you don't know the correct response. Use the following strategies to increase your success on nursing tests or examinations:

- Get sufficient sleep and have something to eat before taking a test. Take deep breaths during the test as needed. Remember, the brain requires oxygen and glucose as fuel. Avoid concentrated sweets before a test, however, to avoid rapid upward and then downward surges in blood glucose levels.
- Read the question carefully, identifying the stem, the 4 options, and any key words or phrases in either the stem or options.
  - Key words in the stem such as "most important" indicate the need to set priorities, since more than one option is likely to contain a statement that is technically correct.
  - Remember that the presence of absolute words such as "never" or "only" in an answer option is more likely to make that option incorrect.
- Determine who is the client in the question; often this is the person with the health problem, but it may also be a significant other, relative, friend, or another nurse.
- Decide whether the stem is a true response stem or a false response stem. With a true response stem, the correct answer will be a true statement, and vice-versa.

- Determine what the question is really asking, sometimes referred to as the issue of the question. Evaluate all answer options in relation to this issue, and not strictly to the "correctness" of the statement in each individual option.
- Eliminate options that are obviously incorrect, then go back and reread the stem. Evaluate the remaining options against the stem once more.
- If two answers seem similar and correct, try to decide whether one of them is more global or comprehensive. If the global option includes the alternative option within it, it is likely that the more global response is the correct answer.

The NCLEX-RN® Licensing Examination

The NCLEX-RN® licensing examination is a Computer Adaptive Test (CAT) that ranges in length from 75 to 265 individual (stand-alone) test items, depending on individual performance during the examination. Upon graduation from a nursing program, successful completion of this exam is the gateway to your professional nursing practice. The blueprint for the exam is reviewed and revised every three years by the National Council of State Boards of Nursing according to the results of a job analysis study of new graduate nurses practicing within the first six months after graduation. Each question on the exam is coded to a *Client Need Category* and an *Integrated Process*.

Client Need Categories. There are 4 categories of client needs, and each exam will contain a minimum and maximum percent of questions from each category. Each major category has subcategories within it. The *Client Needs* categories according to the NCLEX-RN® Test Plan effective April 2007 are as follows:

- Safe, Effective Care Environment
  - Management of Care (13–19%)
  - Safety and Infection Control (8–14%)
- Health Promotion and Maintenance (6–12%)
- Psychosocial Integrity (6–12%)
- Physiological Integrity
  - Basic Care and Comfort (6–12%)
  - Pharmacological and Parenteral Therapies (13–19%)
  - Reduction of Risk Potential (13–19%)
  - Physiological Adaptation (11–17%)

Integrated Processes. The integrated processes identified on the NCLEX-RN® Test Plan effective April 2007, with condensed definitions, are as follows:

- Nursing Process: a scientific problem-solving approach used in nursing practice; consisting of assessment, analysis, planning, implementation, and evaluation.
- Caring: client-nurse interaction(s) characterized by mutual respect and trust and that are directed toward achieving desired client outcomes.
- Communication and Documentation: verbal and/or nonverbal interactions between nurse and others (client, family, health care team); a written or electronic recording of activities or events that occur during client care.

- Teaching and Learning: facilitating client's acquisition of knowledge, skills, and attitudes that lead to behavior change

More detailed information about this examination may be obtained by visiting the National Council of State Boards of Nursing website at http://www.ncsbn.org and viewing the *NCLEX-RN® Examination Test Plan for the National Council Licensure Examination for Registered Nurses.*[1]

[1]Reference: National Council of State Boards of Nursing, Inc. *NCLEX Examination Test Plan for National Council Licensure Examination for Registered Nurses.* Effective April, 2007. Retrieved from the World Wide Web at http://www.ncsbn.org/RN_Test_Plan_2007_Web.pdf.

HOW TO GET THE MOST OUT OF THIS BOOK

Each chapter has the following elements to guide you during review and study:

Chapter Objectives describe what you will be able to know or do after learning the material covered in the chapter.

Objectives

➤ Discuss legal considerations related to maternity nursing.

➤ Delineate ethical issues that influence maternal-newborn nursing practice.

➤ Identify culturally diverse health beliefs that impact the maternity cycle.

➤ Describe a philosophy of care that maintains maternal–newborn safety and fosters family unity.

NCLEX-RN® Test Prep

Use the CD-ROM enclosed with this book to access additional practice opportunities.

Review at a Glance contains a glossary of key terms used in the chapter, with definitions provided up-front and available at your fingertips, to help you stay focused and make the best use of your study time.

Review at a Glance

belief something accepted as true, especially as a tenet or a body of tenets accepted by an ethnocultural group

cultural competency the awareness, knowledge and skills necessary to appreciate, understand and communicate with people of diverse cultural backgrounds

family a group of individuals related by blood, marriage, or mutual goals

family-centered maternity care maternity care that is family oriented and views childbirth as a vital, natural life event rather than an illness

scope of practice legally refers to permissible boundaries of practice for nurses and is defined by statute (written law), rules and regulations, or a combination of the two

Pretest provides a 10-question quiz as a sample overview of the material covered in the chapter and helps you decide in what areas you need the most—or the least—review.

PRETEST

1 The nurse performs a vaginal examination and determines that the fetus is in a sacrum anterior position. The nurse draws which conclusion from this assessment data?

1. The fetal sacrum is toward the maternal symphysis pubis.
2. The fetal sacrum is toward the maternal sacrum.
3. The fetal face is toward the maternal sacrum.
4. The fetal face is toward the maternal symphysis pubis.

Practice to Pass questions are open-ended, stimulate critical thinking, and reinforce mastery of the chapter information.

▶ *Practice to Pass*

The client scheduled for a hysterosalpingogram reports an allergy to shellfish. What should the nurse do?

!

NCLEX Alert identifies concepts that are likely to be tested on the NCLEX-RN® examination. Be sure to learn the information highlighted wherever you see this icon.

Case Study, found at the end of the chapter, provides an opportunity for you to use your critical thinking and clinical reasoning skills to "put it all together." It describes a true-to-life client case situation and asks you open-ended questions about how you would provide care for that client and/or family.

Case Study

A 14-year-old primigravida is admitted in early labor with severe preeclampsia at 42 weeks gestation. The client's blood pressure is 168/102.

1. What other assessment data would you obtain?
2. Describe the complications this client is at risk for.
3. Discuss the medications you expect to administer to this client.
4. What concerns do you have for this fetus? Why?
5. What would you teach this client and her family about her condition?

For suggested responses, see page 343.

Posttest provides an additional 10-question quiz at the end of the chapter. It provides you with feedback about mastery of the chapter material following review and study. All pretest and posttest questions contain comprehensive rationales for the correct and incorrect answers, and are coded according to cognitive level of difficulty, NCLEX-RN® Test Plan category of client need and integrated process.

POSTTEST

1 A client who is a brittle diabetic is seeking to get pregnant. The nursing working in a primary care provider's office suggests that which of the following healthcare providers would be an optimal choice?

1. A certified nurse-midwife
2. A family nurse practitioner
3. An obstetrician
4. A maternal-fetal medicine specialist

NCLEX-RN® Test Prep CD-ROM

For those who want to practice taking tests on a computer, the CD-ROM that accompanies the book contains the pretest and posttest questions found in all chapters of the book. In addition, it contains 30 NEW questions for each chapter to help you further evaluate your knowledge base and hone your test-taking skills. We included some of the newly developed alternate NCLEX Test Items, so these items will give you valuable practice with different types of questions.

Prentice Hall NursingNotes Card

This tear-out card provides a reference for frequently used facts and information related to the subject matter of the book. These are designed to be useful in the clinical setting, when quick and easy access to information is so important!

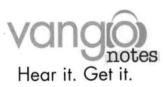

VangoNotes

Study on the go with VangoNotes. Just download chapter reviews from your text and listen to them on any mp3 player. Now wherever you are—whatever you're doing—you can study by listening to the following for each chapter of your textbook:

- **Big Ideas:** Your "need to know" for each chapter
- **Practice Test:** A gut check for the Big Ideas—tells you if you need to keep studying
- **Key Terms:** Audio "flashcards" to help you review key concepts and terms

VangoNotes are **flexible;** download all the material directly to your player, or only the chapters you need. And they're **efficient.** Use them in your car, at the gym, walking to class, wherever. So get yours today. And get studying.

About the Pathophysiology Book

Chapters in this book cover "need-to-know" information about pathophysiology of a wide variety of health problems. They include health problems that relate to the respiratory, cardiovascular, neurological, musculoskeletal, gastrointestinal, endocrine, renal, reproductive, and integumentary systems. Other chapters address immunological, hematological, oncological, and infectious health problems. Finally, the last two chapters review two unique areas, genetically transmitted health problems and multisystem health problems. Mastery of the information in this book and effective use of the test-taking strategies described will help the student be confident and successful in testing situations, including the NCLEX-RN®, and in actual clinical practice.

Acknowledgements

This book is a monumental effort of collaboration. Without the contributions of many individuals, this edition of *Pathophysiology: Reviews and Rationales* would not have been possible. Thank you to all the contributors and reviewers who devoted their time and talents to the previous edition of this book. Their work will surely assist both students and practicing nurses alike to extend their knowledge in the area of pathophysiology.

I owe a special debt of gratitude to the wonderful team at Prentice Hall Nursing for their enthusiasm for this project, as well as their good humor, expertise, and encouragement as the series developed. Maura Connor, Editor-in-Chief for Nursing, was unending in her creativity, support, encouragement, and belief in the need for this series. Danielle Doller, Developmental Editor, devoted many long hours to coordinating different facets of this project, and tirelessly and cheerfully encouraged our efforts as well. Her high standards and attention to detail contributed greatly to the final "look" of this series. Editorial Assistant, Marion Gottlieb, helped to keep the project moving forward on a day-to-day basis, and I am grateful for her efforts as well. A very special thank you goes to the designers of the book and the production team, led by Anne Garcia, Production Editor, and Mary Siener, Designer, who brought the ideas and manuscript into final form.

Thank you to the team at Pine Tree Composition, led by Project Coordinator Jessica Balch, for the detail-oriented work of creating this book. I greatly appreciate their hard work, attention to detail, and spirit of collaboration.

Finally, I would like to acknowledge and gratefully thank my children, who donated time that would have been spent with them, to bring this book to publication. Their love and support kept me energized and motivated.

Mary Ann Hogan

Contributors and Reviewers of the First Edition

Contributors

Karen Hill, PhD, RN
Associate Professor
Southern Louisiana University
Hammond, Louisiana
Consulting Editor; Chapter 1

Julie A. Adkins, RN, MSN, FNP
Family Nurse Practitioner
West Frankfort, Illinois
Chapters 10 and 14

Jana G. Brannan, MN, RN, CNAA
Assistant Professor
Louisiana State University Health
  Science Center
New Orleans, Louisiana
Chapter 17

Carol D. Clark, MS, RN, ANP, GNPC
Associate Professor
Indiana Wesleyan University
Marion, Indiana
Chapter 8

Cathy Cormier, MN, RN, C
Instructor
Southeastern Louisiana University
Hammond, Louisiana
Chapter 5

Mical DeBrow, PhD, RN
Vice President/Healthcare Services
Gulf South Health Plans
Baton Rouge, Louisiana
Chapter 12

Joseann Helmes DeWitt, MSN, RN, C, CLNC
Assistant Professor
Alcorn State University School of
  Nursing
Natchez, Mississippi
Chapter 9

Lynn H. Doyle, RN, MS, CPNP
Assistant Professor Pediatrics
Marian College
Fond du Lac, Wisconsin
Chapter 16

Pam Hamre, RN, MS, CNM
Assistant Professor
College of St. Catherine
St. Paul, Minnesota
Chapter 11

Ann Harley, EdD, RN
Professor
Carson Newman College
Jefferson City, Tennessee
Chapter 3

Sherry Hendrickson, RN, PhD, CS
Assistant Professor of Clinical
  Nursing
The University of Texas at Austin
Austin, Texas
Chapter 4

Barbara Moffett, PhD, RN
Professor
Southeastern Louisiana University
Hammond, Louisiana
Chapter 13

Patsy Rider, RN, MSN, CS
Instructor
The University of Texas at Austin
Austin, Texas
Chapter 4

Diane E. Smith, MSN, RN
Assistant Professor
Baton Rouge, Louisiana
Chapter 6

Susan K. Steele, MN, RN, AOCN
Oncology Clinical Nurse Specialist/
  Assistant Professor
Louisiana State University Health
  Science Center
New Orleans, Louisiana
Chapter 15

Betty Jane Sylvest, BSN, RN, MSN
Instructor
University of Southern Mississippi
Hattiesburg, Mississippi
Chapter 2

Eugenia H. Tickle, RN, MSN, EdD
Associate Professor
Midwestern State University
Wichita Falls, Texas
Chapter 7

Reviewers

Janie Butts, DSN, RN
Assistant Professor
University of Southern Mississippi
Hattiesburg, Mississippi

Christine A. Cannon, RN, PhD
Associate Professor
University of Delaware
Newark, Delaware

Linda Covington, PhD
Associate Professor
Middle Tennessee State University
Murfreesboro, Tennessee

Barbara Daniel, MEd, MS, CRNP
Professor
Cecil Community College
North East, Maryland

Ann M. Findley, PhD
Associate Professor
Department of Biology
University of Louisiana at Monroe
Monroe, Louisiana

Diane Ford, RN, MS, FNP, CS
Assistant Professor
Andrews University
Berrien Springs, Michigan

Wanda Gifford, RN, MSN, CS, FNP
Family Nurse Practitioner/
   Instructor
St. Josephs College
Rensselaer, Indiana

Sandra Smith Huddleston, RN, PhD
Associate Professor
Berea College
Berea, Kentucky

Robin Kirschner, RN, MA, CPAN
Professor
Scottsdale Community College
Scottsdale, Arizona

Jane Koeckeritz, RN, PhD
Professor
University of Northern Colorado
Greeley, Colorado

James A. Metcalf, PhD
Professor
George Mason University
Fairfax, Virginia

Mercy Mammah Popoola, RN, CNS, PhD
Professor
Georgia Southern University
Statesboro, Georgia

Elizabeth Ann Rettew, MSN, RN, FNP-BC
Associate Professor
Malone College
Canton, Ohio

Respiratory Health Problems

1

Chapter Outline

Risk Factors Associated with Respiratory Health Problems

Obstructive Pulmonary Disorders

Restrictive Pulmonary Disorders

Pneumonia

Pulmonary Tuberculosis (TB)

Pleural Effusion

Pleuritis (Pleurisy)

Pneumothorax/Hemothorax

Pulmonary Embolism (PE)

Pulmonary Hypertension

Lung Cancer

Respiratory Failure

Objectives

➤ Define key terms associated with respiratory health problems.

➤ Identify risk factors associated with the development of respiratory health problems.

➤ Explain the common etiologies of respiratory health problems.

➤ Describe the pathophysiologic processes associated with specific respiratory health problems.

➤ Distinguish between normal and abnormal respiratory findings obtained from nursing assessment.

➤ Prioritize nursing interventions associated with specific respiratory health problems.

NCLEX-RN® Test Prep

Use the CD-ROM enclosed with this book to access additional practice opportunities.

Review at a Glance

asthma *an obstructive airflow disorder where narrowing and inflammation of airways cause respiratory distress*

atelectasis *collapse of a portion of lung with limited gas exchange*

bronchiectasis *an irreversible state of bronchial dilation and destruction of bronchial walls*

bronchitis *inflammation of mucous membranes of bronchial airways; another term for chronic bronchitis is "blue bloater" because of hypoxemia that leads to cyanosis*

chronic obstructive pulmonary disease (COPD) *a group of pulmonary diseases involving obstruction of airflow that is chronic and recurrent, usually associated with asthma, emphysema, and bronchitis*

cor pulmonale *a disorder manifested by hypertrophy of right ventricle caused by pulmonary hypertension; manifests as right heart failure*

cystic fibrosis (CF) *autosomal recessive disease of exocrine glands that manifests itself in multiple organs, char-*

acterized by excess production of mucus and COPD in early childhood

emphysema *a chronic disorder of lungs resulting in overinflation of air spaces, loss of elasticity and decreased gas exchange; another term for chronic emphysema is "pink puffer" because client does not become cyanotic until end stages of disease*

flail chest *instability of chest wall usually caused by trauma or fractured ribs with a reverse in chest wall movement from normal; chest wall contracts on inspiration and expands outward on expiration*

hemothorax *collection of blood or fluid in pleural space*

obstructive pulmonary disorders *any respiratory disorder where airflow is hindered to lungs, may be chronic or acute*

pleural effusion *increased accumulation of fluid between visceral and parietal pleura of lung*

pleuritis *inflammation of parietal space of lungs, also known as pleurisy*

pneumonia *inflammation of lungs caused by bacteria, viruses, fungi, or other pathogens*

pneumothorax *collapse of a portion or all of lung due to trapping of air in pleural space*

pulmonary embolism *blockage of a pulmonary artery by an embolus of fat, blood, or other foreign products*

pulmonary hypertension *a sustained elevation of pulmonary artery pressure, greater than 20 mmHg*

restrictive pulmonary disorders *any disease that limits expansion of lungs or chest wall movement*

sleep apnea *having periods of delay or lack of breathing (usually longer than 10 seconds) during sleep*

status asthmaticus *an acute emergency of a prolonged or repetitive asthma attack*

tuberculosis (TB) *infection of lung with an acid-fast bacillus, Mycobacterium tuberculosis*

PRETEST

1 A 67-year-old male client has chronic respiratory acidosis caused by end-stage chronic obstructive pulmonary disease (COPD). Oxygen is delivered at 1 L/min per nasal cannula. Which statement by the nurse best explains to the client's daughter how this therapy prevents respiratory depression?

1. "Your father's breathing effort is driven by lower oxygen levels."
2. "Your father's breathing effort is driven by a low carbon dioxide level."
3. "Your father will retain metabolic acids if the oxygen level is too high."
4. "Your father will breathe best when he has a moderately high oxygen level."

2 A client presents to the Emergency Department with acute respiratory distress and the following arterial blood gases (ABGs): pH 7.35, PCO_2 40 mmHg, PO_2 63 mmHg, HCO_3 23 mEq/L, and oxygen saturation (SaO_2) 93%. The nurse concludes that which of the following represents the best analysis of the etiology of these ABGs?

1. Tuberculosis (TB)
2. Pneumonia
3. Pleural effusion
4. Hypoxia

3 When assessing a client with early impairment of oxygen perfusion from pulmonary embolus, the nurse would expect to find restlessness, dyspnea, and which of the following symptoms?

1. Warm, dry skin
2. Bradycardia
3. Tachycardia
4. Eupnea

4 One day postoperative, the client reports shortness of breath. The respiratory rate (RR) is 35 and slightly labored, and there are no breath sounds in the lower-right base. The nurse would suspect which of the following?

1. Cor pulmonale
2. Atelectasis
3. Pulmonary embolus
4. Cardiac tamponade

5 A client with an acute case of pneumonia has a dry, hacking cough, temperature of 100.6° F, white blood cell (WBC) count of 12,000/mm³, decreased breath sounds, and pain upon deep inhalation or coughing. Which of the following would indicate positive results after a respiratory treatment of normal saline, acetylcysteine (Mucomyst), and albuterol (Proventil)? Select all that apply.

1. Reduced crackles and moderate amount of productive sputum
2. Absent breath sounds in bases and normal breath sounds in upper lobes
3. Wheezing, nonproductive cough
4. Increased coughing but with thinner and easier to expectorate sputum
5. Reduced anxiety and verbalization of improved ability to breathe

6 The nurse prioritizes that which of the following clients needs *immediate* medical attention and emergency intervention?

1. Client reporting sharp pain upon taking a deep breath and excessive coughing
2. Client exhibiting yellow, productive sputum, low-grade fever, and crackles
3. Client with a shift of the trachea to the left, with no breath sounds on the right
4. Client with asthma reporting inability to "catch her breath" after exercise

7 A teenage client newly diagnosed with asthma is being discharged from the hospital after an episode of status asthmaticus. The nurse should include which of the following in discharge teaching?

1. Incidence of status asthmaticus in children and teens
2. Relationship of symptoms to a specific trigger such as physical exercise
3. Limitations in sports that will be imposed by the illness
4. Specific instructions on staying calm during an attack

8 A known cardiac client is experiencing angina at night only, excessive fatigue, and according to the spouse, the client snores excessively. The physician orders a sleep apnea study with and without oxygen. The nurse explains to the client's spouse, who is also a nurse, that a pulmonary source of these symptoms is being investigated at this time for which reason?

1. Sleep apnea is an obstruction of the lower airway that impedes airflow.
2. Clients with sleep apnea have adequate amounts of REM sleep, but snoring contributes to the decrease in oxygen levels.
3. Sleep apnea causes an increase in muscle tone during REM sleep in order to make breathing possible.
4. Excess periods of apnea during sleep and severe drops in oxygen levels can contribute to the angina, which is occurring only at night.

9 The nurse anticipates that a client admitted with newly diagnosed lung cancer would exhibit which of the following most characteristic manifestations?

1. Exertional dyspnea
2. Persistent changing cough
3. Air hunger; dyspnea
4. Cough with night sweats

10 A client is admitted to the nursing unit after being speared by a bull in the right chest wall while repairing a fence in a pasture. The client is diagnosed with a flail chest, and a chest tube is inserted. Which of the following observations indicate that the chest tube is working properly? Select all that apply.

1. Frequent or constant bubbles with decreased breath sounds
2. Fluctuation of the water seal level with respirations
3. Lack of fluctuation and bubbles in the water seal chamber after several days
4. Occasional bubbles in the water seal compartment
5. Collection chamber completely filled with fluid from the pleural space

➤ *See pages 33–35 for Answers & Rationales.*

I. RISK FACTORS ASSOCIATED WITH RESPIRATORY HEALTH PROBLEMS

A. **Obstructive pulmonary disorders** such as asthma, chronic obstructive pulmonary disease (COPD), cystic fibrosis, bronchitis

1. Asthma: allergies, genetic disposition
2. COPD: primarily smoking, exposure to lung irritants, immunological factors
3. Cystic fibrosis: genetic transmission
4. Bronchitis: smoking, exposure to pulmonary irritants, air pollution, exposure to infectious diseases

B. **Restrictive pulmonary disorders** such as atelectasis, acute respiratory distress syndrome (ARDS), flail chest, pulmonary contusion, and sleep apnea

1. Atelectasis: surgery, trauma, pneumonia or other respiratory disorders (COPD), prolonged bedrest, mechanical ventilation
2. ARDS: shock, trauma, smoke inhalation, any cardiac or respiratory event, often unknown; see also Chapter 17
3. Sleep apnea: obesity, COPD, smoking, aging process

C. **Pneumonia:** aging process, compromised respiratory conditions, debilitating diseases, lack of vaccine in at-risk individuals

D. **Tuberculosis:** individuals positive for human immunodeficiency virus (HIV), immigrants and disadvantaged groups, environment (overcrowding, poor ventilation, etc.)

E. **Pleural effusion:** surgery, trauma, inflammation, malignancy, or other respiratory disorder

F. **Pleuritis:** none, usually secondary to other respiratory conditions

G. **Pneumothorax:** smoking, trauma, men (tall, young, thin chest), family history, underlying respiratory diseases (COPD, ARDS, cystic fibrosis, asthma)

H. **Pulmonary embolism:** deep vein thrombosis (DVT) or blood clots in other areas, chronic bedrest, hypercoagulability, surgery, heart conditions (congestive heart failure [CHF], myocardial infarction [MI]), obesity, women taking oral estrogen, hormones, or contraceptives

I. **Pulmonary hypertension:** young women in their 30s to 40s (primary); smoking, chronic lung disease, sleep apnea, obesity, neuromuscular disease, heart conditions leading to hypoxemia (secondary)

J. **Lung cancer:** smoking, lung irritants, family history, air pollution

K. **Respiratory failure:** other respiratory conditions or respiratory dysfunction (COPD, pneumonia)

II. OBSTRUCTIVE PULMONARY DISORDERS

A. Overview

1. Obstructive pulmonary disorders are defined as disorders that obstruct airflow out of lung, primarily impeding expiration
2. Disorders include asthma, emphysema, cystic fibrosis, and bronchiectasis
3. Causes include infection, air pollutants, allergies, smoke inhalation, or genetics

B. Pathophysiology

1. **Asthma** is a chronic inflammatory disorder of airways resulting in reversible bronchoconstriction and air hunger in response to triggers from a variety of sources

   a. This disorder primarily affects bronchial airways and causes mucosal edema, secretion of mucus, and inflammation of airway

   b. When exposed to a trigger, hyperactivity of medium-sized bronchi causes release of leukotrienes, histamine, and other substances from mast cells of lungs; these agents intensify the inflammatory process and cause bronchospasm

   c. *Extrinsic asthma* is triggered by factors such as cold air, high altitude, strong odors, emotional stress, hormone changes, allergens, and exercise

   d. *Intrinsic asthma* is usually from an unknown cause; affects individuals usually after age 40

   e. **Status asthmaticus** is an emergency situation when an asthma attack is prolonged and not responding to usual medications or client is having one asthma attack after another; prompt treatment of this condition is needed to avoid respiratory failure

2. **Chronic obstructive pulmonary disease (COPD)** is a group of pulmonary diseases of a chronic nature characterized by increased resistance to airflow; consists of emphysema, bronchitis, and possibly asthma

   a. **Emphysema** is a break down of the elastin and fiber network of alveoli where the alveoli enlarge or walls are destroyed; alveolar destruction leads to formation of larger than normal air spaces

      1) There is loss of elastic recoil as a result of destruction of elastin and collagen fibers found in lungs; without this recoil, air is trapped in lungs and airways collapse

      2) Air trapping results in hyperinflated lungs, causing a "barrel chest" appearance

      3) The person is able to maintain blood gases by hyperventilating and keeps a pink appearance to skin, thus known as a "pink puffer" early in disease; cyanosis may develop in late stages

   b. Chronic **bronchitis** is an inflammatory response in small and large airways resulting in vasodilation, congestion, mucosal edema, and bronchospasm; a chronic cough and productive sputum for a minimum of 3 months in 1 year for at least 2 consecutive years is the usual method of diagnosis

      1) Bronchial mucosal glands hypertrophy and there is an increase in the number and size of goblet cells accompanied by inflammatory cell infiltration and edema of bronchial mucosa

      2) As bronchial walls thicken, airflow is impeded

      3) Unlike emphysema, an individual with bronchitis cannot increase breathing efforts to maintain blood gases

      4) The presence of cyanosis and edema gives a client with bronchitis a description of "blue bloater"

      5) In the presence of severe chronic hypoxia, the kidneys increase production of red blood cells (RBCs) in an attempt to bring more oxygenated blood to cells, causing polycythemia, increased blood viscosity, and a higher risk for blood clots

    c. Hypercapnia is typical of a client with COPD along with hypoxemia

        1) Arterial blood gases (ABGs) reflect a high carbon dioxide (CO_2) and a low oxygen (O_2)

        2) Therefore, hypoxia is the main stimulus for ventilation rather than the normal increase in CO_2 as a stimulus to breathe

        3) Clients with COPD cannot tolerate high levels of O_2

        4) Hypoxia alone is usually indicated by a partial pressure of arterial O_2 (PaO_2) less than 80 mmHg combined with a low O_2 saturation (SaO_2) (see Box 1-1)

    d. Nailbeds demonstrate clubbing (angle > 160°) or a more flattened, yellow appearance because of chronic hypoxia

  3. Cystic fibrosis (CF) is an autosomal-recessive disorder resulting in excessive production of mucus with chronic obstructive pulmonary disease in early childhood

    a. The lack of a necessary protein needed to transport chloride results in excess absorption of water and sodium

    b. The organs, primarily the lungs, in which this protein is absent, and the deficiency in transporting chloride results in thick, viscous mucous

    c. Because of sodium reabsorption, sweat will have high levels of sodium and chloride

    d. Excess mucus leads to atelectasis, infections, bronchiectasis, and eventually pulmonary hypertension, and **cor pulmonale** (right-sided heart failure due to pulmonary causes)

    e. In older children, the pancreas fails to function properly leading to malabsorption problems and difficulty digesting foods because of a lack of pancreatic enzymes

  4. Bronchiectasis is a permanent enlargement of large bronchi, often associated with respiratory infections

    a. A combination of infection and airway obstruction from this disorder leads to atelectasis, abscesses, destruction, and necrosis of bronchial wall

    b. Usually associated with cystic fibrosis, but can be related to tumors, foreign bodies, tuberculosis, or exposure to lung irritants

    c. Manifested by permanently deformed and dilated distal airways, damage to cartilage and elastic tissue supporting the airways, and fibrosis

C. Nursing assessment

  1. Asthma

    a. Assessment includes complaints of air hunger and chest tightness, anxiety, use of accessory muscles, tachypnea (increased respiratory rate), tachycardia (increased heart rate), and lung sounds (wheezing, long expiratory effort, diminished breath sounds in lower airways)

Box 1-1		
Normal Adult Arterial Blood Gas Values	pH	7.35–7.45
	$PaCO_2$	35–45 mmHg
	PaO_2	80–100 mmHg
	HCO_3^-	21–28 mEq/L
	O_2 saturation (SaO_2)	95–100 %

    b. Diagnostic tests

        1) Pulmonary function studies (PFSs) will show decreased expiratory flow of air: forced expiratory volume (FEV_1) shows amount of expired air, which should be about 80% of client's potential and less than 20% variation over time

        2) Peak expiratory flow (PEF) can be measured at home using a peak flow meter (PFM) to assess amount of expired air before and after treatment

        3) Skin testing is often done to determine problems with allergies and a challenge test using an inhaled histamine or by giving methacholine, followed by a breathing treatment

  2. COPD

    a. Assessment includes cough (productive in bronchitis, dry in emphysema), dyspnea, pursed-lip breathing, use of accessory muscles, orthopnea, nasal flaring, cachectic appearance, adventitious breath sounds (wheezing, rhonchi, or crackles), increased anterior–posterior diameter (barrel chest), prolonged expiration, skin color (pink if emphysema in early stage; cyanotic if later stage or with chronic bronchitis), emphysemic client may have quiet, distant breath sounds, air hunger, fever, chest pain, and tachypnea; symptoms of right-sided heart failure (cor pulmonale) may occur later in disease process

    b. Diagnostic tests: arterial blood gases (ABGs) will usually show hypercapnia and hypoxemia, FEV_1 will be decreased, chest x-ray (CXR) will show flattening of diaphragm, complete blood count (CBC) will show polycythemia

  3. Cystic fibrosis

    a. Assessment includes a complete history of child with particular attention to whether symptoms have changed as child matures

        1) Frequent symptoms include delayed growth and development, frequent respiratory problems (pneumonia, cough with excess mucus production, inability to exercise), clubbing of fingers and toes, barrel chest, crackles, and possibly right-sided heart failure symptoms

        2) Gastrointestinal symptoms include steatorrhea (excess fat in stools), greasy foul-smelling stools, impaired digestion, and abdominal pain

        3) Diabetes mellitus and vitamin K deficiency (from malabsorption) may ensue

    b. Diagnostic tests: sweat chloride test indicates elevated sodium and chloride concentrations; ABGs show hypoxemia, PFSs show reduced air flow and forced vital capacity (FVC_1), CXR may show atelectasis or hyperinflation, stool specimen will show steatorrhea, O_2 saturation will be low

  4. Bronchiectasis

    a. Assessment includes chronic productive cough (foul-smelling, purulent sputum), wheezing or crackles, hemoptysis, dyspnea, weight loss, recurrent respiratory infections, and often right-sided heart failure or cor pulmonale

    b. Diagnostic tests: CXR will show enlarged airways; ABGs will often show hypoxemia; PFS will be similar to bronchitis; CT scan may be used to determine extent of damage

D. Nursing management

  1. Asthma

    a. Medications

        1) Bronchodilators to maintain patency in bronchi

            a) Adrenergics: albuterol (Proventil, Ventolin), salmeterol (Serevent), terbutaline sulfate (Brethine), isoetharine HCL (Bronkosol)

      b) Anticholinergics: ipratropium bromide (Atrovent)

      c) Anti-inflammatory: cromolyn (Intal), nedocromil (Tilade)

      d) Methylxanthine: theophylline (Theo-Dur, Slophyllin, Slo-bid)

    2) Steroids such as beclomethasone (Beclovent, Vanceril), dexamethasone (Decadron), fluticasone (Flonase), budesonide (Rhinocort), and fluticasone propionate (Advair) may be used on short-term basis when exacerbation of attacks occurs or as a maintenance inhaler to suppress the inflammatory process

    3) Nonsteroidal drugs are often used as maintenance inhalers, especially in children

    4) Leukotriene modifiers: zafirlukast (Accolate), montelukast (Singulair)

  b. Educate client about difference between rescue inhalers and maintenance inhalers

    1) Rescue inhalers (used for an acute attack) are drugs such as epinephrine (Adrenalin), isoproterenol solution (Isuprel), isoetharine inhalation (Bronkosol), albuterol (Ventolin, Proventil), metaproterenol (Alupent)

    2) Maintenance drugs/inhalers (used to prevent an attack) include ipratropium (Atrovent), leukotriene antagonists, salmeterol (Serevent), xanthine derivatives, cromolyn (Intal), nedocromil (Tilade), and fluticasone propionate (Advair)

  c. Client teaching about medications includes specific side effects and how to use metered dose inhalers (see Box 1-2) and dry powder inhalers (see Box 1-3)

Box 1-2	
Using a Metered-Dose Inhaler	**Purpose:** To deliver a specific dose of aerosolized medication to be inhaled into the lungs for a local effect. **Expected Outcome:** The client will correctly use an administration technique that results in the medication reaching the lungs.

Client Instructions

1) Insert the medicine canister into the inhaler unit and remove the cover from the mouthpiece. Shake the unit gently according to the manufacturer's recommendations.

2) Hold the inhaler ready for inspiration. Exhale slowly. (Do not breathe into the inhaler; that could clog the inhaler valve.)

3) Place the mouthpiece into your mouth and seal it with your lips. Tilt your head slightly back and keep your tongue away from the mouth of the inhaler. (Alternatively, hold the inhaler 1 to 2 inches in front of your mouth and keep your mouth open. With steroids, do not put the inhaler in your mouth. Ineffective use results from medication bouncing off teeth, tongue, or palate.)

4) Press the top of the canister as you breathe in slowly through your mouth. (Failing to coordinate respiration with inhalation will decrease amount of medication reaching lungs).

5) Remove the inhaler. Hold your breath for 10 seconds, then breathe out slowly through pursed lips.

6) Keep the cap in place between uses to prevent dirt from getting into the inhaler. To clean the inhaler, remove the metal canister and rinse the holder in warm water. Dry the holder thoroughly before using it again.

Source: Harkreader, H. & Hogan, M. (2004). *Fundamentals of nursing: Caring and clinical judgement* (2nd ed). St. Louis: Elsevier Science, p. 858.

Box 1-3	**Purpose:** To deliver a specific dose of dry powder medication to be inhaled into the lungs for a local effect.

Using Dry Dose Inhalers

Purpose: To deliver a specific dose of dry powder medication to be inhaled into the lungs for a local effect.

Rationale: Inhaled medications are easily deposited on the oral mucosa membranes without reaching the lungs if a dry dose powder inhaler is not used properly.

Expected Outcome: The client will correctly use an administration technique that results in the medication reaching the lungs.

Client Instructions — Diskus (see Figure 1-2)

1) Open the diskus.

2) Snap the mouthpiece into position.

3) Breathe out fully, away from the mouthpiece.

4) Place the mouthpiece to the lips and take a steady, deep breath through the mouth.

5) After inhaling, the breath should be held for about 10 seconds.

6) Close the diskus and the counter will count down, showing the number of doses left in the diskus.

7) The diskus should be kept dry at all times.

Client Instructions — Capsule container (see Figure 1-3)

1) Open the container and expose the area to insert the capsule, which should come individually wrapped.

2) After placing the capsule into the appropriate area of the container, close the mouthpiece.

3) Puncture the capsule using the button attached to a needle.

4) Place the mouthpiece to the lips and inhale slowly using a deep breath through the mouth.

5) After inhaling, the breath should be held for about 10 seconds.

6) Open the mouthpiece and discard the used capsule.

7) Close the container until the next use.

8) Keep the container dry at all times.

1) MDIs require attaching a canister to the mouthpiece and delivering one or two "puffs," and rinsing mouth after use (see Figure 1-1); dry powder inhalers such as fluticasone propionate (Advair) require snapping mouthpiece into position and inhaling (see Box 1-3 and Figure 1-2); dry powder inhalers such as tiotropium bromide (Spiriva) require placing a capsule into canister and punching a hole in the capsule provided on the apparatus to release powder (see Box 1-3 and Figure 1-3)

2) Teach children to use steroid inhalers before brushing their teeth to avoid oral infections

3) Steroids can stunt the growth of children, especially under age 12, and can have many side effects if used on a long-term basis

4) Theophylline preparations can reach toxic levels; monitor drug levels and report tremors or jitters to physician; these drugs are not used as frequently anymore

d. Teach client how to identify what triggers an attack and how to avoid these triggers; influenza vaccines are recommended yearly

Figure 1-1

One method for using a
metered-dose inhaler.

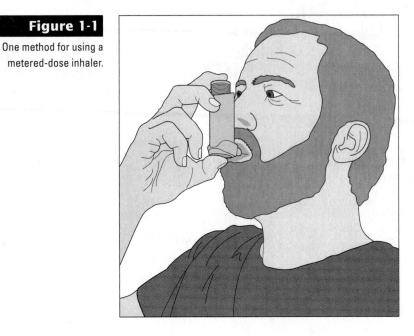

Figure 1-2

Diskus inhaler for dry
powder dose.

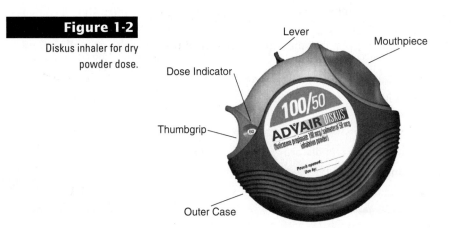

Lever

Mouthpiece

Dose Indicator

Thumbgrip

Outer Case

Figure 1-3

Spiriva applicator.

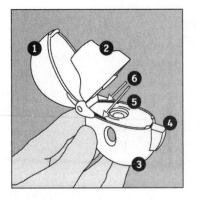

1. dust cap
2. mouthpiece
3. base
4. piercing button
5. center chamber
6. Air intake vents

e. Educate client about disease process and how to avoid anxiety during an attack; client should seek immediate attention if rescue inhaler does not work or status asthmaticus occurs; home portable nebulizers can be purchased

f. Teach children to carry their inhalers at all times; if an attack occurs and an inhaler is not available, drinking two regular caffeinated soda drinks may help until medications are available

g. Inhalers should be checked frequently for fullness; a convenient but not foolproof way to check a canister is to assess whether it floats (empty), sinks (full), or bobs halfway (half-full) when placed in water

h. Monitor VS and breath sounds, offering comfort until the medications take effect during an acute attack

i. Monitor peak flow readings, especially during allergy seasons

   1) Peak flow readings may decrease as much as 24 hours prior to an attack

   2) Medicine used with an attack can be evaluated as effective if peak flow reading after medication use is 80% of client's personal best

j. Use of a dry powder inhaler should be demonstrated to client (see Box 1-3 and Figure 1-2 and 1-3)

2. COPD

   a. Medications

      1) Bronchodilators to maintain patent airways: anticholinergic agents, sympathomimetics, and methylxanthines

      2) Newer bronchodilator (inhaled) is tiotropium bromide (Spiriva)

      3) Steroids (or anti-inflammatory drugs) as needed during exacerbations; prednisone (orally) or inhalers similar to client with asthma; monitor for side effects, especially fluid and sodium retention

      4) Antibiotics as needed during acute infectious periods or prophylactically

      5) Expectorants to help loosen mucus

   b. Instruct clients to maintain their pneumonia and influenza vaccines

   c. Educate client about the following: smoking cessation, maintaining adequate hydration, breathing exercises (pursed-lip breathing to keep airways open by maintenance of positive pressure and abdominal breathing to expand lungs), adequate nutrition, and avoiding other individuals with respiratory infections

   d. Pulmonary hygiene measures may be necessary if secretions are thick: percussion (rhythmic clapping on chest to loosen secretions), postural drainage, suctioning, and respiratory treatments

   e. Use of low-flow O_2 to prevent depression of respiratory drive

   f. Evaluation of a low-profile exercise program

   g. Maintain adequate fluid intake of at least 2 liters/day

3. Cystic fibrosis

   a. Medications

      1) Bronchodilators if airway obstruction is problematic

      2) Antibiotics if an infection is present

      3) Dornase alfa recombinant: this drug hydrolyzes DNA in sputum of clients with CF; as a result, pulmonary function is improved and number of respiratory infections is lessened

      4) Mucolytics to liquefy secretions as needed

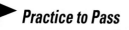

Practice to Pass

A 7-year-old child with asthma is placed on beclomethasone (Vanceril) as a maintenance inhaler. What is the major concern for a child taking this medication?

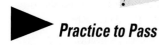

Practice to Pass

An elderly client with chronic obstructive pulmonary disease (COPD) also has a history of congestive heart failure (CHF). What is the major concern for placing this client on an oral dose of a steroid such as prednisone?

    b. Maintain adequate fluid and electrolytes, nutritional status (high in protein, fat, and calories), and adherance to pancreatic enzyme drug therapy

    c. Monitor closely for signs and symptoms of infection

    d. Oxygen therapy may need to be initiated if hypoxemia is present

    e. Pulmonary hygiene measures may be needed to clear airways: postural drainage, positioning, suctioning, percussion, vibration, "huff" cough technique (a valved mask is used for 20 inhalations, followed by 3 to 4 huffs)

    f. Education includes respiratory care techniques, avoidance of respiratory irritants, medication administration, and dietary needs

  4. Bronchiectasis: basically the same as for a client with COPD

    a. Medications include antibiotics as needed for infection and bronchodilators to maintain clear airway

    b. Pulmonary hygiene measures: suctioning as needed, O_2 therapy if hypoxic, percussion, and postural drainage

III. RESTRICTIVE PULMONARY DISORDERS

A. Overview

  1. Restrictive pulmonary disorders are defined as disorders that limit ability of lungs to expand normally in a respiratory cycle

  2. This category includes many disorders

    a. Disorders discussed in this section: atelectasis, flail chest, pulmonary contusion, sleep apnea

    b. Disorders discussed separately: pneumonia, pulmonary tuberculosis, pleural effusion, pneumothorax

    c. Other disorders: Pickwickian syndrome, pulmonary fibrosis, pulmonary edema

  3. Causes include changes in hydrostatic or oncotic forces resulting in accumulation of fluid in pleural spaces, trauma to chest wall, fractured ribs, collapse of lung due to air accumulation in pleural sac, invasion of pathogens (bacterial, viral), reduced lung compliance, scarring and fibrosis of lung parenchyma, musculoskeletal disorders, and neuromuscular disorders

B. Pathophysiology

  1. Atelectasis is the collapse of a lung or an alveolus

    a. Perfusion occurs without ventilation because collapsed alveoli do not participate in air exchange

    b. Without O_2 little if any surfactant (a lipoprotein substance lining alveoli) is produced; surfactant is needed to lower surface tension, which lowers resistance to expansion on inspiration and prevents collapse of alveoli on expiration

    c. Blood flow is not interrupted, but blood travels through airless alveoli; if a large enough area of lung is affected, hypoxemia results

    d. *Primary atelectasis* is often associated with infants who are born with collapsed alveoli at birth; in premature births, a lack of surfactant can cause atelectasis

    e. *Secondary atelectasis* is a collapse of alveoli that were previously expanded and is sub-classified as three types

      1) *Compression atelectasis* is a result of crowding of lung tissue resulting in collapse; may be caused by fluid, tumor, puncture wound, or abdominal distention

    2) *Resorption atelectasis* is a result of blockage to alveolus and can result from mucus buildup, pneumonia, cystic fibrosis, and surgery; alveoli distal to the obstructed bronchus resorb the air and cause collapse of alveolar walls

    3) *Contraction atelectasis* is a result of fibrosis of lung or pleura, it results in inadequate lung expansion

2. Flail chest and pulmonary contusion (bruising of lung tissue) are acute injuries of the chest wall that are usually caused by blunt trauma or penetrating objects; rib fractures and automobile accidents are a common source of chest wall injuries

  a. In flail chest, injury results in instability of chest wall

  b. Negative pressure created within the lung cavity upon inspiration causes chest wall section to collapse

  c. Upon expiration, positive pressure causes chest wall section to expand outward

  d. Penetrating objects also affect pressure within lungs, which leads to collapse of portions or an entire lung

  e. Lack of proper lung expansion causes increased breathing effort, impaired gas exchange, reduced lung compliance, and pain

3. Sleep apnea is a lack of airflow in upper airways for 10 seconds or more; three different forms exist:

  a. *Obstructive sleep apnea* is most common and is caused by an obstruction to airflow while ventilatory efforts continue

    1) As many as 30 apnea periods per hour may occur while sleeping

    2) Normal pharyngeal muscle tone is lost, thus allowing the pharynx to collapse during inspiration

    3) Further obstruction occurs when tongue falls against posterior pharyngeal wall

    4) Client attempts to breathe, but each effort shortens until the obstructive forces are reduced by movement or position change

  b. *Central apnea* is when respiratory center of brain is affected and drive to breathe is inhibited

    1) There is no effort to breathe during a period of apnea

    2) This is thought to occur in sudden infant death syndrome (SIDS)

  c. *Mixed apnea* is a combination of both central and obstructive types of apnea

C. Nursing assessment

  1. Atelectasis

    a. Assessment includes lung sounds (diminished, crackles or gurgles), tachypnea, depth and regularity of breathing, dyspnea, tachycardia, abnormal ABGs (hypoxia), temperature (if infection is suspected as a cause), and coughing

    b. Diagnostic tests: CXR that will usually reveal an area of collapsed lung, and ABGs that will show strain that atelectasis is placing on lung

  2. Flail chest and pulmonary contusion

    a. Assessment includes asymmetry of chest expansion and paradoxical chest movement, pain upon inspiration, dyspnea, tachypnea, lung sounds (diminished, crackles, rhonchi), palpable crepitus (sound of crackling cellophane when skin is touched), and tachycardia

    b. Specific symptoms for pulmonary contusion include symptoms noted above plus copious (often blood-tinged) sputum, restlessness, and apprehension

    c. Diagnostic tests: CXR, ABGs

3. Sleep apnea

   a. Assessment includes changes in behavior and performance (irritability, daytime drowsiness, decreased ability to function, forgetfulness, lethargy), verbal complaints of feeling tired or listless, dark circles under eyes, frequent yawning, changes in posture, loud snoring, cardiac dysrhythmias, angina at night, headaches due to hypercapnia, periods of apnea during sleep, impotence, and respiratory depression (related to certain medications used)

   b. Diagnostic tests: electroencephalography (EEG) to identify stages of sleep, electrocardiogram (ECG) to identify dysrhythmias, polysomnography (overnight sleep study—with and without oxygen); a CBC may be ordered to assess for erythrocytosis (or polycythemia) caused by O_2 needs, and a thyroid function study to rule out hypothyroidism

D. Nursing management

1. Atelectasis

   a. Medications include antibiotics if an infection is suspected as the cause, bronchodilators, and analgesics as necessary

   b. Administer O_2 to enhance oxygenation at alveolar level and monitor oxygen saturation

   c. Elevate head of bed

   d. Encourage turning, coughing, and deep breathing as often as every 1–2 hours

   e. Encourage use of incentive spirometer every 1–2 hours

   f. Encourage adequate fluid intake unless otherwise contraindicated

   g. Encourage ambulation as ordered

2. Flail chest and pulmonary contusion

   a. Medications

      1) Analgesics to maintain control of pain, initially on a *scheduled dosing pattern* rather than as needed; continuous epidural analgesia or even intercostal nerve blocks may be recommended forms of analgesia

      2) Sedatives or neuromuscular blockers to control agitation while on mechanical ventilation

      3) Bronchodilators

      4) Antibiotics as a preventive measure

   b. Administer O_2 as ordered

   c. Internal or external fixation of flail area may be necessary

      1) Use of a sandbag for flail chest may help to stabilize the area through external fixation

      2) Endotracheal intubation and mechanical ventilation with PEEP may support ventilation and provide internal fixation

   d. Maintain adequate hydration while avoiding overhydration

   e. Turn, cough, and deep breathe every 2 hours, yet restrict overall activity to reduce oxygen needs and plan for adequate rest periods

   f. Oral or nasal suctioning as needed

   g. Educate client to use a pillow to splint area during coughing

   h. Maintain bed with head in an elevated position

   i. Monitor VS, O_2 saturation, and level of consciousness (LOC)

      j. Chest tube insertion may be necessary for chest contusions

         1) For chest tubes, assess respiratory status every 2 to 4 hours, maintain a closed system, milk chest tubes only if protocol present, because this increased pleural pressure; check water seal frequently (water level should fluctuate with inspiration and have periodic air bubbles), assess amount, color, consistency of drainage every 4 to 8 hours, and assess water level

         2) Continuous air bubbles usually indicate an air leak; lack of fluctuation indicates inadequate function of system or reinflation of lung

    3. Sleep apnea

      a. Medications

         1) Medroxyprogesterone (Depo-Provera, Provera): stimulates respirations in obese clients who hypoventilate

         2) Theophylline: relaxes smooth muscle of bronchi

         3) Protriptyline (Vivactil): a tricyclic antidepressant

         4) Clonazepam (Klonopin): an anticonvulsant

         5) Fluoxetine hydrochloride (Prozac): an antidepressant

         6) Hypnotics, sedatives, androgens, and alcohol should be completely avoided because of their effects on respiratory system

      b. Implementation of weight reduction plan

      c. Continuous positive airway pressure (CPAP) therapy is most commonly prescribed treatment to force air into back of throat with the use of a compressor and reduce airway occlusion experienced in sleep apnea; a humidifier is often recommended because of drying effect of oxygen treatment

      d. Nosebleeds and nasal congestion may occur while using oxygen and CPAP secondary to dryness

      e. Oxygen supplementation may be recommended

      f. Maintain adequate fluid intake of at least 2 liters/day

      g. Surgery may be recommended including tonsillectomy, adenoidectomy, and uvulopalatopharyngoplasty (removal of tissue contributing to obstruction from soft palate, uvula, and posterior pharyngeal wall)

      h. Oral/dental applications have been tried to reposition mandible with success in some clients

IV. PNEUMONIA

A. Overview

  1. Pneumonia is defined as inflammation of bronchioles, alveoli, interstitial tissues, and on occasion the pleura as a result of infection

  2. Pneumonia may be defined by cause, location, or contributing factors

    a. Cause: bacteria, viruses, fungi, protozoa, or parasites

      1) Common bacteria include *Streptococcus pneumonia* (most common), *staphylococcus, Haemophilus influenzae* and *Pseudomonas* (Gram-negative)

      2) Fungi include *Aspergillus fumigatus, Candida albicans,* and *Pneumocystis carinii*

    b. Location: lobular pneumonia meaning involvement of one lobe, lobar pneumonia meaning involvement of an entire lung, or bronchopneumonia meaning involvement of lobes adjacent to the bronchi

      c. Contributing factors: aspiration pneumonia often occurs with tube feedings; postoperative pneumonia occurs following a surgical procedure; and hospital-acquired pneumonia occurs after admittance to hospital

3. Atypical pneumonia is a type of pneumonia that does not present with usual symptoms or evolve in usual pattern; examples of two types of atypical pneumonia are pneumocystosis, caused by *Pneumocystis carinii* (associated with immunosuppressed clients) or Legionnaires' disease (caused by *Legionella pneumophila*)

      a. Pneumocystosis is a type of pneumoccal pneumonia caused by the parasite *Pneumocystis carinii;* most prominent in clients with AIDS or debilitated or immunosuppressed individuals; symptoms include fever, cough, and dyspnea; has a high mortality rate and is difficult to diagnose; treated with pentamidine isoethionate (Pentam 300)

      b. Legionnaires' disease is an acute bacterial pneumonia; flulike symptoms occur followed by fever, chills, headache, and muscle aches; usually self-limiting and not highly contagious; treated with erythromycin

4. Organisms may enter lung through accidental inhalation, close contact with an infected person, or introduction of organisms through an outside means such as suctioning, intubation, or through the blood; environmental reservoirs may be responsible for Legionnaires' disease

B. Pathophysiology

1. Although normal flora contains many bacteria, which are pathogens by nature, these organisms cause pneumonia when they invade lower respiratory tract

2. Organisms such as *Escherichia coli* or *Pseudomonas aeruginosa* are common in enteric flora but are not a part of upper respiratory tract; these organisms can contaminate lungs via the circulatory system

3. Inflammation within the lung is similar to the inflammatory process anywhere within body

      a. Introduction of bacteria promotes an antigen–antibody response and endo-toxins are released

      b. Air spaces of alveoli become engorged with fluid and red blood cells (RBCs) and exudate forms

      c. The infiltration of lymphocytes, neutrophils, RBCs, and fibrin results in cellular infiltration and massive congestion

      d. Alveoli become airless because of exudate; perfusion accompanied by poor ventilation results

      e. Consolidation of lung tissue results and presents on CXR as white "patchy" infiltrate

      f. Damage may occur to bronchial and alveolar mucous membranes

4. Signs and symptoms of pneumonia include coughing, fatigue, pleuritic pain, dyspnea, chills, fever, elevated white blood cells (WBC), sputum production (rust-colored or purulent), crackles or rales, pleural rub, and tachypnea; elderly clients may present with less dramatic symptoms and may experience changes in mental status or be easily agitated

C. Nursing assessment

1. Assessment

      a. Subjective/objective: cough (productive or nonproductive; effectiveness of cough; if productive, color, amount, and odor); pain with inspiration or cough

Practice to Pass

A client with pneumonia continues to run a temperature of 102 to 103°F even after taking an antibiotic for 3 days. What could account for this and what should be done?

      b. General symptoms: fever

      c. Inspect for dyspnea and tachycardia

      d. Auscultate lung sounds (cracles, rhonchi)

   2. Diagnostic tests: CXR (shows consolidation in affected lobe), CBC (elevated WBC with a shift to left), and culture and sensitivity (C&S) of sputum, possible gram stain, ABGs (expect to see $PaO_2 < 75$ mmHg), pulse oximetry (expect to see 95% or lower), and blood cultures

D. Nursing management

   1. Medications

      a. Antibiotic therapy as indicated by culture and sensitivity within 4 hrs of diagnosis or admission; may begin with a broad-spectrum antibiotic such as one of the penicillins, erythromycins, or cephalosporins until results of C&S are available (see Chapter 13)

      b. Antipyretics

      c. Bronchodilators

         1) Sympathomimetic drugs such as albuterol sulfate (Proventil) or metaproterenol (Alupent)

         2) Methylxanthines such as theophylline and aminophylline

      d. Drugs used to liquefy mucus, such as guaifenesin (Mucinex), acetylcysteine (Mucomyst)

   2. Increase fluid intake to 2,500 to 3,000 mL/day to help liquefy secretions unless contraindicated due to a cardiac or renal condition

   3. Administer O_2 therapy as ordered with monitoring of oxygen saturation by pulse oximetry

      a. Nasal cannula for delivering 24% to 45% O_2 concentration

      b. Face mask for delivering 40% to 60% O_2 concentration

      c. Nonrebreather mask for delivering up to 100% O_2 concentration

      d. Venturi mask for precise measurement of air flow

   4. Chest physiotherapy including postural draining and percussion; during initial stage, lung sounds may worsen and cough may become more productive after chest physiotherapy if congestion is extremely consolidated and if treatment is effective in loosening secretions

   5. Endotracheal suctioning if necessary

   6. Monitor respiratory rate, depth, and use of accessory muscles

   7. Instruct client how to splint chest wall with a pillow to cough more effectively

   8. Monitor for intolerance to exercise or need for assistance with activities of daily living (ADLs)

   9. Encourage client to turn, cough, and deep breathe

  10. Encourage elderly and at-risk clients to have a pneumonia vaccine every 5 years

V. PULMONARY TUBERCULOSIS (TB)

A. Overview

   1. Tuberculosis (TB) is a type of pneumonia caused by *Mycobacterium tuberculosis,* an acid–fast bacillus

2. TB has been fairly controlled until recently; TB in immunosuppressed people has aided in development of resistant strains

3. Primary defense mechanism against these bacilli is a cell-mediated immune response instead of an acute inflammatory reaction

4. Two types exist: *primary infection,* which develops in someone who has not been previously exposed and *secondary tuberculosis,* which means reactivation of dormant bacilli has occurred

5. Although organisms are contracted by airborne droplets from an individual with an active form of the disease, and disease usually affect lungs, it can lie dormant for many years and be reactivated as well as invade other parts of body

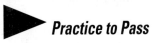

Practice to Pass

A female visits the Emergency Department because of symptoms of gonorrhea. She admits that she practices prostitution and has never been tested for human immunodeficiency virus (HIV). Why would a tuberculosis (TB) skin test be an appropriate order as part of the diagnostic workup?

B. Pathophysiology

1. Organisms carried by airborne droplets enter lungs and multiply in pulmonary alveoli

2. As organisms multiply, they enter lymphatic system and bloodstream, stimulating a cell-mediated response

3. Neutrophils and macrophages are immediately released to lungs to assist in attacking bacilli

4. The bacilli cannot be destroyed, but can be isolated; as macrophages attack the organisms, a granuloma (or tubercle) is formed with inner areas of necrosis; lymphocytes and macrophages form a giant cell known as Langerhans

5. If arrested, these granulomas scar or calcify (called Gohn's complex) and can be identified on a CXR; symptoms of disease may not be present if organisms are arrested early

6. If the cell-mediated response by the body fails, organisms within a calcified granuloma can be reactivated; if immune system is deficient or if the number of organisms is extremely large, damage to lung tissue may occur

7. The *M. tuberculosis* is a rod-shaped bacteria that has a waxy capsule; the waxy capsule requires Gram-staining in order to turn the organism red, and is therefore called an "acid-fast bacillus"

8. Major complications of this disease include poorer diffusion of oxygen and carbon dioxide leading to decreased gas exchange, decreased surface area available for gas diffusion, abnormalities in ventilation-perfusion ratio, hypoxia, and pulmonary hypertension

9. Other complications
   a. Tuberculosis pneumonia, a massive lobular or lobar pneumonia
   b. Pleuritis
   c. Extrapulmonary tuberculosis (often seen in clients with HIV)
      1) Swallowed bacilli may cause tuberculosis in GI tract (small intestines)
      2) Miliary tuberculosis, spreading of tubercle into bloodstream (resemble millet seeds), then are spread to brain, meninges (CSF), liver, kidneys, bone, and joints
   d. Sepsis and respiratory failure

10. Signs and symptoms of tuberculosis include coughing (usually productive in active stage, dry in initial stage), fever in afternoon or night (maybe low-grade), malaise, night sweats, anorexia, weight loss, chest pain, hemoptysis (blood in sputum; later sign), dyspnea, crackles, and enlarged, often painful lymph nodes

C. Nursing assessment

1. Assessment includes: symptom analysis of type and progression of symptoms; color, consistency, and amount of sputum; knowledge of disease; weight pattern; vital signs; description of any pain; palpable lymph nodes; breath sounds; and activity tolerance

2. Diagnostic tests
   a. CXR (shows dense lesions in upper lobes, enlarged lymph nodes, and formation of large cavities)
   b. CBC (presence of leukocytosis)
   c. Fiberoptic bronchoscopy and bronchial washing (for obtaining culture specimens)
   d. Tuberculin skin test should be measured and recorded in millimeters (mm) and not as positive or negative; new guidelines by Centers for Disease Control suggest the following cut points to determine whether a reaction is negative or positive:
      1) Induration of greater than or equal to 5 mm is considered positive in HIV-positive persons; recent contact with TB case persons; persons with changes in CXR consistent with prior TB; organ transplant recipients; immunosuppressed clients receiving corticosteroids
      2) Induration of greater than or equal to 10 mm is considered positive in recent immigrants from countries with high prevalence of TB; drug users of injectable drugs; persons living or working in high-risk settings such as prison, jails, nursing homes, long-term care facilities, homeless shelters, and facilities for AIDS; personnel working in mycobacteriology labatoratories; persons with clinical conditions making them high risk such as diabetes, renal failure, hematologic disorders, malignancies
      3) Induration of greater than or equal to 15 mm is considered positive in persons with no known risk factors for TB
      4) Negative results would be 0 mm or anything below above defined cut points for each category
   e. Clients who have emigrated to United States may have had Bacilli Calmette-Guérin (BCG) vaccine; these individuals will always have a positive skin test and need CXR evaluation
   f. Three early morning sputum collections for acid-fast staining, culture and sensitivity positive for *M. tuberculosis;* results may take up to 10 days

D. Nursing management

1. Medications include *single dose* treatment for prevention or exposure and *at least two* antibacterial medications for an active case of the disease or resistant strains
   a. Prevention of TB requires taking BCG vaccine once for TB or medication for 6 to 12 months for exposure and at least 9 months for clients with HIV
   b. For resistant strains, three or more agents may be combined according to sensitivity report
   c. Medications may be prescribed prophylactically even though symptoms are not present if a positive TB result was obtained
   d. Recommended anti-infective agents: isoniazid (INH), rifampin (Rifadin), ethambutol (EMB), streptomycin (SM), pyrazinamide (PZA)
   e. Secondary agents: para-aminosalicylic acid (PAS), cycloserine (Seromycin), capreomycin (Capastat), ethionamide (Trecator-SC)

2. Hepatotoxicity is a common side effect for many agents, and clients should be monitored closely

3. Compliance is a common problem because of length of therapy; instruct client about compliance needed with medication administration

4. Inform clients of color changes in urine with some agents such as rifampin (Rifadin); this drug causes red-orange urine

5. Once positive, the purified protein derivative (PPD) will remain positive and should not be repeated; a CXR may be ordered to verify exposure versus active disease process

6. Monitor vital signs, noting a pattern of late afternoon low-grade fever

7. Suction as needed for productive cough

8. Maintain adequate hydration and nutritional status; high-protein, high-carbohydrate diet recommended

9. Monitor weight daily for loss

10. Place clients with active cases on airborne precautions (in negative-pressure room)

11. Initiate screening for all family members or close contacts

12. Assist client to turn, cough, and deep breathe

13. Monitor breath sounds every 4 hours

14. Encourage frequent rest periods

VI. PLEURAL EFFUSION

A. Overview

1. Pleural effusion is defined as an excessive amount of fluid located in pleural space between visceral and parietal layers of pleura (tends to accumulate at bases because of effects of gravity)

2. Usually considered a secondary rather than a primary disorder

3. Causes of pleural effusion are either systemic or local

   a. Systemic diseases

      1) Hydrothorax: heart failure, renal failure, liver failure

      2) Empyema (pus in pleural cavity): infections, malignancies, connective tissue disorders

   b. Local diseases

      1) Hemothorax (blood in pleural cavity): chest wall injuries, surgery to chest

      2) Chylothorax: trauma, inflammation (pneumonia, tuberculosis), or malignancy

B. Pathophysiology

1. A pleural effusion results from:

   a. An increase in hydrostatic pressure in pleural capillaries or decreased colloid osmotic pressure in circulatory system that can lead to excess pleural fluid (known as transudative)

   b. An increased capillary permeability as a result of inflammation, infection, or malignancy (known as exudative)

2. Regardless of cause, excess pressure exerted by fluid in pleural space compresses lung and limits its ability to expand, thus compromising gas exchange

3. Amount of fluid in pleural space can become so large as to displace lung tissue and result in a compression atelectasis

4. Decreased lung volume on affected side results in diminished or absent breath sounds

5. Signs and symptoms include dyspnea, diminished or absent breath sounds on affected side, pain, limited chest wall movement, and dull or flat sounds on percussion

C. Nursing assessment

1. Assessment includes symptom analysis of any pain experienced, dyspnea, coughing, vital signs (elevated temperature), respiratory rate and status (shallow respirations, asymmetry), lung sounds (diminished), and percussion for flat or dull sound over area

2. Diagnostic tests: CXR ("white out"—opaque densities of area involved); thoracentesis (aspiration of fluid from pleural space); culture, sensitivity, and cytological examination of fluid if any removed; a CT scan and ultrasonography can determine pleural effusions if needed

D. Nursing management

1. Medications

   a. Antipyretics if fever or pain is present

   b. Antibiotics, parenterally or instillation into pleural space for repeated effusions

2. Goal of treatment should be to resolve the underlying disease process causing the problem and prevention of complications such as atelectasis or pneumothorax

3. Assist with thoracentesis if procedure is done to remove fluid; surgical decortication may be done if recurrent

4. Monitor VS, especially respiratory rate, rhythm, and use of accessory muscles

5. Monitor lung sounds and reports of dyspnea

6. Manage pain if necessary along with bedrest

7. Monitor for signs of changing status: tachycardia, hypotension, increasing shortness of breath (SOB)

VII. PLEURITIS (PLEURISY)

A. Overview

1. Pleuritis (pleurisy) is an inflammation of pleura and is often accompanied by abrupt onset of pain

2. Classifications

   a. Primary or secondary; secondary is typically a result of another respiratory illness such as pneumonia, pleural effusion, or trauma to lung

   b. Unilateral, bilateral, or local; unilateral is most typical

   c. Acute or chronic; acute is most common

   d. Fibrinous or adhesive: fibrinous is characterized by typical symptoms of severe pain without any fluid return upon aspiration; adhesion occurs when parietal pleura adhere to visceral pleura and complete obliteration of pleural space can occur

   e. May be dry or with effusion (pleural effusion); dry is more painful and usually accompanies pneumonia; adhesions may form

B. Pathophysiology

1. Inner visceral layer that lies adjacent to lung and outer parietal layer that lies adjacent to chest wall form a cavity with a thin layer of serous fluid known as the pleural cavity; pressure in the pleural cavity is negative compared to alveolar pressure in order to keep lungs from collapsing

2. Introduction of an infectious process such as pneumonia or viral respiratory diseases can extend to pleura and cause an inflammatory process in the pleural cavity

3. Signs and symptoms of pleuritis

   a. Abrupt pain that is usually unilateral and localized to a specific portion of chest; pain is sharp, stabbing, and may radiate to neck or shoulder; pressure changes caused by breathing, movement, or coughing will intensify pain

   b. Other symptoms may include fever, cough (dry, hacking), localized tenderness, diminished breath sounds, tachypnea, and pleural friction rub

C. Nursing assessment

1. Assessment includes symptom analysis of pain, vital signs, percussion, lung sounds, visual inspection for symmetry of chest wall during respirations

2. Diagnostic tests: CXR (diagnostic purposes only to rule out other pulmonary disorders) and ABGs

D. Nursing management

1. Medications include analgesics or NSAIDs for pain and fever; antibiotics; cough suppressant for nighttime such as codeine (this should be avoided, however, if a productive cough is present)

2. Encourage bedrest

3. Monitor VS, noting fever and respiratory rate

4. Assess respiratory status, percussion, and auscultation of lung sounds

5. Encourage deep breathing and coughing every 1–2 hours and splinting of chest wall when coughing

VIII. PNEUMOTHORAX/HEMOTHORAX

A. Overview

1. Pneumothorax is entrance of air into pleural cavity, resulting in a complete or partial collapse of affected lung

   a. *Spontaneous pneumothorax* is a sudden collapse of lung due to leakage of air into pleural cavity from within lung or from an unknown cause; may occur in tall, thin young men who are healthy or secondary to other disease processes such as COPD, asthma, tuberculosis, emphysema, cystic fibrosis, etc.; smoking and family history of congenital blebs may contribute to this type of pneumothorax

   b. *Traumatic pneumothorax* is usually caused by a traumatic injury to chest wall causing blunt or penetrating trauma; is usually a result of a stabbing, gunshot wound, rib fracture, motor vehicle accident, or a severe fall; may be open or termed a "sucking chest wound" and can be fatal due to severe hypoventilation that occurs from collapse of lung

   c. *Tension pneumothorax* is a dangerous complication and a medical emergency where entering air cannot escape by same route and pressure within pleural cavity increases, resulting in complete collapse of lung; a mediastinal shift to unaffected side and a downward displacement of diaphragm can be observed

   d. *Iatrogenic pneumothorax* is defined as a pneumothorax resulting from a medical intervention, i.e., placement of a catheter, biopsy procedures, cardiopulmonary resuscitation (CPR), mechanical ventilation, or anesthesia

2. Hemothorax is defined as presence of blood in pleural cavity

3. The symptoms, diagnosis, and treatment for all are similar; the severity, type, and size of pneumothorax determine the degree of symptoms experienced by client

B. Pathophysiology

1. The pleural cavity surrounding lungs maintains an airtight seal and has less pressure than within lungs, enabling lungs to remain expanded, known as "negative" pressure; if this negative pressure is lost due to any opening of pleural cavity, lung collapses because of natural contraction of elastic lung tissue; rupture of pleural cavity allows air to flow in and out of space, thus affecting expansion and recoil of lung (see Figure 1-4)

2. In a tension pneumothorax, an added complication hinders lungs even further

   a. Air enters the pleural space on inspiration as seen with a pneumothorax

   b. On expiration, rising pressure in pleural space closes tear or rupture and air is trapped

   c. Each consecutive breath forces more air into pleural cavity and lung collapses completely due to force of pressure being exerted

   d. Pressure is exerted on due to opposite lung and venous return to heart is affected; this condition can be fatal if not treated promptly (refer again to Figure 1-4)

3. Signs and symptoms of a pneumothorax/hemothorax are severe shortness of breath, sharp, intense pain on affected side that may be worse on inspiration, tympanic resonance, absence of breath sounds on affected side, distention on one side of chest, tachypnea, distended neck veins due to pressure in thorax, subcutaneous emphysema (crepitus), hypoxemia, cyanosis, anxiety, and

Figure 1-4 Pneumothorax. *A.* A spontaneous pneumothorax with an air leak from the lung into the pleural space. *B.* A traumatic or open pneumothorax (sucking chest wound) in which air enters the pleural space through a wound in the chest wall. *C.* A tension pneumothorax in which air enters the pleural space during inspiration but is unable to exit during expiration, resulting in rapid lung collapse and a shift of mediastinal structures toward the unaffected side.

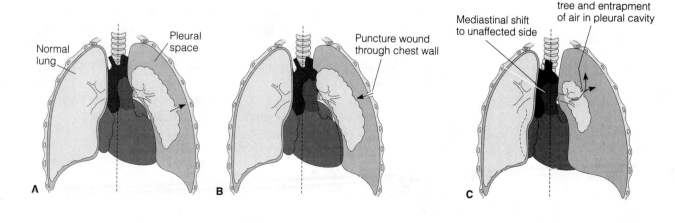

diaphoresis; a shift of mediastinum to unaffected side may be visibly seen in a tension pneumothorax

C. Nursing assessment

1. Assessment includes description of pain and onset, visual inspection (asymmetry of lungs, shift of trachea, and use of accessory muscles), percussion over affected area, auscultation of lung sounds bilaterally, vital signs (tachycardia, hypotension, tachypnea), signs of hypoxemia (ABGs, decreased O_2 saturation, poorer color)

2. Diagnostic tests: CXR (asymmetry of lung expansion, shift in diaphragm or mediastinum, air in pleural cavity), ABGs (decreased PaO_2, decreased pH, increased $PaCO_2$), pulse oximetry (O_2 saturation of less than or equal to 92%), and CBC if hemothorax suspected; thoracentesis may be indicated to assess for fluid in pleural cavity as a treatment or diagnostic tool

D. Nursing management

1. Medications include analgesics and antibiotics (if fluid is present and chest tube is inserted)

2. Administer O_2 as indicated, monitoring pulse oximetry

3. Assist with insertion and maintenance of chest tube, noting fluid drainage, color, consistency, and amount; monitor that water seal is maintained and that tubing is not kinked; monitor insertion site for signs of infection

4. Administer blood transfusion as indicated by orders

5. Assist with thoracentesis (insertion of a needle to withdraw air)

6. Monitor lung sounds and vital sounds

7. Maintain high Fowler's position for ease in breathing

8. Turn and ambulate client, allowing for frequent rest periods

9. Recurrent pneumothorax may require thoracotomy to excise or oversew blebs; provide routine postoperative care

IX. PULMONARY EMBOLISM (PE)

A. Overview

1. Pulmonary embolism is defined as blockage of a pulmonary artery by an embolus or blood clot that has often traveled from a lower extremity

2. Is often a major complication of a deep vein thrombosis (DVT), therefore maintenance heparin therapy is recommended to prevent clot propagation and increased risk of dislodging part of thrombus, which then becomes an embolus

3. Although a lower extremity is usual source of emboli, other sources include a thromboembolism from venous system entering right side of heart, a tumor, or other substances such as fat, air, amniotic fluid, or pieces of tissue

4. PE may manifest itself as several tiny clots, one large clot, or a multitude of showered clots in lung

5. Contributing factors for a pulmonary embolus include venous stasis often associated with prolonged bedrest or surgery, hypercoagulability, obesity, childbirth, use of birth control pills, cardiac diseases, and trauma

B. Pathophysiology

1. A portion of a thrombus dislodges and travels (as an embolus) through venous circulation to right side of heart and enters pulmonary artery, typically lodging there

2. Blocked pulmonary artery causes a decreased blood flow to lung and can result in infarction to lung tissue

   a. Note that lung has two other sources of O_2 to compensate: air from bronchi and O_2 from blood flow from bronchial artery arising from descending aorta

   b. Death can occur if the infarcted section of lung is large enough

3. Embolus may block entire main pulmonary artery (known as a *saddle embolus,* which is lethal) or may block smaller branches of pulmonary circulation, causing pulmonary infarcts (can be asymptomatic or cause pleuritic pain from irritation of pleura); the fibrinolytic mechanism in body often destroys smaller clots

4. The end result of pulmonary embolism is ventilation without perfusion, which decreases oxygenation of body tissues; with pulmonary embolism, alveolar dead space (alveoli not participating in gas exchange) is increased

5. As a result of pulmonary artery blockage, right side of heart is unable to pump blood sufficiently and distends as does proximal portion of pulmonary artery (before the obstruction)

6. Decreased oxygenation of blood and reduced blood flow to left side of heart leads to decreased oxygenation of brain and other vital organs

7. Complications of a pulmonary embolus include pulmonary edema, atelectasis, severe hypoxia, shock, and elevated pulmonary circulation pressures

8. Signs and symptoms include tachypnea, tachycardia, hypotension, sudden acute dyspnea with extreme anxiety, chest or pleuritic pain (sharp, localized), abnormal lung sounds (wheezing, decreased breath sounds or crackles), hypoxemia, respiratory alkalosis, friction rub, diaphoresis, and coughing; petechiae may develop with fat emboli; large clots or more complicated situations include pulmonary hypertension, shock, right heart failure, or sudden respiratory arrest

9. Suspect PE whenever a client presents with *sudden onset* of pleuritic pain, SOB, and extreme anxiety while recovering from a lower extremity surgery, childbirth, major surgery, DVT, or on prolonged bedrest; the anxiety is often described as a feeling of doom, impending death, and is associated with fear of suffocating

C. Nursing assessment

1. Assessment includes analysis of type of pain (increased with inspiration), anxiety level, color (cyanosis), LOC, respiratory status, vital signs, symptoms of DVT (warmth, tenderness, swelling or lower leg or calf), and auscultation of lung sounds

2. Diagnostic tests

   a. CXR: wedge-shaped density (infarcted area), elevated diaphragms, atelectasis, or pleural effusions

   b. ABGs: decreased PaO_2, $PaCO_2$, and elevated pH—respiratory alkalosis

   c. Electrocardiogram (ECG): ST-T wave changes, right axis deviation; performed also to rule out a myocardial infarction

   d. Ventilation-perfusion lung scan or radioisotope lung scan: by injecting radioisotope, peripherally blocked areas will show no blood flow; does not actually diagnose an embolus

   e. Pulmonary angiography: allows direct visualization of pulmonary artery and branches for a definite diagnosis

   f. Ultrasound of legs to locate source of emboli

   g. CT scan

   h. Lab work: decreased partial thromboplastin time (PTT) or prothombin time (PT), elevated bilirubin, elevated lactic dehydrogenase (LDH), elevated fibrin degradation tests

   i. The partial thromboplastin time (PTT) and prothrombin time (PT) will be used to monitor anticoagulant therapy once started and should be 1.5 to 2.0 times the control value for a therapeutic level; monitor client closely for signs of bleeding while on heparin; an international normalized ratio (INR) may be used to monitor oral anticoagulant therapy (2.0–3.0 therapeutic)

D. Nursing management

1. Medications

   a. Anticoagulants: heparin followed by sodium warfarin (Coumadin) for confirmed PE; low molecular weight heparin (LMWH) for prevention after surgery, particularly hip surgery

   b. Thrombolytic therapy if clot is excessively large or needs to be dissolved immediately (tissue plasminogen activator [t-PA], streptokinase)

   c. Analgesics for discomfort or anxiety

   d. Vasopressors if needed for hypotension

2. Administer parenteral fluids as indicated

3. Avoid prolonged bed rest or sitting; limited ambulation may be allowed depending on clot location and size

4. Reassure client often to reduce anxiety

5. Administer O_2 as ordered

6. Apply antiembolism stockings, plexi-pulses or sequential compression devices; these aid in prevention as well as treatment

7. Prevention also includes early ambulation after surgery and leg exercises

8. Monitor ECG for cardiac dysrhythmias

9. Monitor pulmonary artery wedge pressures and cardiac output

10. Monitor vital signs, respiratory assessment, LOC, skin color, and mental status

11. Auscultate heart and lung sounds

12. Monitor lab values and signs of bleeding if on anticoagulant therapy (hematuria, oozing from venipuncture sites or IV lines, bleeding from gums or incisions, excessive bruising)

13. PT or PTT values are not recommended during LMWH therapy

X. PULMONARY HYPERTENSION

A. Overview

1. Pulmonary hypertension is defined as elevated pressures in pulmonary artery usually resulting from pulmonary or cardiac disease

2. Pulmonary artery pressure is normally 12 to 15 mmHg (25 systolic/8 diastolic), a resting mean pressure greater than 20 mmHg constitutes an elevation

3. Usually classified as primary or secondary

   a. *Primary pulmonary hypertension* (PPH) is unrelated to any known cause, has a higher incidence in young women 20 to 30 years of age, is highly uncommon, and can lead to death in 3 to 5 years

    b. *Secondary pulmonary hypertension* is caused by a pulmonary or cardiac disease process including hypoxia, congenital cardiac disease, emboli, COPD, sleep apnea, mitral stenosis, left ventricular failure, and pulmonary emboli

    c. Cor pulmonale, right ventricular hypertrophy and failure result from long-term pulmonary hypertension

B. Pathophysiology

  1. Narrowing of pulmonary vascular bed from major cardiac or pulmonary diseases is a common cause of pulmonary hypertension; vessel destruction, vasoconstriction, or obstruction may all contribute to narrowing of pulmonary vascular bed

  2. The medial (muscular) layer of pulmonary vasculature thickens and extensive intimal fibrosis may occur in severe cases

  3. The pulmonary vascular system usually has low pressure, high blood flow, and low resistance

  4. Pulmonary hypertension can be caused by any condition that results in an exaggerated blood flow in pulmonary bed, a higher resistance to blood flow, or a blockage of blood flow

  5. Complications of pulmonary hypertension include cor pulmonale or pulmonary edema due to inability of pressures in pulmonary artery to be lowered

  6. Signs and symptoms of pulmonary hypertension may not be detected until a significant rise in pulmonary artery pressure occurs and is reflected in a rise in systolic pressure

  7. Clinical manifestations may include fatigue, angina, dyspnea (on exertion and at rest), tachypnea, abnormal breath sounds (distant, decreased, crackles), cyanosis, and dizziness especially upon exertion; in addition, there may be signs of an underlying condition that can mask symptoms of pulmonary hypertension

C. Nursing assessment

  1. Assessment includes symptom analysis of any physical complaints, skin color, signs of edema, vital signs, use of accessory respiratory muscles, breath sounds, and heart sounds

  2. Diagnostic tests: CBC (may show polycythemia), ABGs (hypoxemia), CXR (enlarged right ventricle, dilated pulmonary arteries), ECG (right ventricular hypertrophy, right axis deviation, right bundle branch block), echocardiogram (enlarged right atrium, decreased wall motion), cardiac catheterization (elevated pulmonary artery pressures, decreased cardiac output)

D. Nursing management

  1. Medications

    a. Calcium channel blockers: nifedipine (Procardia), diltiazem (Cardizem) to lower pulmonary vascular resistance

    b. Direct vasodilators: adenosine (Adenocard), inhaled nitric oxide, hydralazine (Apresoline) to decrease afterload

    c. Angiotensin converting enzyme (ACE) inhibitors

    d. Diuretics and digoxin if cor pulmonale occurs

  2. Secondary pulmonary hypertension is aimed at treating underlying disease

  3. Administer O_2 as ordered to assist in treating hypoxemia

  4. Phlebotomy is recommended if polycythemia is present

5. Treatment of cor pulmonale includes fluid restriction, limited salt, and diuretics

6. Monitor activity if intolerance to physical exertion is severe, plan rest periods, and assist with ADLs

7. Monitor vital signs, lung sounds, and heart sounds

8. Assist client in high Fowler's position if needed

9. Encourage coughing and deep breathing

10. Educate client and family about signs of cor pulmonale and pulmonary edema

XI. LUNG CANCER

A. Overview

1. Lung cancer is termed *bronchogenic carcinoma* because tumor usually stems from bronchial mucosa and is defined as cancer of the epithelial lining of lung or lung parenchyma

2. Is a frequently occurring cancer of an internal organ, closely linked to cigarette smoking, and carries a poor prognosis

3. Classification of lung cancer

   a. Non–small-cell lung cancer (NSCLC): squamous cell carcinomas, large cell carcinomas, adenocarcinoma

   b. Small-cell lung cancer (SCLC): oat cell carcinoma

   c. Asbestos lung cancer: caused by exposure to asbestos

   d. Mesothelioma: cancer of lining of lung, also commonly caused by asbestos

B. Pathophysiology

1. Various chemicals and irritants (such as asbestos) act as carcinogens in lung, but those in tobacco smoke are a primary cause

2. Polycyclic hydrocarbons in cigarette smoke are mutagenic and can transform normal cells into malignant ones; the direct effect of these carcinogens on cellular DNA may explain why some individuals who smoke get lung cancer and others do not

3. Combined action of several carcinogens in tobacco may account for the rapid neoplasia that can occur

4. Another theory is that the bronchial epithelium undergoes metaplasia, which is a reversible state initially; in the presence of carcinogenic stimuli, metaplasia progresses to carcinoma

5. Some lung cancer tumors are highly invasive and may extend into mediastinum or spread into pleural cavity; because of highly vascular, network of lung, invasion into lymphatic system occurs early, contributing to metastasis in other areas; distant metastasis may occur in liver, brain, bones, kidneys, and adrenal glands

6. Complications include pneumonia, pleural effusions, Cushing's disease, hypercalcemia, anemia, disseminated intravascular coagulopathy (DIC), syndrome of inappropriate antidiuretic hormone (SIADH), and airway obstruction

7. Signs and symptoms initially may not be present until tumor is large enough to interfere with airway function and cancer is then well advanced

8. Clinical manifestations will then include a persistent productive cough, hemoptysis, frequent lower respiratory tract infections, abnormal breath sounds

(wheezing), angina, pleuritic pain (if pleura is involved), hoarseness and dysphagia (due to pressure from tumor)

9. In advanced stages with metastasis, weight loss, extreme dyspnea, fatigue, bone pain, and various endocrine, neurological, and cardiovascular symptoms are usually present

C. Nursing assessment

1. Assessment includes symptom analysis of any pain being experienced, changes in respiratory function or illnesses, lung sounds, sputum assessment (red or rust color), palpation of lymph nodes or enlarged liver, and weight loss analysis

2. A persistent cough that changes in character is common with lung cancer

3. Diagnostic tests: CXR, magnetic resonance imaging (MRI), CT scan of lung, brain or bone, bronchoscopy, sputum cytology, and lab tests (CBC, liver function, electrolytes, and coagulation studies)

D. Nursing management

1. Medications

   a. Combination chemotherapy: alkylating agents such as mechlorethamine (Mustargen), antibiotics such as doxorubicin (Adriamycin) or other drugs such as cisplatin (Platinol)

   b. Bronchodilators

   c. Antibiotics if an infection is present

   d. Analgesics: non–opioids, NSAIDs, opioids

2. Radiation (use of high-energy radioactive particles for palliative treatment) or surgery (lobectomy—removal of a lobe; pneumonectomy—removal of entire lung; or thoracotomy—incision of chest wall) are also treatment protocols; radiation therapy may be used to decrease tumor size prior to surgery

3. Photodynamic therapy (PDT) is a type of laser therapy that involves injecting a special chemical into bloodstream that remains only in cancer cells; a laser light activates chemical and kills affected cancer cells; often used to treat small tumors or reduce symptoms

4. Administer oxygen therapy as ordered

5. Assess respiratory status and vital signs

6. Auscultate lung and heart sounds

7. Manage pain (around-the-clock) and teach family how to treat pain, especially if client is being discharged; palliative care is essential especially in end-stage disease

8. Assist client to turn, cough, and deep breathe; placing bed in a high Fowler's position may be helpful

9. Provide chest physiotherapy with percussion and postural drainage, suctioning as needed

10. Plan rest periods, especially immediately following an analgesic

11. Assist client and family with grieving process

XII. RESPIRATORY FAILURE

A. Overview

1. Respiratory failure is defined as an inability of lungs to maintain adequate oxygenation and is usually manifested by hypoxemia, hypercapnia, and respiratory acidosis

2. ABGs reveal a PaO_2 less than 60 mmHg, $PaCO_2$ greater than 50 mmHg and pH less than 7.35; it is not a disease process, but a sign of severe dysfunction of respiratory system

3. In a client with COPD, a drop of 10 to 15 mmHg O_2 from *previous levels* indicates respiratory failure

4. Classification
   a. *Acute* (ARF): develops suddenly and can be life-threatening; causes can be pulmonary diseases, cardiac diseases, or non-pulmonary disorders (infections, injuries); ARF can develop in individuals with normal lungs
   b. *Chronic* (CRF): develops slowly or more gradually and is usually a result of chronic bronchitis or emphysema

5. Can also be classified by whether there is impairment of ventilation or diffusion
   a. Impaired ventilation can be caused by airway obstruction (from laryngospasm, foreign body aspiration, or laryngeal/tracheal edema), respiratory diseases (asthma or COPD), neurologic disorders (spinal cord injury, stroke, and neuromuscular diseases), or chest trauma (pneumothorax, flail chest)
   b. Impaired diffusion can be caused by disorders affecting alveoli (pneumonitis, pneumonia), pulmonary edema (near-drowning, acute respiratory distress syndrome [ARDS], cardiac failure), or ventilation-perfusion mismatch (pulmonary embolus)

6. Types include Type I, hypoxemia only; Type II, hypoxemia with hypercapnia; or Type III, hypercapnia caused by hypoventilation

B. Pathophysiology

1. Lungs are unable to remove CO_2 and there is inadequate O_2 inhalation; severe hypoventilation of the lung causes a rise in CO_2 level and respiratory acidosis

2. In chronic respiratory disorders such as emphysema and COPD, breathing becomes more labored, respiratory muscles weaken, and airway resistance is increased

3. Clients with respiratory failure become extremely exhausted and lose energy to breathe; ventilation, diffusion, or perfusion problems may cause respiratory failure (see Figure 1-5)

Figure 1-5

Causes of respiratory failure include ventilation, perfusion, or diffusion problems leading to hypoxemia and/or hypercapnia.

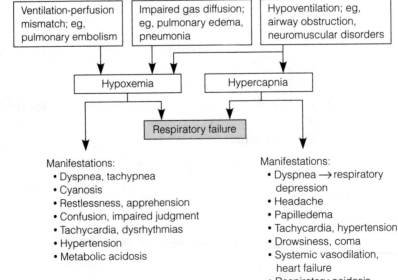

4. Respiratory failure is a cycle that can end in death; as breathing difficulty increases, less oxygen is brought to alveoli, resulting in less production of surfactant and increased resistance to expansion

5. If client is hyperventilating, pCO_2 may be low; if client is hypoxic only, pH will be less than 7.35 and pCO_2 will be normal; if the bicarbonate levels are low, metabolic acidosis can occur

6. Complications include ARDS, cardiac dysrhythmias, and cardiac failure

7. Signs and symptoms include those of underlying disease process along with hypoxemia, hypercapnia, dyspnea, neurological changes (restlessness, apprehension, impaired judgment and motor skills), cyanosis, diaphoresis, cool skin, and initial vital sign changes (tachycardia, hypertension, tachypnea)

8. As fatigue develops and hypoxemia worsens, cardiac output decreases, cardiac dysrhythmias may develop, and vital signs decrease (bradycardia, bradypnea, and hypotension)

C. **Nursing assessment**

1. Assessment includes: LOC, neurovascular assessment, skin color, vital signs, use of accessory respiratory muscles, auscultation of breath sounds, and ECG pattern

2. Diagnostic tests: ABGs (mild hypoxia with PaO_2 of less than 80 mmHg; moderate hypoxia with PaO_2 of less than 60 mmHg; and severe hypoxia with PaO_2 less than 40 mmHg), CXR (shows underlying disease process), ECG (dysrhythmias), hemodynamic monitoring, sputum for C&S

D. **Nursing management**

1. Medications

   a. Bronchodilators: methylxanthines (theophylline derivatives)

   b. Sympathomimetic or anticholinergic drugs in aerosol form for bronchodilation

   c. Corticosteroids

   d. Antibiotics if an infection exists

   e. Sedatives and analgesia while on mechanical ventilation

   f. Benzodiazepines: diazepam (Valium), lorazepam (Ativan), or midazolam (Versed) to decrease respiratory drive

   g. Neuromuscular blocking agents: pancuronium bromide (Pavulon) or vecuronium (Norcuron) to suppress client's ability to breathe while on a ventilator

2. Administer O_2 therapy as ordered (usually low levels) or maintain mechanical ventilation with PEEP; high O_2 levels may cause hypoventilation

3. Administer parenteral therapy, monitor fluid and electrolyte status

4. Administer nebulized inhalation, chest physiotherapy, and suctioning as needed

5. Auscultate breath and lung sounds

6. Assess vital signs, respiratory status, nasal flaring, and use of accessory muscles

7. Assess ECG and hemodynamic monitoring

8. Maintain nutritional support

9. Monitor O_2 saturation by pulse oximetry

Case Study

A 10-year-old boy has just been diagnosed with asthma related to allergies. The nurse working in the clinic is responsible for discharging the child on montelukast (Singulair) 1 tablet every day, albuterol (Ventolin) inhaler as needed for an asthma attack, nedocromil (Tilade) inhaler once a day, and albuterol (Ventolin) drops with saline for use with a nebulizer in the event the rescue inhaler does not work.

1. What discharge instructions should the nurse give the mother about the child's medications?

2. What explanation should the nurse give the mother about asthma?

3. What instructions should the nurse give the mother about when to seek immediate medical attention?

4. What should the child know about an asthma attack?

5. What are triggers and how do they affect asthma?

For suggested responses, see page 532.

POSTTEST

1 A client, who was not wearing a seat belt, was involved in a motor vehicle accident (MVA). The client now exhibits crepitus and decreased breath sounds on the left, reports shortness of breath, and has a respiratory rate of 34/min. Which assessment findings are of most concern to the nurse?

1. Temperature of 102° F and a productive cough
2. Arterial blood gases (ABGs) with a PaO_2 of 92 and $PaCO_2$ of 40 mmHg
3. Trachea deviating to the right
4. Barrel-chested appearance

2 A nurse is teaching a client newly diagnosed with emphysema about the disease process. Which statement that best explains the problems associated with emphysema could the nurse adapt for use in a discussion with the client?

1. "Hyperactivity of the medium-sized bronchi caused by an inflammatory response leads to wheezing and tightness in the chest."
2. "Larger than normal air spaces and loss of elastic recoil cause air to be trapped in the lung and collapse airways."
3. "Vasodilation, congestion, and mucosal edema cause a chronic cough and sputum production."
4. "Chloride is not being transported properly, producing excess absorption of water and sodium and thick, viscous mucus."

3 A sweat test is ordered for a child with respiratory symptoms suggestive of cystic fibrosis (CF). The nurse concludes that which of the following results are consistent with this diagnosis?

1. Chloride 45 mEq/L
2. Chloride 25 mEq/L
3. Chloride 35 mEq/L
4. Chloride 65 mEq/L

4 A client who underwent a hysterectomy experiences shortness of breath when walking. She has never had shortness of breath before. Upon auscultation, no breath sounds are heard in the left lower lobe. All other findings and breath sounds are normal. Which of the following etiologies should the nurse consider as a contributing factor?

1. Pleurisy
2. Pneumonia
3. Atelectasis
4. Pulmonary embolism

5 A client admitted to the medical nursing unit has classic symptoms of tuberculosis (TB) and tests positive on the purified protein derivative (PPD) skin test. Several months later, the nurse who cared for the client also tests positive on an annual TB skin test. The most likely course of treatment if the nurse's chest x-ray (CXR) is negative is to:

1. Repeat a TB skin test in six months.
2. Treat the nurse with an anti-infective agent for six months.
3. Monitor for signs and symptoms within the next year.
4. Follow up every six months with a repeat CXR.

6 The nurse instructs a client with severe sleep apnea to plan frequent rest periods and activities around how well the client feels. When asked by the client how this is will help, the nurse further explains that it is necessary to maximize energy and function because the client may experience which of the following? Select all that apply.

1. Cardiac dysrhythmias or other cardiac problems
2. Daytime fatigue and sleepiness
3. Jaw pain
4. Impaired intellect and memory loss
5. Personality changes and depression

7 A client who smokes cigarettes and has a known history of cardiac problems enters the clinic reporting the sudden onset of sharp, stabbing pain that intensifies with a deep breath. The pain occurs on only one side and can be isolated upon general assessment. The nurse concludes that the client's pain is consistent with which of the following?

1. Pleurisy
2. Pleural effusion
3. Atelectasis
4. Tuberculosis

8 The nurse is delivering post-mortem care to a client who died from a large pulmonary embolus (PE). While reflecting on the client's death, the nurse considers that it was most likely caused by which of the following?

1. Decreased blood flow
2. Decreased alveolar dead space
3. Inefficiency of the heart to pump adequately
4. Infarction of the lung tissue

9 An elderly client recuperating from major abdominal surgery will be in bed for much of the immediate post-operative period. The nurse anticipates that the client will most likely be placed on which medication to prevent a pulmonary embolism (PE)?

1. Tissue plasminogen activator (t-PA)
2. Warfarin (Coumadin)
3. Enoxaparin (Lovenox)
4. Heparin

10 A 50-year-old client with chronic obstructive pulmonary disease (COPD) who has smoked two packs of cigarettes a day is being cared for in the intensive care unit for an acute exacerbation of the disease. Which of the following client data should alert the nurse to the possibility of pulmonary hypertension?

1. Pulmonary artery mean pressure of 30 mmHg
2. Rust-colored sputum
3. Thick, viscous mucus
4. Absent breath sounds

➤ *See pages 35–37 for Answers & Rationales*

ANSWERS & RATIONALES

Pretest

1 **Answer: 1** Clients with COPD tend to have low oxygen (O_2) and high carbon dioxide (CO_2) levels. They cannot tolerate high levels of O_2 because hypoxia is the main stimulus for ventilation in persons with chronic hypercapnia. Increasing the level of oxygen would decrease the stimulus to breathe. It is unlikely that the CO_2 levels will ever be low. High O_2 levels do not directly cause acidemia; rather, acidemia tends to result from retained CO_2 and possibly from metabolic alterations caused by hypoxia.

Cognitive Level: Application **Client Need:** Physiological Integrity: Basic Care and Comfort **Integrated Process:** Teaching/Learning **Content Area:** Adult Health: Respiratory **Strategy:** Note the critical word *chronic* in the stem of the question. Consider the stimulus for ventilation in clients with COPD and use the process of elimination to select the option that reflects the pathophysiology of the disease. **Reference:** Porth, C. M. (2005). *Pathophysiology:*

Concepts of altered health states (7th ed.). Philadelphia, PA: Lippincott Williams & Wilkins, p. 656.

2 Answer: 4 A combined low PO_2 and low SaO_2 represent hypoxia. The pH, PCO_2, and HCO_3 are normal. ABGs will not necessarily be altered in TB or pleural effusion. Initially, in pneumonia, both the PO_2 and PCO_2 are usually low because the hypoxia caused by the infection leads to hyperventilation.
Cognitive Level: Analysis **Integrated Process:** Nursing Process: Analysis **Client Need:** Physiological Integrity: Reduction of Risk Potential **Content Area:** Adult Health: Respiratory **Strategy:** First view the pH, noting that the pH is on the acidotic end of normal. Note the critical word *best* in the question, indicating that more than one option may be plausible but that one is better than the others. Choose option 4 because it fits the clinical picture of the client regardless of the exact underlying etiology. **Reference:** Porth, C. M. (2005). *Pathophysiology: Concepts of altered health states* (7th ed.). Philadelphia, PA: Lippincott Williams & Wilkins, p. 651.

3 Answer: 3 The cardinal signs of respiratory problems and hypoxia are restlessness, diaphoresis, tachycardia, and cool skin. Bradycardia might occur much later in the process when the condition is severe. Eupnea is normal respirations in rate and depth. Warm, dry skin is a normal finding.
Cognitive Level: Application **Client Need:** Physiological Integrity: Physiological Adaptation **Integrated Process:** Nursing Process: Assessment **Content Area:** Adult Health: Respiratory **Strategy:** Note the critical word *early* in the stem of the question. Recall that early signs tend to be milder in nature, although they are abnormal. This enables elimination of options 1 and 4 as normal, and selection of option 3 over option 2 as an expected early compensatory response. **Reference:** Porth, C. M. (2005). *Pathophysiology: Concepts of altered health states* (7th ed.). Philadelphia, PA: Lippincott Williams & Wilkins, pp. 718–719.

4 Answer: 2 Shortness of breath, increased respiratory rate, and slightly labored respirations could be caused by any of the conditions listed. The distinguishing symptom is the lack of breath sounds in the lower-right base when a portion of the lung has collapsed. Atelectasis causes diminished or absent breath sounds since the lung is not expanding with inspiration when a portion of the lower lung has collapsed. This is sometimes a complication of surgery and anesthesia. Pulmonary embolus, cardiac tamponade, and cor pulmonale are not distinguished by absent breath sounds.
Cognitive Level: Analysis **Client Need:** Physiological Integrity: Physiological Adaptation **Integrated Process:** Nursing Process: Analysis **Content Area:** Adult Health: Respiratory **Strategy:** Consider the physiological re-

sponse to and possible etiologies of altered gas exchange in the lungs. Also note that the client in the question is one day postoperative. Recall the risks of surgery and manifestations associated with atelectasis to choose correctly. **Reference:** Porth, C. M. (2005). *Pathophysiology: Concepts of altered health states* (7th ed.). Philadelphia, PA: Lippincott Williams & Wilkins, pp. 639–640, 692–693.

5 Answers: 1, 4, 5 The effects of the respiratory treatment should break up the congestion and cause bronchodilation, thus the improving lung sounds and producing a more productive cough effort. As the pneumonia resolves, the lungs should begin to clear and the cough diminish. The expected effects of the medications are decreased airway resistance and decreased viscosity of mucoprotein strands, producing more sputum and less congestion. Wheezing should improve with bronchodilation. Symptoms of poor gas exchange, such as anxiety and confusion, should improve. The cough will remain productive in the acute stage. Absent breath sounds would suggest a worsening of the condition.
Cognitive Level: Analysis **Client Need:** Physiological Integrity: Physiological Adaptation **Integrated Process:** Nursing Process: Evaluation **Content Area:** Adult Health: Respiratory **Strategy:** Notice that the question asks about an *acute case;* be careful to note the situation in the stem. Watch for opposites in the distracters. **Reference:** Lemone, P., & Burke, K. (2008). *Medical-surgical nursing: Critical thinking in client care* (4th ed.). Upper Saddle River, NJ: Pearson Education, pp. 1275–1276.

6 Answer: 3 The findings in option 3 are consistent with a tension pneumothorax, which is considered a medical emergency. The respiratory system is severely compromised and venous return to the heart is also affected. The mediastinal shift is occurring to the unaffected side. Option 1 outlines symptoms of pleurisy, which is not an emergency situation. Option 2 presents symptoms of bronchitis, which is not an emergency. The client in option 4 should expect difficulty breathing after exercise when asthma is an existing condition, and this client may need immediate attention if the rescue inhaler is ineffective. Although asthma sounds critical, the tension pneumothorax is immediately life threatening and is the better answer.
Cognitive Level: Analysis **Client Need:** Safe, Effective Care Environment: Management of Care **Integrated Process:** Nursing Process: Analysis **Content Area:** Adult Health: Respiratory **Strategy:** The critical word in the stem of the question is *immediate.* Use nursing knowledge and the process of elimination to select tension pneumothorax as the emergency situation. **Reference:** Lemone, P., & Burke, K. (2008). *Medical-surgical nursing: Critical*

thinking in client care (4th ed.). Upper Saddle River, NJ: Pearson Education, p. 1298.

7 **Answer: 2** A young person needs to know the triggers of asthma. Physical exercise in school and as a part of life will be ever-present, and prevention of an attack before exercise is essential at this time in the client's life. Living a productive, normal life should be stressed. Sports do not have to be limited in all asthmatic people. The client may have to use preventive medications before a sport of choice. The fear associated with asthma is common and may take a while to overcome. Instructions on identifying triggers and using the rescue inhalers need to be taught and the fear will eventually subside. Knowledge of the incidence of the disease is not the highest priority for this newly diagnosed teenage client.
Cognitive Level: Application **Client Need:** Physiological Integrity: Physiological Adaptation **Integrated Process:** Teaching/Learning **Content Area:** Adult Health: Respiratory **Strategy:** Consider the developmental stage of the client and the clue words *newly diagnosed*. With these in mind, use nursing knowledge and the process of elimination to make a selection **Reference:** Lemone, P., & Burke, K. (2008). *Medical-surgical nursing: Critical thinking in client care* (4th ed.). Upper Saddle River, NJ: Pearson Education, pp. 1323–1330.

8 **Answer: 4** Clients who have sleep apnea do not get adequate amounts of REM sleep and are often awakened frequently during the night in order to make breathing possible. Sleep apnea is related to decreased muscle tone. Upper airflow obstruction occurs, the CO_2 rises, and cardiac arrhythmias and angina can occur because of the lack of oxygenated blood supply to the heart.
Cognitive Level: Analysis **Client Need:** Physiological Integrity: Physiological Adaptation **Integrated Process:** Teaching/Learning **Content Area:** Adult Health: Respiratory **Strategy:** Recall that progressive asphyxia causes many brief arousals during sleep with resulting physiological effects. Note also that the angina is being experienced only at night. Use this information and knowledge of pathophysiology of sleep apnea to make a selection. **Reference:** Lemone, P., & Burke, K. (2008). *Medical-surgical nursing: Critical thinking in client care* (4th ed.). Upper Saddle River, NJ: Pearson Education, p. 1250.

9 **Answer: 2** The most common sign of cancer of the lung is a persistent cough that changes. Other signs are dyspnea, bloody sputum, and long-term pulmonary infection. Option 1 is common with chronic obstructive pulmonary disease (COPD). Option 3 is common with asthma. Night sweats (option 4) are commonly seen with tuberculosis.
Cognitive Level: Application **Client Need:** Physiological Integrity: Physiological Adaptation **Integrated Process:**

Nursing Process: Analysis **Content Area:** Adult Health: Respiratory **Strategy:** Consider that manifestations are related to the location of the lesion and its possible metastasis. Then eliminate the findings commonly seen with other conditions. **Reference:** Lemone, P., & Burke, K. (2008). *Medical-surgical nursing: Critical thinking in client care* (4th ed.). Upper Saddle River, NJ: Pearson Education, pp. 1309–1311.

10 **Answers: 2, 3, 4** Chest tubes are inserted and attached to a closed drainage system to allow the lung to re-expand while preventing air from entering the pleural space. Periodic bubbles are normal and indicate that the air is being removed from the chest. Fluctuation of the water level in the tube with respiration indicates the system is intact. Fluctuations and bubbles will cease when the lung is expanded. Continuous bubbles may indicate an air leak in the system that could result in collapse of the lung. Decreased breath sounds indicate a deterioration of respiratory status. A full collection system needs to be replaced.
Cognitive Level: Application **Integrated Process:** Nursing Process: Implementation **Client Need:** Physiological Integrity: Physiological Adaptation **Content Area:** Adult Health: Respiratory **Strategy:** Consider principles in working with a closed drainage system. Read carefully for clarifying terms in the options. **Reference:** Lemone, P., & Burke, K. (2008). *Medical-surgical nursing: Critical thinking in client care* (4th ed.). Upper Saddle River, NJ: Pearson Education, p. 1300.

Posttest

1 **Answer: 3** Tracheal deviation toward the unaffected side occurs with mediastinal shift, which indicates a tension pneumothorax when considered in light of the other symptoms in the question. Since the client was involved in an MVA, assessment would be targeted at acute traumatic injuries to the lungs, heart, or chest wall rather than the conditions indicated in the other options. Option 1 is common with pneumonia; values in option 2 are not alarming; and option 4 is typical of someone with chronic obstructive pulmonary disease (COPD).
Cognitive Level: Analysis **Client Need:** Physiological Integrity: Physiological Adaptation **Integrated Process:** Nursing Process: Analysis **Content Area:** Adult Health: Respiratory **Strategy:** Look for the most life threatening condition. Read all the options before making a selection. **Reference:** Lemone, P., & Burke, K. (2008). *Medical-surgical nursing: Critical thinking in client care* (4th ed.). Upper Saddle River, NJ: Pearson/Prentice Hall, pp. 1298–1299.

2 **Answer: 2** Option 2 best describes the pathophysiology behind emphysema. Option 1 explains asthma, option 3 explains bronchitis, and option 4 explains cystic fibrosis.

Cognitive Level: Application **Client Need:** Physiological Integrity: Physiological Adaptation **Integrated Process:** Nursing Process: Analysis **Content Area:** Adult Health: Respiratory **Strategy:** Choose the option that describes the pathophysiology of emphysema. Recall that even a true statement is not the correct option unless it answers the question asked. **Reference:** Lemone, P., & Burke, K. (2008). *Medical-surgical nursing: Critical thinking in client care* (4th ed.). Upper Saddle River, NJ: Pearson/Prentice Hall, p. 1269.

3 **Answer: 4** Cystic fibrosis is diagnosed by a high chloride level on the sweat test. The normal chloride level on this test is less than 60 mEq/L in an adult and less than 50 mEq/L in a child.

Cognitive Level: Application **Client Need:** Physiological Integrity: Reduction of Risk Potential **Integrated Process:** Nursing Process: Analysis **Content Area:** Child Health: Respiratory **Strategy:** Recall that parents of children with cystic fibrosis often report that the child tastes "salty" when kissed. Use this to reason that the chloride level (part of salt) would be high, and choose a high value from the options available. **Reference:** Kee, J.L. (2005). *Laboratory and diagnostic tests with nursing implications* (7th ed.). Upper Saddle River, NJ: Pearson/Prentice Hall, p. 780.

4 **Answer: 3** Resorption atelectasis can occur after surgery and is a common complication. It is manifested by decreased or absent breath sounds in the affected lobe. Pleurisy is incorrect because it would also be accompanied by pain upon inspiration. Pneumonia is common after surgery but would have additional symptoms. Pulmonary embolism is also accompanied by chest pain, acute dyspnea, and severe air hunger with anxiety.

Cognitive Level: Application **Client Need:** Physiological Integrity: Physiological Adaptation **Integrated Process:** Nursing Process: Analysis **Content Area:** Adult Health: Respiratory **Strategy:** Which option stands out from the others and fits the findings described in the stem? **Reference:** Porth, C. M. (2005). *Pathophysiology: Concepts of altered health states* (7th ed.). Philadelphia, PA: Lippincott Williams & Wilkins, pp. 693–694.

5 **Answer: 2** Exposure with a positive TB skin test usually requires six months of prophylactic treatment unless contraindicated. The TB skin test should not be repeated; the results will always be positive. Monitoring will not prevent TB, and the nurse has been exposed. Appropriate therapy is needed to control the spread of TB. A CXR is usually not required annually in the event that the skin test was positive; however, many health care employers require a CXR for employees to verify that the disease has not reactivated.

Cognitive Level: Application **Client Need:** Physiological Integrity: Physiological Adaptation **Integrated Process:**

Nursing Process: Implementation **Content Area:** Adult Health: Respiratory **Strategy:** A positive PPD is a cell-mediated immune response that indicates that the person has mounted an immune response. It does not mean that the disease is active. **Reference:** Lemone, P., & Burke, K. (2008). *Medical-surgical nursing: Critical thinking in client care* (4th ed.). Upper Saddle River, NJ: Pearson/Prentice Hall, pp. 1288–1289.

6 **Answers: 1, 2, 4, 5** Recurrent nocturnal asphyxia due to airway obstruction increases the workload of the heart and may cause cardiac symptoms such as bradycardia or tachycardia. Clients with coronary heart disease may develop ischemia or angina. In some instances, left ventricular function is impaired and heart failure may occur. Any activity increases the need for oxygen, which is already limited in a client with this disorder. The deprivation of oxygen during the night and lack of REM sleep often leaves individuals tired during the day. Personality changes and depression are observed. Jaw pain may be a symptom of myocardial infarction or temporomandibular joint disease (TMJ). Neither of these is directly related to sleep apnea. Recurrent apnea and loss of slow-wave sleep contribute to neurological and behavioral symptoms.

Cognitive Level: Application **Client Need:** Physiological Integrity: Physiological Adaptation **Integrated Process:** Nursing Process: Planning **Content Area:** Adult Health: Respiratory **Strategy:** Which option fits a daytime symptom for a nighttime problem? What ongoing physiologic effects can recurrent apnea and arousal during sleep cause? **Reference:** Lemone, P., & Burke, K. (2008). *Medical-surgical nursing: Critical thinking in client care* (4th ed.). Upper Saddle River, NJ: Pearson/Prentice Hall, p. 1250.

7 **Answer: 1** Pleuritic pain is typically sharp and stabbing. Pleurisy is common in smokers. Pleural effusion can cause pain but usually has other symptoms such as dyspnea and diminished or absent breath sounds. Atelectasis can cause pain but it usually has other symptoms such as dyspnea and diminished or absent breath sounds. Tuberculosis causes chest pain and may cause pleuritis along with other symptoms; however, this is not the first problem suspected when a client presents with the pain described.

Cognitive Level: Application **Client Need:** Physiological Integrity: Physiological Adaptation **Integrated Process:** Nursing Process: Analysis **Content Area:** Adult Health: Respiratory **Strategy:** Rule out the options that are not manifested by the pain described in the stem. **Reference:** Lemone, P., & Burke, K. (2008). *Medical-surgical nursing: Critical thinking in client care* (4th ed.). Upper Saddle River, NJ: Pearson/Prentice Hall, p. 1295.

8 **Answer: 4** If the blockage is large enough and blood flow is hindered to the lung, the tissue will die. This usually occurs when a large clot blocks the entire main pulmonary artery. Option 1 is rather vague because blood flow is decreased to the heart, lung, brain, and other vital organs because of the blockage but the amount of decrease can be variable. Option 2 is incorrect; dead space is increased with PE. Option 3 is correct in pulmonary embolism but is not usually the cause of death. **Cognitive Level:** Application **Client Need:** Physiological Integrity: Physiological Adaptation **Integrated Process:** Nursing Process: Analysis **Content Area:** Adult Health: Respiratory **Strategy:** Eliminate the options known to be wrong. Select the best answer from the remaining choices. Read all the options before choosing the answer. **Reference:** Lemone, P., & Burke, K. (2008). *Medical-surgical nursing: Critical thinking in client care* (4th ed.). Upper Saddle River, NJ: Pearson/Prentice Hall, pp. 1347–1348.

9 **Answer: 3** Without any evidence of a blood clot or PE, a low molecular weight heparin (LMWH) such as enoxaparin is usually used for prevention purposes, especially since the client is elderly and will be in bed for a period of time. Heparin and Coumadin (anticoagulants) are used when a confirmed clot exists. Thrombolytics such as t-PA are used when a clot needs to be immediately dissolved. **Cognitive Level:** Application **Client Need:** Physiological Integrity: Pharmacological and Parenteral Therapies **Integrated Process:** Nursing Process: Implementation **Content Area:** Adult Health: Respiratory **Strategy:** Consider the etiology of pulmonary embolism. Which drugs are therapeutic and which are prophylactic? This situation asks for prevention. **Reference:** Lemone, P., & Burke, K. (2008). *Medical-surgical nursing: Critical thinking in client care* (4th ed.). Upper Saddle River, NJ: Pearson/Prentice Hall, pp. 1349–1350.

10 **Answer: 1** A sustained elevation in the resting mean pressure above 20 mmHg from a pulmonary artery is defined as pulmonary hypertension, which could be caused by the COPD. Rust-colored sputum (option 2) is usually indicative of lung cancer; thick, viscous mucus (option 3) can be significant in a number of disorders; and absent breath sounds (option 4) are present in many pulmonary disorders, such as pneumonia and pneumothorax, but not pulmonary hypertension. **Cognitive Level:** Application **Client Need:** Physiological Integrity: Physiological Adaptation **Integrated Process:** Nursing Process: Assessment **Content Area:** Adult Health: Respiratory **Strategy:** Consider the known history of COPD for a pathophysiologic hint. Note that the critical word *hypertension* in the stem may link to a related word in the correct option (pressure). **Reference:** Lemone, P., & Burke, K. (2008). *Medical-surgical nursing: Critical thinking in client care* (4th ed.). Upper Saddle River, NJ: Pearson/Prentice Hall, pp. 1352–1353.

References

Advair Diskus (2005). Glaxo Smith Kline. Retrieved from http://www.advair.com/asthma_inhaler_instructions.html

Black, J., & Hawks, J. (2005). *Medical surgical nursing: clinical management for positive outcomes* (7th ed.). St. Louis, MO: Elsevier Science.

Centers for Disease Control. *Mantoux TB skin test.facilitator.guide. Appendix D.* Retrieved from http://www.cdc.gov/nchstp/tb/pubs/mantoux/appendix_o.htm

Corbett, J. V. (2004). *Laboratory tests and diagnostic procedures* (6th ed.). Upper Saddle River, NJ: Prentice Hall.

Ignatavicius, D., & Workman, L. (2006). *Medical surgical nursing: Critical thinking for collaborative care* (5th ed.). Philadelphia: W. B. Saunders.

Kee, J. L. (2005). *Laboratory and diagnostic test with nursing implications* (7th ed.). Upper Saddle River, NJ: Reason/Prentice Hall, p. 780.

LeMone, P., & Burke, K. (2008). *Medical-surgical nursing: Critical thinking in client care* (4th ed.). Upper Saddle River, NJ: Prentice Hall, pp. 1041–1069, 1076–1172.

Lewis, S., Heitkemper, M., & Dirksen, S. (2004). *Medical surgical nursing: Assessment and management of clinical problems* (6th ed.). St. Louis, MO: Elsevier Science.

Lung Cancer Treatment Options. Retrieved from http://www.mesothelioma_lung.cancer.org

McCance, K., & Huether, S. (2006). *Pathophysiology: The biologic basis for disease in adults and children* (5th ed.). St. Louis, MO: Elsevier Science.

McKenry, L. Tessier, E., & Hogan, M. (2006). *Mosby's pharmacology in nursing* (22nd ed.). St. Louis, MO: Mosby.

Porth, C. (2005). *Pathophysiology: Concepts of altered health states* (7th ed.). Philadelphia: Lippincott Williams & Wilkins pp. 633–724.

Spiriva Handihaler, (2005). Boehringer Ingelheim Pharmaceuticals, Retrieved from http://www.spiriva.com/spirivaWeb/consumer/index.jsp

Venes, D., Thomas, & Taber, C. (2006). *Taber's cyclopedic medical dictionary* (20th ed.). Philadelphia: F. A. Davis.

Wilson, B., Shannon, M., & Stang, C. (2006). *Nursing drug guide 2006.* Upper Saddle River, NJ: Prentice Hall.

ANSWERS & RATIONALES

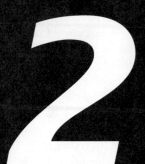

Cardiac Health Problems

Chapter Outline

Risk Factors Associated with Cardiac Health Problems

Coronary Artery Disease (CAD)

Angina Pectoris

Myocardial Infarction (MI)

Congestive Heart Failure (CHF)

Cardiac Dysrhythmias

Inflammatory Diseases of the Heart

Valvular Heart Disease

NCLEX-RN® Test Prep

Use the CD-ROM enclosed with this book to access additional practice opportunities.

Objectives

➤ Define key terms associated with cardiac health problems.

➤ Identify risk factors associated with the development of cardiac health problems.

➤ Explain the common etiologies of cardiac health problems.

➤ Describe the pathophysiologic processes associated with specific cardiac health problems.

➤ Distinguish between normal and abnormal cardiac findings obtained from nursing assessment.

➤ Prioritize nursing interventions associated with specific cardiac health problems.

Review at a Glance

afterload pressure against which heart must pump

angina pectoris chest pain associated with anaerobic metabolism from decreased oxygen supply to myocardium

automaticity ability of a cardiac muscle cell to contract independently, without stimulation

cardiac output amount of blood pumped out of left ventricle each minute; determined by HR × stroke volume

collateral circulation additional outgrowth of tiny vessels that supply heart muscle with oxygenated blood

congestive heart failure (CHF) inability of heart to pump sufficient blood to maintain adequate oxygen and nutrients to tissues

coronary artery disease (CAD) atherosclerotic plaque deposits lining walls of coronary arteries and narrowing these vessels, causing decreased oxygen supply to myocardium

electrocardiogram (ECG or EKG) graphic representation of electrical activity of heart

intermittent claudication cramping in lower extremities, especially when walking or with exercise

ischemia insufficient blood flow that may lead to decreased oxygen supply to tissues causing anaerobic cellular metabolism rather than aerobic metabolism

mitral valve prolapse the mitral valve opens backward toward atrium causing regurgitation of blood from ventricle to atrium

myocardial infarction (MI) death of tissue of myocardium caused by lack of oxygen supply

myocarditis an inflammatory disorder of heart muscle that is unrelated to coronary artery disease or myocardial infarction

pericarditis inflammation of pericardium and/or pericardial sac surrounding heart

preload volume of blood returning to heart, creating "stretch" or tension of myocardial fibers at end diastole

reentry phenomenon blockage of an impulse through one of the bundle branches, causing impulse to retrograde backwards, reenter other side and cause a premature contraction

regurgitation a condition in which blood flows backward through a valve that should be closed but cannot close completely because of damage or disease

stenosis a condition in which valves of heart become hardened and blood does not flow through them adequately

stroke volume amount of blood ejected from left ventricle with each heartbeat

ventricular fibrillation chaotic, irregular quivering of ventricles; a lethal dysrhythmia requiring immediate defibrillation

PRETEST

1 The client experiences chest pain after mowing the lawn. The Emergency Department nurse who receives a telephone call from the client's significant other considers that the pain is most likely the result of which of the following?

1. Pericardial effusion of fluid
2. Pulmonary edema
3. Myocardial ischemia
4. Pulmonary emboli

2 The client who has peripheral edema during the day states he is awakened at night with difficulty breathing. The nurse concludes that the client is most likely experiencing which of the following?

1. Angina pectoris
2. Orthopnea
3. A sinus infection
4. Sleep apnea

3 The client reports onset of shortness of breath, productive cough, tachycardia, and orthopnea. The nurse concludes that these manifestations are frequently consistent with which health problem?

1. Hypertension (HTN)
2. Left ventricular failure
3. Coronary artery disease (CAD)
4. Peripheral vascular disease

4 The client has ST segment depression on the 12-lead electrocardiogram (ECG). The nurse concludes that this ECG change is consistent with:

1. Necrosis.
2. Injury.
3. Ischemia.
4. Nothing significant.

5 The nurse anticipates that left ventricular failure can result in which of the following problems in the client? Select all that apply.

1. Right ventricular failure
2. Diminished left atrial pressures
3. Higher pulmonary pressures
4. Pulmonary edema
5. Decreased perfusion to the brain and peripheral circulation

6 A client undergoing cardiac monitoring by telemetry has sinus rhythm with a heart rate of 54 beats per minute (bpm). The nurse appropriately documents this rhythm as:

1. Sinus bradycardia.
2. Sinus tachycardia.
3. Sinus arrhythmia.
4. Accelerated nodal rhythm.

7 A client with a history of unstable angina is being assessed by the nurse in the Emergency Department. The client demonstrates significant Q waves on the electrocardiogram (ECG). The nurse notifies the physician because this is indicative of:

1. Gangrene.
2. Ischemia.
3. Infection.
4. Infarction.

8 The client in the Emergency Department is diagnosed with acute myocardial infarction (MI). He asks the nurse to explain what this is. The nurse responds that an MI usually occurs because of which of the following?

1. Obstruction of a coronary artery with death of tissue distal to the blockage
2. Spasm of a coronary artery causing temporary decreased blood supply
3. A slow heart rate leading to decreased blood supply to myocardium
4. Dilation of the ventricular wall causing decreased blood supply

9 The nurse is teaching a client about risk factors for the development of atherosclerosis. The nurse should place lowest priority on addressing which of the following risk factors when conducting client teaching?

1. Being female age 59
2. Hyperlipidemia
3. Cigarette smoking
4. Sedentary lifestyle and obesity

10 The client comes to the clinic for a repeat visit following new onset of stable angina. When teaching the client about precipitating causes of angina, such as exercise and stress, what should the nurse include as a way to manage the precipitating causes?

1. Avoid these activities.
2. Perform such activities anyway.
3. Lead a sedentary lifestyle.
4. Use a nitroglycerin (NTG) tablet before the activity.

➤ *See pages 74–76 for Answers & Rationales.*

I. RISK FACTORS ASSOCIATED WITH CARDIAC HEALTH PROBLEMS

A. Coronary artery disease (CAD), angina, and myocardial infarction (MI): smoking, alcohol intake, obesity, sedentary lifestyle, diabetes mellitus, hypercholesterolemia (total cholesterol over 200 mg/dL), hyperlipidemia (LDL over 160 mg/dL); nonmodifiable risk factors include age (over 45 for male and over 55 for female), male gender, family history (genetics), hypertension, stress, race, personality type, elevated triglycerides

B. Congestive heart failure (CHF): anyone with cardiac conditions such as CAD, MI, hypertension (HTN), diabetes mellitus (DM), pericarditis; clients with pulmonary conditions such as chronic obstructive pulmonary disease (COPD), pulmonary HTN, post–coronary bypass clients

C. Cardiac dysrhythmias: clients with known cardiac diseases (CAD, MI, CHF); elderly; electrolyte disturbances; any condition that creates stress on body (fever, hypoxia, etc.)

D. **Inflammatory disease:** environmental and economic factors, damp weather, crowded living conditions, malnutrition, immunodeficiency, decreased access to health care, other illnesses involving development of streptococcal infections or severe stress/trauma to heart; may have genetic tendency; risk factor for myocarditis can be alcohol use, stress, age, and ionizing radiation

E. **Valvular heart disease:** aging process, diseases such as MI, congenital heart defects

F. **Control of risk factors** by effective screening and public education can reduce cardiac morbidity and mortality

II. CORONARY ARTERY DISEASE (CAD)

A. **Overview**

1. **Coronary artery disease (CAD)** is defined as narrowing of coronary arteries causing a decreased lumen and decreased blood flow through those arteries

2. Coronary atherosclerosis is most common cause of CAD

   a. Defined as narrowing of vessel wall by atherosclerotic plaques

   b. The following factors speed development of plaque, which in turn impedes blood flow to myocardium, thereby decreasing oxygen availability to tissue

      1) Elevated cholesterol and triglyceride levels

      2) Elevated blood pressure (BP) by damaging lining

      3) Infection that initiates inflammatory response

      4) Elevated iron levels carry free radicals that cause damage to lining

      5) Elevated homocysteine levels (clients often have vascular disease also)

B. **Pathophysiology**

1. Injury to lining of artery occurs, resulting in increased permeability of endothelial cells, allowing components of plasma to enter

2. An inflammatory reaction occurs, bringing macrophages and platelets to area of injury

3. Hemorrhage into plaque produces thrombi; thrombus formation within arterial lumen is initiated by platelet aggregation

4. Embolization of a thrombus or plaque fragment can occur

5. Cholesterol, fat, and thrombi develop into a plaque formation

6. Progressive narrowing of lumen by plaque enlargement results in **ischemia** (insufficient blood flow leading to decreased oxygen supply to myocardium) due to narrowing of artery lumen

   a. ECG changes (inverted T wave; depressed S-T segment) occur during an acute or severe episode of ischemia (Figure 2-1)

   b. Chest pain or angina pectoris occurs

7. Cholesterol and triglycerides circulate in blood as lipoproteins

   a. High-density lipoprotein (HDL), known as "good cholesterol" is protective against coronary heart disease (CHD) by taking fats away for breakdown

   b. Low-density lipoprotein (LDL) and very low density lipoprotein (VLDL) helps fat remain in cells, known as "bad cholesterol"

8. Signs and symptoms include chest pain, hypertension, increased pulse, increased respirations, pallor of skin, diminished peripheral pulses occasionally;

Figure 2-1

S-T depression suggesting ischemia.

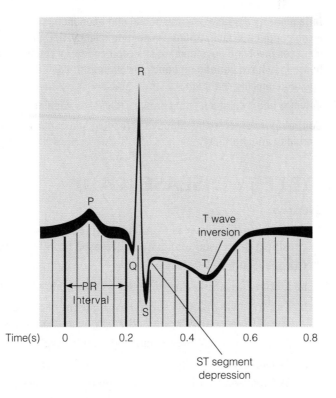

a comparable symptom of atherosclerosis in legs is called **intermittent claudication** (cramping in lower extremities, especially when walking or with exercise)

C. Nursing assessment

1. Assessment

   a. Pain

      1) Location: midsternal, arms, jaw, abdomen, back
      2) Description: heaviness, tightness
      3) Duration: more than 3 minutes
      4) Intensity: rating of 1 to 10 on a verbal rating scale (VRS) or on a visual analog scale

   b. Other: assess vital signs, heart sounds, exercise tolerance, peripheral pulses, skin color

2. Potentiating factors: exercise, stress, cold temperature, anemia, substance abuse, thyrotoxicosis, hyperthyroidism

3. Relieving factors: rest, removal of stressors

4. Diagnostic tests: cholesterol level (HDL [highest], VLDL [lowest], LDL [lower than HDL]), triglyceride level, radiographic studies of arteries (arteriogram, angiogram), ECG

D. Nursing management

1. Medications

   a. Antihyperlipidemic agents and those that lower triglycerides: nicotinic acid (niacin) and HMG-COA reductase inhibitors (also called *statins*) such as atorvastatin (Lipitor) and simvastatin (Zocor)

   b. Antiplatelets: acetylsalicylic acid (aspirin)

► **Practice to Pass**

A client who is diagnosed with coronary artery disease (CAD) states that she did not know she had experienced a heart attack. What should the nurse's response be?

   c. Antihypertensives if necessary

   d. Antianginals: nitroglycerine (Nitrostat; NTG)

   e. Antimicrobials if indicated

2. Teach risk factor management: low-fat diet, regular exercise, regular check-ups, cessation of smoking, stress management

3. Teach person to recognize signs and symptoms of CAD: shortness of breath, chest pain, and dyspnea on exertion; females may have atypical signs

4. Teach person to stop and rest at onset of discomfort

III. ANGINA PECTORIS

A. Overview

1. **Angina pectoris** is defined as chest pain caused by myocardial ischemia from:

   a. Reduced blood flow

   b. Reduced O_2 supply compared to demand by myocardium

   c. Temporary or reversible cause

2. Classified as stable, unstable, or Prinzmetal's angina

3. Causes include CAD, coronary spasms, thrombi, or any condition that creates an imbalance between myocardial O_2 supply and demand

B. Pathophysiology

1. When there is decreased blood flow (O_2 supply) to myocardium (ischemia) and/or increased demand for O_2 that cannot be met, angina occurs; this is body's way of communicating that there isn't enough oxygenated blood; angina is a forewarning that a myocardial infarction (MI) or heart attack may occur

   a. *Reduced oxygen supply* causes a switch from aerobic metabolism to anaerobic metabolism

      1) Anaerobic metabolism causes lactic acid buildup

      2) Anaerobic metabolism affects cell membrane permeability releasing histamine, bradykinins, and specific enzymes that stimulate terminal nerve fibers in myocardium, sending pain impulses to central nervous system (CNS)

      3) Congestive heart failure, congenital heart defects, pulmonary hypertension, left ventricular hypertrophy, and cardiomyopathy also cause decreased O_2 supply to myocardium

      4) Silent ischemia: caused by decreased O_2 supply, just without warning signs of pain

      5) Coronary artery spasm: another form of occlusion and cause of ischemia; occurs from an unknown etiology; causes temporary narrowing of coronary arteries and angina

   b. *Increased O_2 demand* of myocardium results in angina and can be caused by anemia, exercise, thyrotoxicosis, substance abuse (cocaine), hyperthyroidism, and emotional stress

2. Types of angina

   a. Stable angina (most common type)

      1) Caused by specific amount of activity; rather predictable

      2) Relieved with rest and nitrates

      3) No change in cause, amount, or duration of pain over time

    b. Unstable angina (more concerning)

      1) Pain occurring with increasing frequency, severity, and duration over time

      2) Unpredictable and occurs with decreasing levels of activity or stress

      3) May occur at rest

      4) High risk for myocardial infarction

    c. Prinzmetal's (variant) angina

      1) Atypical form occurring without identified precipitating cause

      2) May occur at same time each day or awaken client from sleep

      3) May intensify or worsen over years but does not carry same concern as unstable angina

      4) Usual cause is coronary artery spasm, therefore making it difficult to control

  3. Signs and symptoms include pressure or heaviness in chest, which client may describe using other terms; may be accompanied by sweating, light-headedness, hypotension, pulse changes (low or high), or indigestion; pain may radiate to arms, jaw, abdomen, or back; depressed S-T segment on electrocardiogram

C. Nursing assessment

  1. Assessment includes symptom analysis of pain (location, duration, precipitating factors and relieving factors); vital signs; dyspnea; respiratory pattern; color (pallor); anxiety; heart sounds

  2. Diagnostic tests: **electrocardiogram** (**ECG** or **EKG**) graphic representation of electrical activity of heart, stress test (with and without contrast), radiographic study (angiogram), MUGA scan, troponin T or troponin I, creatinine phosphokinase (CK or CPK) and lactic dehydrogenase (LDH) (with isoenzymes), myoglobin to rule out MI, possible tests for gastric esophageal reflux disease (GERD) to rule out gastric causes

D. Nursing management

  1. Medications

    a. Antianginals: nitroglycerin (Nitrostat, NTG)

    b. Antiplatelet agents

    c. Beta blockers

    d. Calcium channel blockers to decrease **afterload** (pressure against which heart must pump) and spasms

    e. Analgesics for headache (common side effect of NTG)

    f. Thrombolytic therapy if thrombi identified as cause; glycoprotein IIb/IIIa inhibitors

    g. Stool softeners

    h. Class I-A (sodium channel blockers) or I-B or class III (potassium channel blockers; amiodarone) antidysrhythmics may be given prophylactically if premature ventricular contractions (PVCs) occur

  2. Goal is to reduce O_2 demand and improve blood and O_2 supply; primary nursing care is related to education of client

    a. Signs and symptoms of angina pectoris

    b. Use of NTG: take one tablet or one spray every 5 minutes for 3 doses in 15 minutes; report to healthcare provider if no relief

    c. NTG can be used prior to activities that may cause angina (such as sexual activity, work-related activities that cannot be modified, etc.)

3. Administer O_2 as needed
4. Treatment may consist of percutaneous coronary revascularization
   a. Percutaneous transluminal coronary angioplasty (PTCA)
      1) Balloon angioplasty
      2) Stent placement
   b. Coronary artery bypass grafting (CABG)
   c. Minimally invasive coronary artery surgery
      1) Port access coronary artery bypass
      2) Minimally invasive coronary artery bypass
   d. Transmyocardial laser revascularization (TMLR)
5. Monitor vital signs (VS); heart sounds
6. Monitor EKG pattern, heart rate (HR) may increase as a response of sympathetic nervous system (SNS) if blood pressure (BP) drops
7. Instruct client not to strain for bowel movement (BM) or create excess pressure by bending; administer stool softener as needed
8. Help client identify known stressors
9. Begin cardiac exercise program
10. Measure pulse before beta blocker administration and hold if pulse is less than 60 bpm or 50 if ordered by health care provider occasionally; also assess BP as hypotension can occur
11. Check BP before each NTG tablet and record since NTG can cause drastic hypotension; morphine sulfate (MS) may be administered in small doses if BP is below 100 systolic
12. Carefully assess BP during administration of calcium channel blockers

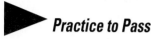

Practice to Pass

The client presents with history of stable angina and asks the nurse "Does this mean I will have a heart attack?" How should the nurse respond?

IV. MYOCARDIAL INFARCTION (MI)

A. Overview

1. **Myocardial infarction (MI)** is defined as death of cells in myocardium, usually related to prolonged or severe ischemia to that area
2. Many MIs are caused by sudden onset of ventricular fibrillation
3. Other causes include embolus, thrombosis, atherosclerotic occlusion, prolonged vasospasm

B. Pathophysiology

1. Cellular injury occurs because of a lack of O_2 over time (ischemia); prolonged (20 to 45 minutes) ischemia can lead to cell death (necrosis)
2. Coronary artery occlusion results in cell death distal to occlusion
3. Scar replaces muscle, but does not contract or conduct an impulse
4. Damage begins at subendocardial layer and progresses to epicardium within 1 to 6 hours
5. Damaged cells cause a decrease in myocardial contractility resulting in:
   a. Decreased **stroke volume** (volume of blood ejected by left ventricle with each heartbeat)
   b. Decreased **cardiac output** (volume of blood ejected from left ventricle each minute)

    c. Decreased BP

    d. Decreased tissue perfusion

6. Myocardial ischemia that reoccurs over time may lead to development of **collateral circulation** (additional outgrowth of tiny vessels), which provides for delivery of O_2 and nutrients to area of ischemia

7. MIs are described by:

  a. Location

    1) Anterior: usually occurring in area supplied by left anterior descending coronary artery (LAD)

    2) Posterior: usually occurring in area supplied by the right coronary artery (RCA)

    3) Lateral: occurring in area supplied by left circumflex artery

  b. Myocardial surface

    1) Transmural infarct: endocardium to epicardium

    2) Subendocardial: endocardial surface into myocardial muscle

    3) Intramural infarction: patchy areas of myocardium

8. Signs and symptoms associated with MI

  a. Pain (typical): midsternal, radiating to jaw, arms, abdomen, or shoulder; tightness, crushing feeling; lasting 15 to 20 minutes; not relieved with NTG or by rest

  b. May be pain-free (silent MI)

  c. Duration of pain important in distinguishing from angina pectoris

  d. Sudden onset of pain, usually not associated with activity, may awaken in middle of night

  e. Tachycardia related to pain and increased need of tissue for O_2

  f. Diaphoresis

  g. Tachypnea, dyspnea

  h. Change in LOC, anxiety, feelings of impending doom

  i. Nausea/vomiting

  j. ECG changes: depressed or *elevated S-T segment* (most common), inverted T wave, formation of Q waves (Figure 2-2)

Figure 2-2

S-T segment suggesting myocardial injury. *A.* S-T segment elevation. *B.* Presence of Q wave.

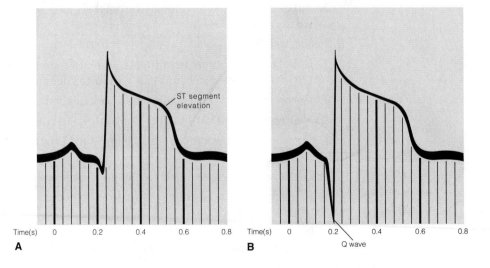

k. Elevated cardiac markers: enzymes are normally present in muscle fibers of body and are not elevated in serum unless injury to muscle occurs; when any muscle is injured, enzymes are released into blood stream as a response to injury; isoenzymes are a breakdown of total enzyme level and when elevated give an indication of which particular muscle has been damaged

  1) Cardiac muscle troponins: proteins are released during a myocardial infarction that are usually indicative of myocardial damage; cardiac-specific troponin T (cT_nT) and cardiac-specific troponin I (cT_nI) are specific to cardiac muscle necrosis and sensitive in detecting small MIs (Table 2-1)

  2) Myoglobin: first cardiac marker to be detectable in blood after an MI; is released quickly after symptoms occur but is not cardiac specific and therefore has limited usefulness

  3) Creatinine phosphokinase (CK or CPK): isoenzymes are CPK I (BB) present in brain tissue and smooth muscle; CPK II (MB) present in heart tissue; and CPK III (MM) present in muscle tissue; therefore, when total CPK level is elevated, assess for an elevated CPK II or MB isoenzyme to determine if an MI has occurred

  4) Lactic dehydrogenase (LDH): isoenzymes are LDH_1 present in cardiac muscle; LDH_2 present in reticuloendothelial system; LDH_3 present in lungs and other tissue; LDH_4 present in placenta, kidneys, and pancreas; and LDH_5 present in liver and striated muscle; normally LDH_1 is less than LDH_2, however in an MI, LDH_1 is greater than LDH_2 (termed a "flipped ratio"); therefore, when the total LDH level is elevated, assess for an elevated LDH_1 isoenzyme to determine if an MI has occurred; this enzyme is less useful due to later elevation by timeframe and usefulness of cardiac markers already listed

Table 2-1	**Enzyme Markers in MI**					
Marker	**Normal Level**	**Primary Tissue Location**	**Significance of Elevation**	**Appears**	**Peaks**	**Duration**
CK (CPK)	Male: 12 to 80 units/L Female: 10 to 70 units/L	Cardiac muscle, skeletal muscle, brain	Injury to muscle cells	3 to 6 hours	12 to 24 hours	24 to 48 hours
CK-MB	0% to 3% of total CK	Cardiac muscle	MI, cardiac ischemia, myocarditis, cardiac contusion, defibrillation	4 to 8 hours	18 to 24 hours	72 hours
cT_nT	<0.2 mcg/L	Cardiac muscle	Acute MI, unstable angina	2 to 4 hours	18 to 24 hours	10 to 14 days
cT_nI	<3.1 mcg/L	Cardiac muscle	Acute MI, unstable angina	2 to 4 hours	18 to 24 hours	7 to 10 days
LDH	45 to 90 units/L	Heart, liver, kidneys, skeletal muscle, brain, RBCs, lungs	MI; pulmonary, liver, renal, RBC, or skeletal muscle disease; CVA; intestinal ischemia; others	24 to 72 hours	3 to 4 days	10 to 14 days

Source. LeMone, P., & Burke, K. (2004). *Medical-surgical nursing: Critical thinking in client care* (3rd ed.). Upper Saddle River, NJ: Prentice Hall, p. 831.

     l. Elevated temperature

     m. Leukocytosis

     n. Cardiac dysrhythmias: premature ventricular contractions (PVCs), ventricular tachycardia caused by irritability

    9. The most common reaction to an MI is to deny symptoms and delay health care

C. Nursing assessment

    1. Assessment includes symptom analysis of chest pain (location, duration, radiation, quality); associated symptomatology (diaphoresis, nausea/vomiting); vital signs; heart sounds (murmur, friction rub, gallop [S_3 or S_4]); a cardiac rhythm; nonverbal cues of discomfort

    2. Diagnostic tests: CPK and LDH with isoenzymes, troponin level, 12-lead ECG, chest x-ray (CXR), angiogram, echocardiogram, stress tests, MUGA scan, arterial blood gases (ABGs), electrolytes, complete blood count (CBC), use pulse oximetry for quick reference of SaO_2

D. Nursing management

    1. Medications

     a. Antianginals: nitroglycerin (Nitrostat, NTG) for vasodilation; anticipate use of sublingual/topical spray, Nitrol drip, and/or Nitrol paste or patch

     b. Analgesics as needed for pain relief; morphine sulfate if BP too low or pain unrelieved by nitrostat; note that morphine may lower BP also

     c. Stool softener

     d. Electrolyte replacement as necessary

     e. Calcium channel blockers

     f. Beta blockers

     g. Angiotensin converting enzyme (ACE) inhibitors

     h. Anticoagulants such as heparin, warfarin (Coumadin) or low molecular weight heparin (LMWH) such as enoxaparin (Lovenox)

     i. Antidysrhythmics may be given prophylactically

      1) Amiodarone hydrochloride (Cordarone): ventricular antidysrhythmics such as PVCs

      2) Atropine: treatment of bradydysrhythmias

      3) Short-acting beta blockers: treatment of tachydysrhythmias

     j. Thrombolytics as indicated

    2. Supplement O_2 via nasal canula at 2 to 5 L/min

    3. Elevate head of bed for respiratory comfort

    4. Maintain intravenous (IV) access site

    5. Monitor bowel movements, encourage client not to strain, and offer stool softener as needed

    6. Provide for physical and psychological rest

    7. Provide emotional support for client and family

    8. Reassess client frequently for pain relief or continued pain; use pain scale to assess quality of pain

    9. Teach client and family when they are ready to listen and absorb information

▶ *Practice to Pass*

The client arrives in the Emergency Department with complaints of midsternal chest pain, diaphoresis, and nausea. The client states "I'm dying." How should the nurse respond?

10. Monitor VS and record with administration of nitrates, beta blockers, and calcium channel blockers: hold if pulse is less than 60 bpm or BP is less than 100 systolic (see Angina, Section D)

11. Begin cardiac rehabilitation program for education and exercise as ordered

12. Monitor for major side effects of medications: hypotension, bradycardia, bleeding, constipation, and depression

V. CONGESTIVE HEART FAILURE (CHF)

A. Overview

1. **Congestive heart failure (CHF)** is defined as heart's inability to pump sufficiently to meet metabolic needs of body, causing decreased tissue perfusion as a result of decreased cardiac output (CO)

2. May be acute (pulmonary edema or cardiogenic shock) or chronic (heart failure); left-sided, right-sided, or both

3. Causes include diseases such as MI, hypertension, CAD, or kidney failure; cardiomyopathies; valve disorders; inflammatory conditions; water intoxication; and side effects of medications such as corticosteroids (Table 2-2)

4. Prognosis is determined by effectiveness of therapeutic regimen

B. Pathophysiology

1. Heart pumps blood to pulmonary and systemic vascular systems in order to maintain an adequate oxygenated blood supply to heart and produce a sufficient CO

2. Cardiac output is regulated by metabolic needs of body

3. Damage to the pump (heart) regardless of cause leads to decreased CO and decreased tissue perfusion

4. Two dysfunctions that contribute to CHF

   a. *Diastolic dysfunction:* when ventricle pumps against an extremely high afterload as in primary hypertension; this effect leads to a decrease in ventricles' ability to comply, decreases ventricular filling (preload), which leads to decreased stroke volume (SV); hypotension can result

   b. *Systolic dysfunction:* when ventricle experiences damage as in MI and ventricle cannot contract effectively; SV decreases, leading to an increased **preload**

Table 2-2	Causes of Heart Failure				
Excess Volume Load	**Excess Pressure Load**	**Increased Metabolic Demand**	**Acute Conditions**	**Altered Function**	**Filling Disorders**
Volume overload Valve regurgitation Left-to-right shunts	Hypertension Aortic stenosis Hypertrophic cardiomyopathy Coarctation of the aorta	Anemias Thyrotoxicosis Pregnancy Infection Fever Physical, emotional, or environmental stressors	Acute hypertensive crisis Aortic valve rupture Massive pulmonary embolism	Cardiomyopathy Myocarditis Rheumatic fever Infective endocarditis Coronary heart disease Dysrhythmias Toxic disorders	Valve stenosis (mitral or tricuspid) Cardiac tamponade Restrictive pericarditis

Source: LeMone, P., & Burke, K. (2004). *Medical-surgical nursing: Critical thinking in client care* (3rd ed.). Upper Saddle River, NJ: Prentice Hall, p. 870.

Table 2-3	Compensatory Mechanisms of Heart Failure		
Mechanism	**Physiology**	**Effect on Body Systems**	**Complications**
Frank-Starling mechanism	The greater the stretch of cardiac muscle fibers, the greater the force of contraction.	Increased contractile force leading to increased CO	Increased myocardial oxygen demand
Neuroendocrine response	Decreased CO causes sympathetic nervous system stimulation and catecholamine release.	Increased HR, BP, and contractility Increased vascular resistance Increased venous return	Tachycardia with decreased filling time and decreased CO Increased vascular resistance Increased myocardial work and oxygen demand
	Decreased CO and decreased renal perfusion stimulate renin angiotensin system.	Vasoconstriction and increased BP	Increased myocardial work Renal vasoconstriction and decreased renal perfusion
	Angiotensin stimulates aldosterone release from adrenal cortex.	Salt and water retention by the kidneys Increased vascular volume	Increased preload and afterload Pulmonary congestion
	ADH is released from posterior pituitary	Water excretion inhibited	Fluid retention and increased preload and afterload Pulmonary congestion
	Atrial natriuretic factor is released.	Increased sodium excretion Diuresis	
	Blood flow is redistributed to vital organs (heart and brain).	Decreased perfusion of other organ systems Decreased perfusion of skin and muscles	Renal failure Anaerobic metabolism and lactic acidosis
Ventricular hypertrophy	Increased cardiac workload causes myocardial muscle to hypertrophy and ventricles to dilate.	Increased contractile force to maintain CO	Increased myocardial oxygen demand Cellular enlargement

Source: LeMone, P., & Burke, K. (2008). *Medical-surgical nursing: Critical thinking in client care* (4th ed.). Upper Saddle River, NJ: Prentice Hall, p. 1024.

(volume of blood returning to heart creating "stretch" or tension of myocardial fibers at end of diastole) and ventricle becomes distended; signs of decreased CO can result

5. Compensatory mechanisms for heart failure (Table 2-3)

   a. Frank-Starling mechanism: force of contraction determined by amount of stretch

   b. Neuroendocrine responses

      1) Sympathetic nervous system (SNS) activation: increase in HR

      2) Renin: angiotensin-aldosterone mechanism activation

   c. Ventricular hypertrophy

6. Decreased CO stimulates aortic baroreceptors, causing release of norepinephrine to increase HR and contractility; this causes vasoconstriction, thereby increasing blood return to heart and increasing CO

7. Decreased CO leads to decreased renal perfusion; remember that kidneys need blood in order to function properly

   a. Decreased renal perfusion leads to release of renin from juxtoglomerular cells

    b. Activation of renin-angiotensin-aldosterone mechanism

        1) Causes vasoconstriction

        2) Stimulates adrenal cortex to produce aldosterone and antidiuretic hormone (ADH) from posterior pituitary gland

            a) Aldosterone causes sodium reabsorption and water retention, thus increasing BP

            b) ADH inhibits water excretion in distal tubules and causes vasoconstriction, thus increasing vascular volume and raising BP

8. Vasoconstriction causes increased blood return to heart (preload), causing greater stretch (Frank-Starling law), and therefore increases CO

9. Atrial stretch stimulates release of atrial natriuretic factor (ANF) or atriopeptin that balances effects of renin and aldosterone, promotes sodium and water excretion and inhibits norepinephrine, renin, and ADH

10. Ventricular hypertrophy results from excess fluid volume and pressure causing cells to enlarge, stiffen, thereby decreasing force of contraction

11. The compensatory mechanisms hasten deterioration of cardiac function and onset of heart failure

    a. Increased HR decreases diastolic filling time, compromises coronary artery perfusion, and increases myocardial O_2 demand; the resulting ischemia leads to decreased CO

    b. Beta-receptors in heart become less sensitive to SNS stimulation, thereby decreasing HR and contractility

    c. Alpha receptors on peripheral blood vessels are increased in sensitivity, which promotes vasoconstriction, thereby increasing afterload and therefore cardiac workload

12. Chronic ventricular dilation leads to ventricular wall thinning, degeneration, and loss of effective contractility

13. Chronic atrial dilation leads to depletion of ANF leaving renin, aldosterone, and norepinephrine to continue unabated; causes increased preload, afterload, and further deterioration of heart failure, thereby decreasing O_2 supply to tissues, leading to further ischemia and tissue death (infarction)

14. Left-sided heart failure (see Figure 2-3)

    a. Left side affected more often than right side

    b. Results from left ventricular wall damage or dilatation

    c. Left ventricular and atrial end-diastolic pressures increase and cardiac output decreases

    d. Impaired left ventricular filling results in congestion and increased pulmonary vascular pressures; remember "**L**"eft and "**L**"ung, the fluid "backs up" to lungs

        1) Increased pulmonary vascular pressure causes shifting of fluid interstitially, leading to alveolar congestion and pulmonary edema

        2) Increased pulmonary artery pressures as measured by a pulmonary artery catheter (normal PA pressure 25/10 mmHg)

    e. Signs and symptoms of left heart failure: fatigue, activity intolerance, dizziness, syncope, dyspnea, shortness of breath, cough, orthopnea, pulmonary crackles on auscultation, S_3 heart sound, tachycardia with possible atrial dysrhythmia, and decreased urine output

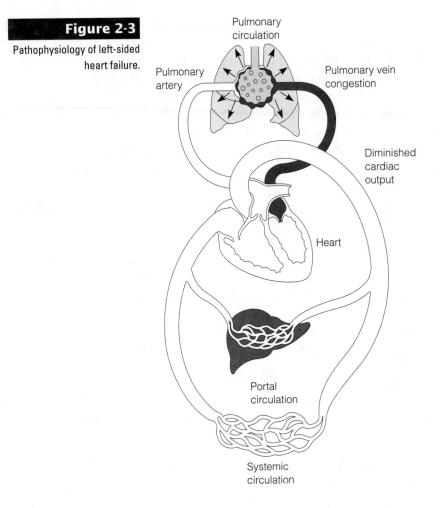

Figure 2-3

Pathophysiology of left-sided heart failure.

Pulmonary circulation

Pulmonary artery

Pulmonary vein congestion

Diminished cardiac output

Heart

Portal circulation

Systemic circulation

15. Right-sided heart failure (see Figure 2-4)

  a. Right heart failure caused by pulmonary hypertension (cor pulmonale) and left heart failure

  b. Right ventricular infarction can cause right-sided heart failure

  c. Pulmonary hypertension causes increased pressure that right ventricle must pump against, so right ventricle cannot empty; hypertrophy and dilation result

  d. Right ventricular distention leads to blood accumulation in systemic veins; remember "**R**"ight and "**R**"est of body, the fluid "backs up" to rest of body

  e. Increased venous pressure causes abdominal organ congestion and peripheral edema

   1) Lower extremity edema occurs in client who is ambulatory

   2) A bedridden client will experience sacral and/or scrotal edema

   3) Liver engorgement will lead to right upper quadrant pain

   4) Anorexia and nausea occur with gastrointestinal (GI) venous congestion

  f. Jugular venous distention occurs

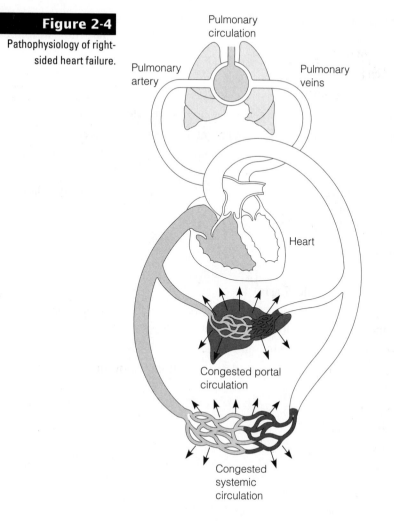

Figure 2-4

Pathophysiology of right-sided heart failure.

16. Biventricular failure; both ventricles fail
    a. Client experiences signs and symptoms of both left and right failure
    b. Paroxysmal nocturnal dyspnea (PND) occurs as peripheral edema is reabsorbed into circulation when client goes to bed and feet are elevated, causing fluid overload and pulmonary congestion
    c. Severe heart failure predisposes client to dyspnea at rest
    d. S_3 and S_4 heart sounds may be heard
    e. Hepatomegaly and splenomegaly result from abdominal engorgement or congestion: increased abdominal pressure, ascites, GI problems (anorexia, nausea, and vomiting), decreased digestion and absorption of nutrients
    f. Dysrhythmias may develop from myocardial distention, causing interference with conduction and lowering cardiac output
    g. Cardiogenic shock or acute pulmonary edema may develop as cardiac function deteriorates

C. **Nursing assessment**
    1. Assessment includes VS; cardiac monitor; heart rhythm; pulse quality (full, bounding, thready); respiratory status (dyspnea, shortness of breath, tachypnea);

lung sounds (crackles, rhonchi, wheezes); heart sounds (S_3 or S_4, murmur or rub); jugular neck vein distention; abdominal assessment (palpation, distention, ascites); edema; activity tolerance

2. Diagnostic tests

  a. Electrocardiogram

    1) Signs of ischemia: depressed S-T segment, inverted T wave

    2) Signs of injury: elevated S-T segment, Q wave development

  b. Atrial natriuretic factor (ANF) or B-type natriuretic peptide (BNP): increase in CHF

  c. Other: electrolytes, liver function tests, ABG analysis, chest x-ray, echocardiogram, O_2 saturation

  d. Tests to rule out an MI may be done if client is having chest pain also

D. Nursing management

  1. Medications

    a. Diuretics: furosemide (Lasix)

    b. Positive inotropic agents: dopamine (Inotropin) — increases urinary output, systemic vasoconstrictor; dobutamine (Dobutex)

    c. Phosphodiesterase inhibitor: amrinone (Inocor)

    d. Analgesics to decrease stress and discomfort and allow decreased oxygen needs

    e. Antihypertensives

    f. ACE inhibitors

    g. Direct vasodilators

    h. Beta blockers

    i. Antidysrhythmics as needed

    j. Cardiac glycosides: digoxin (Lanoxin)

    k. Nitrates

  2. Primary goal is to reduce O_2 demand on myocardium: physical and psychological rest

  3. Manage prescribed medications for reducing cardiac workload, improving contractility, and management of symptoms

  4. Management of decreased CO

    a. Monitor and record VS

      1) Decreased CO stimulates SNS to increase HR and increase diastolic BP; as heart's pumping action deteriorates, BP decreases

      2) Assessment of subtle changes in vital signs may aid in early intervention

    b. Auscultate heart and lung sounds

      1) S_1 and S_2 may be diminished as cardiac function fails

      2) S_3 is an early sign of heart failure (ventricular gallop)

      3) S_4 may also be present (atrial gallop)

      4) Basilar crackles may be heard

      5) Increasing crackles and dyspnea mean worsening of condition

    c. Note level of consciousness (LOC)

        1) Mental changes occur as blood flow to brain decreases

        2) SaO_2 changes may also lead to changes in LOC

    d. Note urine output (UO)

        1) Decreased blood flow to kidneys leads to decreased urine output

        2) Assessing output assists in evaluating effectiveness of some medications used to treat heart failure, such as diuretics and positive inotropic agents

    e. Note color and temperature of skin

        1) Cool, clammy skin frequently present in acute phase of heart failure

        2) Pale and then cyanotic coloring is seen in later stages as cardiac pumping action deteriorates

    f. Monitor client for cardiac dysrhythmias

        1) Sinus tachycardia is usually present

        2) Atrial dysrhythmias are frequently seen in heart failure: atrial fibrillation, atrial flutter, premature atrial contractions (PACs), and atrial tachycardia

        3) Ventricular dysrhythmias will be seen as ventricular hypertrophy and dilation occurs

    g. Supplemental O_2 is given to decrease the effects of hypoxia and ischemia

    h. Place client at rest with head of bed elevated to improve respiratory function and reduce cardiac workload

        1) Assist with personal care needs

        2) Use bedside commode to reduce effort and metabolic energy that would be necessary if bed pan used

        3) Instruct client to avoid Valsalva maneuver

        4) Avoid isometric exercises

    i. Promote psychological rest and minimize anxiety to reduce O_2 consumption and improve cardiac function: maintain quiet environment, allow expression of fear, explain procedures to client's satisfaction

5. Management of fluid volume excess

    a. Assess respiratory status; declining respiratory status indicates worsening left heart failure—shortness of breath, dyspnea, cough, orthopnea, paroxysmal nocturnal dyspnea

    b. Acute pulmonary edema can develop rapidly

        1) Air hunger develops

        2) Client begins to panic

        3) Overwhelming sense of impending doom

        4) Tachypnea

        5) Need to sit straight up in bed

        6) Productive cough with large amounts of pink, frothy sputum occurs

    c. Monitor urinary output closely

        1) Notify physician if output is equal to or less than 30 mL/hr

        2) Use of diuretics reduces circulating volume, producing hypovolemia even in presence of peripheral edema

3) Decreased urinary output could indicate decreased CO and renal ischemia

  d. Weigh client daily at same time, on same scale, and in same clothing

    1) Weight provides objective measure of fluid status

    2) 1 liter of fluid is equal to 2.2 pounds of weight

  e. Assess and record abdominal girth every shift; measure at level of umbilicus; mark area measured for consistency among measurements

    1) Venous congestion leads to development of ascites and may produce GI complaints: nausea, loss of appetite, abdominal discomfort

    2) Increasing girth means increased ascites production (third-spacing)

  f. Keep client on bedrest with head of bed elevated 45 degrees to improve lung expansion and reduce cardiac workload

  g. Assess for signs of deteriorating condition

  h. Monitor hemodynamics (if pulmonary artery catheter in place)

    1) Monitor pulmonary capillary wedge pressures

    2) Monitor pulmonary artery pressure (normal 25/10 mmHg)

    3) Monitor right atrial pressure (CVP)

    4) Systemic vascular resistance

    5) Cardiac output

    6) Cardiac index

  i. Restrict fluids if ordered to decrease fluid overload

6. Management of activity intolerance: minimal or no cardiac reserve for increased activity leads to self-care deficits

  a. Allow adequate rest periods prior to activity

  b. Assess for signs of decreasing activity tolerance

  c. Assist with activities of daily living (ADLs) allowing client to do as much as possible to provide some control to client and reduce feelings of helplessness

  d. Provide passive and active range-of-motion (ROM) to progressively promote improved cardiac function

  e. Teach client about discharge instructions

    1) Low sodium diet

    2) Perform activities as independently as possible

    3) Space meals and activities

    4) Allow time for rest and relaxation

    5) Stop any activity that causes chest pain or shortness of breath

    6) Avoid straining

    7) Begin slowly progressive exercise program

7. Close monitoring and recording of drug therapy should be done by nurse

  a. Monitor apical pulse for one minute prior to administering digoxin (Lanoxin); hold if pulse is less than 60 bpm

  b. Monitor VS and intake and output (I&O) carefully while administering dopamine (Intropin)

    1) Low doses: renal perfusion

    2) Moderate to high doses: elevate BP

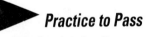

Practice to Pass

The client is being discharged tomorrow after a 6-day hospitalization for heart failure. The client asks when he can return to work. How should the nurse explain the recovery phase?

     c. Close monitoring of I &O with furosemide (Lasix), avoid giving furosemide by intravenous push (IVP) at rate greater than 4 mg/min—ototoxicity can occur

VI. CARDIAC DYSRHYTHMIAS

A. Overview

1. Electrical stimulation of normal heart causes depolarization of myocardium; this depolarization produces a synchronized, rhythmic contraction of myocardium producing a beat; propelling blood through arteries and capillaries

2. Cardiac dysrhythmias are defined as alterations in this stimulation, which can affect synchronized pattern of contractions and affect efficiency of heart

3. Normal sinus rhythm conduction progresses from sinoatrial (SA) node → atrioventricular (AV) node → bundle of His → bundle branches (right bundle branch and left bundle branch) simultaneously → Purkinje fibers, causing contraction of atria and ventricles

4. Cardiac dysrhythmias

    a. May be benign or lethal

    b. Caused by many factors (see Table 2-4)

    c. Any dysrhythmia can affect cardiac function, regardless of cause

    d. Client's response to rhythm determines urgency of treatment

5. Dysrhythmias originate as sinus, atrial, junctional, ventricular, or heart blocks

B. Pathophysiology

1. Altered electrical activity may cause alterations in cardiac function

2. Dysrhythmias may result from internal or external forces

    a. Internal forces

        1) Hypoxia

        2) Electrolyte disturbances

        3) Acidosis

        4) Diseases of myocardium

        5) Atherosclerotic processes

    b. External forces

        1) Stress

        2) Exercise

        3) Pain

        4) Anemia

        5) Hypovolemia

3. Cardiac muscle cells have capability of **automaticity** (ability to fire without stimulation), allowing cell to serve as a pacemaker or cause premature beats

4. Each heartbeat creates distinctive wave forms: P, QRS, and T (see Table 2-5); each QRS should correspond to a pulse

5. An action potential is the electrical activity that occurs in a cell by movement of ions across cell membranes

    a. During resting state, cell is *polarized,* with positive and negative ions equal on either side of cell membrane; maintained by the sodium (Na^+)-potassium (K^+) pump

Table 2-4	Dysrhythmia	Common Causes
Causes of Cardiac Dysrhythmias	Sinus arrhythmia	Increase in vagal tone, digitalis toxicity, or morphine administration
	Sinus tachycardia (ST)	Normal response to any condition that increases the body's need for more oxygen and nutrients: fever, stress, exercise, hypoxia, hypovolemia, anemia, hyperthyroidism, myocardial infarction, heart failure, cardiogenic shock
	Sinus bradycardia (SB)	Increased vagal tone; depressed automaticity; may be normal in athletic heart syndrome or during sleep; other causes include pain, increased intracranial pressure, sinus node disease, myocardial infarction, hypothermia, acidosis, certain drugs such as digoxin (Lanoxin), beta blockers, calcium channel blockers
	Sick sinus syndrome (SSS)	Injury during surgery, ischemia, infarct, fibrosis of conduction fibers associated with aging, drugs such as digitalis (Lanoxin), beta blockers, and calcium channel blockers
	Premature atrial contractions (PAC)	Strong emotions, excessive alcohol intake, tobacco, adrenergic stimulants (caffeine), myocardial infarction, heart failure, pericarditis, valvular disorders, hypoxemia, pulmonary embolism, digitalis toxicity, hypokalemia, hypomagnesemia, metabolic alkalosis
	Atrial tachycardia or paroxysmal supra-ventricular tachycardia	Sympathetic nervous system stimulation, fever, sepsis, hyperthyroidism, heart disease, myocardial infarction, rheumatic heart disease, myocarditis, acute pericarditis
	Atrial flutter	Sympathetic nervous system stimulation, anxiety, caffeine, alcohol intake, thyrotoxicosis, coronary artery disease, myocardial infarction, pulmonary embolism, abnormal conduction syndromes, elderly persons with rheumatic heart disease or valvular disease
	Atrial fibrillation (A-fib)	Congestive heart failure, mitral valve disease, rheumatic heart disease, coronary artery disease, hypertension, hyperthyroidism, thyrotoxicosis
	Junctional rhythm	Digitalis toxicity, quinidine reaction, overdose on beta blockers or calcium channel blockers, hypoxemia, hyperkalemia, increased vagal tone, damage to the AV node, myocardial infarct, congestive heart failure
	Premature ventricular contractions (PVC)	Anxiety or stress, tobacco, alcohol, caffeine use, hypoxia, acidosis, electrolyte imbalances, sympathomimetic drugs, ischemic heart disease, coronary artery disease, myocardial infarct, congestive heart failure, mechanical stimulation of the heart, reperfusion after thrombolytic therapy
	Ventricular tachycardia (V-tach)	Myocardial infarct, ischemia, valvular disease, rheumatic heart disease, cardiomyopathy, anorexia nervosa, metabolic disorders, drug toxicity
	Ventricular fibrillation (V-fib)	Myocardial infarct, ischemia
	First-degree heart block	Myocardial infarct, digitalis toxicity, complications from cardiac surgery, chronic heart disease, effects of certain drugs
	Second-degree heart block, type I, Wenckebach	Myocardial infarction, electrolyte imbalance, acute rheumatic infections, myocarditis, drug toxicity: digitalis (Lanoxin), procainamide (Procan), quinidine sulfate (Quinidine), propranolol (Inderal), verapamil (Isoptin)
	Second-degree heart block, type II, Classical	Myocardial infarction, electrolyte imbalance, acute rheumatic infections, myocarditis, progressive from Type I heart block, drug toxicity from digitalis, procainamide (Procan), quinidine sulfate (Quinidine), propranolol (Inderal), verapamil (Isoptin)
	Third-degree or complete heart block	Ischemia or damage to AV node, frequently associated with inferior or anteroseptal myocardial infarction, degenerative conduction system disease, damage to conduction system during surgery, acute myocarditis, increased vagal tone, digitalis (Lanoxin) or propranolol (Inderal) toxicity, electrolyte imbalance, progression from Type II heart block

	Table 2-5	**Wave Formations on an EKG**	
Configuration		**Wave Form**	**Characteristics**
P wave configuration		P wave	First upright, positive wave; normally smooth, round configuration; one should proceed each QRS; demonstrates atrial contraction
QRS—Q wave configuration		QRS—Q wave	First negative deflection
QRS—R wave configuration		QRS—R wave	First positive deflection after the Q
QRS—S wave configuration		QRS—S wave	Next negative deflection after R wave; called the QRS regardless of the presence of all three waveforms; demonstrates ventricular contraction
T wave configuration		T wave	Large wave form after QRS, upright, positive, round; demonstrates ventricular relaxation
P-R interval configuration		P-R interval	From beginning of P wave to beginning of Q wave; length of time it takes the impulse to travel from SA node through the bundle of HIS; normally 0.12 to 0.20 sec
QRS interval configuration		QRS interval	Beginning of Q wave to end of S wave; length of time it takes the impulse to travel from bundle of HIS to Purkinje fibers; ventricular contraction (depolarization) and beginning of repolarization (resting); normally 0.04 to 0.10 sec
S-T segment configuration		S-T segment	Should be a straight line between the S wave and beginning of T wave (isoelectric); demonstrates beginning and end of ventricular repolarization

b. Depolarization (contraction) requires a change from a negative to positive state; Na^+ ions enter rapidly, opening the Na^+ channels; Calcium (Ca^{++}) is allowed in, K^+ is not allowed to cross

c. A threshold potential is reached when cell becomes less negative, creating an action potential that depolarizes cardiac muscle cells; Ca^{++} enters cell and causes contraction of cardiac muscle

d. Repolarization then occurs to return cell to a polarized state, Na^+ channels close and cell begins to gain negative charge; the Na^+-K^+ pump restores ions to proper concentration

e. Sequence is repeated for each heartbeat

6. A refractory period is a certain stage in conduction cycle where there is resistance to stimulation

a. *Absolute refractory period:* from beginning of Q to middle of T wave; no stimulus of any size can cause another impulse to occur

    b. *Relative refractory period:* from middle of T to end of T wave; a stimulus that is larger than usual stimulus needed to create an impulse can cause muscle cells to contract; an example is when a PVC occurs at same time as a T wave, resulting in ventricular tachycardia or ventricular fibrillation

7. Two major categories of dysrhythmias

    a. Alteration in impulse formation

        1) Rate: tachycardia or bradycardia

        2) Rhythm: regular or irregular

        3) Ectopic beats (extra impulse)

            a) Premature atrial contractions (PAC)

            b) Premature junctional contractions (PJC)

            c) Junctional escape rhythm

            d) Premature ventricular contractions (PVC)

    b. Alteration in conductivity

        1) Heart blocks

        2) **Reentry phenomenon** is blockage of an impulse through a bundle branch, causing impulse to retrograde backwards, reentering other bundle branch and causing a premature beat

8. Cardiac rhythms are classified according to site of impulse formation or site and degree of conduction block (see Table 2-6)

    a. Sinus rhythms

        1) Normal sinus rhythm (NSR): impulse originates at SA node, travels normal pathway; no delays; wave forms are uniform; all waveforms are of a fixed duration; P wave present representing atrial depolarization and waveform is normal, smooth, and upright

        2) Sinus dysrhythmia: sinus rhythm that varies in rate during inspiration (faster) and expiration (slower); common in the very young and very old

        3) Sinus tachycardia (ST)

            a) Same configuration as NSR except rate is greater than 100 bpm

            b) Can be an early warning sign of cardiac dysfunction, such as heart failure

            c) Client may be asymptomatic; symptoms experienced may be "racing" feeling, syncope, dyspnea

        4) Sinus bradycardia (SB)

            a) Same configuration as NSR except rate is less than 60 bpm

            b) Clients may be asymptomatic; if not tolerating the bradycardia, may experience decreased LOC, syncope, and hypotension

        5) Sinus arrest or sinus block

            a) All configurations are normal; drop one or more complete complexes

            b) Sinus block: measurement of R-R will be exact, even with missing complex

            c) Sinus arrest: measurement of R-R will not be exact with missing complex

            d) Symptoms may not be present unless pause is great enough to decrease CO; client will experience same signs and symptoms as bradycardia

Table 2-6	ECG Characteristics of Selected Cardiac Rhythms and Dysrhythmias	
Rhythm/ECG Appearance	**ECG Characteristics**	**Management**

Supraventricular Rhythms

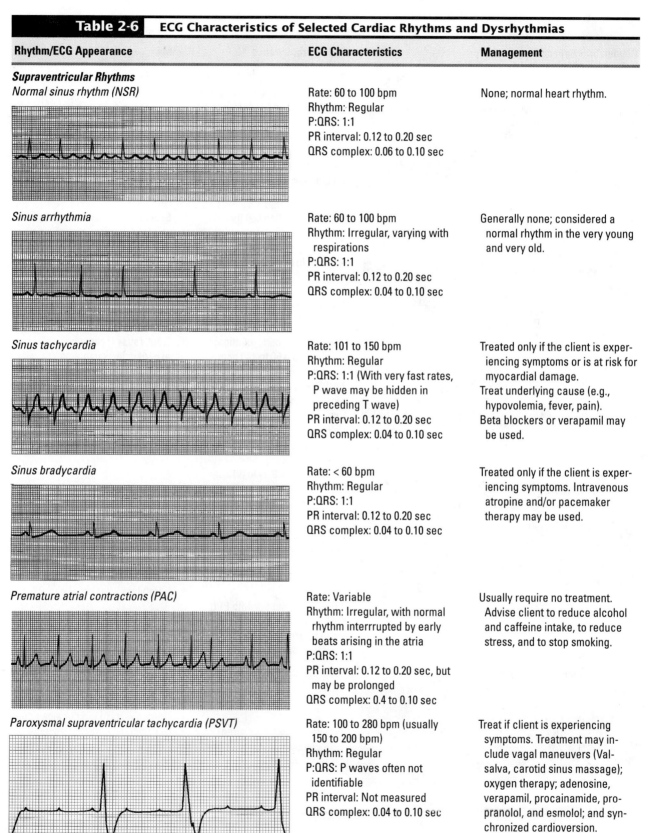

Normal sinus rhythm (NSR)

Rate: 60 to 100 bpm
Rhythm: Regular
P:QRS: 1:1
PR interval: 0.12 to 0.20 sec
QRS complex: 0.06 to 0.10 sec

None; normal heart rhythm.

Sinus arrhythmia

Rate: 60 to 100 bpm
Rhythm: Irregular, varying with
   respirations
P:QRS: 1:1
PR interval: 0.12 to 0.20 sec
QRS complex: 0.04 to 0.10 sec

Generally none; considered a
   normal rhythm in the very young
   and very old.

Sinus tachycardia

Rate: 101 to 150 bpm
Rhythm: Regular
P:QRS: 1:1 (With very fast rates,
   P wave may be hidden in
   preceding T wave)
PR interval: 0.12 to 0.20 sec
QRS complex: 0.04 to 0.10 sec

Treated only if the client is experiencing symptoms or is at risk for
   myocardial damage.
Treat underlying cause (e.g.,
   hypovolemia, fever, pain).
Beta blockers or verapamil may
   be used.

Sinus bradycardia

Rate: < 60 bpm
Rhythm: Regular
P:QRS: 1:1
PR interval: 0.12 to 0.20 sec
QRS complex: 0.04 to 0.10 sec

Treated only if the client is experiencing symptoms. Intravenous
   atropine and/or pacemaker
   therapy may be used.

Premature atrial contractions (PAC)

Rate: Variable
Rhythm: Irregular, with normal
   rhythm interrrupted by early
   beats arising in the atria
P:QRS: 1:1
PR interval: 0.12 to 0.20 sec, but
   may be prolonged
QRS complex: 0.4 to 0.10 sec

Usually require no treatment.
   Advise client to reduce alcohol
   and caffeine intake, to reduce
   stress, and to stop smoking.

Paroxysmal supraventricular tachycardia (PSVT)

Rate: 100 to 280 bpm (usually
   150 to 200 bpm)
Rhythm: Regular
P:QRS: P waves often not
   identifiable
PR interval: Not measured
QRS complex: 0.04 to 0.10 sec

Treat if client is experiencing
   symptoms. Treatment may include vagal maneuvers (Val-
   salva, carotid sinus massage);
   oxygen therapy; adenosine,
   verapamil, procainamide, propranolol, and esmolol; and synchronized cardioversion.

(continued)

| **Table 2-6** | **ECG Characteristics of Selected Cardiac Rhythms and Dysrhythmias (cont.)** |

Rhythm/ECG Appearance	**ECG Characteristics**	**Management**
Atrial flutter 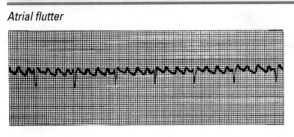	Rate: Atrial 240 to 360 bpm; ventricular rate depends on degree of AV block and usually is < 150 bpm Rhythm: Atrial regular, ventricular usually regular P:QRS: 2:1, 4:1, 6:1; may vary PR interval: Not measured QRS complex: 0.04 to 0.10 sec	Synchronized cardioversion; medications to slow ventricular response such as a beta blocker or calcium channel blocker (verapamil), followed by quinidine, procainamide, flecainide, or amiodarone.
Atrial fibrillation 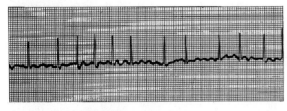	Rate: Atrial 300 to 600 bpm (too rapid to count); ventricular 100 to 180 bpm in untreated clients Rhythm: Irregularly irregular P:QRS: Variable PR interval: Not measured QRS complex: 0.04 to 0.10 sec	Synchronized cardioversion; medications to reduce ventricular response rate: verapamil, propranolol, digoxin, anticoagulant therapy to reduce risk of clot formation and stroke.
Junctional escape rhythm 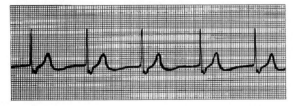	Rate: 40 to 60 bpm; junctional tachycardia 60 to 140 bpm Rhythm: Regular P:QRS: P waves may be absent, inverted and immediately preceding or succeeding QRS complex, or hidden in QRS complex PR interval: < 0.10 sec if P wave is prior to QRS complex QRS complex: 0.04 to 0.10 sec	Treat cause if client is experiencing symptoms.
Ventricular Rhythms *Premature ventricular contractions (PVC)* 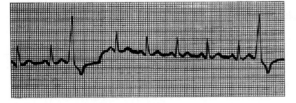	Rate: Variable Rhythm: Irregular, with PVC interrupting underlying rhythm and followed by a compensatory pause P:QRS: No P wave noted before PVC PR interval: Absent with PVC QRS complex: Wide (> 0.12 sec) and bizarre in appearance; differs from normal QRS complex	Treat if client is experiencing symptoms. Advise against stimulant use (caffeine, nicotine). Drug therapy includes intravenous lidocaine, procainamide, quinidine, propranolol, phenytoin, bretylium.
Ventricular tachycardia (VT or V tach) 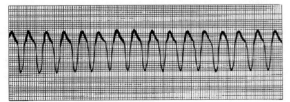	Rate: 100 to 250 bpm Rhythm: Regular P:QRS: P waves usually not identifiable PR interval: Not measured QRS complex: 0.12 sec or greater; bizarre shape	Treat if VT is sustained or if the client is experiencing symptoms. Treatment includes intravenous procainamide or lidocaine and/or immediate defibrillation if the client is unconscious or unstable.

| Table 2-6 | ECG Characteristics of Selected Cardiac Rhythms and Dysrhythmias (*cont.*) | |

Rhythm/ECG Appearance	ECG Characteristics	Management
Ventricular fibrillation (VF, V fib) 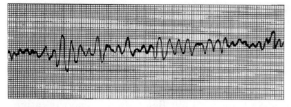	Rate: Too rapid to count Rhythm: Grossly irregular P:QRS: No identifiable P waves PR interval: None QRS: Bizarre, varying in shape and direction	Immediate defibrillation.
First-degree AV block 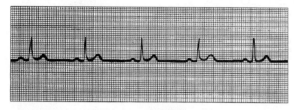	Rate: Usually 60 to 100 bpm Rhythm: Regular P:QRS: 1:1 PR interval: > 0.20 sec QRS complex: 0.04 to 0.10 sec	None required.
Second-degree AV block, type I (Mobitz I, Wenckebach) 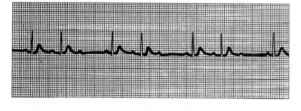	Rate: 60 to 100 bpm Rhythm: Atrial regular; ventricular irregular P:QRS: 1:1 until P wave blocked with no subsequent QRS complex PR interval: Progressively lengthens in a regular pattern QRS complex: 0.04 to 0.10 sec; sudden absence of QRS complex	Monitoring and observation; atropine or isoproterenol if client is experiencing symptoms.
Second-degree AV block, type II (Mobitz II) 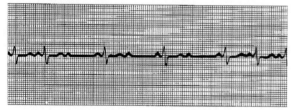	Rate: Atrial 60 to 100 bpm; ventricular < 60 bpm Rhythm: Atrial regular; ventricular irregular P:QRS: Typically 2:1, may vary PR interval: Constant PR interval for each conducted QRS complex QRS complex: 0.04 to 0.10 sec	Atropine or isoproterenol; pacemaker therapy.
Third-degree AV block (Complete heart block) 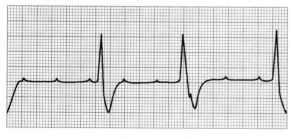	Rate: Atrial 60 to 100 bpm; ventricular 15 to 60 bpm Rhythm: Atrial regular; ventricular regular P:QRS: No relationship between P waves and QRS complexes; independent rhythms PR interval: Not measured QRS complex: 0.04 to 0.10 sec if junctional escape rhythm; > 0.12 sec if ventricular escape rhythm	Immediate pacemaker therapy.

6) Sick sinus syndrome (SSS)

   a) From diseases that affect SA node; often found in older clients

   b) Dysfunctions that cause problems with formation, transmission, or conduction of impulse

   c) Electrocardiographic characteristics of SSS are changes in type of rhythm, pacemaker site and/or rate; client may alternate between: sinus bradycardia or sinus arrhythmia; sinus pauses or sinus arrest; atrial tachydysrhythmias such as atrial fibrillation, atrial flutter, or atrial tachycardia; brady-tachy syndrome (alternating periods of bradycardia and tachycardia)

   d) Signs and symptoms of SSS: dizziness, light-headedness, syncope, fatigue or other signs of decreased CO

b. Atrial dysrhythmias

   1) Impulse originates in atrial tissue (ectopic) outside normal conduction system (SA node)

   2) Premature atrial contraction (PAC)

   a) Ectopic beat that comes early in cycle with same configuration as normal beats

   b) Usually asymptomatic and benign

   3) Atrial tachycardia (AT) or paroxysmal supraventricular tachycardia (PSVT)

   a) Fast rate with unidentifiable, normal P wave or P wave with a different configuration

   b) Sudden onset, sudden termination

   c) Usually related to reentry mechanism around AV node

   d) Seen more often in females

   e) Signs and symptoms: palpitations, "racing" heart, anxiety, dizziness, dyspnea, angina pain, diaphoresis, extreme fatigue, polyuria

   4) Atrial flutter

   a) Usually regular rhythm (but may be irregular) with saw-toothed waves instead of P waves

   b) Thought to be result of intra-atrial reentry mechanism

   c) Signs and symptoms: may be asymptomatic, palpitations or "fluttering" in chest, if rapid ventricular response is present, signs of decreased CO are present because of loss of "atrial kick" and decreased ventricular filling time

   5) Atrial fibrillation (A-fib)

   a) Chaotic atrial activity causing atria to quiver instead of contract normally

   b) Rapid impulses firing from atrial wall bombard AV node, resulting in a wavy baseline between R-R, no visible consistent P waves, and an irregular ventricular response pattern

   c) May be intermittent or a chronic rhythm disturbance

   d) Clinical signs and symptoms depend on ventricular response: signs and symptoms of decreased CO, hypotension, shortness of breath, fatigue, angina, syncope, heart failure; peripheral pulses will be irregular and variable in quality

e) High risk for thromboemboli formation due to pooling of blood in atria and absence of "atrial kick"; should be managed aggressively

c. Ventricular dysrhythmias

1) Originate in ventricles (idioventricular rhythm); inherent rate 20 to 40 bpm

2) Denoted by wide and bizarre QRS complexes that are greater than 0.12 second in duration with an increased amplitude, abnormal S-T segment, and a T wave that has an opposite deflection from QRS complex

3) P wave will have no relationship to QRS complex

4) Premature ventricular contraction (PVC)

   a) Most common dysrhythmia

   b) Occurs early in cardiac cycle

   c) Frequent, recurrent, or multifocal PVCs indicate myocardial irritability; may precipitate lethal dysrhythmias

   d) Incidence greatest following myocardial ischemia, infarction, hypertrophy, or infection

   e) Common and usually clinically insignificant in older adults

   f) May be unifocal (coming from one site) or multifocal (coming from different sites in ventricular wall)

   g) May come in patterns: bigeminy—every other beat is a PVC; trigeminy—every third beat is PVC; couplets—two beats together; triplets—three beats together; salvo—three to six beats in a row

   h) Signs and symptoms: may be asymptomatic; client may feel "skipped beats," chest discomfort, dyspnea, or dizziness; hypotension can occur

5) Ventricular tachycardia (V tach or VT)

   a) Rapid ventricular rhythm disturbance defined as three or more consecutive PVCs; can be short burst or sustained rhythm; usually regular with a rate greater than 100 bpm

   b) Reentry mechanism usual cause

   c) Signs and symptoms: fluttering in chest, palpitations, shortness of breath, signs of decreased CO, hypotension, loss of consciousness, no palpable pulses, may soon deteriorate into lethal rhythm

6) **Ventricular fibrillation (VF, V-fib)**

   a) Rapid chaotic ventricular rhythm causing ventricles to quiver; heart does not pump; cardiac arrest occurs

   b) Without effective treatment death occurs

   c) Effective treatment: defibrillation and cardiopulmonary resuscitation (CPR)

   d) ECG shows chaotic irregular bizarre complexes with no discernable rate or rhythm

7) Idioventricular rhythm

   a) Normal complexes are not present; P waves, if present, are not associated with QRS; QRS wide and bizarre like a PVC; overall rate slow (20 to 40)

   b) Lethal arrhythmia, may follow defibrillation, V-fib or V tach

   c) Signs and symptoms: decreased CO, usually unconscious

    d. Atrioventricular conduction blocks (heart blocks)

      1) Conduction defects that delay or block transmission of sinus impulse through AV node

        a) May be from injured or diseased SA node or AV node

        b) May occur because of increased vagal tone

        c) May be benign or severe

        d) Should be monitored for progression to a more severe level of block

      2) First-degree AV block

        a) Benign condition and is not considered a true block

        b) Prolonged but constant PR interval (greater than 0.20 sec) in duration, otherwise normal sinus rhythm (see Table 2-7)

        c) Usually asymptomatic; can progress to higher level block

      3) Second-degree AV block: Mobitz Type I (Wenckebach)

        a) Tip to remember: "W"enckebach and "w"eird pattern

        b) Cyclic pattern of complexes with a progressively prolonging PR interval until one QRS is totally blocked or dropped (see Table 2-7)

        c) Signs and symptoms: asymptomatic; if rate drops, then signs and symptoms of decreased CO would occur

      4) Second-degree AV block: Mobitz Type II or classical

        a) Usually seen in coronary artery disease and anterior wall MI

        b) Nonconducted impulses usually occurring in a regular manner

        c) Must have more than one P wave to every QRS complex (can have several Ps to each QRS)

        d) PR interval is constant (see Table 2-7)

        e) Signs and symptoms depend on ventricular rate

      5) Third-degree AV block (complete heart block)

        a) SA node fires, P waves are regular but do not conduct through to AV node; ventricular rhythm (QRS) will be regular but in no way related to P wave

        b) No relationship between P waves and QRS complexes; may or may not have more Ps than QRS complexes

        c) PR interval constantly varies (see Table 2-7)

        d) Signs and symptoms associated with bradycardia and decreased co: light-headedness, confusion, syncope

        e) Requires intervention, can be life-threatening

  C. Artificial pacemaker rhythms (following pacemaker insertion)

    1. Can be atrial (pace atrium), ventricular (pace ventricle) or A-V sequential (pace dual atrial and ventricular chambers)

Table 2-7	PR Interval Is Constant	PR Interval Is NOT Constant
Determining the Type of Heart Block	First-degree heart block—PR interval > 0.20	Second-degree heart block—Type I, Mobitz I, Wenckebach
	Second-degree heart block—Type II, Mobitz II, Classical	Third-degree heart block

2. Demand pacemaker most common: set at a rate that is individualized for each client; should begin to fire when client's own HR drops to or below set rate

3. Types

   a. Atrial pacemaker: spike occurs before each P wave while in demand mode

   b. Ventricular pacemaker: spike occurs before each QRS wave while in demand mode

   c. A-V sequential: two spikes occur while in demand mode; one before P wave and one before QRS

4. Problems encountered

   a. Failure to sense or undersensing: pacemaker does not sense client's own rhythm and continues to send an impulse; ECG will show spike at regular intervals throughout client's regular rhythm

   b. Failure to pace or oversensing: pacemaker fails to begin firing when HR drops below set rate; ECG may show whatever rhythm occurred that caused the need for the pacer

   c. Noncapture (pacemaker fires in a regular pattern but ventricle does not depolarize; ECG shows spikes without any QRS

D. **Nursing assessment**

1. Nursing assessment includes VS, symptoms of decreased CO; analysis of monitor pattern for rate, rhythm, assessment of P wave morphology, calculation of intervals; assessment of S-T segment, determination of rhythm

2. Diagnostic tests: 12-lead ECG; single-lead telemetry (usually lead II); electrophysiologic studies

   a. No specific laboratory test for cardiac dysrhythmias

   b. Laboratory tests may be helpful in determining cause of dysrhythmia, such as hypoxia, electrolyte imbalances, acid-base imbalances, or drug levels

E. **Nursing management**

1. Medications: antidysrhythmic drugs (see Table 2-8); magnesium if level is low

2. Recognize NSR as well as knowledge of dysrhythmias

3. Observe monitoring system and use rapid decision making process

4. Engage in collaborative care with health care provider; standing orders are needed for lethal dysrhythmias

5. Administer O_2 as necessary

6. Countershock

   a. Used to interrupt cardiac rhythms that compromise CO

   b. Causes total depolarization of all cardiac cells wiping out the dysrhythmia and allowing the SA node to resume its normal rhythm

   c. Two types of countershock

      1) Defibrillation: emergency treatment for ventricular fibrillation; the quicker the delivery of the shock, the higher the survival rate; place paddles or pads at base and apex of heart

      2) Synchronized cardioversion: countershock synchronized with R wave so that heart is totally depolarized to allow all cells to repolarize at same time so SA node can resume sinus rhythm; also used as an electric procedure for treatment of tachydysrhythmias (atrial fibrillation, atrial flutter, supraventricular tachycardia, stable ventricular tachycardia)

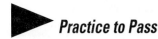

Practice to Pass

The client is on telemetry monitoring showing a normal sinus rhythm with a rate of 82 bpm. The alarm sounds and the monitor shows chaotic activity on the screen. What should the nurse's actions include?

Table 2-8	Antidysrhythmic Drug Classifications		
Class	Group	Action	Common Drugs
I	Sodium channel blockers Class I-A	Prolong action potential, reduce automaticity	Quinidine sulfate (Quinidine), procainamide hydrochloride (Pronestyl), disopyramide phosphate (Norpace), quinidine poly-galacturonate (Cardioquin)
	Class I-B	Decrease refractory period, slow conduction velocity	Xylocaine hydrochloride (Lidocaine), mexiletine hydrochloride (Mexitil), tocainide hydrochloride (Tonocard), phenytoin (Dilantin)
	Class I-C	Decrease automaticity and conduction through the AV node	Flecainide (Tambocor), propafenone hydro-chloride (Rythmol)
II	Beta blockers	Decrease automaticity and conduction through the AV node, lower BP	Esmolol hydrochloride (Brevibloc), propranolol hydrochloride (Inderal), acebutolol (Sectral)
III	Potassium channel blockers	Prolong repolarization and refractory period and decrease intraventricular conduction	Sotalol (Betapace), amiodarone hydrochloride (Cordarone), dofetilide (Tikosyn)
IV	Calcium channel blockers	Block calcium influx across the myocardial cell; negative dromotropic effect, lower BP and HR	Verapamil hydrochloride (Isoptin), nifedipine (Procardia), diltiazem (Cardizem)
V	Miscellaneous antidysrhythmics	Decrease automaticity, slow conduction through AV node	Adenosine (Adenocard), digoxin (Lanoxin), ibutilide (Corvert)

7. Implantable cardioverter-defibrillator (ICD) can be surgically implanted to detect life-threatening changes in rhythm; the device will automatically deliver an electric shock to convert the rhythm; ICDs are useful in preventing sudden death due to ventricular fibrillation

8. Pacemakers

   a. Temporary pacemakers are used after surgery, particularly CABG or during a code situation for emergency pacing; an external pulse generator is used

   b. Permanent pacemakers are surgically implanted to treat acute and chronic conduction defects; these are primarily used for bradyarrhythmias, but are available for use with tachyarrhythmias

VII. INFLAMMATORY DISEASES OF THE HEART

A. Overview

1. Inflammatory diseases of the heart are defined as inflammation of any layer of cardiac tissue (endocardium, myocardium, pericardium) that can damage valves, muscle, or pericardial lining

2. Conditions include rheumatic heart disease, endocarditis, myocarditis, and pericarditis

3. Causes

   a. Rheumatic heart disease: *Beta-hemolytic streptococcus* bacteria

   b. Infective endocarditis: bacterial infection or abnormal immunological reaction

   c. Myocarditis: viral, bacterial, or fungal infection, often *Coxsackievirus*

   d. Pericarditis: cardiac trauma, MI, infection, neoplasm, kidney disease, rheumatic fever

B. Pathophysiology

1. Rheumatic heart disease (RHD)

    a. A chronic condition characterized by valvular deformity, which slowly progresses; follows an acute or repeated episode of rheumatic fever (inflammatory disease from a *Beta-hemolytic streptococcus*)

    b. In acute stage, valves become red, swollen, and inflamed with lesions developing on leaflets

    c. In chronic stage, scar tissue develops, leaflets become rigid and deformed; stenosis or regurgitation may develop

    d. Left heart valves are affected more often; mitral valve most often

    e. Signs and symptoms

       1) Precordial chest discomfort

       2) Tachycardia

       3) Evidence of heart failure

       4) Pericardial friction rub

       5) S_3 (atrial gallop) or S_4 (ventricular gallop)

       6) Murmur from mitral or aortic regurgitation may be noted

       7) Cardiomegaly

       8) Pericardial effusion

2. Infective endocarditis

    a. Defined as inflammation of lining of heart; involves any part of endothelial lining of heart, most often mitral valve

    b. *Staphylococcus aureus* is usual infective organism

    c. Acute and subacute classifications exist

    d. Begins with platelet–fibrin vegetation on healthy valves (acute) and on damaged valves or endocardial tissue (subacute)

    e. Signs and symptoms of infective endocarditis: murmur, cough, shortness of breath, anorexia, abdominal pain, anemia, splenomegaly, fever (greater than 101.5°F), chills, night sweats, flu-like symptoms, joint pain, and petechiae

3. **Myocarditis**

    a. Defined as an inflammatory disorder of heart muscle that is unrelated to CAD or MI

    b. Infection can be caused by viruses, bacteria, or protozoa; immunologic response can be due to effects of radiation, chemical poisons, drugs, burns, or *Coxsackie B enterovirus* (most common in United States)

    c. Inflammatory process causing local or diffuse swelling and damage to myocardial cells, abscesses in interstitial tissue from infectious agents; pinpoint hemorrhage in layers of heart

    d. If condition deteriorates, could lead to dilated cardiomyopathy

    e. Results in weakening of heart muscle and decreased contractility

    f. Signs and symptoms depend on degree of cardiac damage

       1) May be asymptomatic at first

       2) Signs of inflammation: fever, chills, fatigue, malaise, dyspnea, palpitations, arthralgias

       3) Signs of heart failure: tachycardia, dysrhythmias, S_3 or S_4 gallop, systolic murmur, transient pericardial friction rub, cardiomegaly, and ECG abnormalities

4. Pericarditis

    a. Defined as an inflammation of pericardium (fluid-filled sac surrounding heart)

    b. May be primary or secondary to other disease processes; usually viral; affects more men than women

    c. Frequent complication of end stage renal failure; frequently seen after MI or following cardiac surgery

    d. When inflammatory mediators are released, vasodilatation occurs causing hyperemia (increased blood flow) and edema

    e. Increased capillary permeability allows plasma proteins and fibrinogen to gather in pericardial space

    f. Exudate is formed that may contain RBCs or be purulent if infective

    g. Fibrosis and scarring may restrict heart's ability to function effectively; pericardial effusions may develop

    h. Chest pain occurs due to inflammation of nerve fibers in pericardium

    i. Acute pericarditis lasts 2 to 6 weeks

    j. Signs and symptoms

        1) Sharp chest pain (rapid onset) worsening with deep breath, cough or change in position; pain improves if elevated or sits up

        2) Dyspnea

        3) Dry cough

        4) Fever (low grade)

        5) Pericardial friction rub (leathery, grating sound) heard most commonly on expiration

    k. Complications include cardiac tamponade or pericardial effusions

C. Nursing assessment

  1. Assessment

    a. Rheumatic fever: VS, lung sounds, heart sounds, apical pulse, symptom analysis of any chest discomfort

    b. Infective endocarditis: VS, symptom analysis of complaints, nutritional status, palpate spleen, skin assessment for bleeding; heart sounds, peripheral pulses, capillary refill

    c. Myocarditis: VS, symptom analysis of complaints and pain, ECG pattern, heart sounds

    d. Pericarditis: VS, symptom analysis of pain and what worsens or relieves it, lung sounds, respiratory status

  2. Diagnostic tests

    a. Rheumatic fever: CBC, C-reactive protein (show inflammation), erythrocyte sedimentation rate (ESR), antistreptolysin (ASO) titer

    b. Infective endocarditis: CBC, immune testing, blood cultures, urine (increased creatinine, hematuria, and increased protein), ECG

    c. Myocarditis: ESR, CBC, antiviral antibodies, ECG, heart catheterization with biopsy of heart muscle, serum immunoglobulins, cultures

    d. Pericarditis: ESR, ECG, echocardiogram, hemodynamic monitoring, CXR, CT scan, and MRI

D. Nursing management

1. Medications

   a. Rheumatic fever: antibiotics (penicillin, erythromycin [EES], clindamycin [Cleocin], amoxicillin [Amoxil]); salicylates (aspirin); or corticosteroids for inflammation and joint pain

   b. Infective endocarditis: antibiotics (may use multiple drugs—oxacillin [Bactocill], penicillin, ampicillin [Ampicin], gentamicin sulfate [Gentamycin], cefazolin sodium [Ancef], vancomycin hydrochloride [Vancocin]); antipyretics, antiinflammatory agents

   c. Myocarditis: antipyretics, antidysrhythmics, anticoagulants, digoxin (Lanoxin) if heart failure occurs, corticosteroids or immunosuppressive drugs, antimicrobial agents

   d. Pericarditis: non-narcotic analgesics, NSAIDs, antipyretics, corticosteroids

2. Provide supportive care, emotional rest

3. Prevent complications and future recurrences; IV therapy if indicated

4. Monitor VS, heart sounds, ECG pattern, respiratory status

5. Priorities of nursing care

   a. Assess and treat pain

   b. Assist with ADLs; allow rest periods

   c. Provide diversional activity

   d. Monitor for signs of infection

   e. Monitor for signs of decreased CO

   f. Teach client importance of compliance and taking antibiotics until completed

   g. Teach client effective coping mechanisms

6. With myocarditis, client needs to decrease workload and increase O_2 supply to heart

7. Pericarditis may require a pericardiocentesis (removal of fluid) or surgery

8. Administer O_2 as needed

VIII. VALVULAR HEART DISEASE

A. Overview

1. Valvular heart disease is defined as diseases or conditions that interfere with unidirectional blood flow in heart

2. Can be acquired from either acute (endocarditis or calcium deposits) or chronic (rheumatic heart disease) conditions

3. Occurs as **stenosis** (inability of leaflets to open and close properly) or **regurgitation** (backflow of blood through a valve that cannot close properly due to damage or disease)

4. Other causes include MI and congenital heart defects

B. Pathophysiology

1. Stenosis

   a. Involves fusion of valve leaflets producing a narrow opening and rigidity

   b. Fusion may result from scarring of valves caused by:

      1) Endocarditis

2) Myocardial infarction

3) Calcification

c. Blood flow is impeded resulting in decreased CO, impaired ventricular filling, ejection fraction and stroke volume

d. Can affect mitral, tricuspid, aortic, or pulmonary valve

2. Regurgitation

   a. Caused by insufficient or incompetent valves causing incomplete closure, allowing backflow of blood

   b. Result from deformity or erosion of valve by vegetative lesions of bacterial endocarditis; scarring or tearing from MI; cardiac dilation—as heart enlarges, valves stretch; leaflets no longer meet causing regurgitation

3. Hemodynamic changes occur

   a. Blood volume and pressure are reduced in front of affected valve

   b. Volume and pressure increase behind affected valve

4. Chambers behind affected valve hypertrophy due to increased pressure of blood flow; CO falls as compensatory mechanisms become ineffective; heart begins to fail

   a. Increased muscle size leads to increased O_2 demand

   b. Decreased blood supply to enlarged muscle leads to heart failure

   c. Infarction occurs and loss of functional muscle

5. Affect aortic and mitral valve; **mitral valve prolapse** occurs when the mitral valve prolapses back into atrium causing regurgitation of blood from ventricle to atrium

6. Signs and symptoms

   a. Stenosis: pulmonary congestion, dyspnea, pulmonary hypertension, dizziness, fatigue, tachycardia, murmur or rub, S_3 or S_4 heart sound, angina; pulmonary stenosis may cause venous distention and swelling of ankles

   b. Regurgitation

      1) Mitral: dyspnea, pulmonary hypertension, decreased CO, dizziness and fatigue, tachycardia, angina, murmur or rub, S_3 or S_4 heart sound

      2) Aortic: wide pulse pressure, hyperkinetic (strong, bounding) peripheral pulses, signs and symptoms of CHF, angina

C. Nursing assessment

1. Assessment includes: VS, heart sounds, lung sounds, symptom analysis of complaints and pain, respiratory status, exercise tolerance, presence of edema, peripheral pulses

2. Diagnostic tests: ECG, echocardiogram, CXR, cardiac catheterization

D. Nursing management

1. Medications include digitalis (Lanoxin), diuretics, Class I or III antidysrhythmic, prophylactic antibiotics prior to invasive procedures

2. Close observation for progression of disease, angina that might occur

3. Monitor prophylactic therapy to prevent infection of diseased valves

4. Observe for signs and symptoms of CHF; treat as necessary

5. Pre- and postoperative teaching when medical treatment no longer effective and surgical intervention is necessary

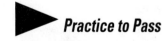

Practice to Pass

The client has been diagnosed with mitral prolapse. What should the nurse teach the client regarding treatment plans?

6. Teach client not to abruptly stop taking beta blockers or symptoms may return

7. Prepare client for and monitor following percutaneous balloon valvuloplasty

Case Study

M. J. presents to the emergency department with complaints of substernal crushing chest pain radiating to his left arm. He is a 58-year-old executive. He was having dinner with a client when the pain began. He states the pain started 2 hours ago and has been increasing in intensity since that time.

1. What type of assessment should the nurse do?

2. What parts of his past medical history would be important?

3. What diagnostic studies should the nurse anticipate the health care provider ordering?

4. What medications should the nurse anticipate being ordered for his chest pain?

5. What ECG changes should the nurse look for?

For suggested responses, see pages 532–533.

POSTTEST

1 The client on a telemetry unit exhibits regular cardiac rhythm strip complexes of normal duration and a heart rate of 82 beats per minute (bpm). In assessing the client, the nurse notes that for each complex there is a corresponding palpable pulse. The nurse concludes that the:

1. Ventricles are contracting regularly.
2. Ventricles are in fibrillation.
3. Client has ventricular tachycardia.
4. Atria are not contracting.

2 The client arrives in the Emergency Department with a heart rate of 130. The client appears anxious and is tachypneic. The nurse interprets that what physiological mechanism is most likely responsible for the increased heart rate?

1. Parasympathetic nervous system (PNS) activity
2. Sympathetic nervous system (SNS) activity
3. Increase in circulating acetylcholine
4. Decrease in circulating catecholamines

3 The client arrives in the Emergency Department with a diagnosis of right-sided heart failure. What clinical manifestations should the nurse expect to assess in this client? Select all that apply.

1. Distended neck veins
2. Pitting edema in the feet and ankles
3. Crackles in the lungs
4. Abdominal ascites
5. Reflex bradycardia with activity

4 A client with a history of angina pectoris is given nitroglycerin (NTG) 0.4 mg by the sublingual route for chest pain. Prior to the NTG, the blood pressure was 110/78. After five minutes, the client says the chest pain is better but not gone. The nurse should first:

1. Give another NTG.
2. Check the pulse rate.
3. Give morphine sulfate instead of NTG.
4. Check the blood pressure (BP).

5 A client with congestive heart failure has digoxin (Lanoxin) ordered every day. Prior to giving the medication, the nurse assesses that the digoxin level is 1.2 ng/mL and auscultates a one-minute apical pulse rate of 62. The nurse should:

1. Withhold the digoxin.
2. Withhold the dose and request an order for a potassium level.
3. Notify the physician.
4. Give the digoxin as ordered.

POSTTEST

6 Which of the following clients is at high risk for developing coronary artery disease (CAD) that may not be responsive to diet and exercise alone? A client who:

1. Has diabetes mellitus.
2. Has a strong family history of cardiovascular disease.
3. Is overweight and 55 years old.
4. Had a hemorrhagic stroke at age 40.

7 The client presents to the Emergency Department with substernal chest pain and is diagnosed with a subendocardial myocardial infarction (MI). The client asks the nurse what that means. The nurse should respond that the damage is:

1. On the anterior wall of the left ventricle.
2. On the posterior wall of the left ventricle.
3. Involving the full thickness of the wall.
4. Involving the inner layer of the heart.

8 The client is admitted to the coronary care unit (CCU) with a diagnosis of left-sided heart failure. When listening to the lung sounds, the nurse hears crackles bilaterally. The nurse concludes that this is an expected finding because left ventricular failure leads to:

1. Increased coronary artery perfusion.
2. Pulmonary emboli.
3. Increased peripheral resistance.
4. Pulmonary congestion.

9 The client with a diagnosis of anterior wall myocardial infarction (MI) begins to show dysrhythmias on the cardiac monitor. The nurse anticipates that the client is most at risk for which dysrhythmias based on the location of the MI? Select all that apply.

1. Ventricular fibrillation
2. AV block
3. Atrial fibrillation
4. Premature ventricular contractions
5. Sinus bradycardia

10 The client who experienced a myocardial infarction (MI) is being discharged from the hospital. What important self-care measures should the nurse teach the client to reduce the risk of reinfarction?

1. Compliance with ongoing thrombolytic therapy
2. Increase exercise to include activities like high-intensity aerobics
3. Consume a low-fat, low-sodium diet
4. Decrease the number of cigarettes smoked daily

➤ *See pages 76–78 for Answers & Rationales*

ANSWERS & RATIONALES

Pretest

1 **Answer: 3** Angina pectoris is the term for chest pain related to myocardial ischemia (not enough oxygen supply to the tissue for the demand). Any activity that increases the need for oxygen without an adequate available supply can cause angina. Pain from a pulmonary embolus would be abrupt in onset and not necessarily related to activity. Pulmonary edema would cause acute onset of dyspnea and pain might or might not be a predominant feature. Pain from pericardial effusion would not be caused by activity.
Cognitive Level: Application **Client Need:** Physiological Integrity: Physiological Adaptation **Integrated Process:** Nursing Process: Assessment **Content Area:** Adult Health: Cardiovascular **Strategy:** Consider the activity of the client at the time of the pain. Narrow the choices by eliminating some of the options in which pain is not associated with exertion. **Reference:** Porth, C. M. (2005). *Pathophysiology:*

Concepts of altered health states (7th ed.). Philadelphia, PA: Lippincott Williams & Wilkins, p. 545.

2 **Answer: 2** Orthopnea is shortness of breath caused by the movement of fluid back into the vasculature when the client lies down. The client may have beginning signs of congestive heart failure and should be checked. Sleep apnea may cause orthopnea but not edema; angina pectoris does not necessarily cause edema but chest pain would be a hallmark of this health problem. Sinus infections do not cause edema.
Cognitive Level: Application **Client Need:** Physiological Integrity: Physiological Adaptation **Integrated Process:** Nursing Process: Analysis **Content Area:** Adult Health: Cardiovascular **Strategy:** Note the critical word *edema* and use knowledge of concepts of fluid movement and cardiovascular system to answer this question. Note that the question focuses on respiratory manifestations. Consider the interrelationship between the cardiovascular and respiratory systems to aid in making a selection.

Reference: Porth, C. M. (2005). *Pathophysiology: Concepts of altered health states* (7th ed.). Philadelphia, PA: Lippincott Williams & Wilkins, p. 611.

3 **Answer: 2** Left ventricular failure impedes the flow of blood from the pulmonary blood vessels into the left side of the heart. This leads to pulmonary congestion and increased pressure in the blood vessels of the lungs, which then increases cardiac workload as the right side of the heart must pump against higher pulmonary pressures. The overall increase in cardiac workload and incomplete ventricular emptying leads to tachycardia as a compensatory mechanism. Orthopnea and cough are manifestations of the pulmonary congestion that occurs as part of the pathophysiology. Hypertension is often silent (option 1). CAD often manifests with chest pain called angina pectoris (option 3). PVD is characterized by leg pain while walking.

Cognitive Level: Application **Client Need:** Physiological Integrity: Physiological Adaptation **Integrated Process:** Nursing Process: Assessment **Content Area:** Adult Health: Cardiovascular **Strategy:** Remember Left and Lung—the two Ls go together; two of the symptoms deal with respiratory symptoms and none of the other answers are related to a diagnosis affecting the lungs. **Reference:** Porth, C. M. (2005). *Pathophysiology: Concepts of altered health states* (7th ed.). Philadelphia, PA: Lippincott Williams & Wilkins, pp. 610–611.

4 **Answer: 3** Depressed ST segments and inverted T waves represent myocardial ischemia in the leads that correspond with the area of the heart affected. Necrosis (option 1) would be accompanied by pathological Q waves. Injury (option 2) usually is accompanied by ST segment elevation. Option 4 represents a failure to understand the significance of the findings.

Cognitive Level: Application **Client Need:** Physiological Integrity: Physiological Adaptation **Integrated Process:** Nursing Process: Analysis **Content Area:** Adult Health: Cardiovascular **Strategy:** Read the question carefully, noting the critical words *ST segment depression.* Apply principles of electrocardiography to determine the etiology. **Reference:** Porth, C. M. (2005). *Pathophysiology: Concepts of altered health states* (7th ed.). Philadelphia, PA: Lippincott Williams & Wilkins, p. 548.

5 **Answer: 1, 3, 4, 5** The initial failure may be left sided but long term failure usually involves both sides of the heart. Left ventricular failure results in inability to pump effectively enough to empty the blood in the left ventricle, leading to increased left atrial pressures, increased pulmonary pressures and pulmonary edema. The forward effect of heart failure is a decrease in peripheral arterial blood flow.

Cognitive Level: Analysis **Client Need:** Physiological Integrity: Physiological Adaptation **Integrated Process:** Nursing Process: Analysis **Content Area:** Adult Health: Cardiovascular **Strategy:** Consider the pathophysiology of left-sided heart failure. When the blood does not move from the left side, what is the chain of events? **Reference:** Porth, C. M. (2005). *Pathophysiology: Concepts of altered health states* (7th ed.). Philadelphia, PA: Lippincott Williams & Wilkins, pp. 609–610.

6 **Answer: 1** Normal sinus rhythm has a rate of 60 to 100 bpm. A rate below 60 bpm but originating in the sinus node is termed sinus bradycardia. Tachycardia is defined as a rate greater than 100 bpm. Sinus arrhythmia is an irregularity to the rhythm, which is normal in children and some young adults but is abnormal in adults and older adults. The normal rate of firing of the AV node is 40–60 bpm, so an accelerated nodal rhythm would be a rhythm that has a rate greater than 60 up to 100 bpm.

Cognitive Level: Application **Client Need:** Physiological Integrity: Physiological Adaptation **Integrated Process:** Communication and Documentation **Content Area:** Adult Health: Cardiovascular **Strategy:** Consider the features of each rhythm represented in the options and make an association between the critical data *54 bpm* and the word *bradycardia* in the correct option. **Reference:** Porth, C. M. (2005) *Pathophysiology: Concepts of altered health states* (7th ed.). Philadelphia, PA: Lippincott Williams & Wilkins, p. 590.

7 **Answer: 4** Clients with unstable angina are at risk for myocardial infarction. Since Q waves are seen with acute MI (infarction), immediate attention is needed for this client. Gangrene (option 1) and infection (option 3) are irrelevant to the question. Ischemia (option 2) would show on ECG as inverted T waves in the affected area.

Cognitive Level: Application **Client Need:** Physiological Integrity: Physiological Adaptation **Integrated Process:** Nursing Process: Assessment **Content Area:** Adult Health: Cardiovascular **Strategy:** Review ECG and physiologic changes following acute myocardial infarction. One option best fits the pathophysiology of MI even if the ECG changes are unfamiliar. **Reference:** Porth, C. M. (2005) *Pathophysiology: Concepts of altered health states* (7th ed.). Philadelphia, PA: Lippincott Williams & Wilkins, p. 548.

8 **Answer: 1** Occlusion of a coronary artery blocks the blood flow and prevents oxygen getting to the myocardium. Option 2 indicates ischemia; option 3 could be bradycardia or an atrioventricular (AV) heart block; option 4 could be hypertrophy.

ANSWERS & RATIONALES

Cognitive Level: Application **Client Need:** Physiological Integrity: Physiological Adaptation **Integrated Process:** Nursing Process: Analysis **Content Area:** Adult Health: Cardiovascular **Strategy:** Only one option describes the pathophysiology of MI. Use knowledge of this pathophysiology and the process of elimination to make a selection. **Reference:** Lemone, P., & Burke, K. (2008). *Medical-surgical nursing: Critical thinking in client care* (4th ed.). Upper Saddle River, NJ: Pearson/Prentice Hall, pp. 982–984.

9 **Answer: 1** Hyperlipidemia (option 2), cigarette smoking (option 3), and lifestyle (option 4) may be changed by modifying behaviors, which is why they are collectively called modifiable risk factors. These risk factors should be stressed and plans made for how to change them. Since age and gender cannot be changed (nonmodifiable), this option is the lowest priority when considering the learning needs of the client.

Cognitive Level: Analysis **Client Need:** Health Promotion and Maintenance **Integrated Process:** Nursing Process: Planning **Content Area:** Adult Health: Cardiovascular **Strategy:** Note the presence of the critical words *lowest priority* in the stem, which means the correct option is one that is either the least significant option or cannot be changed. Use this information and the process of elimination to make a selection. **Reference:** Lemone, P., & Burke, K. (2008). *Medical-surgical nursing: Critical thinking in client care* (4th ed.). Upper Saddle River, NJ: Pearson/Prentice Hall, pp. 959–960.

10 **Answer: 4** NTG can be taken as a preventive measure prior to activities that trigger angina. This is especially helpful with sexual activity or work-related activities that may need to be continued. Modifying such activities may be necessary, but clients with cardiac disease should not become restricted by their condition and lead sedentary lifestyles.

Cognitive Level: Application **Client Need:** Physiological Integrity: Physiological Adaptation **Integrated Process:** Nursing Process: Planning **Content Area:** Adult Health: Cardiovascular **Strategy:** Choose a client-centered answer that allows the client to manage the disease. **Reference:** Lemone, P., & Burke, K. (2008). *Medical-surgical nursing: Critical thinking in client care* (4th ed.). Upper Saddle River, NJ: Pearson/Prentice Hall, pp. 967–968.

Posttest

1 **Answer: 1** Depolarization of the myocardium results in contraction (systole) and that produces the palpable pulse and the corresponding QRS complex on the cardiac rhythm strip. This heart is beating regularly at 82 bpm. Ventricular fibrillation (option 2) and standstill (option 4) do not produce a pulse. Atrial activity cannot be assessed from the information given.

Cognitive Level: Application **Client Need:** Physiological Integrity: Reduction of Risk Potential **Integrated Process:** Nursing Process: Analysis **Content Area:** Adult Health: Cardiovascular **Strategy:** Identify equally plausible options and eliminate them because the correct answer must be an option that is better than the others. **Reference:** LeMone, P., & Burke, K. (2008). *Medical-surgical nursing: Critical thinking in client care* (4th ed.). Upper Saddle River, NJ: Pearson/Prentice Hall, pp. 997–999.

2 **Answer: 2** Stimulation of the SNS increases heart rate, blood pressure, and respiratory rate. The SNS is mediated by epinephrine and norepinephrine. The PNS is mediated by acetylcholine and decreases the heart rate. **Cognitive Level:** Application **Client Need:** Physiological Integrity: Physiological Adaptation **Integrated Process:** Nursing Process: Analysis **Content Area:** Adult Health: Cardiovascular **Strategy:** Note that the client has both rapid breathing (tachypnea) and rapid pulse (tachycardia). Remember the fight-or-flight response is mediated by the SNS and this increases the heart rate. **Reference:** LeMone, P., & Burke, K. (2008). *Medical-surgical nursing: Critical thinking in client care* (4th ed.). Upper Saddle River, NJ: Pearson/Prentice Hall, p. 1000.

3 **Answers: 1, 2, 4** Right-sided heart failure leads to backward venous congestion, resulting in jugular vein distention, peripheral edema, and portal hypertension leading to abdominal venous congestion and ascites. Crackles are found in left-sided heart failure. Reflex bradycardia with activity does not occur with either left or right heart failure; instead, the heart rate would increase with activity because of increased myocardial demand. **Cognitive Level:** Application **Client Need:** Physiological Integrity: Physiological Adaptation **Integrated Process:** Nursing Process: Assessment **Content Area:** Adult Health: Cardiovascular **Strategy:** Remember "R"ight means "R"est of the body, whereas "L"eft means "L"ung in identifying where fluids stagnate. **Reference:** LeMone, P., & Burke, K. (2008). *Medical-surgical nursing: Critical thinking in client care* (4th ed.). Upper Saddle River, NJ: Pearson/Prentice Hall, pp. 1026–1027.

4 **Answer: 4** The client needs another dose of NTG if the chest pain is still present; however, a BP should be assessed *first*. Vasodilation may lower the blood pressure and this client's pressure started at 110/78. If the systolic is greater than 100, another NTG can be given. If the systolic is less than 100, the physician should be consulted. Morphine sulfate is often given in this case. The heart rate is not necessarily changed by the NTG.

Cognitive Level: Analysis **Client Need:** Physiological Integrity: Pharmacological and Parenteral Therapies **Integrated Process:** Nursing Process: Implementation **Content Area:** Adult Health: Cardiovascular **Strategy:** Note the initial blood pressure and the clue word *first*. This tells you that more than one option may contain a correct action but that a proper sequence of activities is appropriate. **Reference:** LeMone, P., & Burke, K. (2008). *Medical-surgical nursing: Critical thinking in client care* (4th ed.). Upper Saddle River, NJ: Pearson/Prentice Hall, p. 973.

5 **Answer: 4** The therapeutic serum range for digoxin is 0.5 to 2.0 ng/mL. The dose should be given as ordered since the apical pulse rate is greater than 60 per minute. The dose of digoxin should be withheld for a pulse rate less than 60, unless a different specific parameter is ordered by the prescriber. It is not necessary to notify the physician or to request an order for a potassium level with the information in the question.
Cognitive Level: Application **Client Need:** Physiological Integrity: Reduction of Risk Potential **Integrated Process:** Nursing Process: Implementation **Content Area:** Adult Health: Cardiovascular **Strategy:** Apply nursing standards for administering medications. Compare the heart rate and digoxin level in the stem of the question to normal parameters. **Reference:** LeMone, P., & Burke, K. (2008). *Medical-surgical nursing: Critical thinking in client care* (4th ed.). Upper Saddle River, NJ: Pearson/Prentice Hall, pp. 1032–1034.

6 **Answer: 2** Family history (genetics) is a non-modifiable risk factor. Although proper diet and exercise are encouraged, these may not be sufficient to lower cholesterol and prevent CAD. Diabetes mellitus or overweight status may relate to risk of CAD but these risks may be more amenable to reduction with diet and exercise. A hemorrhagic stroke can occur because of hypertension, neurological factors such as intracranial aneurysm or arteriovenous malformation, and may not actually relate to development of CAD.
Cognitive Level: Analysis **Client Need:** Physiological Integrity: Physiological Adaptation **Integrated Process:** Nursing Process: Analysis **Content Area:** Adult Health: Cardiovascular **Strategy:** The core issue of the question is identification of the client whose risk factors for CAD may not easily be reduced. Interpret the information in the question to indicate that the answer is a non-modifiable risk factor. **Reference:** LeMone, P., & Burke, K. (2008). *Medical-surgical nursing: Critical thinking in client care* (4th ed.). Upper Saddle River, NJ: Pearson/Prentice Hall, pp. 962–964.

7 **Answer: 4** The inner layer of the heart is referred to as the endocardium and thus an MI that affects this layer is termed an endocardial MI. Options 1 and 2 would be called an anterior MI or posterior MI, respectively. An MI that affects the full thickness of the myocardial wall (option 3) is called a transmural MI.
Cognitive Level: Application **Client Need:** Physiological Integrity: Physiological Adaptation **Integrated Process:** Nursing Process: Analysis **Content Area:** Adult Health: Cardiovascular **Strategy:** Use knowledge of anatomy and physiology and look for a clue word that indicates the area of the heart involved. **Reference:** LeMone, P., & Burke, K. (2008). *Medical-surgical nursing: Critical thinking in client care* (4th ed.). Upper Saddle River, NJ: Pearson/Prentice Hall, pp. 961–962.

8 **Answer: 4** Left ventricular failure leads to pulmonary congestion. When the left ventricle fails and has inadequate emptying, congestion occurs in the lungs because blood from the lungs cannot flow freely into the left atrium and ventricle. Coronary perfusion would be decreased rather than increased (option 1). Pulmonary emboli (option 2) typically arise from thrombi in the legs (most common), fat from a bone fracture, air, or amniotic fluid. Increased peripheral vascular resistance (option 3) may be associated with increased blood pressure.
Cognitive Level: Application **Client Need:** Physiological Integrity: Physiological Adaptation **Integrated Process:** Nursing Process: Analysis **Content Area:** Adult Health: Cardiovascular **Strategy:** The question asks for a response to left CHF, not an etiology. Distinguish between CHF and pathophysiology because of respiratory or other conditions. **Reference:** LeMone, P., & Burke, K. (2008). *Medical-surgical nursing: Critical thinking in client care* (4th ed.). Upper Saddle River, NJ: Pearson/Prentice Hall, pp. 1026–1027.

9 **Answers: 1, 4, 5** The ischemia causing the MI can also cause the cardiac muscle cells to become irritable and fire early, causing ventricular dysrhythmias. PVCs are common when the anterior wall is affected, and ventricular fibrillation is a dangerous complication. Sinus bradycardia may occur because of ischemia to the sinoatrial (SA) node. Sinus tachycardia has many causes, including exercise, caffeine or nicotine intake, fever, and physiological stressors such as MI. AV block is more likely to occur when there is ischemia to the AV node, which is more common in clients with an inferior wall MI, with blockage of the right coronary artery that also supplies the AV node in most people.
Cognitive Level: Application **Client Need:** Physiological Integrity: Physiological Adaptation **Integrated Process:** Nursing Process: Assessment **Content Area:** Adult Health:

Cardiovascular **Strategy:** Recall the pathophysiology of MI and link this to the underlying anatomy to determine which cardiac dysrhythmias are most likely to occur with an anterior wall MI. **Reference:** LeMone, P., & Burke, K. (2008). *Medical-surgical nursing: Critical thinking in client care* (4th ed.). Upper Saddle River, NJ: Pearson/Prentice Hall, pp. 997–999.

10 **Answer: 3** A low-fat, low-sodium diet aids in the reduction of cholesterol and/or triglycerides that could cause atherosclerosis and subsequent development of MI. A client who has had an MI should not participate in heavy exercise (option 2); a moderate exercise program with daily walking would be sufficient. Anticoagulant therapy with aspirin, not thrombolytics (option 1), may be recommended, and clients with an MI should stop smoking completely (option 4).

Cognitive Level: Application **Client Need:** Physiological Integrity: Physiological Adaptation **Integrated Process:** Nursing Process: Implementation **Content Area:** Adult Health: Cardiovascular **Strategy:** Read the question carefully and note critical words that modify or change the meaning of an option (such as *thrombolytic* in option 1, *high-intensity* in option 2, and *decrease* in option 4). Use knowledge of self-care after discharge and the process of elimination to make a selection. **Reference:** LeMone, P., & Burke, K. (2008). *Medical-surgical nursing: Critical thinking in client care* (4th ed.). Upper Saddle River, NJ: Pearson/Prentice Hall, p. 994.

References

Adams, M., Josephson, O., & Holland, L. (2005). *Pharmacology for nurses: A pathophysiologic approach.* Upper Saddle River, NJ: Prentice Hall Health, pp. 284–311, 328–343.

Black, J., & Hawks, J. (2005). *Medical surgical nursing: Clinical management for positive outcomes* (7th ed.). St. Louis, MO: Elsevier Science.

Ignatavicius, D., & Workman, L. (2006). *Medical surgical nursing: Critical thinking for collaborative care* (5th ed.). Philadelphia, PA: W. B. Saunders.

Lewis, S., Heitkemper, M., & Dirksen, S. (2007). *Medical surgical nursing: Assessment and management of clinical problems* (7th ed.). St. Louis, MO: Elsevier Science.

McCance, K., & Huether, S. (2006). *Pathophysiology: The biologic basis for disease in adults and children* (5th ed.). St. Louis, MO: Elsvier Science.

LeMone, P., & Burke, K. M. (2008). *Medical-surgical nursing: Critical thinking in client care* (4th ed.). Upper Saddle River, NJ: Pearson Education.

Porth, C. M. (2005). *Pathophysiology: Concepts of altered health states* (7th ed.). Philadelphia, PA: Lippincott Williams & Wilkins, pp. 545, 548, 590, 609–611.

Venes, D., & Thomas, C. (2006). *Taber's cyclopedic medical dictionary* (20th ed.). Philadelphia, PA: F. A. Davis.

Walraven, G. (2006). *Basic arrhythmias* (6th ed.). Upper Saddle River, NJ: Prentice Hall Health.

Wilson, B. A., Shannon, M. T., & Stang, C. L. (2006). *Nursing drug guide: 2006.* Upper Saddle River, NJ: Prentice Hall Health.

ANSWERS & RATIONALES

Vascular Health Problems

3

Chapter Outline

Risk Factors Associated with Vascular Health Problems

Hypertension

Peripheral Vascular Disease

Aneurysms

Thrombophlebitis

Varicose Veins

Arteriospastic Disease (Raynaud's Syndrome)

Thromboangiitis Obliterans (Buerger's Disease)

Objectives

➤ Define key terms associated with vascular problems.

➤ Identify risk factors associated with the development of a vascular health problem.

➤ Explain the common etiologies of vascular health problems.

➤ Describe pathophysiologic responses associated with specific vascular health problems.

➤ Distinguish between abnormal and normal vascular findings obtained from nursing assessment.

➤ Prioritize nursing interventions associated with specific vascular health problems.

NCLEX-RN® Test Prep

Use the CD-ROM enclosed with this book to access additional practice opportunities.

Review at a Glance

aneurysm a dilatation or an outpouching of the wall of an artery or vein that can occur anywhere in body

arterial steal a phenomenon that occurs when arterioles are maximally dilated because of hypoxia; in order to meet metabolic needs of tissues, these arterioles steal from cutaneous and peripheral vessels, causing client to be aware of a "pins and needles" sensation in affected area(s)

chronic venous insufficiency chronic failure of venous valves to function, resulting in interference with venous blood return to heart and production of generalized systemic edema

diastolic pressure of blood against arterial walls when ventricles of heart are at rest

embolus a foreign object such as a piece of a thrombus floating in bloodstream until such time as it becomes trapped in a vessel

hemodynamics a study of movement of blood within body

hypertension a blood pressure that is greater than normal, usually greater than 140 systolic and 90 diastolic

ischemia a deficiency in supply of oxygenated blood caused by a circulatory obstruction to a body part; client experiences considerable pain in affected part

orthostatic hypotension syncope or dizziness with sudden position changes, usually from supine to upright position, because of a drop in blood pressure

peripherial vascular resistance (PVR) sum of all resistances that body has within vascular system

pheochromocytoma a tumor that originates in neural crest cells of sympathetic nervous system and is responsible for about 0.1 to 2.0% of cases of hypertension; tumor cells release catecholamines that cause episodic and sustained heart palpitations, sweating, headaches, fainting, and hypertensive emergencies

primary hypertension an elevated blood pressure from unknown causes that occurs in about 95% of diagnosed hypertensive clients; also known as idiopathic hypertension or essential hypertension

primary varicose veins dilated superficial veins; seldom involves communicating veins; if valvular breakdown occurs, it is caused by hereditary factors

pulse pressure difference between systolic and diastolic blood pressure readings; range of difference is usually 30 to 40 mmHg

secondary hypertension an elevated blood pressure associated with pulmonary, circulatory, endocrine, and renal diseases such as hyperaldosteronism, pheochromocytoma, Cushing's syndrome, diabetes mellitus, coarctation of aorta, and hyperthyroidism

secondary varicose veins veins that are characterized by venous stasis and chronic venous insufficiency; occurs in deep and communicating veins

systolic pressure of blood against arterial walls when ventricles of heart are contracted

thrombophlebitis inflammation of a vein with clot formation within that vein

thrombus a collection of fibrin, platelets, clotting factors, and cellular elements of blood that attach to interior wall of artery or vein; sometimes, it will occlude a vessel

varicose veins dilated, tortuous leg veins

vasospasm spasm or constriction of a blood vessel

white coat phenomenon hypertension that occurs in a normotensive client when a healthcare professional approaches to take his or her blood pressure; differentiation between white coat hypertension and secondary hypertension is essential for effective therapy to begin

PRETEST

1 A client at the local health clinic has a systolic blood pressure (BP) of 164 mmHg. The nurse tells the client that it could be caused by:

1. An increase in the heart's electrical activity, causing hypertrophy of the left ventricle.
2. Failure of the elastic tissue or the side effects of antihypertensive medications.
3. Use of over-the-counter medications or increased intake of salt.
4. Anaphylactic shock or increased electrical activity of the heart causing hypertrophy of the heart muscle.

2 The nurse makes it a priority to assess the client's pulse and blood pressure (BP) as part of the administration of which of the following drugs?

1. Sulfinpyrazone (Anturane) and calcitonin (Calcimar)
2. Propranolol (Inderal) and clonidine (Catapres)
3. Glucagon (GlucaGen) and pyridostigmine bromide (Regonol)
4. Hydroxyzine (Vistaril) and prazosin hydrochloride (Minipress)

3 The nurse should discuss which of the following as non-modifiable risk factors influencing hypertension?

1. Ethnicity and stress
2. Obesity and substance abuse
3. Nutrition and occupation
4. Family history and gender

4 When examining an adult client with a possible diagnosis of hypertension, the nurse should gather data using which of the following methods?

1. Blood pressure from one arm only
2. Orthostatic blood pressure with one minute between each reading
3. Blood pressure from both arms taken five minutes apart
4. Cuff and doppler blood pressure in both arms

5 The nurse is teaching a client with Buerger's disease. Which measure in managing the disease is of highest priority for the nurse to include in discussions with this client?

1. Wear gloves if the extremities are cold and painful
2. Avoid wearing flat-heeled shoes
3. Report severe pain that may require analgesics
4. Cessation of smoking

6 A hypertensive client exhibits non-adherence to the care regimen after hospital discharge. The home care nurse considers that this client's behavior is likely to be influenced by which of the following factors? Select all that apply.

1. Medication not working as indicated by the client statement, "I don't feel any different."
2. Antihypertensive drug causes unpleasant side effect
3. Many lifestyle changes needed in diet, exercise, and smoking patterns seem overwhelming
4. Client has helped in planning goals and treatment
5. Client often does not feel symptoms of high blood pressure and does not know pressure is elevated

7 Which of the following clients has the greatest risk of developing a thromboembolism?

1. 20-year-old client
2. Client with a cardiac disease
3. Female client who is Jewish
4. Client with known kidney disease

8 The nurse anticipates that the management of deep vein thrombosis (DVT) in an assigned client will include which of the following?

1. Orders for anticoagulant therapy to inhibit clotting factors
2. Keeping the client's legs in any position of comfort
3. Using low molecular weight heparin (LMWH) once confirmed diagnosis exists
4. Elevating head of the bed six inches on wooden blocks

9 An elderly gentleman enters the Emergency Department with reports of back pain and fatigue. Upon examination, his blood pressure is 200/110, pulse is 120, and hematocrit and hemoglobin are both low. The nurse palpates the abdomen, which is soft and non-tender, but notes a pulsating mass and auscultates an abdominal bruit. The nurse concludes that the client's manifestations are compatible with which of the following?

1. Secondary hypertension
2. Aortic aneurysm
3. Congestive heart failure (CHF)
4. Buerger's disease

10 The nurse is caring for a client with Raynaud's disease. Which of the following outcomes concerning medication regimen is a priority? Select all that apply.

1. Relaxing smooth muscle to avoid vasospasms
2. Relieving the pain if vasospasms occur
3. Avoiding lesions on the feet
4. Preventing major disabilities that may occur
5. Discontinuing medication as soon as symptoms disappear

➤ *See pages 101–103 for Answers & Rationales.*

I. RISK FACTORS ASSOCIATED WITH VASCULAR HEALTH PROBLEMS

A. Hypertension (HTN)

1. Risk factors that cannot be modified
   a. Family history
      1) Multifactorial and multiple genes may be involved
      2) Family incidence of elevated intracellular sodium levels with an associated lower potassium-sodium ratio
      3) Clients who have parent(s) with HTN are at higher risk at a younger age
   b. Age
      1) Primary HTN: usually appears between ages of 30 and 50 years
      2) Clients over 50 years of age have a higher incidence of HTN; clients over 60 years of age have a 50% to 60% chance of having BP over 140/90
      3) Blood pressure (BP) readings are a good predictor for potential stroke, coronary heart disease, heart failure, and renal disease
   c. Mortality caused by HTN according to ethnicity indicates a higher risk of mortality in blacks than whites, especially black females
   d. Gender
      1) Men have a higher incidence of HTN until about age 55
      2) Men and women are approximately equal between ages of 55 and 74
      3) After 74 years of age, women are at greater risk for HTN
2. Factors responding to physiological modification
   a. Stress
      1) Environmental stressors, such as noise, heat, and cold
      2) Personality characteristics, such as responses to life events and/or life-changing events
      3) Physiological events, such as pain, decrease in blood O_2 concentration, drugs, and obesity
      4) Food choices
         a) High sodium intake may induce high amounts of atrial natriuretic peptide (ANP) hormone to be released, suggesting a possible link to increasing BP
         b) Low intake of potassium, calcium, and magnesium
         c) Being overweight and distribution of fat, particularly to upper body
         d) High consumption of alcohol, legal and illegal drugs
         e) Smoking: nicotine from cigarette smoking immediately raises blood pressure

5) Caffeine consumption: coffee, soda with caffeine, and chocolate are stimulants and are associated with a rise in BP

B. Peripheral vascular disease

1. Arterial

   a. Diseases such as atherosclerosis, autoimmunity

   b. Clotting problems: **embolus** (a foreign object such as a piece of a thrombus floating in bloodstream), **thrombus** (collection of fibrin, platelets, clotting factors, and cellular elements of blood that attach to interior wall of an artery or vein)

   c. Trauma, inflammation

   d. **Vasospasm** (spasm or constriction of blood vessel)

   e. Obesity

2. Venous

   a. Over 40 years of age

   b. Surgery longer than 30 minutes using general anesthesia, spinal anesthesia, or epidural anesthesia

   c. Venous stasis caused by prolonged travel, bedrest, cerebrovascular accident (CVA or stroke)

   d. History of previous deep vein thrombosis (DVT), family history of blood clotting disorder

   e. Cardiac disease such as heart failure, myocardial infarction, cardiomyopathy, malignancy

   f. Pregnancy, estrogen therapy, and oral contraceptives

   g. Obesity

C. Aneurysms: clients with HTN and/or atherosclerosis

D. Thrombophlebitis: diseases causing venous stasis, surgery, oral contraceptives, varicose veins, obesity, pregnancy, prolonged immobility

E. Raynaud's disease: gender (female, 18 to 40); heredity

F. Buerger's disease: smoking, gender (males), Asian or Eastern European descent

II. HYPERTENSION

A. Overview

1. Hypertension is defined as a sustained BP that is greater than normal, usually greater than 140 mmHg **systolic** (pressure of blood against arterial walls when ventricles of heart are contracted) and 90 mmHg **diastolic** (pressure of blood against arterial walls when ventricles of heart are at rest); however, age specifics need to be considered

2. Two types

   a. **Primary hypertension,** also known as *idiopathic hypertension* or *essential hypertension* (an elevated BP from unknown causes, which occurs in about 95% of diagnosed hypertensive clients)

   b. **Secondary hypertension** (an elevated BP associated with a disease process or abnormality)

      1) Cause can usually be identified: pulmonary, circulatory, endocrine, renal diseases, medicines such as volume expanders, increased sodium (Na^+) intake

      2) Examples: hyperaldosteronism, **pheochromocytoma** (tumor that releases catecholamines and causes hypertensive emergencies), Cushing's syndrome, diabetes mellitus, hyperthyroidism

   3. **White coat phenomenon:** client is normotensive except when BP is measured by a health professional

   4. Isolated systolic HTN: a systolic BP over 140 mmHg and a diastolic BP of less than 90 mmHg; this phenomena has a higher incidence with advancing age

   5. Labile HTN is extreme elevation of BP at one time with a normal BP later without other noted causes; limited physiological changes; changes do occur over time in heart, brain, and kidneys; should be closely monitored

   6. Pregnancy-induced hypertension: a complication of pregnancy with increasing BP, proteinuria, and edema

      a. This diagnosis is made if BP increase is 30 mmHg systolic and 15 mmHg diastolic over baseline BP on two assessments with a minimum of 6 hours between readings, as well as confirmed presence of proteinuria and edema

      b. This condition is most frequently present in third trimester of pregnancy and must be treated promptly; if untreated, condition may lead to eclampsia, a dangerous condition

   7. Malignant HTN is a progressive, rapidly developing HTN that causes vascular damage and possibly death; persistent severe diastolic HTN of over 110 to 120 mmHg; often occurs after anesthetic drugs are given

   8. HTN is called a "silent killer" because many clients do not have symptoms

   9. Diagnosis should be made after three or more consistent BP readings are taken after a 5-minute period of rest because BP can vary from day to day, within different periods of same day, and because of many factors

B. Pathophysiology

   1. Regulation of BP

      a. Is continually influenced by cardiac output (CO) and **peripheral vascular resistance** (PVR) (sum of all resistances that the body has within the vascular system)

      b. Regulated by management of arterioles, venules, heart, and kidneys

      c. Blood Pressure = Cardiac Output × Peripheral Vascular Resistance (BP = CO × PVR)

      d. Regulation of cardiac output

         1) Autonomic nervous system (ANS)

         2) Heart rate (HR) and stroke volume (SV)

         3) Fluid volume, which is influenced by mineralocorticoids, sodium, and water

      e. Peripheral resistance

         1) A smaller diameter of vessel will cause changes in vascular resistance, causing BP to rise

         2) A decrease in vascular resistance will cause BP to fall

         3) Increases in peripheral resistance may be caused by increased activity of sympathetic nervous system, angiotensin and catecholamines (elements controlling autoregulation), and thickening of blood vessel walls from atherosclerosis

      f. Neurohormonal mediators

         1) Arterial baroreceptor: monitors arterial pressure

         2) Baroreceptors are located in carotid sinuses and wall of left ventricle; these monitor arterial BP and counteract rising pressure by vasodilation through stimulation of vagus nerve

         3) Chemoreceptors: are located in medulla and carotid and aortic bodies

            a) Sensitive to changes in blood pH produced by variations in concentrations of carbon dioxide (CO_2), oxygen (O_2), and hydrogen ions

            b) A major reflex response is caused by changes in body's O_2 saturation, but to a lesser extent changes in blood pH and CO_2 concentration

    g. Body fluid volume

         1) Excess concentration of Na^+ and water: as systemic fluid volume increases, result is an increase in BP and rise in kidney filtration pressure, causing diuresis

         2) BP is altered through loss of salt and water and an over-production of sodium-retaining hormone

    h. Increased activity of the renin/angiotensin/aldosterone (RAA) system

         1) Renin: is released under control of central neural influence; leading to a decrease in blood flow to kidneys, a fall in BP, and a decreased concentration of tubular Na^+

         2) Angiotensin I combines with renin to form a nonpressor form of angiotensin I

            a) It is converted in lungs to angiotension II (a potent vasoconstrictor) by angiotensin converting enzyme, which because of its potency can elevate BP

            b) Angiotensin II causes a release of aldosterone, leading to reabsorption of Na^+ and water, leading to HTN

         3) Additional explanations concerning HTN

            a) Inability of kidneys to increase excretion of Na^+ in response to an elevated systolic BP

            b) Failure of the normal sodium-potassium or sodium-calcium transport mechanism within intracellular space

    i. Vascular autoregulation

         1) Blood viscosity: blood flow resistance increases as blood becomes thicker, and blood flow resistance decreases as viscosity decreases

         2) Autoregulation is aided through kinins by:

            a) Relaxing arteriolar smooth muscle, which increases capillary permeability as well as constriction of venules

            b) Prostaglandins producing either vasoconstriction or vasodilation

2. Primary HTN

    a. Primarily caused by an increased peripheral vascular resistance (PVR)

    b. PVR results from vasoconstriction or narrowed peripheral blood vessels

    c. In HTN, left ventricle must work harder to overcome resistance met when emptying (afterload); a constant increased workload and more pressure within left ventricle leads to hypertrophy (known as left ventricular hypertrophy or LVH)

    d. Initially, LVH is a compensatory mechanism by heart to regulate BP; later LVH is a complication because more O_2 and blood flow is needed for muscle to meet workload demands

      e. Initially, arterioles increase resistance to blood flow, leading to increased PVR and HTN

      f. Later, kidneys become involved by activating RAA system

  3. Secondary HTN

      a. Multiple system involvement with direct or indirect impact on renal system

      b. Aldosterone, cortisol, and catecholamines in excess

      c. Chronic stress: prolonged excess of catecholamines

  4. Signs and symptoms

      a. May be asymptomatic

      b. Headache is the most common symptom if any are felt

      c. Severe HTN: dizziness, nausea, vomiting, confusion (can signify encephalopathy), visual disturbances, renal insufficiency, aortic dissection, hypertensive crisis

  5. Complications include stroke, congestive heart failure (CHF), ventricular hypertrophy, damage to retina, renal insufficiency, aortic dissection, and hypertensive crisis

C. Nursing assessment

  1. Assessment

      a. Complete health, nutritional, medication, and social history

      b. Client's understanding of plan of care

      c. Assess for the following

        1) Occipital headache (HA) in the morning and length of time HA occurs

        2) Periods of dizziness: frequency, when it occurs, its duration, and relationship to any activity

        3) Tinnitus: have client describe characteristics of this phenomenon

        4) Pounding in chest: frequency, duration, and when it last happened

        5) Assess client's BP: obtain BP in each arm using three positions—lying down, sitting, standing (orthostatic BP)

          a) Record findings, identifying client's position for each reading

          b) An average amount of time between each reading should be a minimum of 1 minute, and is usually 2 minutes

          c) When client is seated, arm is supported at level of heart

          d) Note **pulse pressure** (difference between systolic and diastolic BP reading; range of difference is 30 to 40 mmHg)

        6) A physical examination, with emphasis on cardiovascular and associated systems

          a) Abdominal masses: may be pulsating, describe location and size

          b) Bruits: where they are found and whether they are bilateral or unilateral

          c) Characteristics of Cushing's syndrome

          d) Signs of pheochromocytoma

          e) Funduscopic eye examination

          f) Cardiac, vascular, and extremity examination

          g) Pulmonary examination

2. Diagnostic tests

   a. Urinalysis and tests for renin, cortisol, urine catecholamines; 24-hr urine collection

   b. Blood chemistries (potassium [K$^+$], Na$^+$, fasting glucose, complete blood count [CBC], blood urea nitrogen [BUN], creatinine, and lipid profile), serum calcium (Ca^{++}), and magnesium (Mg^{++})

   c. Other: electrocardiogram (ECG), echocardiogram, and possible vascular studies to determine significance of end-organ involvement

   d. Measurement of BP with appropriate cuff size for a week

D. Nursing management

   1. A change in lifestyle is always recommended *first:* diet control, weight loss, increased activity, and decreasing stress

   2. Medications include diuretics (combination, loop and potassium-sparing), beta blockers, calcium channel blockers, and ACE inhibitors

      a. Clients are usually started on diuretics or beta blockers initially; if managed on one drug, no further action is taken

      b. Clients not responding to one drug may have another added; ACE inhibitors are being combined with many drugs successfully

      c. Management of HTN follows guidelines of Joint National Committee on Prevention, Detection, Evaluation, and Treatment of High Blood Pressure (JNC–7); see Table 3-1

   3. Discuss client's nutritional needs

      a. Assess amount of Na$^+$ consumption and recommend no more than 2 to 6 grams of Na$^+$ daily

      b. Blood cholesterol of less than 200 mg/dL

Table 3-1

Management of Hypertension

Blood Pressure Classification	Systolic/Diastolic Blood Pressure (mm Hg)	Initial Antihypertensive Therapy	
		Without Compelling Indication*	**With Compelling Indication***
Normal	119/79 or less	No antihypertensive indicated	No antihypertensive indicated
Prehypertension	120–139/80–89		
Stage 1 hypertension	140–159/90–99	Thiazide diuretic (for most patients)	Other antihypertensives, as needed
Stage 2 hypertension	160 or higher/100 or higher	Two-drug combination antihypertensive (for most patients)	

*Compelling indications include heart failure, post myocardial infarction, high risk for coronary artery disease, diabetes, chronic kidney disease, and recurrent stroke prevention.
Source: JNC-7 Express: The Seventh Report of the Joint National Committee on Prevention, Detection, Evaluation and Treatment of High Blood Pressure by National High Blood Pressure Education Program, National Heart, Lung & Blood Institute, 2003, www.nhlbi.nih.gov. In Abrams, M., Josephson, D., and Holland, L. (2005). *Pharmacology for nurses: A pathophysiologic approach.* Upper Saddle River, NJ: Prentice Hall, p. 263.

    c. Reduction of calories and weight: body mass index (BMI) should be less than 25; otherwise a weight reduction plan should be investigated

4. Monitor vital signs (VS) and intake and output (I&O); test for edema

5. Monitor weight daily at same time, in same amount of clothing, on same scale; preferably is done upon arising from sleep and after voiding

6. Emphasize compliance with food, medications, and risk involved in not keeping BP in appropriate range; factors to be considered include:

    a. High cost of medication(s), unpleasant side effects, interference with lifestyle, and lack of understanding need to take medications when feeling well; also males may have sexual side effects

    b. Because HTN is an asymptomatic disease, its seriousness can be underestimated by client and significant others

    c. Some lifestyle changes prescribed for client are difficult to accept and implement; support groups may be of assistance

7. Teach client how to check own BP at home

    a. Help client plan a realistic schedule for measuring and recording BP

    b. Teach client and the significant others when it is necessary to call the health care professional because of an unusually high or low reading

8. Monitor heart rate (HR) and BP prior to administration of antihypertensives

    a. Hold if systolic BP is less than 100 mmHg and HR is less than 50 to 60 bpm as determined by healthcare provider

    b. Always check BP and pulse before taking beta blockers

    c. Monitor for **orthostatic hypotension** (syncope or dizziness with sudden position changes because of a drop in BP)

9. Discuss importance of medical follow-up for a lifetime

10. Discuss over-the-counter (OTC) medications that client is taking; educate about avoiding cold remedies that can increase BP

11. Health maintenance program should include an individualized aerobic exercise program, monitored by using a self-reporting system or within an organized club

    a. Client reports the following: heart rate during exercise, sensations of reduced physical and emotional stress, and reduction in systemic BP

    b. Guidelines for aerobic exercise are 20 to 30 minutes, 5–6 times per week, but these are dependent on age and physical condition of client

    c. Maximal heart rate (MHR) is determined by subtracting client's age from 220

    d. Prior to beginning rehabilitation, an exercise physiologist must conduct a detailed performance evaluation

12. Avoid smoking cigarettes or cigars, or using chewing tobacco or alcohol

13. Monitor drug effectiveness, especially in elderly who may experience fluid shifts, which can change distribution

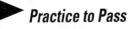

Practice to Pass

A client was diagnosed 3 months ago with essential hypertension. The client states to the nurse, "It doesn't matter if I forget to take my medicine. I just take the make-up dose at the next medication time." How should the nurse answer?

III. PERIPHERAL VASCULAR DISEASE

A. Overview

1. Peripheral vascular disease (PVD) is defined as those conditions resulting in interference in blood flow to or from extremities

Table 3-2		Arterial	Venous
Comparison of Arterial and Venous Insufficiency	**Description of Pain**	Intermittent claudication, relieved by dependent position	Aching, cramping, relieved by elevation
	Pulse Assessment	Diminished or absent	Present
	Ulcer Characteristics	Deep, pale; located on toes, feet, or other area of skin	Superficial, pink; over inner or outer ankle
	Skin Characteristics	Dependent rubor; pallor upon elevation; dry, shiny skin; cool or cold temperature; edema mild if present at all	Thick and tough; brawny (brown) pigment; skin normal temperature; may have edema
	Complications	Gangrene	Poor healing

2. Can be arterial or venous in origin (Table 3-2)
   a. Peripheral arterial occlusive disorders: partial stenosis or complete occlusion
   b. Venous disorders
      1) Acute, such as thromboembolism
      2) Chronic, such as **varicose veins** (dilated, tortuous leg veins) and **chronic venous insufficiency** (chronic failure of venous valves to function, resulting in interference with venous blood return to heart)
3. Causes include cardiovascular disease, thrombi, prolonged immobility, excess standing, pulmonary diseases

B. **Pathophysiology**
   1. Arterial
      a. Any alteration of blood supply compromises O_2 supply and alters demand
      b. Prolonged change in blood flow or decreased blood perfusion to large areas will start a sequence of vasodilation; this in turn will promote development of collateral arterial pathways, as well as use of anaerobic mechanisms to meet O_2 demands of cells
      c. The vasodilation has a limited effect, as arteries deprived of O_2 become maximally dilated and **arterial steal** occurs (when arterioles are maximally dilated because of hypoxia, they steal from cutaneous and peripheral vessels, which causes client to be aware of a "pins and needles" sensation in affected area)
      d. Of concern is the risk for development of tissue acidosis; this occurs when large amounts of lactic acid and pyruvic acid build up quickly; these acids are very toxic to body
      e. If compensatory mechanisms prove inadequate, client will experience pain called intermittent claudication
         1) Symptoms occur when a muscle is forced to contract without an adequate amount of blood supply to meet activity needs
         2) All muscles of body may claudicate, however, this often refers to lower extremities
      f. Lower limbs are most susceptible to arterial occlusive disorders and atherosclerosis because of limitation in collateral circulation
      g. Signs and symptoms
         1) Intermittent claudication
         2) Dusky, purplish discoloration when feet are dependent

3) White, pale color when legs are elevated

4) Thickened toenails

5) Ulcers on legs (see Table 3-2)

6) Venous refilling when foot is dependent

7) Decreased or absent pedal pulse

8) Numbness and cold, tingling feeling in extremity

h. Progression of symptoms from onset is slow, beginning from age 20 to 40 years; some clients have an associated severe coronary artery disease (CAD) and symptoms are influenced by body's use and speed of O_2 consumption in legs

2. Venous

a. Blockage within venous system may occur in system of superficial veins or deep veins

b. Causes of thrombus formation

1) Venous stasis from immobility, prolonged travel, obesity, pregnancy, and heart disease

2) Hypercoagulability from conditions causing dehydration and blood dyscrasias may cause platelet counts to rise, decrease fibrolysis, increase clotting factors, thus changing blood viscosity; in addition, oral contraceptives and hematologic disorders may increase blood coagulability

3) Injury to vessel wall may be caused by trauma of an intravenous infusion, fractures, contusions, and chemical injury from sclerosing agents and from Buerger's disease (thromboangiitis obliterans)

a) Injury to venous wall attracts platelets and debris gathers

b) With low blood flow, a hypercoagulable state occurs with resulting formation of a thrombus

c. Signs and symptoms

1) Discoloration of lower extremities

2) Edema over tibia

3) Ulcers (see Table 3-2)

4) Tenderness in legs

5) Positive Homan's sign (nonspecific; could occur in any painful condition of calf)

C. Nursing assessment

1. Assessment

a. Arterial

1) Symptom analysis of reason for seeking medical help

2) Activity tolerance and presence of pain

3) Skin color

4) Palpation of arterial pulses; use a doppler if necessary to detect them and document whether each is palpated or auscultated

5) Other circulatory assessments: capillary refill, temperature and presence of venous refilling

6) Observe sitting position of client for crossing of legs at knees or ankles, use of garters or knee stockings, and foot, leg, or ankle edema

    b. Venous

       1) Identify clients who are at high risk for thrombophlebitis

       2) Assess client's legs for discoloration, edema, and tenderness

       3) Measure and record leg circumference

       4) Determine amount of discomfort client is experiencing by asking about location, intensity, and duration

       5) Assess for Homan's sign

  2. Diagnostic tests

    a. Cholesterol and lipid panel

    b. Arteriogram

    c. Doppler ultrasonic flow study to identify blood flow through arteries

    d. Digital subtraction angiography to identify arteries in specific areas

    e. Oscillometry to determine volume of a pulse

    f. Stress testing

    g. Coagulation studies: partial thromboplastin time (PTT) for heparin; prothrombin time (PT) or INR for warfarin (Coumadin)

D. Nursing management

  1. Medication

    a. Pentoxifylline (Trental) to decrease blood viscosity and increase microcirculation

    b. Vasodilator: prostaglandins

    c. Anticoagulant or thrombolytic therapy for a thrombus

    d. Antiplatelet drugs: cilostazol (Pletal)

  2. Risk reduction through management of body weight for overweight clients using a low-fat, low-cholesterol diet with fruits and vegetables

  3. Risk reduction through physical exercise: encourage clients to walk 30 to 60 minutes each day if no skin alterations are present; clients need to have individualized physical exercises modified for them

  4. Educate on smoking cessation and harmful effects of nicotine; refer client to a support group

  5. If client has hyperlipidemia, evaluate need for reduction of total calorie intake, total fat intake, and other sources of cholesterol; in some cases where genetics are a major risk factor, the only management is a pharmacological regime

  6. Discuss with client reasons to avoid standing in one spot for a long period of time; if intermittent claudication occurs, stop, rest and then continue activity; avoid long car trips or air travel (if these are necessary, use frequent rest stops or position changes)

  7. Recommend to client to wear light warm clothing in order to prevent vasoconstriction of vessels of lower legs

  8. Inform client to avoid crossing legs or ankles because this decreases rate of perfusion and to elevate legs when sitting in a chair or when in bed

IV. ANEURYSMS

A. Overview

  1. An aneurysm is defined as a permanent dilatation of an artery or an outpouching of an arterial wall

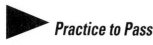

Practice to Pass

A client with a peripheral vascular disease (PVD) asks the nurse why it is essential to follow the health care provider's plan of care to reduce his cardiovascular risk. What should the nurse tell this individual?

    2. Most aortic aneurysms are situated below level of renal arteries; other sites are at bifurcation of aorta or within the structure of an artery or vein anywhere in body

    3. Classified as true or false aneurysm

        a. *True aneurysm* is a result of weakening of vessel wall over time and is usually a result of high BP or atherosclerosis

        b. *False aneurysm* is usually a result of a traumatic break in vascular wall instead of a weakening seen in a true form

    4. Aneurysms vary in pathophysiology, clinical findings, and treatment depending on where aneurysm is located

    5. They may occur in either an artery or vein

    6. Causes of aneurysms include HTN, trauma, atherosclerosis, or infections

B. Pathophysiology

    1. Morphology

        a. Fusiform aneurysm is cylindrical and involves entire circumference of vessel

        b. Saccular aneurysm is an outpouching of a sac on vessel; example: berry aneurysm

        c. Pseudoaneurysm: wall of aneurysm is not the original wall of the aorta; the mass is made up of connective tissue and structures surrounding extravasated blood

    2. Etiology: aneurysms may be classified according to cause

        a. Atherosclerotic aneurysm: caused by atherosclerosis

        b. Mycotic aneurysm: caused by bacterial infection

        c. Luetic aneurysm: caused by syphilis

    3. Location: type of aneurysm is determined by its location

        a. Thoracic aorta

            1) Progresses rapidly and often ruptures

            2) Symptoms include pain in back, neck and substernal areas; respiratory problems (stridor, dyspnea, cough); hoarseness

        b. Superior vena cava: accompanied by distended neck veins, facial edema

        c. Abdominal aorta

            1) Most develop below level of renal arteries; are most frequent

            2) Often asymptomatic with audible pulsation in abdomen or pulsating mass in abdomen

            3) Other symptoms can include: mild to severe abdominal and back pain, cool extremities, claudication

        d. Dissecting aneurysms

            1) A medical emergency

            2) Hemorrhage occurs because of a tear in aorta intima

            3) Often occurs in high pressure areas such as ascending aorta

            4) Symptoms include pain (abrupt, severe), elevated BP, undetectable pulses, syncope, heart failure

    4. An aneurysm of 5 cm may be palpable in a non-obese client

    5. Treatment of an abdominal aneurysm is surgery (Figure 3-1)

Figure 3-1

Surgical Repair of Aneurysm
A. Clamping of aorta and
visualization of clot within the
vessel. B. Graft within the
vessel used for repair.

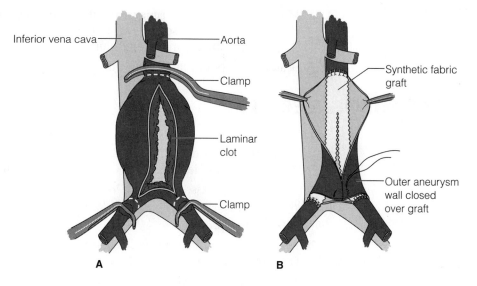

A

B

Practice to Pass

A 70-year-old client with an
abdominal aortic aneurysm
needs an MRI every 6
months. The aneurysm cur-
rently measures 4.5 cm. The
physician tells the family
surgery is usually not done
until it is greater than 5 cm,
as long as there is no evidence of growth or hemor-
rhage. The family asks the
nurse why surgery can't be
performed now. How should
the nurse respond?

C. Nursing assessment

1. Assessment includes characteristics of client's pain (intense pain in abdomen, back, flank, and scrotum); auscultation of abdomen; palpation (rigid because of accumulation of blood); VS; signs of hemorrhagic shock

2. Diagnostic tests

   a. Ultrasonography

   b. CT scan or MRI

   c. Chest x-ray (CXR)

   d. Renal function studies

D. Nursing management

1. Medications

   a. Antihypertensives

   b. Beta adrenergic blockers

   c. Anticoagulants and antibiotics postsurgery

   d. Analgesics

2. Monitor for complications following a major surgical procedure

   a. Underlying coronary artery disease (CAD) and chronic obstructive pulmonary disease (COPD)

   b. Postoperative atelectasis

   c. Decreased toleration of changes in **hemodynamics** (movement of blood within body) such as low blood volume and fluid shifts

   d. Myocardial infarction

   e. Kidney function: reflects integrity of cardiovascular system

   f. Emboli

3. Postoperative care

   a. Monitor for fluid volume deficit from insufficient intravenous fluids or hemorrhage

    b. Monitor client for increasing pulse rate, decreasing BP, clammy skin, anxiety, changing levels of consciousness (LOC), oliguria, pallor, and thirst as signs of shock from reduced circulating volume

  4. Educate client about compliance with measures to control HTN

V. THROMBOPHLEBITIS

A. Overview

  1. Thrombophlebitis is defined as an inflammation of vein with a clot formation made up of various elements in blood supply trapped in a fibrin mesh

  2. Causes are usually associated with Virchow's triad

    a. Injury to vessel wall: mechanical trauma, thermal injury, septic states, or an autoimmune problem

    b. Blood stasis: thrombus forms in an area of static blood flow and in valve cusps of veins

    c. Hypercoagulability, change in blood concentration, or blood coagulation factors; deficiency of naturally occurring antithrombins; and factors that assist in increasing blood viscosity

B. Pathophysiology

  1. Injury to intimal lining of vein causes a decrease in circulation and stimulates aggregation of platelets as well as other inflammatory mediators

  2. A protrusion from this site begins to occlude vessel and may partially or completely block blood flow

  3. Inflammatory mediators (leukocytes, lymphocytes, and fibroblasts) gather, causing congestion within vessel wall

  4. Thrombi may occur in any vessel, but are more prominent in veins because blood flow is more sluggish than in an artery

  5. Emboli can break away from thrombi and travel to different parts of body, most commonly to pulmonary circulation

  6. Signs and symptoms

    a. Small- and medium-sized veins may produce no symptoms

    b. Larger vessels: temperature (102°F)

    c. Superficial veins: redness, pain, tenderness, and swelling

    d. Deep vein thrombosis (DVT): calf pain, tenderness in calf muscle, positive Homan's sign (is nonspecific)

    e. Iliofemoral vein: thigh and/or groin pain, edema (may be pitting), cyanotic appearance to leg, fever, tachycardia; brawny edema (skin is thick, hard, has "orange-peel" appearance, and edema)

C. Nursing assessment

  1. Assessment includes neurovascular status of affected part (capillary refill, temperature, pulses, sensation, color of skin); VS; symptom analysis of pain; positive Homan's sign

  2. Diagnostic tests

    a. Blood cultures and CBC

    b. Phlebography (assess location of clot using a contrast medium)

    c. Doppler ultrasound

       d. Venous pressure measurement

       e. Plethysmography (measure changes in fluid volume passing through a vessel)

D. Nursing management

    1. Medications include anticoagulants, low-molecular weight heparin (LMWH), antiplatelets, anti-inflammatory agents, thrombolytics, and antibiotics

    2. Elevate foot of bed 6 to 8 inches on blocks or elevate affected part

    3. Maintain client on bedrest

    4. Administer moist heat to involved extremity; if warm moist soaks are prescribed to affected area, frequency prescribed is usually every 4 to 6 hours for 30 minutes; an aquathermia pad may be applied over a moist towel

    5. Listen to client's concerns; use community referrals as needed

    6. Monitor intravenous infusions carefully

    7. Encourage client to rest affected part

    8. Monitor effect of medications and treatments used; teach client about effects of medications and potential side effects

VI. VARICOSE VEINS

A. Overview

    1. A varicose vein is defined as a superficial vein that is twisted and enlarged

    2. May involve any part of body but occur most often in lower extremities and esophagus

    3. Types

       a. Primary: involving superficial veins and not communicating veins

       b. Secondary: involve deep communicating veins

    4. Causes

       a. Primary varicose veins frequently are familial and predispose client to loss of elasticity of vein wall and subsequent incompetent valves

       b. Secondary varicose veins occur with trauma, deep vein thrombosis, and inflammation/damaged valves

B. Pathophysiology

    1. Chronic venous insufficiency results from incompetent valves that cause:

       a. Reduction in venous return

       b. Increase in venous pressure

       c. Venous stasis

    2. Excessive dilation of vein causes spreading of valve cusps

    3. This causes valvular incompetency and produces a reflux of blood from superficial veins to enter deep veins by muscular pump

    4. Signs and symptoms appear after veins have been chronically engorged and tortuous

       a. Distended veins that may be bluish in color and bulging

       b. Pain in feet and ankles; heaviness or feeling of heat in legs

       c. Swelling of lower extremities

       d. Stasis ulcers

       e. Itching of skin over affected extremity

C. Nursing assessment

1. Assessment includes inspection of lower extremities for edema, discoloration, tenderness or discomfort (location and intensity), positive Homan's sign, signs of pulmonary embolism (anxiety, dyspnea, increased respiratory rate, "air hunger," tachycardia, diaphoresis, chest pain); bowel habits for constipation

2. Diagnostic tests
   a. Tourniquet tests: determine location of incompetent valves
   b. Doppler ultrasonic flow tests
   c. Angiographic studies
   d. Plethysmography

D. Nursing management

1. Medications are not recommended unless OTC analgesics are needed

2. If client is a smoker, discuss value and need to stop smoking; may refer client to a support group

3. Encourage client not to stand in one position for a long period of time; to take a walk each day for 30 to 60 minutes; and to rest if intermittent claudication occurs

4. A referral to Bureau of Vocational Rehabilitation would be helpful if client's position cannot be accommodated by employer

5. Suggest to client that light warm clothing is essential to prevent vasoconstriction of blood vessels in lower extremities

6. Assist client in learning about not crossing legs or ankles when sitting and to elevate legs when in a supine position

7. Prevent constipation or straining

VII. ARTERIOSPASTIC DISEASE: RAYNAUD'S SYNDROME

A. Overview

1. Arteriospastic disease: Raynaud's syndrome is defined as a condition of small arteries and arterioles of the fingers and skin that constrict in response to cold or emotional upsets (Table 3-3)

2. Raynaud's syndrome is termed Raynaud's disease if symptoms persist for 3 years with intermittent attacks

3. May be associated with autoimmune disorders, such as systemic lupus erythematosus, genetic tendency, or unknown cause

4. Primarily a disease of young women

B. Pathophysiology

1. Raynaud's syndrome causes color changes in hands when hands are exposed to causative stimuli

2. Digital arteries go into spasm, and hands change color, becoming very pale

3. This may occur after exercise

4. Tissue hypoxia occurs causing arteries to dilate slightly

5. Fingers appear bluish because they are now carrying mostly deoxygenated blood; this may occur in one or both hands

6. A rubor (redness) will occur when arterial spasms have stopped

7. One digit may demonstrate severe **ischemia** (deficiency in supply of oxygenated blood) with other digits demonstrating good blood flow

Table 3-3	Comparison of Raynaud's Disease and Buerger's Disease	
	Raynaud's Disease	**Buerger's Disease**
Definition	Condition of small arteries and arterioles of the fingers and skin; constriction in response to cold or emotional upsets	An inflammatory occlusive vascular disease involving the medium-sized arteries and veins
Causative Factors	Autoimmune disorders such as systemic lupus erythematosus; genetic tendency; unknown etiology	Genetic disposition; smoking; tobacco allergy; autoimmune response
Population Affected	Primarily affects young women	Primarily men of Asian and Jewish or Eastern European descent, under age 40, history of heavy smoking
Pathophysiology	Causative stimuli leads to color changes in hands; digital artery spasm; tissue hypoxia causes arteries to dilate; rubor occurs when spasms cease	Thrombi develop; vessel is blocked; lesion becomes fibrotic; vasospasms obstruct flow of blood
Signs and Symptoms	Red-white-blue syndrome of digits; pallor or cyanosis that is bilateral or unilateral; normal pulse; sensory changes in extremities; pain	Pain at rest; intermittent claudication; decreased or absent pulses; rubor and cyanosis of extremities; signs of decreased circulation
Characteristics	Triggers include exercise, long-term exposure to cold, stress; lesions can progress to gangrene	Triggered by smoking, cold, and emotional stress Most commonly affects hands and feet; upper extremities may be affected also; has periods of exacerbations and remissions; gangrene is a complication

8. Stenosis may cause an absence of pulse and a localized bruit
9. Main difference between Raynaud's disease and Raynaud's syndrome is there is less involvement in Raynaud's syndrome
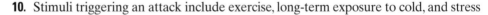
10. Stimuli triggering an attack include exercise, long-term exposure to cold, and stress
11. Signs and symptoms
    a. Raynaud's disease: known as blue-white-red disease (digits turn blue, then white, then red as spasms resolve)
    b. Other: pallor or cyanosis that is bilateral or unilateral; normal pulse; sensory changes (tingling, stiffness, pain, decreased sensation)
    c. Long-term: fingertips thicken because of lack of O_2 and nails become brittle (trophic change); gangrene is a serious complication

C. **Nursing assessment**
    1. Assessment
        a. Complete a careful history from a client who is presenting with hand(s) that have discomfort and are demonstrating changes in color
        b. Palpate distal pulses bilaterally noting rate and volume
        c. Assess pain levels, noting frequency of pain, its duration, intensity, location and current pain treatment; determine if present medication management is sufficient to control pain
        d. Assess all extremities for edema, lesions, and gangrene
        e. If lesions are present, measure circumference of each extremity; measure and document location of any lesion
        f. Assess client's use of medications
        g. Assess if client is continuing to smoke
    2. Diagnostic tests: diagnosis is determined by symptoms and ruling out other causes of decreased circulation

D. Nursing management

1. Medications include: vasodilators; a low-dose calcium channel blocker such as nifedipine (Procardia); nitrates (transdermal nitroglycerine or long-acting oral forms); analgesics for pain

2. If client is a smoker, discuss importance of quitting; consider a referral to a smoker support group or to a healthcare provider for nicotine patches or other medications

3. Clothing must be loose and warm to aid in maintenance of circulation: includes warm gloves, wool or heavy socks, comfortable, supportive shoes, and a warm hat

4. Teach client relaxation techniques to reduce effects of stress

VIII. THROMBOANGIITIS OBLITERANS: BUERGER'S DISEASE

A. Overview

1. Buerger's disease is defined as an inflammatory occlusive vascular disease involving medium-sized arteries and veins (see Table 3-3)

2. Primary clients are men (Asian and Eastern European) who are less than 40 years of age and have a history of heavy smoking

3. Commonly affects legs and feet, but may affect upper extremities as well

4. Known for periods of exacerbations and remissions; long-term effects include more intense and longer episodes with ulcerations and gangrene as complications

5. Causes include genetic disposition; smoking (primary); tobacco allergy; autoimmune response

B. Pathophysiology

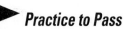

Practice to Pass

How should the nurse explain to a client the difference between Raynaud's syndrome and Buerger's disease?

1. Characteristic problems in this disease are development of panarteritis (inflammation of coats of one or more arteries) and panphlebitis (inflammation of veins)

2. Thrombi develop on vessel wall, which subsequently block vessel, and lesion becomes fibrotic; arteriosclerosis is not noted in lesion

3. Vasospams occur commonly and may obstruct blood flow

4. Primary result is arterial occlusion but veins may become involved

5. Signs and symptoms

   a. Pain (most common) at rest or intermittent claudication; may be triggered by smoking, cold, emotional stress

   b. Intolerance to cold

   c. Decreased pulses (even absent), cool or cold temperature in feet

   d. Rubor and cyanosis of extremities

   e. Loss of hair and thin, shiny skin in extremities

   f. Thick nails

   g. Signs of decreased circulation in extremities; changes with position changes

C. Nursing assessment

1. Symptom analysis of pain including toes and forefoot when client is at rest

2. Assess lower extremities and foot muscles for claudication

    3. Assess for migratory thrombophlebitis in a variety of veins

    4. Assess for development of gangrene in foot or feet

    5. Assess foot for fulminating digital ischemia (temperature, capillary refill, pulses)

D. Nursing management

!   **1.** Medications

        a. To offer some relief: antibiotics, corticosteroids, vasodilators, and anticoagulants

        b. Calcium channel blockers: diltiazem (Cardizem) and verapamil (Isoptin)

        c. Antiplatelets: pentoxifylline (Trental)

!   **2.** Non-surgical treatment of a client with Buerger's disease is to stop smoking; if smoking is stopped, symptom relief is expected

    3. Surgical treatment of a client with Buerger's disease is amputation of affected limb

    4. Educate client to avoid drugs that decrease circulation or diminish blood supply to extremities

    5. Educate client on triggers and to avoid extreme temperature changes

    6. Instruct client to inspect feet frequently; keep clean and dry and use soft padding if necessary

    7. Avoid standing in one position for long periods of time and avoid tight or restrictive clothing/shoes

    8. Use a bedcradle to relieve pressure from linens if necessary

Case Study

A 65-year-old female has been diagnosed with essential hypertension. She attends the local Council on Aging (COA) and sees a different health care provider at a local clinic whenever necessary. She has her blood pressure (BP) monitored at the COA monthly by a volunteer nurse. She takes a beta blocker and a diuretic, and her BP ranges from 130–140/70–90. She is compliant with her diet, doesn't smoke, and watches her weight. During the autumn, she has a few colds and begins to experience an increase in her BP, ranging from 190–210/100–120. The COA arranges for her BP to be checked more frequently, and she is referred to her health care provider. The doses of her beta blocker and diuretic are increased, and she continues to have high BP readings. Concerned about risk of stroke, her family is notified and a copy of the last month's BP readings is given to the family. She is again referred by the nurse to her health care provider, who places her on an ACE inhibitor.

1. What information should the health care provider gather concerning the client's present state of health and history data?

2. What education does the family need?

3. What is the essential information for clients to know concerning self-administration of their pharmacological regime?

4. What are the nursing priorities of care for this client? What is the plan for the implementation of this client's care?

5. How should the nurse explain the diagnosis of essential hypertension to the client and family?

For suggested responses, see page 533.

POSTTEST

1 In teaching a group of middle-aged men concerned about hypertension, the nurse should emphasize which of the following? Select all that apply.

1. Eat a diet rich in fruits and vegetables and low in salt and saturated fat
2. Alcohol consumption should not exceed five ounces per day
3. Smoking contributes to high blood pressure
4. Remain active with activities like walking several days a week
5. A sedentary lifestyle is best to keep the blood pressure lower

2 The nurse is teaching a pregnant female who has been diagnosed with hypertension. Which statement about secondary hypertension would be most useful for this client?

1. "Hypertension in pregnancy is expected and is not a cause for alarm."
2. "The renin-angiotensin system raises the blood pressure when the blood volume is increased."
3. "Hypertension in pregnancy needs to be controlled to reduce the health risks to you and the baby."
4. "White coat hypertension is a secondary hypertension because the cause has been identified."

3 The nurse suggests a dietary sodium reduction to help lower the blood pressure in an obese sedentary client. What rationale should the nurse share for reducing sodium intake?

1. "A low sodium diet has been shown to reduce the systolic and diastolic blood pressure."
2. "The blood volume will be decreased after a high intake of sodium."
3. "Reduced salt makes food taste less appealing so you will lose weight."
4. "Salt intake and smoking go together so reducing one helps with the other."

4 The nurse reviews the results of which laboratory results ordered for a client newly diagnosed with hypertension that are helpful in evaluating the etiology of the hypertension? Select all that apply.

1. International normalized ratio (INR)
2. Hematocrit
3. Cholesterol level
4. Serum creatinine
5. Troponin

5 Which of the following clients is at highest risk for developing a deep vein thrombosis (DVT)?

1. 25-year-old male who is a smoker with hypertension
2. 67-year-old overweight female recovering from a hip replacement (1st day post-op)
3. 22-year-old female with a history of Raynaud's disease in the family
4. 72-year-old male with a history of arthritis and bypass surgery

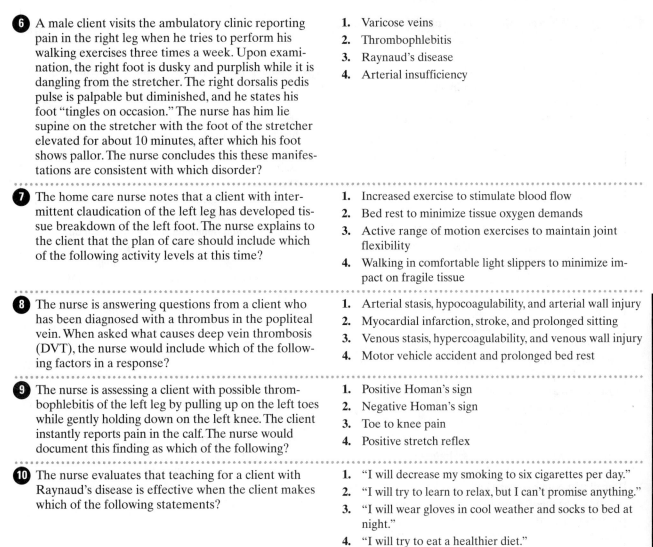

6 A male client visits the ambulatory clinic reporting pain in the right leg when he tries to perform his walking exercises three times a week. Upon examination, the right foot is dusky and purplish while it is dangling from the stretcher. The right dorsalis pedis pulse is palpable but diminished, and he states his foot "tingles on occasion." The nurse has him lie supine on the stretcher with the foot of the stretcher elevated for about 10 minutes, after which his foot shows pallor. The nurse concludes this these manifestations are consistent with which disorder?

1. Varicose veins
2. Thrombophlebitis
3. Raynaud's disease
4. Arterial insufficiency

7 The home care nurse notes that a client with intermittent claudication of the left leg has developed tissue breakdown of the left foot. The nurse explains to the client that the plan of care should include which of the following activity levels at this time?

1. Increased exercise to stimulate blood flow
2. Bed rest to minimize tissue oxygen demands
3. Active range of motion exercises to maintain joint flexibility
4. Walking in comfortable light slippers to minimize impact on fragile tissue

8 The nurse is answering questions from a client who has been diagnosed with a thrombus in the popliteal vein. When asked what causes deep vein thrombosis (DVT), the nurse would include which of the following factors in a response?

1. Arterial stasis, hypocoagulability, and arterial wall injury
2. Myocardial infarction, stroke, and prolonged sitting
3. Venous stasis, hypercoagulability, and venous wall injury
4. Motor vehicle accident and prolonged bed rest

9 The nurse is assessing a client with possible thrombophlebitis of the left leg by pulling up on the left toes while gently holding down on the left knee. The client instantly reports pain in the calf. The nurse would document this finding as which of the following?

1. Positive Homan's sign
2. Negative Homan's sign
3. Toe to knee pain
4. Positive stretch reflex

10 The nurse evaluates that teaching for a client with Raynaud's disease is effective when the client makes which of the following statements?

1. "I will decrease my smoking to six cigarettes per day."
2. "I will try to learn to relax, but I can't promise anything."
3. "I will wear gloves in cool weather and socks to bed at night."
4. "I will try to eat a healthier diet."

➤ *See pages 103–105 for Answers & Rationales.*

ANSWERS & RATIONALES

Pretest

1 Answer: 3 Systolic hypertension may occur after the use of over-the-counter (OTC) cold remedies containing an adrenergic drug as a decongestant. A warning is placed on OTC medications, cautioning clients with hypertension to consult a physician first. Renal diseases contribute to hypertension, and salt causes fluid volume retention, which increases the BP. Increases in the electrical activity of the heart will cause a variety of arrhythmias, not systolic hypertension (option 1). The failure of the elastic tissue is frequently seen in the skin of the elderly and side effects of antihypertensives would most likely cause systolic hypotension (option 2). Anaphylactic shock or an increased electrical activity of the heart would lead to hypotension (option 4).

Cognitive Level: Application **Client Need:** Physiological Integrity: Physiological Adaptation **Integrated Process:** Nursing Process: Analysis **Content Area:** Adult Health: Cardiovascular **Strategy:** Consider the etiology or risk factors for hypertension and eliminate the wrong options. **Reference:** Porth, C. M. (2005). *Pathophysiology: Concepts of altered health states* (7th ed.). Philadelphia, PA: Lippincott Williams & Wilkins, pp. 503–516.

2 Answer: 2 When administering propranolol (Inderal), the client's apical pulse and BP must be assessed. Propranolol is a beta blocker used to treat hypertension and tachycardia. The drug should not be given if the apical pulse is below 60 beats per minute (bpm), if there has been a significant drop in the BP, or if the systolic BP is below 100 mm Hg. Side effects include bradycardia, congestive heart failure, pulmonary edema, hypotension and edema, depression, memory loss, insomnia, drowsiness, and dizziness. Clonidine (Catapres) is an alpha blocker prescribed to control mild to moderate hypertension. Side effects are drowsiness, nightmares, nervousness, depression, hypotension, and bradycardia. Sulfinpyrazone (Anturane) is a medication used to manage long-term gout, while calcitonin (Calcimar) is used in the treatment of Paget's disease by decreasing the rate of bone destruction (option 1). Glucagon (GlucaGen) is used to manage hypoglycemia when glucose is not appropriate (option 3). Hydroxyzine (Vistaril) is used in the treatment of anxiety, pruritus caused by allergies, psychiatric and emotional emergencies, nausea and vomiting (excluding the nausea and vomiting of pregnancy), as a preoperative and postoperative sedation, and as antepartum and postpartum adjunct therapy (option 4).
Cognitive Level: Application **Client Need:** Physiological Integrity: Pharmacological and Parenteral Therapies **Integrated Process:** Nursing Process: Implementation **Content Area:** Adult Health: Cardiovascular **Strategy:** Recall that both parts of a multiple part option must be correct to be the right answer. Eliminate any option where one part is wrong. **Reference:** Lemone, P., & Burke, K. (2008). *Medical-surgical nursing: Critical thinking in client care* (4th ed.). Upper Saddle River, NJ: Pearson/ Prentice Hall, pp. 1161–1162.

3 Answer: 4 Family history and gender cannot be modified as risk factors in any form of hypertension. Current research suggests there are several genes influencing the development of hypertension. Ethnicity is a non-modifiable risk factor; however, stress can be modified if the interruption of the stressor is undertaken (option 1). Obesity and substance abuse are risk factors that may be managed through behavioral modification and support groups (option 2). Nutrition and occupation are both modifiable with assistance (option 3).
Cognitive Level: Application **Client Need:** Health Promotion and Maintenance **Integrated Process:** Nursing Process: Implementation **Content Area:** Adult Health: Cardiovascular **Strategy:** The critical word in the question is *non-modifiable.* Focus on options that refer to factors that cannot be changed and use the process of elimination to make a selection. **Reference:** Lemone, P., & Burke, K. (2008).

Medical-surgical nursing: Critical thinking in client care (4th ed.). Upper Saddle River, NJ: Pearson/Prentice Hall, pp. 1156–1157.

4 Answer: 2 Blood pressure readings from three different positions are helpful in ruling out the presence of hypertension. The difference between each of these readings should be less than 5 mmHg. If the reading difference is higher, repeat readings should be within the follow-up plan for this client. Options 1, 3, and 4 will not provide enough data to determine if a problem exists.
Cognitive Level: Application **Client Need:** Physiological Integrity: Physiological Adaptation **Integrated Process:** Nursing Process: Assessment **Content Area:** Adult Health: Cardiovascular **Strategy:** Think about which option gives the most comprehensive data. **Reference:** Porth, C. M. (2005). *Pathophysiology: Concepts of altered health states* (7th ed.). Philadelphia, PA: Lippincott Williams & Wilkins, pp. 517–518.

5 Answer: 4 Smoking is the primary etiological factor identified with clients diagnosed with Buerger's disease. Emphasis should be placed on cessation of smoking. Option 1 is usually required with clients with Raynaud's disease, although clients with Buerger's should protect the extremities from cold injury as well. Clients with Buerger's disease should wear comfortable shoes that will not cause blisters or sores, but they do not necessarily have to be flat (option 2). Although pain is present, the use of opioids is usually not indicated (option 3).
Cognitive Level: Analysis **Client Need:** Health Promotion and Maintenance **Integrated Process:** Nursing Process: Implementation **Content Area:** Adult Health: Cardiovascular **Strategy:** Differentiate between Raynaud's and Buerger's disease to eliminate option 1. Choose option 4 over the other options recalling that cigarette smoking is the chief risk factor. **Reference:** Porth, C. M. (2005). *Pathophysiology: Concepts of altered health states* (7th ed.). Philadelphia, PA: Lippincott Williams & Wilkins, p. 489.

6 Answers: 2, 3, 5 Frequently, clients perceive themselves as helpless when confronted with multiple lifestyle changes. The healthcare team and the client need to determine the most significant lifestyle modification needed and begin to work with this one. Many times the therapeutic action of the medication will not cause the client to feel or perceive any difference in his or her well-being. Client education, a concern for the nurse, can help to enlighten a client about the need for lifelong therapy. Antihypertensive drugs may cause unpleasant side effects while the disease often has no symptoms. If the client is a partner in the plan, it has a better chance of compliance.
Cognitive Level: Application **Client Need:** Health Promotion and Maintenance **Integrated Process:** Nursing Process: Im-

plementation **Content Area:** Adult Health: Cardiovascular **Strategy:** Note that the wording of the question indicates that the correct option is one that promotes poor adherence to therapy. With this in mind, eliminate any option that actually aids in compliance. **Reference:** Lemone, P., & Burke, K. (2008). *Medical-surgical nursing: Critical thinking in client care* (4th ed.). Upper Saddle River, NJ: Pearson/Prentice Hall, pp. 1164–1165.

7 Answer: 2 Cardiac diseases such as congestive heart failure, myocardial infarction, and cardiomyopathy are conditions that coexist with thromboembolism. Each of these conditions creates the possibility of thrombus occurring because of ineffective emptying of the heart during its pumping action. Thromboembolism generally occurs in clients over the age of 40. Gender usually does not play a role in embolism; a male who is Jewish and over the age of 40 is more prone to Buerger's disease (option 3). Kidney disease has not been identified as a cause of emboli (option 4). **Cognitive Level:** Analysis **Client Need:** Health Promotion and Maintenance **Integrated Process:** Nursing Process: Assessment **Content Area:** Adult Health: Cardiovascular **Strategy:** Recall that thromboembolism is most likely to occur when blood flow is sluggish from inadequate cardiac pumping action or when blood is viscous. Use this information and the process of elimination to make a selection. **Reference:** Lemone, P., & Burke, K. (2008). *Medical-surgical nursing: Critical thinking in client care* (4th ed.). Upper Saddle River, NJ: Pearson/Prentice Hall, pp. 1180, 1186.

8 Answer: 1 Part of the medical regime will include anticoagulant therapy. The rationale for this is to prevent the development or extension of thrombi by inhibiting the synthesis of the clotting factors or through deactivation of the mechanism. The client's legs need to remain in an elevated position for comfort and to facilitate venous circulation to prevent the development of emboli and thrombi in the lower extremities (option 2). Low molecular weight heparin (LMWH) is usually used as a preventive agent in clients prone to thrombophlebitis, not as a treatment with a confirmed diagnosis (option 3). The head of the bed may be elevated for activities such as eating and bathing but not continually (option 4). **Cognitive Level:** Application **Client Need:** Physiological Integrity: Physiological Adaptation **Integrated Process:** Nursing Process: Planning **Content Area:** Adult Health: Cardiovascular **Strategy:** Recall that thromboembolism involves abnormal clotting and use this knowledge to select the option that most effectively interferes with abnormal clotting. **Reference:** Lemone, P., & Burke, K. (2008). *Medical-surgical nursing: Critical thinking in*

client care (4th ed.). Upper Saddle River, NJ: Pearson/Prentice Hall, pp. 1188–1189.

9 Answer: 2 The symptoms exhibited by the client are typical of an abdominal aortic aneurysm. The most significant sign is the audible pulse in the abdominal area. If hemorrhage were present, the abdomen would be tender and firm. There isn't enough information to determine if the hypertension is secondary or essential (option 1). There is no evidence of congestive heart failure (CHF) in the client (option 3). Signs of Buerger's disease involve the extremities (option 4). **Cognitive Level:** Analysis **Client Need:** Physiological Integrity: Physiological Adaptation **Integrated Process:** Nursing Process: Analysis **Content Area:** Adult Health: Cardiovascular **Strategy:** Analyze the abdominal assessment findings and use the process of elimination to make a selection. **Reference:** Lemone, P., & Burke, K. (2008). *Medical-surgical nursing: Critical thinking in client care* (4th ed.). Upper Saddle River, NJ: Pearson/Prentice Hall, pp. 1171–1173.

10 Answers: 1, 2 The major task of the health care team is to medicate the client with drugs that produce smooth muscle relaxation, which will decrease the vasospasm and increase the arterial flow to the affected part. The drugs used are calcium antagonists. Frequently, the client will be medicated during the cold months when vasoconstriction is a physiological response to the environmental temperature. Relieving pain is also a concern. If the medications work, pain will be reduced and blood flow maintained (thus lesions prevented). Raynaud's disease does not usually cause major disabilities. A client may develop gangrene of the skin of the tips of the digits, but these are in the upper extremities. **Cognitive Level:** Analysis **Client Need:** Physiological Integrity: Physiological Adaptation **Integrated Process:** Nursing Process: Planning **Content Area:** Adult Health: Cardiovascular **Strategy:** Note the diagnosis in the question and recall that this is caused by inadequate circulation to the upper extremities, often accompanied by vasospasm, to choose the correct options. **Reference:** Lemone, P., & Burke, K. (2008). *Medical-surgical nursing: Critical thinking in client care* (4th ed.). Upper Saddle River, NJ: Pearson/Prentice Hall, pp. 1182–1183.

Posttest

1 Answers: 1, 3, 4 The healthcare provider must be sure that clients are aware of the need to eat sufficient amounts of calcium, magnesium, and potassium. Foods high in magnesium are green leafy vegetables, seafood, wheat bran, milk, legumes, bananas, oranges, grapefruit, and chocolate. Foods high in calcium are milk, cottage cheese, cheese, yogurt, rhubarb, broccoli, collard greens, spinach, tofu, canned sardines, and salmon. Potassium-rich foods are fruits and fruit juices, vegetables and vegetable juices, meats, and milk products. The consumption of alcohol is limited to one ounce per day; however, with some anti-hypertensive medications, the recommendation is that the client should not consume any alcohol (option 2). Aerobic exercise, such as walking, 3 to 5 days a week reduces stress and blood pressure. Smoking is not part of a healthy lifestyle. **Cognitive Level:** Analysis **Client Need:** Health Promotion and Maintenance **Integrated Process:** Nursing Process: Implementation **Content Area:** Adult Health: Cardiovascular **Strategy:** Consider healthy lifestyle recommendations for middle-aged men and choose these options since the wording of the question indicates the correct answer(s) will be true statements. **Reference:** Lemone, P., & Burke, K. (2008). *Medical-surgical nursing: Critical thinking in client care* (4th ed.). Upper Saddle River, NJ: Pearson/Prentice Hall, pp. 1158–1160.

2 **Answer: 3** By definition, secondary hypertension has some underlying physiological cause. Approximately 10 percent of all pregnant women develop this condition, which places both the mother and baby at risk. The renin-angiotensin system is triggered by low blood volume. A client with white coat hypertension is normotensive except when the BP is measured by a health care professional (option 4). **Cognitive Level:** Application **Client Need:** Physiological Integrity: Physiological Adaptation **Integrated Process:** Communication and Documentation **Content Area:** Adult Health: Cardiovascular **Strategy:** The wording of the question indicates the correct option is a true statement. Evaluate each option as to its accuracy and use the process of elimination. **Reference:** Porth, C. M. (2005). *Pathophysiology: Concepts of altered health states* (7th ed.). Philadelphia, PA: Lippincott Williams & Wilkins, pp. 522–524.

3 **Answer: 1** Increased salt intake has been suspected as an etiology in hypertension. Results from using the low sodium DASH (Dietary Approaches to Stop Hypertension) diet have shown reduced blood pressure. More fluid is retained to balance a high sodium intake so the blood pressure is not lowered. There is no known link between smoking and salt intake or salt intake and anorexia. **Cognitive Level:** Application **Client Need:** Health Promotion and Maintenance **Integrated Process:** Communication and Documentation **Content Area:** Adult Health: Cardiovascular **Strategy:** Do not be fooled by distracting information in the stem. Look for a physiologic rationale. **Reference:**

Porth, C. M. (2005). *Pathophysiology: Concepts of altered health states* (7th ed.). Philadelphia, PA: Lippincott Williams & Wilkins, pp. 515–516.

4 **Answers: 2, 3, 4** An elevated cholesterol level would suggest hypertension related to atherosclerosis. Creatinine is the most specific test of kidney function (a cause of hypertension) and is not affected by foods as would be the blood urea nitrogen (BUN). A lowered hematocrit could indicate fluid overload, which could account for hypertension also. Cardiac enzymes such as troponin and INR do not give information related to hypertension. **Cognitive Level:** Analysis **Client Need:** Physiological Integrity: Reduction of Risk Potential **Integrated Process:** Nursing Process: Analysis **Content Area:** Adult Health: Cardiovascular **Strategy:** Recall the contributing factors that lead to elevation of the blood pressure and consider which of these is evidenced in the laboratory tests listed. **Reference:** Porth, C. M. (2005). *Pathophysiology: Concepts of altered health states* (7th ed.). Philadelphia, PA: Lippincott Williams & Wilkins, pp. 513–520.

5 **Answer: 2** An overweight client on bed rest from a hip surgery is at higher risk because of the two risk factors (obesity and immobility). Even though the client will be ambulated and progressively increase weight bearing, the potential exists because of the immobility. Hypertension does not increase the risk, nor does smoking (option 1). Raynaud's is not a factor (option 3); option 4 is vague about the cardiac history and further information is needed. **Cognitive Level:** Analysis **Client Need:** Physiological Integrity: Physiological Adaptation **Integrated Process:** Nursing Process: Analysis **Content Area:** Adult Health: Cardiovascular **Strategy:** Look for the situation that has the highest risk. In this question each option contains two parts, so the correct answer is the one in which both elements represent a risk for DVT. **Reference:** Porth, C. M. (2005). *Pathophysiology: Concepts of altered health states* (7th ed.). Philadelphia, PA: Lippincott Williams & Wilkins, pp. 496–498.

6 **Answer: 4** The signs and symptoms are consistent with arterial insufficiency. The diagnosis is supported by the pallor noted when the feet are elevated for 10 minutes. The pulse is diminished because this is an arterial occlusion and not venous. Pain and itching are usually felt with varicose veins (option 1). Thrombophlebitis is associated with redness, warmth, and swelling of an extremity (option 2). Raynaud's is more involved with the digits of both the hands and feet (option 3). **Cognitive Level:** Analysis **Client Need:** Physiological Integrity: Physiological Adaptation **Integrated Process:** Nursing Process: Analysis **Content Area:** Adult Health:

Cardiovascular **Strategy:** Recall that gravity affects blood flow to extremities. Evaluate the described findings in terms of how gravity influences blood flow and eliminate the options that do not fit the expected findings. **Reference:** Porth, C. M. (2005). *Pathophysiology: Concepts of altered health states* (7th ed.). Philadelphia, PA: Lippincott Williams & Wilkins, pp. 487–490.

7 **Answer: 2** Whenever there is tissue breakdown associated with intermittent claudication, the client will be confined to bed so the body can meet the oxygen requirements for the damaged tissues. Activity in any form (options 1, 3, and 4) raises the amount of oxygen required to sustain both healthy and diseased tissues to a point where deficits will occur and healing will be delayed. When the client is ready to resume ambulation, the shoe of choice is a supportive, comfortable shoe. **Cognitive Level:** Application **Client Need:** Physiological Integrity: Physiological Adaptation **Integrated Process:** Nursing Process: Implementation **Content Area:** Adult Health: Cardiovascular **Strategy:** Recall that options that are similar cannot be correct. The option that is different is the one that does not involve activity and increased tissue demand for oxygen. **Reference:** Lemone, P., & Burke, K. (2008). *Medical-surgical nursing: Critical thinking in client care* (4th ed.). Upper Saddle River, NJ: Pearson/Prentice Hall, pp. 1178–1180.

8 **Answer: 3** The factors in option 3 are known as Virchow's triad and are the most commonly associated reasons for a thrombosis. A thrombus usually involves the venous system, not arterial (option 1). Situations that contribute to venous stasis are myocardial infarction and prolonged sitting; however, a stroke is not classified in this manner (option 2). Injury may or may not cause thrombi, while continued bed rest can contribute (option 4). **Cognitive Level:** Application **Client Need:** Physiological Integrity: Physiological Adaptation **Integrated Process:** Nursing Process: Assessment **Content Area:** Adult Health: Cardiovascular **Strategy:** Recall that when there are mul-tiple parts to an option, all the parts of that option must be correct for the option to be the correct answer. **Reference:** Porth, C. M. (2005). *Pathophysiology: Concepts of altered health states* (7th ed.). Philadelphia, PA: Lippincott Williams & Wilkins, pp. 496–498.

9 **Answer: 1** Pain felt in the calf while pulling up on the toes is abnormal and indicates a positive Homan's sign. If the client feels nothing or just feels like the calf muscle is stretching, this is a normal finding and Homan's sign is considered negative. **Cognitive Level:** Application **Client Need:** Physiological Integrity: Physiological Adaptation **Integrated Process:** Nursing Process: Assessment **Content Area:** Adult Health: Cardiovascular **Strategy:** When two options are opposite, there is an increased likelihood that one of them is correct. With this in mind, eliminate options 3 and 4. Choose option 1 based on knowledge that pain would be a positive finding. **Reference:** Porth, C. M. (2005). *Pathophysiology: Concepts of altered health states* (7th ed.). Philadelphia, PA: Lippincott Williams & Wilkins, pp. 496–498.

10 **Answer: 3** A client with Raynaud's disease needs to be taught to protect the digits from extreme cold by using warm clothing, gloves, and socks. Use of gloves is essential any time the digits may be cold (such as at night). Smoking should be stopped completely (option 1). Relaxation and stress management are essential (option 2). Diet is not associated with Raynaud's disease (option 4). **Cognitive Level:** Analysis **Client Need:** Health Promotion and Maintenance **Integrated Process:** Nursing Process: Evaluation **Content Area:** Adult Health: Cardiovascular **Strategy:** The wording of the question tells you that the correct option also contains a true statement. Which client statement follows the treatment regime for Raynaud's disease? **Reference:** Lemone, P., & Burke, K. (2008). *Medical-surgical nursing: Critical thinking in client care* (4th ed.). Upper Saddle River, NJ: Pearson/Prentice Hall, pp. 1185–1186.

References

Adams, M., Josephson, D., & Holland, L. (2005). *Pharmacology for nurses: A pathophysiologic approach.* Upper Saddle River, NJ: Prentice Hall, pp. 260–283.

Black, J., & Hawks, J. (2005). *Medical surgical nursing: Clinical management for positive outcomes* (7th ed.). St. Louis, MO: Elsevier Science.

Guyton, A., & Hall, J. E. (2001). *Textbook of medical physiology* (10th ed.). Philadelphia, PA: W. B. Saunders.

Ignatavicius, D., & Workman, L. (2006). *Medical surgical nursing: Critical thinking for collaborative care* (5th ed.). Philadelphia, PA: W. B. Saunders.

JNC–7 Express: The Seventh Report of Joint National Committee on Prevention, Detection, Evaluation, and Treatment of High Blood Pressure. National High Blood Pressure Education Program, National Heart, Lung, & Blood Institute (2003). Retrieved from http://www.nhlbi.nih.gov

Kozier, B., Erb, G., Berman, A. J., & Snyder, S. (2007). *Fundamentals of nursing: Concepts, process, and practice* (8th ed.). Upper Saddle River, NJ: Prentice Hall.

LeMone, P., & Burke, K. M. (2008). *Medical surgical nursing: Critical thinking in client care* (4th ed.). Upper Saddle River, NJ: Prentice Hall.

ANSWERS & RATIONALES

Lewis, S., Heitkemper, M., & Dirksen, S. (2007). *Medical surgical nursing: Assessment and management of clinical problems* (7th ed.). St. Louis, MO: Elsevier Science.

McCance, K. L., & Huether, S. (2006). *Pathophysiology: The biologic basis for disease in adults and children* (5th ed.). St. Louis, MO: Mosby.

NHLBI, "Issues New Clinical Advisory on Systolic Blood Pressure." From: National Institutes of Health. May 4, 2000. (http://www. nhlbi.nih.gov/new/press/may04-00.htm)

NHLBI, "Stops part of study—High blood pressure drug performs no better than standard treatment." From: National Institutes of Health, Wednesday, March 8, 2000. (http://www. nhlbi.nih.gov/new/press/mar08-00.htm)

Porth, C.M. (2005). *Pathophysiology: Concepts of altered health states* (7th ed.). Philadelphia, PA: Lippincott Williams & Wilkins, pp. 496–498, 503–516, 522–524

Smith, S., Duell, D., & Martin, B. (2007). *Clinical nursing skills: Basic to advanced skills* (7th ed.). Upper Saddle River, NJ: Prentice Hall, p. 361.

Neurological Health Problems

4

Chapter Outline

Risk Factors Associated with Neurological Health Problems

Increased Intracranial Pressure (ICP)

Intracranial Hematomas

Cerebrovascular Accident (CVA)/Stroke

Spinal Cord Injuries

Encephalitis

Meningitis

Seizures

Guillain-Barré Syndrome

Myasthenia Gravis

Parkinson's Disease

Multiple Sclerosis (MS)

Amyotrophic Lateral Sclerosis (ALS)

Pain

Alzheimer's Disease

Objectives

➤ Define key terms associated with neurological health problems.

➤ Identify risk factors associated with the development of neurological health problems.

➤ Explain the common etiologies of neurological health problems.

➤ Describe the pathophysiological processes associated with specific neurological health problems.

➤ Distinguish between normal and abnormal neurological findings obtained from nursing assessment.

➤ Prioritize nursing interventions associated with specific neurological health problems.

➤ Describe the pathophysiology of pain.

➤ Prioritize nursing interventions used to treat pain.

NCLEX-RN® Test Prep

Use the CD-ROM enclosed with this book to access additional practice opportunities.

Review at a Glance

anterior cord syndrome complete paralysis below level of lesion; hyperaesthesia below level of lesion; hypalgesia below level of lesion; preservation of touch, position, pressure, and vibration

automatism automatic action or behavior without conscious knowledge; repetitive, semi-purposeful, patterned movement such as lip smacking

autonomic dysreflexia a life-threatening involuntary response of sympathetic nervous system to a noxious stimulus when there is injury above T6

Brown-Séquard's syndrome hemi-section of the spinal cord; ipsilateral motor loss below level of lesion; ipsilateral loss of position and vibration sense below level of lesion; contralateral loss of pain and temperature sensation below level of lesion

Brudzinski's sign flexion of neck causes neck pain and hip and knee to flex

bulbocavernous reflex contraction of bulbocavernosis muscle on percussing dorsum of penis

central cord syndrome greatest percentage of incomplete injuries; motor loss in upper extremities greater than loss in lower extremities; spasticity in lower extremities; variable degree of sensory loss; variable degree of bladder dysfunction

cogwheel rigidity manual manipulation of body parts may take on feel of a cogwheel

decerebrate extensor posturing indicating brainstem injury

decorticate flexor posturing indicating corticospinal tract lesions

diplopia double vision

equianalgesic chart shows pain relief obtained with different drugs, doses, and routes

hematomyelia hemorrhage within spinal cord

hydrocephalus brain substance expanded into a watery sac protruding through a cleft in cranium

Kernig's sign flexion of hip and knee and then extension of leg causes hamstring pain

lead-pipe rigidity cataleptic condition during which limbs remain in any position in which placed; smooth, stiff movement

Monro-Kellie hypothesis as volume of one brain component increases, volume of another decreases, to a limit

nuchal rigidity muscle contraction in nape of neck

neurogenic pulmonary edema an extremely rapid discharge of nerve impulses from a cerebral injury disrupting vascular permeability

paresthesia localized sensation of numbness, tingling, and heightened sensitivity

phantom pain sensation that pain exists in a removed part

spinal shock a neurophysiologic cessation of all or nearly all reflexes below level of injury

status epilepticus intense, repetitive seizures with very short periods of calm between them

PRETEST

1 Which of the following items would be a high priority for the nurse who is preparing the room for a client to be admitted with a new C7 level spinal cord injury?

1. Special kinetic bed
2. Halo brace device
3. Ventilator on stand-by
4. Catheterization tray

2 Upon return from the radiology department after a CT scan, a client with closed head injury is positioned on the side with the head of bed elevated 30 degrees and with a towel roll placed vertically under the pillow. The nurse explains to the client that this unique positioning facilitates:

1. Prevention of pulmonary embolism.
2. Venous drainage from the brain.
3. Airway management.
4. Intracranial pressure (ICP) readings.

3 After regaining consciousness, a male client reports a tremendous headache as he was taken by ambulance from the site of a motorcycle accident. The wife is unprepared when arriving at the hospital to find he had become comatose. The nurse explains the cause as which of the following?

1. Expanding epidural hematoma
2. Reticular activating system concussion
3. Diffuse axonal injury
4. Expanding pericardial hematoma

4 Following a grand mal seizure, the client is unconscious and unresponsive when the nurse tries to awaken the client. The nurse implements which of the following actions?

1. Calls the rapid response team
2. Notifies the physician
3. Administers the next dose of phenytoin (Dilantin) IV instead of by mouth
4. Allows gradual awakening

5 The nurse assesses the client's understanding of discharge needs and goals after experiencing a cerebrovascular accident (CVA). Which client statement indicates further information and teaching will be necessary? Select all that apply.

1. "I'm getting a lifetime supply of adult disposable briefs."
2. "I will never have another stroke."
3. "I've got to find a walking buddy."
4. "I'm getting a rail installed in my tub."
5. "I'll be glad to get home and have a cigarette."

6 When developing a plan of care for a client newly hospitalized with meningitis, the nurse determines that which of the following areas should be the major focus of nursing care?

1. Enhancing coping skills
2. Providing cognitive stimulation
3. Assessing risk for injury and preventing complications
4. Increasing cardiac output

7 The client comes to the Emergency Department with weakness that has been progressing upward in both legs for two days. The nurse, suspecting Guillain-Barré syndrome, begins care by doing which of the following? Select all that apply.

1. Taking medical history, noting recent viral influenza
2. Giving the client orange juice for fatigue and low blood glucose
3. Assessing neurological and respiratory function
4. Evaluating for petit mal seizures
5. Assessing vital signs

8 Which of the following items would be of priority for the nurse to include in a teaching plan for a client with myasthenia gravis?

1. Exercise to increase peripheral circulation
2. Plan important activities for late afternoon
3. Identify signs of and action during crisis
4. Eat three well-balanced meals a day

9 The client with Parkinson's disease tells the nurse that the resting tremor present in the right hand is very frustrating. The nurse advises the client to do which of the following?

1. Practice deep-breathing for relaxation
2. Take a warm bath to aid microcirculation to the extremities
3. Hold an object in that hand to control hand movements
4. Take diazepam (Valium) as needed for relaxation of muscles

10 On the first postoperative day after abdominal surgery, a male client rates his pain as 9 on a scale of 0 (no pain) to 10 (worst pain). He is laughing and talking with visitors at this time. In reviewing the client's orders and plan of care, the nurse notes that the client has defined a pain level of 5 as his comfort level goal and he has an order for analgesics every three hours. His last dose was three hours ago with no untoward effects. The nurse should do which of the following at this time? Select all that apply.

1. Record his pain level at 5
2. Administer a dose of the analgesic
3. Telephone the physician for an order for patient-controlled analgesia
4. Reassess the pain 30 minutes after analgesic is administered
5. Ask client if he can wait a while longer for medication since his behavior does not reflect acute pain

➤ *See pages 150–152 for Answers & Rationales.*

I. RISK FACTORS ASSOCIATED WITH NEUROLOGICAL HEALTH PROBLEMS

A. **Increased intracranial pressure:** stroke, tumor, head trauma, inflammation, and neurological conditions such as meningitis

B. **Intracranial hematomas:** males (adolescent to young adulthood), injury, radiation, jobs or incidents where electrocution is a possibility, outside employment where weather can be severe or falls are a high probability

C. **Stroke:** diseases (hypertension [HTN], sickle cell anemia, polycythemia, atherosclerosis, cardiac valvular disease, diabetes), valve and organ replacement, anticoagulant therapy, atrial fibrillation, cardioversion, oral contraceptives, drug abuse, smoking, high salt or alcohol intake, sedentary lifestyle

D. **Spinal cord injury:** athletes, drug and/or alcohol abuse, employment where falls are a high probability, diseases such as tumors, syringomyelia, degenerative diseases

E. **Encephalitis:** populations living with an abundance of mosquitoes, especially if cattle and horses are nearby; individuals drinking goat's milk; exposure to ticks; metal poisonings; recent immunizations and illnesses such as German measles or chickenpox

F. **Meningitis:** impaired immune function as in very old or very young clients or those with human immunodeficiency virus (HIV) or on chemotherapy, those with otitis media, sinusitis, basal skull fracture, neurosurgery, systemic sepsis, or crowded living conditions (college dorms, military institutions, and prisons)

G. **Seizures:** brain tumors, family history, head injury, or neurological disorders

H. **Guillain-Barré Syndrome:** viral infections, recent immunizations

I. **Myasthenia gravis (MG):** family or previous history of autoimmune diseases

J. **Parkinson's disease (proposed theories only):** cerebral anoxia, advancing age, genetic factors, and factors toxic to dopaminergic cells

K. **Multiple sclerosis (MS):** individuals living in colder climates; genetic or family history of MS or autoimmune illnesses; age

L. **Amyotrophic lateral sclerosis (ALS):** possibly genetics

M. **Pain:** work requiring strenuous lifting or bending, individuals with poor posture, stage of life factors, chronic diseases, arterial or ischemic wounds

N. **Alzheimer's disease:** aging, head trauma, family history, trauma, presence of risk gene (APO–E4)

II. INCREASED INTRACRANIAL PRESSURE (ICP)

A. **Overview**

1. Defined as a rise in pressure of cerebrospinal fluid (CSF) that maintains subarachnoid space between skull and brain; nondistendable bone and meninges surround brain; a balance among volumes of content (brain 80%, blood 10%, CSF 10%) of cranial vault usually exists

2. Increased ICP is an ICP greater than 15 mmHg

3. A significant increase is termed intracranial hypertension

4. Causes:

   a. Increases in tissue volume

      1) Neoplasm

      2) Cerebral edema: interstitial; vasogenic seen in tumor, trauma; cytotoxic in hypoxic-ischemic injury; infarction; and infection or other disease state

    b. Abscess

    c. Increases in blood volume: hemorrhage and hematoma formation, increased arterial inflow, and decreased venous return

    d. Increases in CSF volume

        1) Obstruction of CSF pathways produces **hydrocephalus** (brain substance expanded into a watery sac)

        2) Deficient CSF absorption: usually caused by blockage of arachnoid villi or idiopathic as in normal pressure hydrocephalus (post-bleed)

        3) Overproduction of CSF

    e. Other causes: congenital or developmental, metabolic, or pseudotumor cerebri (benign intracranial hypertension)

B. Pathophysiology

    1. Monro-Kellie hypothesis: as volume of one component (brain tissue, blood, CSF) increases, volume of another decreases, to a limit

        a. Controlled by autoregulation: cerebral arterioles change diameter to maintain blood flow when ICP increases

        b. Brain tissue unable to compensate (decrease volume)

    2. Maximal compensation occurs after volume increases; ICP begins to increase

    3. ICP values

        a. ICP value alone is not a reliable measure of brain's compliance: ICP may be in normal range (< 15 mmHg); but client is still in danger of herniation because of poor compliance

        b. Changes in ICP in response to stimuli may be predictive of compliance; decreased compliance indicated by: sustained increases in ICP in response to stimuli; large increases in response to non-noxious stimuli

    4. Physiology

        a. Cerebral blood flow (CBF): normally 750 mL/min

        1) Hypercarbia: $PaCO_2$ greater than 45 mmHg produces vasodilation; increases ICP by increasing volume

        2) Hypocarbia: $PaCO_2$ less than 25 mmHg produces rebound cerebral vasodilation, loss of autoregulation

        b. Cerebral perfusion pressure (CPP)

        1) Normal CPP ranges from 60 to 100 mmHg; determines CBF

        2) Hyperperfusion and increased ICP occur with CPP greater than 100 mmHg

        3) Hypoperfusion and cerebral ischemia: with CPP 40 to 60 mmHg

        4) Irreversible ischemia and infarction: with CPP less than 40 mmHg

        5) Brain death: with CPP 0–40 mm Hg

    5. Compensatory mechanisms

        a. Activated when increase in ICP occurs to balance volumes within cranial vault to protect brain

        b. Dependent upon rate of expansion of brain volume

        c. Rapidly increasing volume prevents activation of compensatory mechanisms

        d. Compensatory mechanisms involve CSF changes

        1) Normal shunting of CSF into spinal subarachnoid space to reduce pressure (most common)

2) Increased absorption of CSF

3) Decreased secretion of CSF

e. Venous blood may also be shunted to allow more room for expansion

6. Failure of compensatory mechanisms causes ischemia, hypoxia, herniation, and brain death

a. As ICP approaches systemic arterial pressure, CPP and CBF decrease

b. When ICP equals systemic arterial pressure, CBF ceases and brain death ensues

c. Elevated range

1) Moderate: 20 to 40 mmHg

2) Severe: greater than 40 mmHg

3) Effect of elevation on circulation determined by CPP with mean arterial pressure (MAP) a primary influence; MAP is the average pressure in arteries during a cardiac cycle (influenced by elasticity of arterial walls and mean volume of arterial blood)

7. Signs and symptoms

a. Gastrointestinal: ulceration and bleeding

b. Cardiovascular: elevation or depression of S-T segments; large positive or negative U waves; prolonged Q-T or Q-U intervals; Q waves in both standard and precordial leads; deeply inverted or tall spiky upright T waves; dysrhythmias

c. Cushing's triad/response

1) A response involving three classic signs: widening pulse pressure, elevated systolic pressure, and bradycardia; respirations may become irregular

2) The brainstem reflects the final effort to maintain cerebral perfusion

3) Caused by rapidly expanding lesions such as epidural hematoma or lesion in posterior fossa

4) Seen when ICP is greater than 45 mmHg or when ICP approaches systemic diastolic BP

5) Pressure on brainstem causes ischemia of vasomotor center of medulla

6) Systolic BP increases while diastolic remains the same causing widened pulse pressure

7) Increased BP: sensed in baroreceptors of carotid arteries and aortic arch; causes vagal response of bradycardia

d. **Neurogenic pulmonary edema** is an extremely rapid discharge of nerve impulses from an injured brain disrupting vascular permeability

e. Intracranial effects

1) Increase in ICP decreases microvascular CBF leading to tissue hypoxia and causing respiratory center dysfunction

2) Hypoventilation develops causing increased $PaCO_2$ and decreased blood pH

3) Hypercarbia causes cerebral vessel vasodilation and edema

4) ICP increases resulting in herniation, cerebral ischemia, and brain death

8. Herniation syndromes occur, which are displacement of a portion of brain through or around linings of brain or openings within the intracranial cavity

a. Mechanism is categorized as supratentorial, infratentorial, or extracranial

1) Caused by increased pressure in one or all compartments; usually occurs when a pressure difference exists between supratentorial and infratentorial (posterior fossa) compartments

2) Supratentorial herniation syndromes: herniation of structures normally lying above tentorium cerebelli; include cingulated herniation; uncal herniation; and transtentorial or central herniation

3) Infratentorial herniation syndrome: herniation of structures lying below tentorium cerebelli; include upward transtentorial herniation and downward cerebellar or tonsillar herniation

4) Extracranial herniation syndrome: occurs when opening in skull allows intracranial contents under pressure to herniate outward; may occur through open wound, surgical incision, ICP monitor site or through fractures of ear or nose; resulting decrease in volume lowers ICP and possibly prevents intracranial herniation

b. Results: compression, laceration, distortion, or necrosis of brain structures; vascular compromise; blocked flow of CSF; brain compression and death

C. Nursing assessment of increased ICP

1. Assessment

a. Airway patency and breathing patterns: central nervous system dysfunction is associated with decreased level of consciousness (LOC), hypercapnia, and potential for pulmonary edema

b. Pupillary dysfunction (early sign): compression of oculomotor nerve (CN III) results in dilation of ipsilateral pupil, sluggish or no response to light, inability to move eye upward, and ptosis (drooping) of eyelid; note that a nonreactive, dilated pupil is a late sign and a neurological emergency heralding transtentorial brain herniation

c. Changes in vital signs (late sign): Cushing's triad of increased systolic pressure, bradycardia, and an irregular respiratory pattern is seen with sustained and elevated ICP; fever is possible as compensatory measures fail

d. Visual abnormalities: decreased or blurred vision or extraocular movements

e. Papilledema: swelling of optic disc, as seen with an ophthalmoscope; indicative of long-standing increased ICP

f. Motor function: contralateral hemiparesis or hemiplegia may be seen; no movement or flaccidity is the least favorable sign; localization to a painful stimulus may result in an effort to produce movement

1) Decorticate: flexor posturing indicating corticospinal tract lesions (see Figure 4-1A)

2) Decerebrate: extensor posturing indicating brainstem injury (see Figure 4-1B)

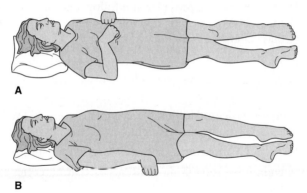

Figure 4-1

Abnormal posturing seen in head injuries: A. Decorticate; B. Decerebrate.

A

B

    g. Headache: unusual, seen with slowly increasing ICP, worse with straining and position changes, especially on awakening

    h. Emesis: projectile vomiting without nausea

  2. Diagnostic tests: arterial blood gases (ABGs), complete blood count (CBC), CSF cultures, CT scan, serum osmolality

D. Nursing management

  1. Medications include: stool softeners, diuretics (osmotics, loop), corticosteroids: dexamethasone (Decadron), antipyretics: acetaminophen (Tylenol), H_2 receptor antagonists, antiepileptics if seizures occur

  2. Secure airway patency and clearance

    a. Hyperventilate and oxygenate with 100% O_2 using sigh mode on ventilator prior to suctioning; avoid suctioning for longer than 10 seconds

    b. Auscultate lungs and clear any secretions

    c. Position client side to side to decrease aspiration risk in case of emesis

    d. Promote normal breathing pattern: monitor arterial carbon dioxide pressure ($PaCO_2$) to stay within 25 to 30 mmHg, avoiding cerebral vasodilation

  3. Optimize cerebral perfusion

    a. Monitor signs and symptoms of pulmonary edema including: increasing restlessness, anxiety, dyspnea, weak and rapid pulse, and blood-tinged, frothy fluid

    b. Position client to avoid extreme rotation or flexion of neck resulting in raising jugular venous pressure and ICP; a neutral or midline position aids cerebral venous drainage

    c. Avoid or greatly reduce extreme hip flexion causing an increase in intra-abdominal and intrathoracic pressure, producing increased ICP

    d. Provide high-fiber diet to decrease use of Valsalva maneuver; assist with bowel movements using bedpan

    e. Avoid physiological and environmental stimuli

    f. Monitor nursing care to keep ICP below 25 mmHg and to promote return to baseline levels within five minutes

  4. Monitor for symptoms prior to herniation

    a. Report and treat per protocol signs of acutely increasing ICP: decreasing Glasgow Coma Scale (GCS) score, behavioral changes, disorientation, difficulty in following simple commands, speech changes, less purposeful response to painful stimuli, posturing movements, loss of or abnormal (i.e., positive Babinski) reflexes

    b. Notify health care provider and follow unit protocol for pupil and eye changes: blurred vision, **diplopia** (double vision), extraocular movement (EOM) abnormalities, and nystagmus

  5. Prevent infection

    a. Adhere to written protocols for care of client with an intracranial pressure monitoring device

    b. Monitor indicators of infection: white blood cell (WBC) counts, positive cultures, fever, chills, nuchal rigidity and changes in vital signs

    c. Inspect ICP monitoring site and connections for leaking CSF or drainage

  6. Avoid administration of medications such as narcotics that can mimic signs of increased ICP

7. Support family: encourage family to visit client; provide information to optimize decision making when clients are unable to make treatment choices; anticipate grieving and identify sources of community support

III. INTRACRANIAL HEMATOMAS

A. Overview

1. Defined as a break in a blood vessel within cranium or skull that leads to swelling caused by hemorrhage
2. Peak occurrence during evening and night hours on weekends
3. Pathological mechanisms
   a. Direct impact
      1) Acceleration: rapidly moving object strikes relatively stationary head
      2) Deceleration: coming to a sudden, abrupt stop, as when head strikes an immobile object/static surface (more severe damage because of effects on brain stem)
      3) Rotation: lateral blow rotates brain, contusing brain stem and disrupting white matter
   b. Indirect stresses: trauma not to head but involves brain; rotational displacement of head on extreme motion of neck causes shear, tensile strains and compressive forces transmitted to brain; landing on buttocks or feet from a height transmits force through spinal column to base of brain
   c. Systemic: chronic alcoholism, cerebral atrophy, anticoagulants, long history of hypertension
4. Mechanisms of injury: blunt (closed, non-penetrating); penetrating (open); and compression: skull compressed between two forces causing a crush effect on brain
5. Types of injury
   a. Scalp injuries
   b. Skull fractures
   c. Dural integrity injury
      1) Open: dura torn by laceration; compound, depressed fractures, penetrating objects
      2) Closed: dural continuity maintained; simple, linear fracture may be present
6. Intracranial hemorrhage classified as epidural, subdural, or intracerebral
7. Common causes: vehicular accidents (automobiles, motorcycles), falls, violence, sports-related injuries, ingestion of alcohol and/or drugs, other (intrauterine and birth injury, radiation, electrocution, heat stroke, lightning)

B. Pathophysiology

1. *Epidural* hematoma: cerebral artery bleed above dura mater; usually in middle fossa caused by laceration of middle meningeal artery; constitute 2 to 6% of head injuries
   a. Signs of brain stem compression usually occur within 24 hours
   b. Signs and symptoms
      1) Short period of unconsciousness followed by a lucid interval
      2) Lucid interval followed by progressive depression of consciousness
      3) Focal signs: ipsilateral pupil dilation, weakness of contralateral extremities

2. *Subdural* hematoma: bleeding into subdural space of brain with disruption of cortical veins; most often over parietal areas; 29% of head injuries

   a. Acute: symptomatic within 24 to 72 hours

      1) Majority of clients deteriorate quickly, become deeply comatose, with brain unable to compensate from rapid compression; often associated with severe brain trauma and high mortality; may mimic epidural hematoma

      2) Signs and symptoms include depressed LOC, usually from time of injury; ipsilateral pupil dilation and contralateral weakness

   b. Subacute: symptomatic within 2 to 10 days

      1) Better prognosis than acute, still 25 to 35% mortality

      2) Signs and symptoms include headaches; decreased LOC and focal signs of compression; failure to show improvement

   c. Chronic: symptomatic occurring after 10 days (elusive, nonspecific, and fluctuating)

      1) Gradual clot formation allows brain time to accommodate; traumatic etiology may be unclear, minor, forgotten; prognosis good (mortality rates 10%); may reaccumulate

      2) Signs and symptoms include slowly progressive change in behavior (apathy) or personality, headaches; variable LOC; lethargy, confusion, motor weakness with loss of upward gaze, dysphasia, urinary or bowel incontinence

3. *Intracerebral* hematoma: bleeding from small arteries or veins in subcortical white matter

   a. Lucid interval followed by decreased LOC

   b. Focal signs based on location

   c. Signs and symptoms include possible headache, hemiplegia, ipsilateral pupil dilation, progressing ICP with potential for herniation; petechiae common, usually seen with contusion, edema; majority occur in frontal and temporal lobes; signs and symptoms according to location

4. Subarachnoid hemorrhage

   a. Bleeding between pia mater of covering of brain and spinal cord and arachnoid membrane

   b. Signs and symptoms include severe headache and restlessness; **nuchal rigidity** (muscle contraction to nape of neck), fever, and a positive **Kernig's sign** (flexion of hip and knee and then extension of leg causes hamstring pain), (see Figure 4-2); positive **Brudzinski's sign** (flexion of neck causes flexion at hip;

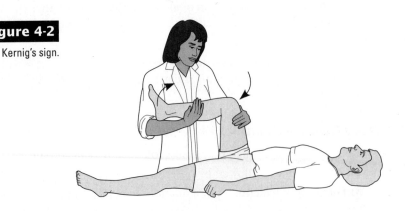

Figure 4-2

Kernig's sign.

Figure 4-3

Brudzinski's sign.

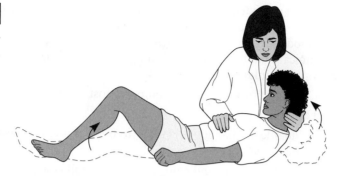

see Figure 4-3); positive Babinski sign (dorsiflexion of great toe upon stimulating sole of feet)

C. Nursing assessment

1. Assessment

   a. Airway and breathing pattern

   b. Assess vital signs (VS), LOC, pupils, and motor responses; document baseline and monitor for subtle, sudden changes

   c. Observe for clinical indications of expanding lesions

      1) Localized/focal signs: hemiplegia, visual field defect, eye deviation, cerebellar signs, cranial nerve signs

      2) Generalized signs of increased ICP: headache, restlessness, irritability

   d. Gather data about traumatic event from family, witnesses including: details and time of injury; change in consciousness (lucid period, duration of unresponsiveness); and seizure activity

   e. Assess signs and symptoms of increased ICP, which may occur suddenly, resulting in tentorial herniation and sudden respiratory arrest

2. Diagnostic tests: CT scan, MRI, ABGs, CBC

D. Nursing management

1. Surgical intervention is the recommended treatment; no specific medications are recommended

2. Maintain adequate airway and cerebral perfusion: monitor respiratory pattern, breath sounds, cyanosis, restlessness, and use of accessory muscles; monitor ICP readings; prepare for O_2 administration, intubation or tracheostomy; prepare for possible cranial surgery if unable to maintain perfusion

3. Advocate for client rest periods between frequent VS and neurological assessments

4. Provide seizure precautions because of risk for seizures secondary to increased ICP (when dura interrupted)

5. Support client and family in understanding assessment and management issues

IV. CEREBROVASCULAR ACCIDENT (CVA)/STROKE

A. Overview

1. Defined as an abrupt loss of consciousness with resulting paralysis that may be temporary or permanent

2. Often preceded by transient ischemic attacks (TIAs), which mimic a stroke without permanent paralysis; cause is a temporary interference in cerebral blood flow causing neurological dysfunction from focal or retinal ischemia with clinical symptoms typically lasting less than one hour and without evidence of an acute infarction

3. Causes of stroke include thrombus (most common), embolus, and hemorrhage

B. Pathophysiology

1. Cellular level changes begin four to five minutes after blood flow and oxygenation of neurons are reduced

2. The sodium pump and neurotransmitters fail as a result of anaerobic glycolysis, resulting in cerebral edema as sodium (Na^+) draws water into brain

3. Cerebral blood vessel walls swell, circulation is compromised, and vasospasm combined with blood viscosity reduces cerebral perfusion

4. Outcomes of decreased cerebral perfusion: cerebral anoxia caused by interruption of blood supply to brain; cerebral infarction if anoxia lasts longer than 10 minutes, which results in irreversible changes; cerebral edema causing secondary damage; contralateral deficits when stroke is in cerebral hemisphere; permanent deficit reflecting locality of stroke

5. Signs and symptoms include altered consciousness or unconsciousness, stertorous breathing, unequal pupils (larger pupil noted on same side as stroke), paralysis of one side, perspiration, aphasia (abnormal or absent speech), blank stare, dysphagia, inability to make decisions, loss of memory, and gait instability

C. Nursing assessment

1. Assessment
   a. Nursing history: interview client and family; history of risk factors; client and family's understanding of illness
   b. Assessment: airway obstruction and hypoxia if decreased LOC; neurological deficits; vital sign stability; urine output; fluid and caloric needs; visual impairment (corneal abrasions, eye discomfort, diplopia); loss of sensation and functional ability of mouth, face and swallowing ability; bowel and bladder function; immobility issues; communication; perceptual deficits; psychosocial needs; and understanding of therapeutic regimen

2. Diagnostic tests: electrolytes, CT scan, MRI, ABGs, arteriography, ultrasound of carotid arteries, lumbar puncture, coagulation studies such as prothrombin time (PT), partial thromboplastin time (PTT), international normalized ratio (INR)

D. Nursing management

1. Medications include stool softeners, anticoagulants or thrombolytics, antiplatelet agents, calcium channel blockers, diuretics (if increased ICP exists), antiepileptics if seizures occur; monitor effects of drugs

2. Monitor neurological status
   a. Hyperthermia: maintain temperature within normal limits
   b. Neglect syndrome: provide care around perceptual deficits
   c. Seizures: promote safety and cerebral perfusion
   d. Agnosia: support recognition of previously known subject
   e. Communication deficits: consult with speech therapist, use communication board
   f. Visual: provide care with recognition of hemianopia, diplopia, or decreased acuity; placing a patch over one eye reduces double vision

    g. Cognitive changes: create plan of care with health care team to address memory loss, poor attention span, distractibility, judgment, problem solving difficulty, and disorientation

    h. Behavioral changes: educate family as to causes and approaches to use with labiality, loss of inhibitions, fear, anger, and depression

    i. Increased ICP: monitor closely for any changes in LOC

3. Respiratory status

    a. Brainstem damage: test for decerebrate posturing as a response to noxious stimuli as one indicator of brainstem involvement

    b. Airway obstruction: suction per assessment, after oxygenating and with goal of preventing increased ICP; monitor ABGs

    c. Poor cough and gag reflexes: intermittent positive pressure breathing (IPPB) therapy and position client on side to decrease risk of aspirating own secretions

    d. Pulmonary emboli: mobilize client as soon as tolerated; administer anticoagulant therapy, monitoring appropriate lab values

4. Monitor gastrointestinal system

    a. Dysphagia (difficulty swallowing): provide swallow evaluation before instituting feeding

    b. Constipation: provide stool softeners and bowel routine

    c. Stool impaction: encourage roughage, high fiber, and mobility to prevent impaction; increase fluid intake; remove any fecal impaction and document

5. Monitor genitourinary system

    a. Incontinence: evaluate behavioral, pharmacological, and supportive devices to create a plan with client for long-term maintenance but discourage dependency on adult disposable briefs early in stroke

    b. Urgency: offer bedpan, urinal, or commode use every two hours; avoid caffeine

    c. Retention: avoid in-dwelling urinary catheters because of risk for infection; develop intermittent catheterization schedule; use bladder scan device or straight catheterization to detect post-void residuals

    d. Renal calculi: keep urine dilute (at least 2000 mL per day), prevent urinary stasis and infection; teach clients a prevention diet that is low in oxalate-rich foods and purines; monitor fluid and nutritional status

6. Monitor musculoskeletal system

    a. Hemiplegia: apply pneumatic compression device or elastic hose to reduce deep vein thrombosis; instruct family on range of motion (ROM) exercises of joints from shoulder to ankle; initiate physical therapy for gait training

    b. Contractures: create positioning schedule of two hours on unaffected side, 30 minutes on affected side, 30 minutes prone, indicating schedule in charting; use high top tennis shoes or therapeutic boots to prevent foot drop

    c. Atrophy: begin ROM exercises early, combined with stretching at least 4 times a day, instructing family as able

    d. Dysarthria (difficulty and defective speech caused by impairment of tongue or other muscles essential to speech): use communication board, avoid frustration; keep communication simple; consult with speech pathology for motor relearning plan

    e. Osteoporosis: facilitate weight-bearing activity, screen for progression of condition

    f. Sensory deprivation: create plan to optimize balance in sensory stimulation; provide appropriate repetition for learning

    g. Self-image: provide positive feedback; encourage grooming and street attire; begin rehabilitation as soon as tolerated

    h. Sexual dysfunction: encourage open communication among partners; inform client/partner of options; introduce topic before discharge from acute care

7. Monitor safety: explore what life will be like in home setting with new deficits; provide safety assessment for home setting, identifying areas to modify based on fall risk; create plan with client and family to optimize return to community, identify support services, and recognize warning signs of another stroke event

▶ **Practice to Pass**

A client who had a stroke is preparing for transfer to a rehabilitation setting. What would support the client and family's transition?

V. SPINAL CORD INJURIES

A. Overview

1. Defined as a fracture or injury (twisting, compression, pulling) of bones of spinal column; damage may involve part of or all of spinal cord

2. Incidence is more prominent in young males (18 to 30); is increasing in young females; increases with use of alcohol and/or drugs

3. Types of injury

    a. Level of injury: cervical (most common site); thoracic (least common site); and lumbar

    b. Upper and lower motor neuron damage (see Table 4-1)

        1) Upper motor neurons (UMN) drive voluntary movement; UMNs originate in cerebral cortex and end at anterior horn cell of cord resulting in spastic paralysis and reflexes

        2) Lower motor neuron (LMN) begins at anterior horn cell; LMNs become part of peripheral nerve to muscle, motor side of reflex arc; usually present in cauda equina injuries; areflexia results in flaccid paralysis; these neurons are responsible for innervation and contraction of skeletal muscles

4. Mechanism of injury: hyperextension (usually with rotation), hyperflexion (usually with rotation), vertical compression (axial loading), cord contusion without vertebral disruption (fracture, dislocation), and penetrating wounds

5. Types of vertebral injury

    a. Fractures: spinous, lateral and/or articular processes, body, pedicles

        1) Odontoid fractures: Types I, II, III

        2) Hangman's fracture: bilateral arches of axis, with or without dislocation of axis on C3

        3) Jefferson: burst fracture of atlas

        4) Occiput-atlanto dislocation

    b. Dislocation: unilateral or bilateral facets, vertebral body

    c. Subluxation: facets

    d. Compression: burst or wedge fractures

    e. Fracture: dislocation

6. Common causes: motor vehicle crashes; falls and falling objects; athletics (diving, football, skiing, boating); penetrating wounds: gunshot, stabbing

Table 4-1	Degrees of Motor and Sensory Loss in Spinal Cord Injury
Level of Lesion	**Degree of Motor and/or Sensory Loss**
Central cord syndrome, greatest percentage of incomplete injuries	Motor loss in upper extremities greater than loss in lower extremities; spasticity of lower extremities Variable degree of sensory loss Variable degree of bladder dysfunction Associated with hyperextension injuries of cervical spine, especially in osteoarthritis of spine
Anterior cord syndrome, associated with flexion injuries of cervical spine	Complete paralysis below level of lesion Hyperesthesia below level of lesion Hypalgesia below level of lesion Preservation of touch, position, pressure, and vibration **Paresthesia** (localized sensation of numbness, tingling, and heightened sensitivity) may be present
Brown-Séquard's syndrome, (hemi-section of the cord) associated with open penetrating wounds to the cord	Ipsilateral motor loss below level of lesion Ipsilateral loss of position and vibration sense below level of lesion Contralateral loss of pain and temperature senses below level of lesion
Posterior cord syndrome (rare)	Loss of light touch and proprioception below level of lesion Motor function of extremities, pain, and temperature remain intact Associated with cervical hyperextension
Sacral sparing	Preservation of sensation in genitals and saddle area (S_3–S_5) Can occur in presence of profound motor and sensory loss Characteristic of central and anterior cord syndromes
Cauda equina lesions	Sparing of function unpredictable: unilateral or bilateral, motor, sensory, or both Indirect trauma to peripheral nerves associated with fractures Potential for regrowth and recovery

B. Pathophysiology

1. Influencing factors
   a. Spinal cord is located in a relatively small space
   b. Peculiarities of spine: canal space varies
      1) Wider in children: fewer children with traumatic cervical injuries become quadriplegic; wide canal allows cord more space to move without compression
      2) Narrower with congenital anomalies, cervical spondylosis, age, osteoarthritic changes
   c. Variability of vascular supply
   d. Presence of osteophytes
2. Mechanisms
   a. Concussion: pressure waves propagated through cord, resulting in transient loss of function with immediate flaccid paralysis and complete recovery in minutes to hours
   b. Compression: bone, ligaments, extruded disc material and hematoma
   c. Contusion: results in edema, petechial hemorrhages, neuronal changes, inflammation
   d. **Hematomyelia:** hemorrhage within cord
   e. Transection: actual (rare) or functional

       f. Overstretching: causing disruption of tissue

       g. Edema: produces further impairment of capillary circulation and venous return

       h. Ischemia: interruption of blood flow of anterior or posterior arterial system by compression

   3. Necrosis of spinal cord substance

       a. Vascular pathology: ischemia is implicated as causing reduction or interruption of blood supply, leading to necrosis

         1) Injury to spinal cord causes increase in permeability of blood vessels which leads to edema formation, causing a decrease in blood flow to area

         2) Further ischemia leads to necrosis with vascular stasis, causing thrombosis, which leads to further decrease in blood flow and the vicious cycle continues, leading eventually to traumatic hemorrhagic necrosis of gray matter (within 4 to 48 hours)

       b. Neuronal pathology

         1) Injury alters electrophysiology of affected neurons, causing sodium leakage into cells, creating a negative resting potential

         2) This results in spinal shock stage, where there is a neurophysiologic cessation of all or nearly all reflexes below level of injury

       c. Biochemical pathology

         1) Accumulated vasoactive amines (norepinephrine, serotonin, dopamine, histamine) are released or transported to wounded tissue after injury

         2) Induces maximal toxic vasospasm, impedes microcirculation, diminishes local oxygenation, and produces necrosis of vessels and neurons

       d. Disintegration of myelin sheath and axis cylinder

       e. Spinal cord may liquefy in severe disruption

   4. Hematomyelia and edema of the cord may ascend above level of initial injury; syringomyelia (progressive, chronic spinal cord disease) may develop as a result

   5. Degree of functional impairment of spinal cord

       a. Complete: total sensory/motor loss and autonomic disruption below level of lesion, reflecting irreversible spinal cord damage

         1) Tetraplegia or quadriplegia: occurs in cervical region; loss of leg function with variable loss of arm function depending on level of injury

         2) Paraplegia: occurs in thoracic region and lumbar 1 and 2 region; loss of leg function

       b. Incomplete and variable degrees of motor and/or sensory loss below level of lesion, reflecting sparing of certain tracts

   6. Horner's syndrome

       a. Incomplete cord transection involving cervical sympathetic nerves

       b. Ipsilateral ptosis of eyelid, constricted pupil, and lack of facial sweating (anhidrosis)

   7. Spinal cord segmental level: functional loss depends on degree of spinal cord damage, may not correspond to vertebral level, particularly in thoracolumbar and sacral level (see Table 4-2)

   8. **Spinal shock:** loss of all reflex activity below level of injury

       a. Duration: two days to several months

       b. Associated with hypotension and bradycardia

Table 4-2		Functional Loss According to Spinal Cord Segmental Level
Spinal Column	**Vertebrae**	**Functional Loss**
Cervical	C 1–2	Total tetraplegia and respiratory paralysis
	C 3–4	Total tetraplegia, weak diaphragm, absent intercostals
	C 5–6	Tetraplegia with gross arm movements; diaphragm may be impaired initially
	C 6–7	Tetraplegia with biceps and deltoid function; no triceps
	C 7–8	Tetraplegia with triceps function; no intrinsic hand function
Thoracic	T 1–5	Paraplegia often with diaphragmatic breathing; arm function intact; loss of leg function, bladder, bowels; sensation present down to nipple line
	T 6–12	Paraplegia with no abdominal reflexes present at T12; usually spastic paralysis of lower limbs; at level of T12, sensation is present down to groin area
Below T12	Conus medullaris	Bowel and bladder sphincter dysfunction; may have lower leg weakness; sacral dermatome hyperaesthesia or anesthesia, back pain
	Cauda equina	Asymmetric, atrophic, areflexic paralysis (lower motor neuron); sensory root loss; outer aspect legs, ankles, posterior lower limbs, and saddle area; sphincter dysfunction
Sacral	S 1–5	Loss of bladder, bowel, sex function; some foot displacement may be present; no paralysis of leg muscle from S3 to S5; loss of sensation involves saddle area, scrotum, perineum, penis, anal area, and upper third of posterior aspect of thigh

    c. Bulbocavernous reflex (contraction of bulbocavernous muscle on percussing dorsum of penis) is an early sign of resolving spinal shock: absence of this spinal reflex arc implies there is no physiological continuity between lower spinal cord and supraspinal centers

    d. Appearance of involuntary spastic movement and positive deep tendon reflexes below level of injury indicate spinal shock has resolved

  9. Degree of functional loss: depends on level and amount of damage to spinal cord; myelopathy refers to cord damage; radiculopathy refers to dysfunction of nerve roots; may have some sparing or eventual return, as part of the peripheral nervous system

  10. Early intervention (within first few hours after injury) reduces or minimizes cellular damage leading to better prognosis for function

  11. Prognosis for degree of bladder, bowel, and sexual function varies with level of lesion: related to upper or lower motor neuron lesion; if sacral nerve roots are damaged, prognosis for any reflex activity of these functions is very poor

  12. Late stage: spinal cord may become fibrotic, and pathological changes may extend above and below damaged segment

  13. Signs and symptoms include hypotension, loss of motor control and sensation below level of injury, decreased or absent reflexes, urinary retention, stool and urinary incontinence, neurogenic bladder, impotence, muscle spasms, muscle atrophy, paraplegia, tetraplegia, decreased chest expansion, decreased cough reflex, hypercalcemia, cardiac dysrhythmias, pain (note: manifestations will depend on level of injury)

  14. Complications from a spinal cord injury: stress ulcers, paralytic ileus, pressure ulcers, stool impaction, decreased venous return, pathologic fractures caused by bone demineralization and joint contractions

C. Nursing assessment

1. Assessment

   a. Emergency assessment at scene or in emergency department

      1) Suspect cervical spine injury until proven otherwise; all head injuries are also considered spinal cord injuries until ruled out by diagnostic methods, such as C-spine X-rays

      2) Maintain airway (using chin lift/jaw thrust method), breathing, and circulation

      3) Maintain neck in neutral position, palpate cervical spine region

      4) Assess movement and sensation in extremities: if *conscious,* ask client to move toes, feet, legs, fingers, hands, arms; ask if client can feel touch on toes, feet, legs, fingers, hands, arms; test for reflex withdrawal; if *unconscious,* observe any spontaneous movements by client; use stimuli to elicit more purposeful voluntary movements or reflex withdrawal

   b. Physical examination

      1) Precise level of motor and sensory findings include sacral sparing, voluntary toe flexion

      2) Presence/absence of all deep tendon and superficial reflexes

      3) Tenderness or gaps between spinous processes

      4) Deformities, swelling, limitation of movement particularly in neck

      5) Evidence of other trauma: head, chest, abdomen, extremities

   c. Establish early, accurate baseline: motor and sensory function of all extremities; breathing pattern; presence of sweating; subjective reports of pain; bladder function, distention, voiding reflex; presence of bowel sounds, anal reflex; vital signs; neuro exam, including cognition level; and sexuality

   d. Assess abdomen for distention; ileus is common

   e. Assess for trauma to other systems; note lacerations, abrasions, etc.

   f. Collect pertinent data to assist in formulation of care plan: previous health problems, allergies; health programs (include medications, treatments); and psychosocial data (include previous hospital experience)

   g. Assess for **autonomic dysreflexia** (a life-threatening involuntary sympathetic response of central nervous system to a noxious stimuli) with injury above T6

      1) Occurs after spinal shock is resolved

      2) Precipitated by bowel or bladder distention or other noxious stimuli

      3) Symptoms: severe and sudden hypertension, bradycardia, headache, profuse sweating above level of injury and pale, cold, dry skin below injury

   h. History: type of accident; speed, site of impact; symptoms at time of injury (drugs/alcohol, hypoxia, hypotension, arrest)

2. Diagnostic tests

   a. Multiple spine films specific to area of suspected injury

   b. Cervical spine films to rule out fracture; C7 to T1 difficult to view; may need "swimmer's" view

   c. Computerized tomography, with or without contrast

   d. Laminar tomography, useful to identify injuries at cervicothoracic junctions

   e. Myelography rarely used but may be useful with progression of deficit

   f. Clients with head injury generally require cervical spine films

   g. Lab: CBC, electrolytes, ABGs

D. Nursing management

1. Medications include: stool softeners, H_2 antagonists or antacids, low-dose anticoagulant therapy, vasopressor drugs if hypotensive, topical antibiotics if halo brace applied, corticosteroids, antispasmodics, a non-steroidal antiinflammatory drug (NSAID) as analgesic, and/or antidepressants

2. Emergency management at scene or in emergency department: secure an airway without flexing, extending or rotating neck; immobilize neck before moving client, transport supine with forehead taped to stretcher to prevent movement; administer O_2 or place on ventilator, and monitor cardiovascular stability

3. Promote optimal breathing

   a. Observe client, consult with health care team to treat decreasing vital capacity and ABGs

   b. Suction bronchial and pharyngeal secretions with care to avoid vagal nerve irritation leading to bradycardia and potential cardiac arrest

   c. Provide percussion or appropriate chest physiotherapy for weak cough

   d. Plan routine breathing exercises with client to support accessory muscles of inspiration

   e. Hydrate client and ensure humidification to thin pulmonary secretions

   f. Create cough during exhalation by pushing in and up between umbilicus and xiphoid process

4. Prevent and treat autonomic dysreflexia

   a. Prevent fecal impaction, bladder distention, or other triggering stimuli

   b. Raise head of bed immediately and remove compression stockings to decrease venous return, and assess BP

   c. Catheterize immediately; remove impaction after antihypertensive medication given

   d. Continue to assess BP while medicating, until stable

   e. Assess client's knowledge of prevention and management

5. Report any deterioration in neuro function; do not turn until treatment plan has been established; monitor LOC, pupillary reaction, possibility of head injury; note affect, reaction to information and events

6. Check motor and sensory level hourly or as ordered; sensory level may be marked on client's skin

7. Monitor cardiovascular function: interruption of sympathetic function leads to wide fluctuations of BP, hypotension, and dysrhythmias

8. Prevent hazards of immobility

   a. Maintain dorsal or supine body alignment until placement of halo brace if appropriate (cervical injuries)

   b. Reposition and turn every 2 hours, monitoring clients with mid-thoracic or higher lesions for hypotension

   c. Provide client with passive ROM exercises and instruct family members how to assist in preventing contractures and atrophy within 48 to 72 hours after injury

   d. Initiate deep vein thrombosis and pulmonary embolism precautions: low-dose anticoagulation therapy and pneumatic compression devices

    e. Reduce hypotensive episodes: slowly change positions, use abdominal corset if appropriate before sitting upright, thigh-high elastic stockings and vasopressor drugs

9. Maintain skin integrity: inspect skin, pad or lubricate bony prominences, and reposition every 2 hours, using circular motion massage to increase circulation; apply skin barrier ointment/spray to perineum before irritation begins; teach and encourage client and family to prevent pressure ulcers

10. Promote urinary elimination

    a. Involve client and family in intermittent catheterization routine addressing prevention of distention and infection

    b. Encourage client and family to track fluid intake to assure adequate fluids and to assess voiding pattern and characteristics of urine

    c. Teach client to practice trigger voiding technique prior to straight catheterization: stroking inner thigh, pulling pubic hair, tapping on abdomen over bladder, and pouring warm water over perineal area in female clients

    d. Explain that successful stimulation of parasympathetic nerve fibers causes reflex activity; this triggered voiding should be followed by catheterization for residual urine during bladder retraining; less than 80 mL of residual urine is acceptable

11. Optimize bowel function

    a. Check for residual amounts of tube feeding, and client tolerance of gastric feedings after bowel sounds resume

    b. Offer a high-calorie, high-protein, high-fiber diet, gradually increasing oral amounts as tolerated

    c. Institute a bowel retraining program; use stool softeners, rectal suppositories with digital stimulation as needed after meals

    d. Manual removal of stool on a routine timetable may be required for client with LMN injury lacking a defecation reflex

12. Halo brace care

    a. Prevent infection at pin sites by clipping hair around pins to facilitate inspection; clean with ½-strength peroxide, normal saline, and topical antibiotic ointment, or soap and water in accordance with hospital or agency protocol

    b. Maintain integrity of halo device by inspecting pins and traction bars for tightness, report loosened parts to physician

    c. Cleanse client's skin under sheepskin liner of vest per protocol; do not use powder or allow vest to become wet

    d. Change sheepskin vest when soiled and per protocol

    e. Maintain client position so that back of head is free of pressure point, massaging gently and with care not to move neck

    f. Keep wrench with vest and know how to release if cardiopulmonary resuscitation is needed

13. Provide sexuality information: offer accurate information on sexual function; discuss alternatives to intercourse if not physically possible and strategies for initiating or maintaining a sexual relationship; secure sexual counseling for client as needed

14. Support optimal self-esteem: keep open communication lines, encourage client self-awareness; encourage decision making and progressive self-care; identify

with client strategies to address goals; refer to support groups and family counseling

15. Prepare for discharge

    a. Reassess and update baseline data in terms of self-care

    b. Explore mobility issues

    c. Facilitate preparation of home setting

    d. Plan for ongoing psychological support

    e. Identify community resources

    f. Evaluate client and family's knowledge of medications, activities of daily living, use of assistive devices, and caregiver respite

VI. ENCEPHALITIS

A. Overview

    1. Defined as a central nervous system (CNS) disorder with inflammation of brain tissue; if both brain and meninges are affected, it is termed meningoencephalitis

    2. Viral encephalitis is more serious than meningitis; can be fatal or cause long-term neurologic disability

    3. Termed as: Western equine encephalitis (occurs in West and in horses); Eastern equine encephalitis (occurs in East and in horses); St. Louis and California encephalitis (not limited to those geographic areas); herpes encephalitis (usually fatal); Japanese encephalitis (similar to St. Louis); Russian spring-summer encephalitis (tick-borne)

    4. Outbreaks are usually in summer and fall when mosquito (vector) is most active

    5. Causes include transfer of arthropod-borne virus (arbovirus) from animals (particularly horses) to humans by mosquitoes; following diseases (rabies, German measles, chickenpox, herpes virus, smallpox); post-vaccination; can be caused by viruses, bacteria, rickettsia, parasites, and fungi; exposure to toxins such as lead poisoning

B. Pathophysiology

    1. Organism (usually virus) enters body and makes its way to the CNS through cerebral capillaries and choroid plexus, then affecting specific cells and producing a wide variety of effects

    2. Damage to CNS results in invasion and lysis of cells, demyelination and selective lysis, an immune response to viral antigens; and destruction of cells without inflammation

    3. Effects of viral encephalitis vary with client's age and may include general symptoms, focal impairment, movement limitations, brain stem involvement, mental and personality changes, cerebral edema, hemorrhage, and even coma

    4. Signs and symptoms include cerebral edema, headache, photophobia, high fever (always present), confusion, seizures, restlessness, hemiparesis, asymmetry of reflexes, positive Babinski's sign, ataxia, difficulty in speaking or understanding, facial weakness, ocular palsies, mental deterioration, muscle stiffness, malaise, sore throat, upper respiratory tract problems, nuchal rigidity, projectile vomiting, pupil irregularities, changes in VS, ptosis, diplopia, strabismus, and abnormal sleep patterns

C. Nursing assessment

1. Assessment includes neurovascular assessment, fluid status, symptom analysis of pain or discomfort, reflexes, ambulation, coordination, VS, cranial nerves
2. Diagnostic tests: lumbar puncture for CSF (increased pressure, increased proteins, normal glucose and chloride); CBC, electrolytes, MRI, CT scan

D. Nursing management

1. Medications include antipyretics, antiviral agents, corticosteroids, anticonvulsants if seizures occur, sedatives, analgesics, stool softeners
2. Monitor fluid balance, measure intake and output (I&O)
3. Monitor nutritional status, measure weight
4. Monitor for signs of increasing ICP
5. Keep environment conducive to rest and decrease stimulation (lights low, limit visitors)
6. Protect client from injury if seizures occur
7. Reposition client frequently, positioning neck for comfort and to decrease joint stiffness
8. Physical therapy should be initiated for ROM exercises
9. Offer assurance to client and family, especially if a child is involved

VII. MENINGITIS

A. Overview

1. Meningitis is defined as an inflammation of meninges (pia mater and arachnoid membrane) surrounding brain and spinal cord
2. Classifications
   a. Viral meningitis (aseptic meningitis) is usually self-limiting with complete recovery
   b. Bacterial meningitis (septic) may leave residual effects or lead to death
3. Higher incidence occurs in fall, winter, and early spring with children more susceptible because they have more upper respiratory tract infections
4. Causes include bacterial or viral infection, often after an upper respiratory tract infection; fungi or toxins may also be causes
5. Preventive public education includes information on meningococcal vaccine

B. Pathophysiology

1. Infection occurs when pathogen crosses blood-brain barrier and migrates throughout CNS
   a. Bacterial meningitis is most often preceded by *Neisseria meningitis* (meningococcal), *Streptococcus pneumoniae,* or *Haemophilus influenzae*
   b. Viral meningitis often occurs after mumps or herpes zoster, herpes simplex, or cytomegalovirus (CMV) infection
2. An inflammatory response causes increased CSF, as well as pressure and purulent exudate that spreads quickly throughout brain and spinal cord in bacterial meningitis
3. Signs and symptoms
   a. Acute infection with inflammation: high fever, nausea, vomiting, chills, malaise, tachycardia

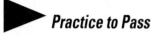

Practice to Pass

A client has bacterial meningitis caused by *Streptococcus pneumoniae.* What measures should the nurse institute to protect the client, healthcare professionals, and others?

    b. Irritated meninges (nuchal rigidity and photophobia)

        1) Stiff/sore neck

        2) Positive Kernig's sign (refer back to Figure 4-2)

        3) Positive Brudzinski's sign: flexion of neck causes neck pain and the hip and knee to flex (Figure 4-3)

    c. Signs of increased ICP

    d. Vascular problems

        1) Thrombophlebitis of cerebral vessels may lead to infarction, seizures, and stroke

        2) Septic emboli may block small vessels of hands and feet leading to gangrene

        3) Fibrinolysis occurring in bacteremia may lead to disseminated intravascular coagulopathy (DIC), a generalized response to injury associated with septic shock with simultaneous bleeding and clotting

C. Nursing assessment

    1. Assessment includes pain (especially neck); reflexes (Brudzinski's, Kernig's sign); mental assessment (LOC, neurovascular); VS, peripheral neurovascular status of all extremities (cool pale to cyanotic extremities with decreased pulses and sensation may indicate emboli); fluid status, respiratory status, nutritional status

    2. Diagnostic tests: lumbar puncture with CSF analysis (high protein, low glucose, positive for bacteria); culture & sensitivity of CSF; CT scan, magnetic resonance imaging (MRI) (swelling and sites of necrosis), blood urea nitrogen (BUN), creatinine (CR), electrolytes, ABGs, C&S of throat, blood, urine, sputum; urine specific gravity

D. Nursing management

    1. Medications include broad-spectrum antibiotics (penicillins, third-generation cephalosporins) until cultures return, analgesics, antipyretics, antiemetics if nausea occurs, antiepileptics if seizures occur, diuretics for cerebral edema

    2. Essential to nursing management of client with meningitis is careful assessment and supportive intervention as needed for acute infection, irritated meninges and increased ICP; elderly clients should receive their pneumonia and flu vaccines per recommended schedules

    3. Administer medications as prescribed and monitor for client's response; avoid narcotics such as opioids that further depress CNS and mask changes in symptoms; clients should be instructed to take complete course of antibiotics to avoid relapse

    4. Carefully monitor VS, neurological and peripheral neurovascular status for changes

        a. Signs of increasing ICP such as changes in LOC (early) or widening pulse pressure, bradycardia, bounding pulse (late)

        b. Signs of peripheral vascular compromise: cool, pale, decreased sensation, faint to absent pulses

        c. Severe headache

        d. Seizures

        e. Cranial nerve dysfunction

    5. Carefully monitor fluid and electrolyte status: strict I&O, daily weights, condition of mucous membranes, skin turgor, urine specific gravity

6. Promote effective airway clearance and exchange: monitor O_2 saturation levels, ABGs; turn every 2 hours, perform chest physiotherapy; suction if needed; elevate head of bed to 30 degrees

7. Relieve hyperthermia; apply cooling blanket or tepid sponge baths as needed

8. Relieve pain: maintain a quiet, dark environment, administer analgesics, encourage gentle ROM, back rub and massage, arrange care/visitors to promote periods of rest

9. Protect from injury: have oral airway, O_2 and suction equipment available; keep side rails up, bed in low position; rails padded; record seizure: event, length, head and eye deviations, interventions, postictal state; monitor for generalized bleeding

10. Maintain adequate nutrition via nasogastric tube feeding if needed, high protein, high calorie, in small frequent feedings

11. Promote health maintenance: instruct client in all medications; instruct to take complete course of all antibiotics; instruct client and close contacts to seek exposure care for fever, headache, irritability, neck stiffness, with prophylactic antibiotic therapy; refer as needed for rehabilitation of residual effects

VIII. SEIZURES

A. Overview

1. Seizures are defined as uncontrolled discharge of neurons of cerebral cortex that interfere with normal function; may be associated with involuntary muscle contractions; may originate as aura or sensory experience before clinical signs are evident

2. **Status epilepticus** can develop during seizure activity; seizures become continuous with very short periods of calm between intense, repetitive seizures; the cumulative effect is life-threatening

3. Epilepsy is defined as recurrent paroxysmal disorder of cerebral function characterized by sudden, brief attacks of altered consciousness, motor activity, or sensory phenomena

4. Classifications of seizures

   a. Partial (focal): simple or partial (Jacksonian), complex

   b. Generalized: tonic-clonic (grand mal) or absence (petit mal), myoclonic, atonic, tonic, or clonic

5. Causes

   a. Genetic tendency/chromosomal abnormalities

   b. Structural factors: head trauma, infections (encephalitis, meningitis, brain abscess, opportunistic lesions from acquired immunodeficiency syndrome [AIDS]); cerebrovascular disorders: hemorrhage, embolism, ischemia; space-occupying lesions: primary and metastatic tumors, neurofibromatosis, arteriovenous malformation (AVM), subdural hematoma

   c. Metabolic-nutritional factors

      1) Electrolyte and water imbalance, hyponatremia, hypocalcemia, hypocapnia, hypoglycemia

      2) Hypoxia

      3) Acidosis

      4) Pyridoxine (Vitamin B_6) deficiency

        5) Fat and amino acid metabolism disorder

        6) Toxins and toxic factors: heavy metals

        7) Systemic disorders: uremia, toxemia

        8) Drugs: "street" drugs, theophylline overdose

        9) Withdrawal: alcohol, barbiturates, antiepileptic drugs, diazepam (Valium)

    d. Idiopathic: no known etiology, possible genetic tendency

B. Pathophysiology

  1. Excessive synchronous discharge of neurons

  2. Neurons in epileptogenic focus recruit other neurons to fire synchronously in adjacent and more distant areas

  3. Abnormal electrical discharge may occur without clinical manifestations

  4. Clinical manifestations occur when sufficient number of neurons are excited

  5. Resulting clinical manifestations depend upon part of brain from which discharge originates and path of spread

  6. Classification and clinical characteristics

    a. Partial seizures (involve part of brain)

        1) Simple partial seizures (consciousness not impaired), with motor symptoms: "Jacksonian" march, spread topographically (systematically); limited to one part of body

        2) Simple partial seizures, with sensory or somatosensory symptoms: may be somatic sensory phenomena only, e.g., tingling, numbness of body part; may have visual, auditory, olfactory or taste symptoms only; dizzy spells may be seizure manifestations

        3) Complex partial seizures (impaired consciousness): begin as simple partial and progress to impairment of consciousness; impairment of consciousness at onset: most commonly involves **automatisms** (automatic actions or behavior without conscious knowledge; repetitive, semi-purposeful, patterned movements such as lip smacking); may include antisocial or aggressive behavior especially if forcefully restrained

        4) Partial seizures secondarily generalized: may spread from original discharge site to other parts of brain and become generalized; generalized seizure preceded by specific aura is partial seizure that becomes generalized

    b. Generalized seizures (involving whole brain at onset) are classified as tonic-clonic, tonic, absence, myoclonic, tonic, or infantile spasms

        1) Absence—simple (petit mal): staring spell; usually lasts less than 15 seconds, during which client is unaware of surroundings; diagnosed by a three cycle/second (C/S) spike and wave on electroencephalogram (EEG); usually present only in children

        2) Absence—atypical: staring spell accompanied by myoclonic jerks and automatisms such as chewing and smacking of lips; atypical spike wave pattern on EEG

        3) Myoclonic—single jerk of one or more muscle groups; lasting only a second

        4) Atonic—drop attack; sometimes associated with myoclonic seizure

        5) Clonic—jerking of muscle groups

        6) Tonic—stiffening of muscle groups

7) Tonic clonic (grand mal): starts with tonic or stiffening phase followed by clonic or jerking phase, unconsciousness, possible bowel and bladder incontinence, may have only tonic or only clonic phase, may bite tongue, reduced consciousness during postictal recovery

8) Metabolic or toxin induced seizure activity—usually generalized; usually does not recur as long as underlying cause remains corrected

c. Status epilepticus: continuing or immediately recurring seizures, recovery between attacks incomplete, usually lasts 30 minutes or more

7. Precipitating factors (unique for each individual)

a. Physical: specific sensory stimuli (flashing lights and certain sounds); fever (children under 5 years of age at risk); injury; physical exhaustion; sleep deprivation; inadequate nutrition; drugs, alcohol, other addictive substances; and hyperventilation

b. Psychosocial: family and environmental stress, coping, shock

8. Signs and symptoms include partial or complete loss of consciousness, falling, incontinence of bowel and bladder, aura before event, muscular contractions, tonic-clonic convulsions of all extremities, facial movements, tongue biting, salivation, a postictal stage (decreased LOC, decreased VS), headache, and fatigue

C. Nursing assessment

1. Assessment

a. History: description of seizure from client or witness; antecedent events; precipitating factors and postictal events; frequency and duration; past history of illness, trauma, infection; alcohol or drug use; family history of seizures; perinatal history, growth and development

b. Physical and neurological examination: seizure activity (length, progression of jerking, time started and other associated signs, such as incontinence), presence of oral bleeding, postictal stages, vital signs, posturing

c. Assess client's knowledge of lifestyle and factors that may trigger seizures

2. Diagnostic tests

a. Serum electrolytes: hyponatremia, hypocalcemia (especially in children), hypoglycemia

b. BUN

c. ABGs: hypoxia and acidosis

d. CSF analysis: infection and/or hemorrhage

e. Drug screen: toxicity of sedatives, hypnotics, heavy metals, drug interactions, "street" drugs, theophylline, and antiepileptic drug levels

f. EEG

1) May be normal between seizures

2) Activation techniques may elicit epileptic discharge: hyperventilation, photo stimulation, or sleep deprivation

3) Nasopharyngeal or sphenoidal leads used to localize temporal lobe focus

g. Initial studies may include computed tomography (CT) scan or magnetic resonance imaging (MRI), or positive emission tomography (PET) scan

D. Nursing management

1. Medications

   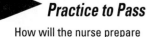
   a. Antiepileptics: phenytoin (Dilantin), carbamazepine (Tegretol), valproic acid (Depakene), ethosuximide (Zarontin), clonazepam (Klonopin), gabapentin (Neurontin)

   b. Diazepam (Valium), lorazepam (Ativan), phenytoin (Dilantin) or phenobarbital may be used for status epilepticus

2. Document details of seizure: date, time of onset, duration of seizure; activity of client at time of onset; precipitating factors, if any; aura; seizure activity (body parts involved and sequence); character of movements (tonic, clonic, head or eye deviation, behavior)

3. Monitor autonomic signs: pupil size and reactivity, respirations, cyanosis, diaphoresis, incontinence, salivation

4. Record and evaluate LOC during and after seizure: arousability, duration of reduced consciousness, awareness of and memory for event

5. Monitor postictal state (period immediately following termination of a seizure; usually lasts 30 to 90 minutes): confusion, exhaustion, sleepiness, difficulty to arouse, muscle soreness, headache, weakness, aphasia, inability to maintain airway if not arousable, partial paralysis

6. Inspect for presence of injury, especially head or tongue: lacerations or bruises

7. Provide safety management during seizure

   a. Protect from injury

   b. Do not force hard object between teeth

   c. Do not restrain

   d. Turn to side to keep airway open during postictal period

8. Monitor serum drug levels to determine if antiepileptic drug (AED) in therapeutic range; dosage depends on pharmacokinetics, individual metabolism and degree of seizure control; clarify that AED must be taken on a continuous basis; if adverse effects occur, dose is lowered or different drug is tried

9. Control precipitating factors

10. Surgical intervention may be a treatment option: cortical resection of epileptic focus may be indicated if criteria met

11. Maintain large vein access while hospitalized for treatment of status epilepticus

> ### ▶ *Practice to Pass*
>
> How will the nurse prepare a client who is newly diagnosed with seizures for his first EEG?

IX. GUILLAIN-BARRÉ SYNDROME

A. Overview

1. Defined as an acute (sudden onset), rapidly progressing inflammation of peripheral motor and sensory nerves characterized by:

   a. Variable motor weakness and paralysis

   b. Paralysis that ascends symmetrically from lower extremities in most cases

   c. With excellent care, has a 96% complete recovery

2. Occurs most commonly between ages of 30 to 50 years, equally in both genders

3. Causes include unknown etiology, autoimmune attack; are common after viral infections, immunizations, febrile illness, injury, or surgery

B. Pathophysiology

1. A cell-mediated immune reaction is triggered by a viral illness or immunization
2. Instead of normal antibody role of preventing invading organism from causing harm, the antibody formed has a damaging effect on peripheral nerve myelin; an IgM antimyelin antibody exists, lymphocytes are sensitized and aid in damaging myelin
3. With demyelination, nerve impulses are slowed or stopped and muscles lose innervation and begin to waste without exercise
4. During recovery, remyelination occurs in descending order over a period of a few months to a couple of years
5. Signs and symptoms include weakness/paresis (partial paralysis), paralysis progressing upward from lower extremities to total paralysis requiring ventilatory support; paresthesias (numbness and tingling) and pain; muscle aches, cramping, and nighttime pain; respiratory compromise and/or failure: dyspnea, diminished vital capacity, breath sounds, decreasing O_2 saturation, abnormal blood gases; cranial nerve involvement: impaired extraocular eye movements, dysphagia, diplopia, difficulty speaking; and autonomic dysfunction: orthostatic hypotension (lowered BP and dizziness with sudden position changes), hypertension, change in heart rate (bradycardia, heart block, asystole or tachycardia), bowel and bladder dysfunction, flushing and diaphoresis

C. Nursing assessment

1. Includes onset and chronology of symptoms including any illnesses in previous 1 to 8 weeks; head to toe muscle strength testing (see Tables 4-3 and 4-4); head-to-toe sensory assessment; cranial nerve involvement, respiratory status, fluid balance, skin integrity, bladder and bowel control
2. Diagnostic tests: electrolytes, ABGs, nerve conduction tests, lumbar puncture for CSF (elevated protein)

D. Nursing management

1. Medications and treatment
   a. IV immunoglobulins: may cause low-grade fever, muscle aches, headache, acute renal failure (rare), retinal necrosis
   b. Plasmapheresis: plasma is removed and separated from whole blood and blood cells are returned without the plasma to remove antibodies responsible for disease; monitor for complications
      1) Loss of clotting factors, bleeding
      2) Fluid and electrolyte imbalance
   c. Adrenocorticoid hormone (ACTH) and corticosteroids or antiinflammatory drugs
   d. Other: stool softeners, antacids or H_2-receptor antagonists, analgesics

Table 4-3		
Muscle Strength Scale	0	No visible muscle contraction: paralysis
	1	Trace: slight contraction but no movement
	2	Poor: ROM with gravity eliminated
	3	Fair: ROM against gravity
	4	Good: ROM against gravity with some resistance
	5	Normal: full ROM and full resistance

Table 4-4	Ocular and lids	Close eyes tightly
Head-to-Toe Muscle Strength Testing	Facial	Puff cheeks, stick out tongue
	Neck	Bend head forward and back
	Deltoid	Hold arms up
	Biceps	Flex arm
	Triceps	Extend arm
	Wrists	Flex and extend
	Finger	Grip examiner's crossed plexor and second finger
	Hip	Raise straight leg from supine
	Gluteal and leg	Cross legs
	Ankle and foot	Flex and extend

2. Care is supportive with attention to function of all systems, especially respiratory and cardiac

    a. Monitor respiratory status: rate, depth, breath sounds, vital capacity, note secretions and check gag, cough, and swallowing reflexes

    b. Monitor cardiac status: heart rate, BP, dysrhythmias

3. Administer chest physiotherapy and pulmonary hygiene measures

4. Maintain adequate nutrition as appropriate: administer tube feeding, parenteral nutrition or assisted small frequent feedings of soft foods; weigh client weekly; check electrolyte status, give mouth care every two hours

5. Monitor bowel and bladder function: assess bowel sounds and frequency, amount, color of bowel movements; offer bed pan; check for distention and residuals in client who cannot void spontaneously; perform intermittent catheterization as needed; encourage fluid intake to 3,500 mL/day unless contraindicated by concurrent cardiac or renal disease

6. Prevent complications of immobility

    a. Encourage use of weak extremities as able

    b. Work with physical therapy to plan passive and active ROM to all extremities

    c. Protect immobile extremities with use of:

        1) Air mattress or special bed

        2) Elbow and heel protectors

    d. Turn and position in good body alignment

    e. Elevate extremities to prevent dependent edema

    f. Use antiembolic compression devices/stockings

7. Provide eye care for client unable to close eyelids completely: instill artificial tears, cleanse eyes as needed, use eye shields and tape eyes closed as needed

8. Provide comfort and analgesics as needed: assess pain with VS; administer analgesics before painful activities; log roll and move client gently; use imagery, relaxation, distraction, humor, music as appropriate; pain is common, and nocturnal pain is reported as more severe

9. Promote communication, encouragement, and support to client and family

    a. If client is on ventilator or is unable to communicate because of weak speech muscles, collaborate with speech therapist to develop a communication system

    b. Explain all care with rationale and provide information about progression of disease

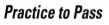

Practice to Pass

List nursing diagnoses in order of priority for the client with Guillain-Barré syndrome who is in the acute phase experiencing tetraplegia (quadriplegia).

      c. Encourage client and family to express feelings and participate in care as much as possible

    10. Begin to plan for discharge needs upon admission to acute care setting

X. MYASTHENIA GRAVIS

A. Overview

1. Myasthenia gravis is a chronic progressive disorder of peripheral nervous system affecting transmission of nerve impulses to voluntary muscles, causing muscle weakness and fatigue that increases with exertion and improves with rest; eventually leads to fatigue without relief from rest

2. Varies from mild disturbance of ocular movement to respiratory failure from weakness of the diaphragm and muscles of respiration; 3 types exist and are labeled as ocular, bulbar, and generalized

3. Characterized by unpredictable remissions and exacerbations

4. Affects women three times more than men until after age 50 with onset usually between ages 20 and 30 years

5. Causes include unknown etiology, family history of autoimmune disorders, thyroid tumors

B. Pathophysiology

1. An autoimmune process triggers formation of autoantibodies that decrease the number of acetylcholine receptors and widen gap between axon ending and muscle fiber in the neuromuscular junction; muscle contraction is hindered because IgG autoantibodies prevent acetylcholine from binding with receptors; destruction of receptors at the neuromuscular junction occurs

2. Associated with continued production of autoantibodies by thymus gland in 75% of cases

3. Onset is usually slow but can be precipitated by emotional stress, hormonal disturbance (pregnancy, menses, thyroid disorders), infections/vaccinations, trauma and surgery, temperature extremes, excessive exercise, drugs that block or decrease neuromuscular transmission (opioids, sedatives, barbiturates, alcohol, quinidine, anesthetics), and thymus tumor

4. Signs and symptoms include: mild diplopia (double vision) and unilateral ptosis (eyelid drooping) caused by weakness in extraocular muscles; may also involve face, jaw, neck, and hip; complications arise when severe weakness affects muscles of swallowing, chewing, and respiration; respiratory distress manifested by tachypnea, decreased depth, abnormal ABGs, O_2 saturation less than 92%, decreased breath sounds; bowel and bladder incontinence, paresthesias, and pain in weak muscles

5. Myasthenic crisis: sudden motor weakness; risk of respiratory failure and aspiration; most often caused by not enough medication or an infection

6. Cholinergic crisis: severe muscle weakness; caused by overmedication; signs are cramps, diarrhea, bradycardia, and bronchial spasm with increased pulmonary secretions and risk of respiratory compromise

C. Nursing assessment

1. Assessment

    a. Progression and severity of fatigue; which body parts are affected; effect on ADLs; adequacy of coping skills

    b. Cranial nerve dysfunction

      1) Ocular: diplopia and ptosis; test for ptosis by asking client to look upward for 2 to 3 minutes; eyelid droop will increase so that eye can hardly be held open; after rest, eyes can open

      2) Facial: smile may be a snarl, jaw may need to be propped closed

      3) Laryngeal and pharyngeal: voice may be weak with a nasal twang, may have dysphagia (difficulty swallowing), and difficulty chewing with some choking

    c. Other muscle weakness

      1) Test all muscle groups (see Table 4-3): flexors of neck, shoulder, and hip may be affected: difficulty holding head up, difficulty climbing stairs, lifting, raising arms over head, difficulty holding, sitting, standing posture

      2) Bowel and bladder incontinence

    d. Respiratory distress from weakness of diaphragm and respiratory muscles and difficulty swallowing secretions; lung sounds, respiratory rate (RR) and depth

  2. Diagnostic tests: ABGs, pulmonary function tests

    a. Electromyography (EMG) shows decreased amplitude when motor neurons are stimulated

    b. Confirmation of clinical diagnosis can be made by IV administration of edrophonium chloride (Tensilon), which allows voluntary muscle contraction; Tensilon allows acetylcholine to bind with its receptors, which temporarily improves symptoms; weakness returns after effects of Tensilon wear off

D. Nursing management

  1. Medications and treatment

    a. Anticholinesterases: neostigmine (Prostigmin), pyridostigmine (Mestinon); give medications on time or client may be too weak to swallow

    b. Immunosuppressants: corticosteroids, azathioprine (Imuran), cyclosporine (Cytoxan)

    c. Anti-inflammatory drugs

    d. Thymectomy (removal of thymus gland)

    e. Plasmapheresis: removes IgG antibodies

    f. Atropine sulfate (Atropine) for cholinergic crisis

  2. Monitor client response and side effects to medications; give medications on time to maintain blood levels and thus muscle strength during essential activities and eating

  3. Maintain effective breathing pattern and airway clearance

    a. Thoroughly assess for respiratory distress

    b. Monitor meals and teach client to bend head slightly forward while eating/drinking

    c. Teach client to avoid exposure to infections, especially respiratory

    d. Teach client effective coughing, use chest physiotherapy and incentive spirometry

    e. Have oral suction available and teach client how to use it

    f. Have intubation equipment on hand

  4. Provide adequate nutrition

    a. Schedule medications 30 to 45 minutes before eating for peak muscle strength while eating

  b. Offer food frequently in small amounts that are easy to chew and swallow; soft or semisolid as needed

  c. Administer IV fluids and nasogastric tube feedings if client is unable to swallow

5. Instruct in alternative methods of communication if needed: eye blink, finger wiggle for yes or no; flash cards, communication board; teach to support lower jaw with hands to assist with speech

6. Promote improved physical mobility

  a. Refer to physical therapy/occupational therapy

  b. Instruct client to plan rest periods and to conserve energy

   1) Plan major activities early in day

   2) Schedule activities during peak medication effect

  c. Passive and active ROM

  d. Instruct client to avoid extremes of hot and cold, exposure to infections, emotional stress and medications that may worsen or precipitate an exacerbation (alcohol, sedatives, local anesthetics)

  e. Instruct client in signs of crisis and differences between causation of myasthenic and cholinergic crises

  f. Encourage client to wear a Medic alert bracelet

7. Provide eye care: instill artificial tears, use a patch over one eye for double vision; wear sunglasses to protect eyes from bright lights

8. Promote positive body image and coping skills

  a. Encourage participation in treatment plan

  b. Set aside time for active listening and encourage client to express feelings

  c. Reinforce progress and explain all care

  d. Provide low energy diversional activities

  e. Refer to myasthenia gravis self-help group

XI. PARKINSON'S DISEASE

A. Overview

1. Defined as a progressive gradual neurological degenerative disorder of brain characterized by: "resting" (nonintentional) tremors; bradykinesia (slow, sometimes frozen movement); and muscle rigidity or stiffness

2. Affects mostly older adults between ages of 50 and 60 years

3. Classified as primary or secondary (caused by other disorders)

4. Causes: primary—unknown; secondary—linked to infection; neoplasms; encephalitis; intoxication with carbon monoxide, manganese, and mercury; use of some drugs (reserpine, methyldopa, haloperidol, phenothiazines); and hypoxia and cerebral ischemia

B. Pathophysiology

1. Affects brain centers that control and regulate movement

2. Neurons in substantia nigra and corpus striatum in midbrain degenerate and become deficient in production and storage of the neurotransmitter dopamine

3. When dopamine levels that inhibit motor activity deplete, acetylcholine is not inhibited, allowing increased excitation that is the basis for symptoms of Parkinson's disease

4. Signs and symptoms include weight loss, constipation, dysphagia, depression, and dementia

   a. Tremors

      1) Mild "pill-rolling": nonintentional tremor of thumb and first finger as if rotating a small object

      2) May begin in one hand with tremor spreading to arm, then other arm, and later head

      3) Usually lessens with purposeful movement

   b. Bradykinesia and loss of automatic movement characterized by: mask-like face with staring gaze; soft, monotone voice; drooling of saliva; impaired balance and loss of righting reflex (correcting posture when changing positions); stooped posture; difficulty initiating movement; and unsteady shuffling propulsive gait

   c. Rigidity

      1) Cogwheel: manual manipulation of body parts may take on the feel of a cogwheel; increased resistance to passive ROM with jerky catches when joint is moved

      2) Lead pipe: cataleptic condition during which limbs remain in any position in which placed; smooth, stiff movement

   d. Autonomic dysfunction: insomnia, oily skin, sweating, heat intolerance, orthostatic hypotension

C. Nursing assessment

   1. Assessment includes onset and progression of disease; changes in function throughout day and in response to medication (difficulty dressing, eating, walking, writing); movement (tremors, bradykinesia, rigidity), bowel function, nutritional status, mental status (forgetfulness, long-term and short-term memory), reflexes, and memory

   2. Diagnostic tests: no specific tests are diagnostic, based on signs and symptoms; glucose may be tested because of side effects of drugs

D. Nursing management

   1. Medications

      a. Dopaminergics: levodopa (L-dopa), carbidopa–levodopa (Sinemet), amantadine (Symmetrel), pramipexole dihydrochloride (Mirapex)

      b. Dopamine agonists: bromocriptine (Parlodel), pergolide (Permax)

      c. Anticholinergics: trihexyphenidyl hydrochloride (Artane), benztropine mesylate (Cogentin)

   2. Monitor for symptom control and adverse reactions to medications such as anemia, dystonia (prolonged muscle contraction that may cause twisting and repetitive movements or abnormal posture), nausea, darkened urine and sweat, orthostatic hypotension, changes in mentation and vision, tachycardia, urinary retention, dry mouth, constipation, and impaired glucose tolerance

   3. Encourage mobility with daily exercise directed by physical therapy; use of assistive devices as needed

      a. Spring-loaded chair/straight-backed chair with arms and slight elevation of back legs

      b. Elevated toilet seat

      c. Slip-on shoes or Velcro-fastened shoes

  d. Velcro fasteners on clothes

  e. Canes, splints, braces as needed

  f. Rope tied to foot of bed to assist getting to sitting position

  g. Instruct client who "freezes" to think about stepping over something

  h. Instruct client to lift legs and take big steps when walking to offset shuffling, propulsive gait

  i. Instruct client to hold an object to decrease resting tremors

  j. Instruct client to "look at horizon" when walking to prevent lowering of head that increases risk of falls

4. Provide a safe environment

  a. Remove throw rugs and excess furniture

  b. Provide grab bar in bathroom, handrails on both sides of stairs

  c. Ensure adequate lighting in home

5. Promote a well-balanced diet

  a. Assess client's nutritional status, ability to feed self and swallow

  b. Consult with dietician, speech and occupational therapists to develop individual interventions

  c. Provide food of proper consistency to prevent aspiration as determined by client's swallowing function

  d. Provide stabilized dishes and utensils, flexible straw for drinking

  e. Offer small frequent meals and snacks

  f. Encourage high fiber and 3,000 mL of water intake a day under additional fluids contraindicated by concurrent renal or cardiac disease

6. Promote adequate rest

  a. Assess client's perception of adequacy of rest, sleep pattern and existing conditions, medications that might impact sleep

  b. Avoid exercise or napping close to bedtime

  c. Limit caffeine and alcohol intake; drink milk before bedtime

  d. Provide a firm mattress with a small pillow, sheepskin or air mattress

  e. Darken bedroom and decrease noise

7. Allow client to participate in own care; client should be treated respectfully and not made to feel left out

8. Maintain an unhurried environment to allow sufficient time for client to attempt own ADLs

► *Practice to Pass*

A client with Parkinson's disease has dysphagia (difficulty swallowing). What mealtime interventions should the nurse consider to prevent aspiration and ease swallowing?

XII. MULTIPLE SCLEROSIS (MS)

A. Overview

1. Defined as a chronic disorder of CNS where myelin and nerve axons in brain and spinal cord are destroyed

2. Most prominent in women and European Americans

3. Four forms based on rate of progression: benign, relapsing-remitting, primary progressive, and secondary progressive

4. Four syndromes based on which nerve tract is originally affected: corticospinal syndrome, brain stem syndrome, cerebellar syndrome, and cerebral syndrome; symptoms will usually be suggestive of one of these areas

5. Exacerbations of illness can be precipitated by stress, pregnancy, illness, fever, fatigue

6. Causes: unknown etiology, possibly an autoimmune or genetic basis; childhood viral infections also suggested

B. Pathophysiology

1. Destruction of myelin and nerve axons causes a temporary, repetitive, or sustained interruption in conduction of nerve impulses that causes symptoms of MS

2. Plaque formation occurs throughout white matter of CNS, which also affects nerve impulses; disorder affects optic nerves, cervical spinal cord, and thoracic and lumbar spine

3. Inflammation occurs around plaques as well as normal tissue; astrocytes (gliosis) appear in lesions and scar tissue forms, replacing axons and leading to permanent disability; the term *gliosis* leads to the term *sclerosis,* which means scarring

4. The immune response

a. Helper T-cells are elevated in CSF at onset of disease

b. T-suppressor cells are decreased in serum before and during an exacerbation of illness

c. Immunocompetent cells are present within plaques

d. Antibody production is evident intrathecally

5. Types (based on rate of progression of disease)

a. *Benign*—nervous system dysfunction will occur in different episodes, full recovery follows

b. *Relapsing-remitting* (most common)— neurological exacerbations occur but improvement can be seen with either complete or partial recovery

c. *Primary progressive*—sudden loss of neurological function occurs, which may not resolve; leaves severe functional impairments; these may actually worsen over time; no remission follows

d. *Secondary progressive*—starts similar to relapsing-remitting; changes to a primary progressive form; no remission follows

6. Signs and symptoms include visual disturbances or blindness (retrobulbar neuritis), sudden, progressive weakness of one or more limbs, spasticity of muscles, nystagmus, tremors, gait instability, fatigue, bladder dysfunction (UTIs, incontinence), depression

C. Nursing assessment

1. Assessment includes symptoms analysis of complaints, neurovascular assessment, movement, mental assessment, and eye exam

2. Diagnostic tests: lumbar puncture for CSF (clonal IgG bands present), MRI, CT scans, PET scans, muscle testing of evoked potentials

D. Nursing management

1. Medications include immunomodulators (interferon alpha and beta) and glatiramer acetate (Copaxone), antiviral drugs, corticosteroids, antibiotics for UTIs, anticholinergic drugs, antispasmodics, immunosuppressants, and muscle relaxants (baclofen [Lioresal], dantolene [Dantrium], and diazepam [Valium])

2. No cure is available, supportive care should be maintained; may include intrathecal baclofen (Lioresal), or dorsal rhizotomy for intractable spasms

3. Maximum support to client and family is usually needed

> ! ▸ 4. Client education should include medications, symptoms, bladder training, self-intermittent catheterization, sexual functioning, avoiding complications, and possible triggers
>
> 5. Safety should be assessed in home and work environments

XIII. AMYOTROPIC LATERAL SCLEROSIS (ALS)

A. Overview

1. Defined as a degenerative disease of upper and lower motor neurons of cerebral cortex, brain stem, and spinal cord that results in total paralysis (except for cranial nerves III, IV, and VI); also known as Lou Gehrig's disease

2. Occurs in fourth or fifth decade of life; more common in men; usually fatal in 3 to 5 years

3. Causes include unknown etiology, viral infections, metabolic disorders, and trauma; familial patterns and autoimmune responses have been implicated

B. Pathophysiology

1. Motor neurons in cortex, brain stem, and spinal cord are lost; disease is noninflammatory; axon degeneration causes demyelination

2. Effect on UMN function leads to spastic, weak muscles and increased deep tendon reflexes

3. Effect on LMN function causes muscle atrophy and flaccid paralysis

4. Only one muscle group may be affected initially; clinical symptoms will vary according to muscle groups involved; loss of muscle innervation → muscle atrophy → decrease in muscle mass → increasing fatigue

! ▸ 5. The difficulty of ALS is that mentation, cognitive ability, vision, hearing, and sensation are not lost; client loses control of function without losing mental awareness

! ▸ 6. Signs and symptoms

   a. Musculoskeletal: weakness, fatigue, loss of fine motor control, spasticity, paresis, hyperreflexia, atrophy, paralysis; fasciculations of tongue, slurred speech and facial muscles

   b. Respiratory: dyspnea, ineffective airway clearance, upper respiratory infection (URI), respiratory failure

   c. Nutritional: dysphagia, inability to chew, malnutrition

   d. Other: depression, impotence, loss of bowel and bladder control

C. Nursing assessment

1. Assessment includes coordination, muscle stiffness and wasting, gait, signs of atrophy, dysarthria, dysphagia, dyspnea, decreased reflexes, decreased respiratory function; and changes in VS, weight, and bowel function

2. Diagnostic tests: creatinine phosphokinase (CPK) (elevated), CSF (elevated protein), myelography, CT scan, muscle biopsy, electromyelogram, nerve conduction studies

D. Nursing management

1. Medications: anticholinesterase agents, steroids, antibiotics, muscle relaxants

! ▸ 2. Administer O_2 and ventilatory support as needed; suction as needed

3. Monitor cardiac status and VS

4. Monitor fluid status and offer nutritional support

5. Initiate physical therapy

6. Auscultate breath sounds

7. Encourage client to administer own ADLs as long as possible

8. Monitor bowel and bladder function, avoid constipation

9. Turn every two hours as needed; encourage ambulation; avoid strenuous exercise and plan rest periods

10. Encourage client and family to ventilate feelings

11. Involve client in support group; refer to ALS center to minimize cost and maximize effectiveness

12. Client education should include avoiding complications, importance of ongoing outpatient care, need to maintain physical mobility, use of assistive devices

13. Counseling for advance directives with decision about use of ventilator for respiratory support

XIV. PAIN

A. Overview

1. Pain is a subjective feeling, an individual response to noxious stimuli on sensory nerve endings

2. Components of pain are affective (emotional), behavioral (behavioral responses), cognitive (beliefs, attitudes), sensory (perceptual), and physiological

3. Unrelieved pain has harmful effects that slow healing; stimulation of stress response causes increased muscle tension, local vasoconstriction, increased myocardial activity and O_2 consumption

   a. Pain tolerance is the degree of pain an individual can withstand; differences in affect, behavioral response, and cognitive factors vary from one person to the next

   b. Pain threshold is the point of pain recognition; it varies somewhat from person to person also

4. Pain can be classified according to source, speed, duration, and if "referred pain"

   a. Sources of pain

      1) Cutaneous: from skin and subcutaneous tissue

      2) Deep somatic: from muscles, tendons, joints

      3) Visceral/splanchnic: from abdominal organs; contractions, distention, colic

      4) Psychogenic/functional: pain of unknown physical cause

   b. Speed

      1) Fast: carried by A-delta fibers that are myelinated and carry sharp, bright, well-localized pain

      2) Slow: carried by C-fibers, which are unmyelinated and carry dull, burning, aching diffuse sensations

   c. Duration is considered either acute or chronic with different times and physiological and/or psychological responses

      1) Acute pain: defined as pain for 6 months or less, usually of sudden onset with localization in affected area; physiological response (often see in autonomic sympathetic "flight or fight" response), psychological response (heightened emotional response with anxiety, fear)

2) Chronic pain: defined as pain for 6 months or greater, persists over an indefinite period, is poorly localized, often diffuse; physiological response (may be none or may be a fatigued autonomic response with depressed vital signs); psychological response (characterized by attention to pain as all-consuming and signs of depression such as a sleeping disorder, anorexia or overeating, crying, flat or sad affect, and withdrawal)

    d. Referred pain is pain that is perceived at a site different from its origin

5. Phantom pain (pain that exists in a removed part) occurs in an amputated body part or limb, possibly caused by spontaneous firing of spinal cord neurons that have lost their normal sensory input

6. Intractable pain or malignant pain is chronic progressive pain that is unrelenting and severely debilitating

7. Causes of pain include surgery, injury, trauma, chronic diseases (cancer, arthritis, AIDS, etc.), strenuous work, hormone shifts (migraines, menstruation), pregnancy, earache, toothaches, and infections

B. Pathophysiology

1. Nociception is the process of how pain is recognized consciously and can be considered conceptually in four steps: transduction, transmission, perception, and modulation

    a. Transduction: conversion of a stimulus to an action potential at site of tissue injury

        1) Chemicals are released with cellular damage from such things as burns, radiation, pressure, tears, and cuts

        2) These chemicals sensitize primary afferent nociceptors (PANs), fibers that carry painful stimuli; PANs are: A-delta (fast pain); C-fibers (slow pain)

        3) Analgesics that work to block transduction by interfering in production of chemicals that sensitize PANs to begin the action potential and send signals to spinal cord include: corticosteroids, which block the formation of arachidonic acid; NSAIDS (nonsteroidal antiinflammatory drugs), which block formation of prostaglandins

    b. Transmission: a neuronal action potential is transmitted to and through CNS so that pain can be perceived

        1) Impulse is projected to spinal cord

        2) It is processed in dorsal horn

        3) It is then transmitted to brain

        4) Analgesics that work at level of transmission stabilize membranes by inactivating sodium channels, thus inhibiting the action potential

        5) Referred pain occurs when nerve fibers from visceral areas and somatic areas that converge in the same area in the dorsal horn are processed in such a way that they are perceived as originating in an area of somatic sensory A-delta fibers rather than visceral C-fibers (e.g., myocardial ischemia is perceived as pain in left arm)

        6) Gate control theory of pain offers an explanation for why such interventions as TENS (transcutaneous electrical nerve stimulator), heat and cold, and massage are effective

            a) There are theoretical gates in dorsal horn

            b) Small-diameter nerve fibers carry pain impulses through a gate, but large-diameter sensory nerve fibers going through same gate can close gate and inhibit transmission

      c. Pain perception (the experience of pain) occurs in cerebral cortex; may occur at a basic level in thalamus

      d. Modulation, inhibition of nociception

         1) Efferent fibers descending from brain stem modulate or alter pain; mechanisms include:

            a) Endogenous opioids (naturally occurring, morphine-like chemicals) made in CNS inhibit transmission of pain by binding to opioid receptors in CNS to block transmission of nociceptive signals (e.g., endorphin, norepinephrine, enkephalin)

            b) Endogenous analgesia center in midbrain produces profound analgesia when stimulated

         2) Many analgesics modulate pain by mimicking endogenous neuromodulators; examples include tricyclic antidepressants that block serotonin reuptake (work well for neuropathic pain that is dull, aching, burning); synthetic opioids [e.g., morphine sulfate, meperidine (Demerol), hydromorphone (Dilaudid)]; the variability of individual endorphin levels may explain how pain thresholds to same stimulus are different from person to person

         3) Surgical treatment of intractable pain (chronic, progressive pain that is unrelenting and severely debilitating) interrupts pain pathways; types include: nerve block (destroys nerve roots chemically with phenol or alcohol); rhizotomy (destroys sensory nerve roots at level of entry into spinal cord); and cordotomy (transects spinal pain pathway before impulses ascend spinothalamic tracts)

   2. Signs and symptoms include elevated BP, increased HR, increased RR, grimacing, crying, sweating, posturing, depression, dilated pupils, anxiety and/or agitation, hypermotility

C. Nursing assessment

   1. Assessment

      a. Sensory components of pain (location, character or quality, pattern, duration, quantity or severity)

         1) Location: Where is the pain? Is the pain on the surface or deep? Can you put your finger on it? Does it radiate or spread?

         2) Character or quality: Describe how it feels (aching, burning, shooting, stinging, constant, intermittent, sharp, dull)

         3) Pattern: How often does it come? Is it different at different times? Does anything make it start, make it worse or better?

         4) Duration: How long have you had the pain?

         5) Intensity or severity: Can you rank the pain on a scale of 0 to 10, with 0 as no pain and 10 as the worst possible?

      b. Affective, behavioral, and cognitive components of pain; emotion will influence pain; expression of pain and beliefs about pain will vary from culture to culture; questions to ask include:

         1) What does the pain mean to you? Does it interfere or hinder you in any way?

         2) What do you think is causing the pain?

         3) What do you think will make it better?

         4) What home remedies or herbal agents have you tried or are you using?

         5) What prescription or over-the-counter (OTC) medications have you tried or are you using to treat the pain?

2. Diagnostic tests: not recommended generally; rating scale of 1 to 10 and symptom analysis of complaints are used; specific diagnostic tests to determine cause of pain are used according to reports voiced and location of pain

D. Nursing management

1. Medications include OTC analgesics such as acetaminophen (Tylenol), NSAIDs such as ibuprofen (Motrin), opioid analgesics such as morphine or hydrocodone, anticonvulsants for chronic pain (such as gabapentin [Neurontin]), and antiemetics

2. General principles in nursing management of pain

   a. Establish a trusting nurse-client relationship

   b. Always listen; believe and respect client

   c. Clarify responsibilities, collaborate with client to promote control and participation: discuss client's role in reporting pain, client's acceptable level of pain and nurse's commitment when client reports pain

   d. Be with client during pain; offer support, concern, empathy and reassurance

   e. Explain all interventions for pain and how they work

3. Intervene to relieve pain

   a. Administer pain medications as ordered early in pain episode to achieve client's acceptable pain level

   b. Consider round-the-clock administration of pain medication if pain is present most of day

   c. If client has patient-controlled analgesia (PCA) (intravenous delivery of opioid by pump that allows client to deliver analgesia on demand with preset dose and frequency limits and option of preset continuous dosage):

   1) Instruct in concept and demonstrate

   2) Emphasize that client controls the device, not the family

   d. If client has an epidural catheter, assess for orthostatic hypotension and inspect insertion site for infection

   e. Assess pain with using an analgesic scale each time VS are taken, after each administration of medication and with peak effect

   f. Assess for side effects of pain medications and symptoms that aggravate pain: sedation, nausea, constipation, respiratory depression, urinary retention, and hypotension

   g. Clients taking opioids should be on a bowel management program, using a stool softener or laxative

   h. Include pain management in discharge teaching

4. Promote rest and relaxation; implement nondrug pain treatments (alternative or complementary therapies) as appropriate; these include:

   a. Cognitive strategies, such as distraction (music, TV, reading, humor), guided imagery, and positive suggestion; suggest the desired effect will be obtained when administering medications and alternative therapies; use words like "episode" and "experience" instead of "attack," and use "comfort" instead of "pain"

   b. Behavioral approaches such as rhythmic, slow breathing

   c. Therapeutic touch

   d. Cutaneous stimulation such as pressure, acupressure, heat and cold therapy, and massage

   e. Lower lights and reduce noise

   f. Reposition, support body parts, encourage mild activity such as gentle ROM

   g. Plan care and schedule visitors to provide uninterrupted rest periods

5. Chronic pain requires a comprehensive approach to manage it effectively; assess how pain affects client's ability to perform ADLs and consider this in developing plan of care

6. Monitor constraints to effective pain management including these misconceptions:

   a. Use of opioids (formerly narcotics) for management of acute pain will lead to addiction (compulsive drug-seeking): research indicates that only 0.1% of persons using opioids for acute pain management during postoperative period will become addicted; addiction should *not* be confused with:

      1) Physical dependence: experience of physiological withdrawal symptoms with rapid discontinuance of opioids

      2) Tolerance: a need for increasing amounts of opioids to achieve same level of pain relief

   b. It is better to wait until pain peaks to take analgesics: less analgesic is needed and better relief is obtained when analgesic is given at onset of pain

   c. Oral analgesics do not work as well as intravenous or intramuscular routes: if an **equianalgesic chart** (same pain relief obtained with different drugs, doses, and routes) is used, the oral route is equally effective; amount of drug needed is increased because of first-pass effect of liver

7. Intervene to alter the affective and cognitive components of pain

   a. Encourage client to discuss factors that may impact and contribute to pain experience such as sociocultural influences, economic stress, and past experiences with pain

   b. Assist client to identify previously effective coping strategies

   c. Refer to appropriate health care resources for counseling and therapy such as the psychologist, occupational therapist, physical therapist, or social worker as needed

XV. ALZHEIMER'S DISEASE

A. Overview

1. Defined as a chronic, progressive form of dementia (cognitive impairment from organic syndrome) with cerebral degeneration

2. Occurs most often after age 65 (senile dementia); but can occur between 40 to 60 years of age (presenile dementia)

3. Causes include unknown etiology but has been linked to genetic tendency

B. Pathophysiology

1. Plaques, pathological changes, and neuronal tangles occur in brain; within these plaques are dying nerve terminals, possible aluminum deposits, and abnormal protein fragments

2. Theories as to cause:

   a. An abnormal processing of a protein known as amyloid precursor protein (APP) allows part of protein to kill cells

   b. Inheritance of a gene coding for apolipoprotein E (APO-E4), which causes neuronal cell death

3. The number of functioning neurons is decreased, which accounts for decline in cognition, memory, and thought

> **4.** Signs and symptoms include:
>> **a.** Forgetfulness, decreased judgment, personality changes, behavioral changes, loss of short-term memory, and speech and language problems
>> **b.** In terminal stages, loss of ability to perform ADLs, seizures, delusions, paranoia, depression, and inability to recognize loved ones
>> **c.** Death usually results from complications of immobility

C. Nursing assessment

1. Assessment includes: mental status, memory (short- and long-term), ability to make decisions or plans, ability to calculate, speech, energy level, mood, sleep patterns, initiative and motivation, VS, indications of gastrointestinal (GI) or urinary problems (anorexia, dysphagia, urinary or fecal incontinence); emotional status; skin assessment for trauma

2. Diagnostic tests: no specific tests are available for diagnosis, MRI, positron emission tomography (PET), and single photon emission computed tomography (SPECT) scans support diagnosis

D. Nursing management

1. Medications include acetylcholinesterese inhibitors such as tacrine (Cognex), donazepil hydrochloride (Aricept), galantamine (Reminyl), and rivastigmine (Exelon)

2. Client education should include memory aids, diet, and safety

3. Plans should be made with family present for support measures and safety issues

4. Assist with reality orientation: repeat caregivers' names on a regular basis, use written instructions and directions, large-face clocks, orient client as needed, use familiar objects and memory aids

5. Be consistent, use simple instructions, avoid rushing

6. Allow client to perform ADLs as long as possible, assisting as necessary

7. Monitor fluid and nutritional status

8. Involve family and multidisciplinary team to determine whether client can safely remain at home or when placement in a specialty setting, such as an Alzheimer's unit, is needed

Case Study

F. J. is an elderly man with newly diagnosed Parkinson's disease who has just been admitted to an extended-care facility. He is admitted, reluctantly, by his family who cannot care for him at home where he lives alone. F. J. does not feel he needs to be admitted and wants his family to leave him alone.

1. What signs and symptoms should the nurse anticipate?

2. What nursing diagnosis will be the highest priority?

3. When will be the best time to schedule his physical therapy session?

4. When it takes him a long time to get dressed in the morning, the nurse offers assistance. He becomes very upset. How should the nurse handle this?

5. What are some specific instructions the nurse should give him to assist with his mobility problems?

For suggested responses, see page 534.

POSTTEST

1 A young female diagnosed with multiple sclerosis (MS) has just discovered she is also pregnant. She and her husband have been trying to conceive for several years and are very excited. What client education should the nurse provide to the client concerning her disease and pregnancy?

1. Immediately report weakness that progresses upward in the extremities
2. Report a change in level of consciousness, severe headache, or slow pulse
3. Recognize that a sore/stiff neck and pain when the neck is flexed are critical signs to report
4. Immediately report spasticity, weakness, or visual changes

2 A client has seizure activity that is continuous in nature. The seizures subside and then immediately resume and continue. The client's color is getting worse. The nurse has standing orders and identifies the need to treat this client as ordered for:

1. Anticonvulsant syndrome.
2. Status epilepticus.
3. Brain herniation.
4. Syphilitic posturing.

3 Which of the following assessment findings should concern the nurse in a 35-year-old client with an intracranial hematoma? Select all that apply.

1. Hamstring pain when the hip and knee are flexed and then extended
2. Dorsiflexion of the big toe and fanning of the other toes when stroking the bottom of the foot upward
3. Muscle aches and cramping, especially at night
4. Cogwheel and lead pipe rigidity
5. Headache, drowsiness, and confusion

4 After a client undergoes magnetic resonance imaging (MRI) to rule out an expanding brain lesion, the nurse prepares the client for a lumbar puncture. The nurse would include which information in discussion with the client?

1. Risk of paralysis because the needle is inserted through the spinal cord
2. Maintaining a full bladder in case a catheterized specimen is needed
3. Maintaining bed rest for a few hours after procedure
4. Directions to straighten the legs slowly during procedure

5 The ambulatory clinic nurse assesses a client who reports the presence of a pounding headache. The client is known to have a T4 level spinal cord injury that occurred some time ago. The nurse should first assess for:

1. Sinus infection.
2. Spinal shock.
3. Upper motor neuron deficit.
4. Autonomic dysreflexia.

6 The nurse plans to prevent corneal abrasion in the client with myasthenia gravis by taking which of the following actions?

1. Applying saline soaks every shift
2. Instilling artificial tears in the eyes every one to two hours
3. Ensuring the client's contact lenses are on while awake
4. Providing sunglasses when sunlight is entering the room

7 To reduce risks for meningitis, the nurse's best instruction to an older adult client is to do which of the following?

1. Avoid being in any situations in which there are large crowds
2. Get pneumococcal pneumonia, influenza, and meningococcal vaccinations
3. Drink at least 2,000 mL fluids per day
4. Exercise 15 to 30 minutes most days of the week

8 The nurse working on a neurological nursing unit overhears that a client will be scheduled for plasmapheresis. The nurse concludes that this discussion is most likely applying to clients with which of the following diagnoses? Select all that apply.

1. Meningitis
2. Parkinson's disease
3. Myasthenia gravis
4. Amyotrophic lateral sclerosis
5. Guillain-Barré syndrome

9 The client with newly diagnosed Parkinson's disease states, "I just don't think I can handle having Parkinson's disease." The nurse's best first response is:

1. "You are really feeling overwhelmed, aren't you?"
2. "I am sure you can. A lot of other people do."
3. "What do you think will be the hardest thing to handle?"
4. "The entire health care team will help you manage the disease."

10 A client is admitted to the Emergency Department with acute onset of loss of sensation and weakness in the left side. What other symptoms would alert the nurse to the presence of a stroke (cerebrovascular accident or CVA) or transient ischemic attack (TIA)? Select all that apply.

1. Difficulty speaking
2. Hyperglycemia and history of type 2 diabetes
3. Loss of coordination and trouble walking
4. Sudden difficulty with vision
5. Facial weakness and an asymmetrical smile

➤ *See pages 152–153 for Answers & Rationales.*

ANSWERS & RATIONALES

Pretest

1 **Answer: 3** Although a ventilator is not absolutely required for spinal cord injury below the level of C3, the innervation of intercostal muscles is affected. Hemorrhage and cord swelling extends the level of injury and deficit, making it likely that this client could need a ventilator temporarily. The client will also need to be on cervical traction but may not yet be ready for a halo brace. A kinetic bed is not the priority at this time. A catheterization tray will be needed but that has lesser priority than the ventilator to maintain an airway when planning care.
Cognitive Level: Analysis **Client Need:** Physiological Integrity: Physiological Adaptation **Integrated Process:** Nursing Process: Planning **Content Area:** Adult Health: Neurological **Strategy:** Focus on the level of spinal cord injury and recall that cervical injury increases the risk of airway impairment. Anticipate this type of complication as life threatening to choose the option that protects the airway over the others. **Reference:** LeMone, P., & Burke, K. (2008). *Medical-surgical nursing: Critical thinking in client care* (4th ed.). Upper Saddle River, NJ: Pearson/ Prentice Hall, p. 1604.

2 **Answer: 2** Keeping the head of the bed elevated to 30 degrees promotes venous drainage from the brain, which is important in decreasing intracranial pressure (ICP). Alignment of the head prevents obstruction of the jugular veins. Obstruction would impede venous drainage and raise the ICP. Although the airway is also maintained, it is not the reason for the positioning. This position does not prevent pulmonary embolism. The client would not be positioned on the side to obtain ICP readings.
Cognitive Level: Application **Client Need:** Physiological Integrity: Physiological Adaptation **Integrated Process:**

Teaching/Learning **Content Area:** Adult Health: Neurological **Strategy:** Recall that proper positioning of a client often involves principles of gravity, particularly when it affects blood flow. With this in mind, select the option that reflects this theme. **Reference:** LeMone, P., & Burke, K. (2008). *Medical-surgical nursing: Critical thinking in client care* (4th ed.). Upper Saddle River, NJ: Pearson/ Prentice Hall, p. 1541.

3 **Answer: 1** Momentary loss of consciousness followed by a lucid period and rapid deterioration is a classic picture resulting from a torn cerebral artery, producing an epidural bleed. This pattern of symptoms is not displayed with the conditions listed in options 2, 3, and 4.
Cognitive Level: Application **Client Need:** Physiological Integrity: Physiological Adaptation **Integrated Process:** Nursing Process: Implementation **Content Area:** Adult Health: Neurological **Strategy:** Use the history of head trauma as a clue. Eliminate wrong options using pathophysiology and the pattern of symptoms presented.
Reference: Porth, C. M. (2005). *Pathophysiology: Concepts of altered health states* (7th ed.). Philadelphia, PA: Lippincott Williams & Wilkins, p. 1238.

4 **Answer: 4** The period after the clonic phase of a seizure is the postictal period. Typically, the client slowly regains consciousness, moving from a relaxed, quiet state to confusion or disorientation on awakening. The nurse does not change a medication dose without an order (option 3). Although it is appropriate to notify the physician of seizure activity, it is unnecessary to do so regarding a postictal state (option 2). It is unnecessary to call the rapid response team, since the client's condition is not quickly deteriorating (option 1).
Cognitive Level: Application **Client Need:** Safe, Effective Care Environment: Management of Care **Integrated Process:** Nursing Process: Implementation **Content Area:**

Adult Health: Neurological **Strategy:** Recall the usual findings in a client following a tonic-clonic (grand mal) seizure to make the appropriate selection. **Reference:** LeMone, P., & Burke, K. (2008). *Medical-surgical nursing: Critical thinking in client care* (4th ed.). Upper Saddle River, NJ: Pearson/Prentice Hall, p. 1549.

5 Answers: 1, 2, 5 Protective pads/undergarments should be used only after all other treatment modes have been tried. Early dependency on incontinence products may decrease motivation to seek evaluation and treatment. The client, with the same risks as for the first stroke, may have another. Teaching is needed to control the modifiable risk factors, such as cigarette smoking. Walking and safety measures are desirable.

Cognitive Level: Application **Client Need:** Health Promotion and Maintenance **Integrated Process:** Nursing Process: Evaluation **Content Area:** Adult Health: Neurological **Strategy:** The wording of the question indicates the correct options will be incorrect statements. Note the presence of critical words such as *lifetime supply* in option 1 and *never* in option 2 and select these options. Then note that cigarette smoking adds to the risk of recurrence of stroke to select this option also. **Reference:** LeMone, P., & Burke, K. (2008). *Medical-surgical nursing: Critical thinking in client care* (4th ed.). Upper Saddle River, NJ: Pearson/Prentice Hall, pp. 1591–1592.

6 Answer: 3 Clients with meningitis will be less able to protect themselves from both internal and external injury. Providing cognitive stimulation and increasing cardiac output are contraindicated with meningitis. Enhancing coping skills may be a focus if the client has residual effects from meningitis but is not a major focus during the acute phase.

Cognitive Level: Application **Client Need:** Safe, Effective Care Environment: Safety and Infection Control **Integrated Process:** Nursing Process: Planning **Content Area:** Adult Health: Neurological **Strategy:** Use Maslow's hierarchy of needs to address physiological needs before psychosocial needs to eliminate option 1. Use knowledge of factors that increase intracranial pressure to eliminate options 2 and 4. **Reference:** LeMone, P., & Burke, K. (2008). *Medical-surgical nursing: Critical thinking in client care* (4th ed.). Upper Saddle River, NJ: Pearson/Prentice Hall, p6. 1564,1567–1569.

7 Answers: 1, 3, 5 Predisposing events to Guillain-Barré syndrome are often a viral infection or immunization (option 1). Lower extremity weakness or paralysis that progresses upward is classic in Guillain-Barré syndrome. Preventing problems from immobility and altered respiratory function is important (option 3). Autonomic nervous system involvement may be manifested by bradycardia and hypotension (option 5). Fa-

tigue and low blood glucose (option 2) are not usually seen, nor are tremors or seizures (option 4).

Cognitive Level: Analysis **Client Need:** Physiological Integrity: Physiological Adaptation **Integrated Process:** Nursing Process: Assessment **Content Area:** Adult Health: Neurological **Strategy:** Begin the nursing process with assessment to eliminate option 2 first. Note that the paralysis is ascending upward to eliminate option 4, which involves the brain. **Reference:** LeMone, P., & Burke, K. (2008). *Medical-surgical nursing: Critical thinking in client care* (4th ed.). Upper Saddle River, NJ: Pearson/Prentice Hall, pp. 1653–1655.

8 Answer: 3 The client should know the signs of crisis and should report them immediately. There is often more fatigue and weakness later in the day than in the morning, so the client should plan important activities for early in the day. It may be easier to eat three small meals with snacks because chewing may cause fatigue.

Cognitive Level: Application **Client Need:** Physiological Integrity: Physiological Adaptation **Integrated Process:** Nursing Process: Implementation **Content Area:** Adult Health: Neurological **Strategy:** The critical word in the stem of the question is *priority*. Use nursing knowledge and the process of elimination noting the corresponding critical word *crisis* in the correct option. **Reference:** LeMone, P., & Burke, K. (2008). *Medical-surgical nursing: Critical thinking in client care* (4th ed.). Upper Saddle River, NJ: Pearson/Prentice Hall, pp. 1647–1652.

9 Answer: 3 The resting or nonintentional tremor may be controlled with purposeful movement, such as holding an object. Deep-breathing, a warm bath, and diazepam will promote relaxation but are not specific interventions for the tremor.

Cognitive Level: Application **Client Need:** Physiological Integrity: Physiological Adaptation **Integrated Process:** Teaching/Learning **Content Area:** Adult Health: Neurological **Strategy:** Note that three options are focused on relaxation. The correct option is different. **Reference:** LeMone, P., & Burke, K. (2008). *Medical-surgical nursing: Critical thinking in client care* (4th ed.). Upper Saddle River, NJ: Pearson/Prentice Hall, pp. 1640–1642.

10 Answers: 2, 4 It is important to always believe the client's report and rating of pain. The client tolerated the last full dose of medication so he should be given a dose now without delay. The nurse would reassess the client's pain level within 30 minutes of administering pain medication depending on peak action time of the drug. The pain level would be recorded at 9, not 5. It is unnecessary to initiate PCA because the analgesic last used was effective.

Cognitive Level: Analysis **Client Need:** Safe, Effective Care Environment: Management of Care **Integrated Process:**

Nursing Process: Implementation **Content Area:** Adult Health: Neurological **Strategy:** The level of pain is subjective data. Follow the order for the drug if it is safe for the client and appropriate. Identify the opposite options as incorrect and eliminate the PCA option as unnecessary with the information in the question. **Reference:** LeMone, P., & Burke, K. (2008). *Medical-surgical nursing: Critical thinking in client care* (4th ed.). Upper Saddle River, NJ: Pearson/Prentice Hall, p. 181.

Posttest

1 **Answer: 4** Stresses such as pregnancy can increase the chance of an exacerbation of MS. Signs of an exacerbation are spasticity, weakness, or visual changes. Option 1 indicates Guillain-Barré syndrome; option 2 indicates increased intracranial pressure or hematoma; option 3 indicates meningitis.
Cognitive Level: Analysis **Client Need:** Physiological Integrity: Physiological Adaptation **Integrated Process:** Teaching/Learning **Content Area:** Adult Health: Neurological **Strategy:** Eliminate the options that are appropriate for neurological problems other than MS. **Reference:** LeMone, P., & Burke, K. (2008). *Medical-surgical nursing: Critical thinking in client care* (4th ed.). Upper Saddle River, NJ: Pearson/Prentice Hall, pp. 1626–1627.

2 **Answer: 2** When seizure activity becomes continuous and repetitive, respirations are affected and the progression to a state of status epilepticus is life-threatening. Nursing interventions address prevention of hypoxia, acidosis, hypoglycemia, hyperthermia, and exhaustion.
Cognitive Level: Application **Client Need:** Physiological Integrity: Physiological Adaptation **Integrated Process:** Nursing Process: Analysis **Content Area:** Adult Health: Neurological **Strategy:** Make an association between the term *seizure* in the stem of the question and *epilepticus* in the correct option. **Reference:** LeMone, P., & Burke, K. (2008). *Medical-surgical nursing: Critical thinking in client care* (4th ed.). Upper Saddle River, NJ: Pearson/ Prentice Hall, p. 1549.

3 **Answers: 1, 2, 5** A positive Kernig's sign, described in option 1, is common in intracranial hematomas. Option 2 is a positive Babinski, expected with a hematoma. Option 5 is indicative of acute subdural hematoma. Option 3 is common in many illnesses; option 4 is specific to Parkinson's disease.
Cognitive Level: Analysis **Client Need:** Physiological Integrity: Physiological Adaptation **Integrated Process:** Nursing Process: Assessment **Content Area:** Adult Health: Neurological **Strategy:** Choose options that reflect an acute central nervous system problem. With this in mind, eliminate option 3 because it is vague and is worse at night, and option 4, which is classic for Parkin-

son's syndrome. **Reference:** LeMone, P., & Burke, K. (2008). *Medical-surgical nursing: Critical thinking in client care* (4th ed.). Upper Saddle River, NJ: Pearson/ Prentice Hall, pp. 1558, 1561.

4 **Answer: 3** The spinal needle is inserted into the area below the spinal cord eliminating the likelihood of paralysis. The client must maintain the knees to chest position until completion of the lumbar puncture. Because cerebrospinal fluid (CSF) has been removed during the lumbar puncture, time must be allowed for production and replacement of the CSF. Smaller gauge needles are now used for lumbar punctures, reducing the loss of CSF and allowing the client to move and ambulate sooner with less risk of headache.
Cognitive Level: Application **Client Need:** Physiological Integrity: Reduction of Risk Potential **Integrated Process:** Nursing Process: Implementation **Content Area:** Adult Health: Neurological **Strategy:** Note that the wording of the question indicates that the correct answer is also a true statement. Use nursing knowledge and the process of eliminate to make a selection. Recall that bed rest with the head positioned according to the type of dye used (oil or water based) will help minimize meningeal irritation and subsequent headache. **Reference:** LeMone, P., & Burke, K. (2008). *Medical-surgical nursing: Critical thinking in client care* (4th ed.). Upper Saddle River, NJ: Pearson/Prentice Hall, pp. 1515–1516.

5 **Answer: 4** Spinal cord injury at or above the level of T6 can experience an exaggerated sympathetic response, seen only after recovery from spinal shock. Autonomic dysreflexia is a clinical emergency. Without prompt treatment severe hypertension progresses and coma or death can occur.
Cognitive Level: Analysis **Client Need:** Physiological Integrity: Physiological Adaptation **Integrated Process:** Nursing Process: Assessment **Content Area:** Adult Health: Neurological **Strategy:** Assessment for life-threatening complications such as autonomic dysreflexia is always a priority. Note the critical words *some time ago* to discriminate between the correct option and spinal shock. **Reference:** Porth, C. M. (2005). *Pathophysiology: Concepts of altered health states* (7th ed.). Philadelphia, PA: Lippincott Williams & Wilkins, p. 1222.

6 **Answer: 2** Corneal abrasion in the client with myasthenia gravis is caused by dryness of the cornea from inability to close the eyelids and blink. It can be prevented by application of artificial tears every one to two hours. Saline soaks and use of contact lenses or sunglasses are of no use.
Cognitive Level: Application **Client Need:** Physiological Integrity: Physiological Adaptation **Integrated Process:** Nursing Process: Planning **Content Area:** Adult Health:

Neurological **Strategy:** Apply the pathophysiology of muscle weakness to the face and eyelids. Determine which action best prevents corneal trauma. **Reference:** LeMone, P., & Burke, K. (2008). *Medical-surgical nursing: Critical thinking in client care* (4th ed.). Upper Saddle River, NJ: Pearson/Prentice Hall, pp. 1647–1652.

7 **Answer: 2** Meningitis bacteria or viruses often gain entry into the cerebrospinal fluid secondary to an upper respiratory tract infection. Options 1, 3, and 4 are generally healthy practices for the elderly client but not specific health promotion for prevention of meningitis. Immunizations are recommended.
Cognitive Level: Application **Client Need:** Health Promotion and Maintenance **Integrated Process:** Teaching/Learning **Content Area:** Adult Health: Neurological **Strategy:** Note which action specifically prevents the infection. Keep in mind the age of the client and the presence of the word *any* in option 1. **Reference:** LeMone, P., & Burke, K. (2008). *Medical-surgical nursing: Critical thinking in client care* (4th ed.). Upper Saddle River, NJ: Pearson/ Prentice Hall, pp. 1567–1569.

8 **Answers: 3, 5** Plasmapheresis is performed to remove autoantibodies that attack the myelin sheaths of motor and sensory nerves in Guillain-Barré and attack the acetylcholine receptors at the neuromuscular junction in myasthenia gravis. The health problems listed in the other options have not been identified as being autoimmune disorders.
Cognitive Level: Analysis **Client Need:** Physiological Integrity: Physiological Adaptation **Integrated Process:** Nursing Process: Implementation **Content Area:** Adult Health: Neurological **Strategy:** The core issue of the question is knowledge of plasmapheresis as a treatment option and the underlying pathophysiology of the health

problems listed. Use this information and the process of elimination to make a selection. **Reference:** LeMone, P., & Burke, K. (2008). *Medical-surgical nursing: Critical thinking in client care* (4th ed.). Upper Saddle River, NJ: Pearson/Prentice Hall, pp. 1651, 1654.

9 **Answer: 1** The nurse should first encourage the client experiencing a loss to express his feelings. Option 1 acknowledges the client's feelings, is open-ended, and promotes further discussion.
Cognitive Level: Analysis **Client Need:** Psychosocial Integrity **Integrated Process:** Communication and Documentation **Content Area:** Adult Health: Neurological **Strategy:** First recall information about the course of Parkinson's disease. Then apply therapeutic communication techniques and note the clue word *first* in the stem of the question. **Reference:** LeMone, P., & Burke, K. (2008). *Medical-surgical nursing: Critical thinking in client care* (4th ed.). Upper Saddle River, NJ: Pearson/Prentice Hall, pp. 1640–1642.

10 **Answers: 1, 3, 4, 5** Weakness, numbness, confusion, difficulty speaking, trouble with coordination and ambulation, and visual difficulties are warning signs of a CVA or TIA. Although uncontrolled type 2 diabetes increases the risk of stroke, its presence does not indicate a stroke.
Cognitive Level: Application **Client Need:** Physiological Integrity: Physiological Adaptation **Integrated Process:** Nursing Process: Assessment **Content Area:** Adult Health: Neurological **Strategy:** Identify the neurological manifestations of a cerebral problem and use the process of elimination to make your selection(s). **Reference:** LeMone, P., & Burke, K. (2008). *Medical-surgical nursing: Critical thinking in client care* (4th ed.). Upper Saddle River, NJ: Pearson/Prentice Hall, pp. 1582–1583.

References

Adams, M., Holland, L., Bostwick, P. (2008). *Pharmacology for nurses: A pathophysiologic approach* (2nd ed.). Upper Saddle River, NJ: Prentice Hall.

Ball, J., & Binder, R. (2006). *Pediatric nursing: Caring for children* (4th ed.). Upper Saddle River, NJ: Prentice Hall.

Black, J., & Hawks, J. (2005). *Medical-surgical nursing: Clinical management for positive outcomes.* Philadelphia: W.B. Saunders, pp. 2073–2201.

Corbett, J. V. (2004). *Laboratory tests and diagnostics procedures* (6th ed.). Upper Saddle River, NJ: Prentice Hall.

Ignatavicius, D., & Workman, M. (2006). *Medical-surgical nursing: Critical thinking for collaborative care* (5th ed.). Philadelphia: W.B. Saunders.

LeMone, P., & Burke, K. M. (2008). *Medical-surgical nursing: Critical thinking in client care* (4th ed.). Upper Saddle River, NJ: Prentice Hall.

Lewis, S. M., Heitkemper, M. M., & Dirksen, S. R. (2004). *Medical surgical nursing: Assessment and management of clinical problems* (6th ed.). St. Louis, MO: Mosby, pp. 1491–1631.

McCaffery, M. (1999). *Pain: Clinical manual* (2nd ed.). St. Louis, MO: Mosby, pp. 15–34, 36–102, 121–122.

McCance, K. L., & Huether, S. E. (Eds.). (2006). *Pathophysiology: The biologic basis for disease in adults and children* (5th ed.). St. Louis, MO: Mosby.

Porth, C. M. (2005). *Pathophysiology: Concepts of altered health states* (7th ed.). Philadelphia, PA: Lippincott Williams & Wilkins.

Venes, D., & Thomas, C. L. (2006). *Taber's cyclopedic medical dictionary* (20th ed.). Philadelphia: F.A. Davis.

ANSWERS & RATIONALES

5

Musculoskeletal Health Problems

Chapter Outline

Risk Factors Associated with Musculoskeletal Health Problems

Osteoarthritis (OA)

Rheumatoid Arthritis (RA)

Gouty Arthritis

Osteomyelitis

Paget's Disease (Osteitis Deformans)

Muscular Dystrophy (MD)

Fibromyalgia

Bone Tumors

Systemic Lupus Erythematosus (SLE)

Scleroderma (Systemic Sclerosis)

Fractures

Compartment Syndrome

Osteoporosis

NCLEX-RN® Test Prep

Use the CD-ROM enclosed with this book to access additional practice opportunities.

Objectives

➤ Define key terms associated with musculoskeletal health problems.

➤ Identify risk factors associated with the development of musculoskeletal health problems.

➤ Explain the common etiologies of musculoskeletal health problems.

➤ Describe the pathophysiologic processes associated with specific musculoskeletal health problems.

➤ Distinguish between normal and abnormal musculoskeletal findings obtained from nursing assessment.

➤ Prioritize nursing interventions associated with specific musculoskeletal health problems.

Review at a Glance

ankylosis joint immobility or fixation secondary to an underlying disease process

articular cartilage connective tissue covering the epiphysis where joint surfaces meet; it acts as a cushion between joint surfaces

bone remodeling formation of new bone by osteoblasts and removal of old bone by osteoclasts; this process is regulated by actions of parathyroid hormone, calcitonin, and vitamin D

Bouchard's node formation of hard nodules in proximal interphalangeal (PIP) joints resulting in joint deformity characteristic of osteoporosis

bouttonière deformities joint deformity associated with rheumatoid arthritis, characterized by flexion of PIP joint and hyperextension of distal interphalangeal (DIP) joint

calcinosis abnormal deposits of calcium salts on skin

diaphysis long portion or shaft of long bones; inner portion of diaphysis contains medullary cavity which is comprised of bone marrow; this is surrounded by cortical bone

epiphysis proximal and distal end of long bones, comprised of cancellous bone surrounded by cortical bone

fascia fibrous connective tissue responsible for supporting and connecting structures of musculoskeletal system

Heberden's node formation of a hard nodule in distal interphalangeal (DIP) joints resulting in joint deformity characteristic of osteoarthritis (OA)

metaphysis located in area of flaring between epiphysis and diaphysis of long bones; it contains growth plates that are responsible for longitudinal growth of bones during growth years

osteolysis softening and breakdown of bone

osteophytes outgrowth of bony tissue commonly referred to as spurs

pannus vascular granulation tissue that forms in synovial membrane of clients with rheumatoid arthritis (RA); is responsible for destruction of bones and surrounding tissue in affected joints

periosteum membrane covering bone, except in areas where articular cartilage is present; it contains nerve, lymph, and blood vessels

rheumatoid nodules subcutaneous masses found in 20% of clients with rheumatoid arthritis (RA); characterized as firm, nontender masses usually found on olecranon bursae or along extensor surface of forearm

scleradactyly scleroderma that is localized within fingers

swan neck joint deformity associated with rheumatoid arthritis (RA), characterized by hyperextension of PIP joint with flexion of DIP joints

telangiectasis small, dilated blood vessels with a bright-red center point and spiderlike branches that may occur in clients with scleroderma

ulnar drift joint deformity characteristic of rheumatoid arthritis (RA)

PRETEST

1 The nurse has completed instructions on health maintenance for a client diagnosed with osteoarthritis. The nurse concludes that the client understood the instructions if the client states that participation in which of the following sports would be beneficial?

1. Tennis
2. Jogging
3. Swimming
4. Volleyball

2 The nurse would document which of the following expected health history and physical assessment data findings on an adult client with rheumatoid arthritis (RA)? Select all that apply.

1. Heberden's nodes
2. Morning stiffness lasting longer than 30 minutes
3. Asymmetric joint swelling
4. Swan neck deformities
5. Weight loss, anorexia, fatigue, and weakness

3 A client with a diagnosis of gouty arthritis is receiving medications to treat an acute attack. What action by the nurse will facilitate the excretion of urates and help prevent uric acid renal calculi?

1. Encourage client to eat acid-forming foods to acidify the urine
2. Give liberal fluids as tolerated to maintain a urine output of 2000 mL or more
3. Restrict fluids to 1000 mL in 24 hours
4. Keep client on bed rest with the affected joint elevated

4 Which of the following interventions may be included by the nurse in a plan of care for a client with acute osteomyelitis? Select all that apply.

1. Apply heat compresses to affected area
2. Immobilize affected area in functional position
3. Administer narcotic analgesics as ordered for severe pain
4. Administer acetaminophen (Tylenol) as ordered for mild pain
5. Maintain strict handwashing practices

5 The nurse would interpret that which laboratory or diagnostic test data would be most significant in the client with Paget's disease?

1. Elevated white blood count (WBC)
2. Elevated erythrocyte sedimentation rate (ESR)
3. Positive tissue biopsy for *Staphylococcus*
4. Elevated serum alkaline phosphatase

6 The nurse considers that which of the following clients seen in the ambulatory clinic is at greatest risk for developing an osteosarcoma?

1. Male, age 42
2. Female, age 59
3. Female, age 35
4. Male, age 15

7 The nurse makes it a priority to take a drug history in a client with systemic lupus erythematosus (SLE), making note of use of which of the following drugs?

1. Procainamide (Procan SR)
2. Acetylsalicylic acid (aspirin, ASA)
3. Diazepam (Valium)
4. Azathioprine (Imuran)

8 To prevent occurrences of Raynaud's phenomenon, what instructions should the nurse give to a client diagnosed with systemic sclerosis (scleroderma)?

1. Wear gloves if the temperature is cold
2. Perform range-of-motion exercises daily
3. Limit sodium intake
4. Avoid warm temperatures

9 A client, viewing X-rays of a healing bone fracture, asks the nurse if the bone will ever be normal again. The nurse's response will be based on what knowledge of the remodeling phase of bone healing?

1. Callus formation occurs
2. Callus is replaced with mature bone
3. Osteoclasts resorb excess callus to return the bone to its original shape
4. Proliferation of osteoblast and fibroblasts occurs within the hematoma at the fracture site

10 The nurse is caring for a client who had a cast applied to immobilize a tibia that sustained a fracture six hours ago. The client reports severe pain in the leg that is unrelieved by the opioid analgesic. The nurse suspects that what cycle of events may be causing compartment syndrome and jeopardizing the limb?

1. Increased pressure within tissues results from excessive edema at fracture site, compressing the vascular network
2. Nerves are damaged by trauma, and narcotics will not relieve pain
3. Peripheral pulses will become accelerated to compensate for inadequate oxygen supply to injured tissue
4. Injured fascia is elastic and expands with fluid so the cast becomes too tight, causing pain and compromising circulation

➤ *See pages 182–183 for Answers & Rationales.*

I. RISK FACTORS ASSOCIATED WITH MUSCULOSKELETAL HEALTH PROBLEMS

A. **Osteoarthritis (OA):** obesity, age, gender (affects genders equally up to age 55, incidence increases in women after this time), heredity

B. **Rheumatoid arthritis (RA):** gender (occurs 2 to 3 times more frequently in females); age (onset usually occurs during middle age; however, it can occur at any time); possible genetic link

C. **Gouty arthritis:** gender (increased frequency in men, may occur postmenopausal or in women with a genetic link), obesity, heavy alcohol intake, familial trait, disease states (malignancies, diabetes mellitus [DM], kidney disease, hypertension [HTN], acidosis); clients taking the following medications may experience drug-induced gout—thiazide diuretics, cytotoxic drugs, low-dose acetylsalicylic acid (aspirin), and ethambutol (Myambutol)

D. **Osteomyelitis**

1. Hematogenous: children under age 10 with recent history of throat, ear, or skin infections; debilitated clients with recurrent upper respiratory infection (URIs), urinary tract infections (UTIs), and skin infections; and intravenous (IV) drug-abusers

2. Direct entry: recent history of puncture wound, gunshot wound, fracture, surgery

E. **Paget's disease:** adults over 40 years of age, more common in males

F. **Muscular dystrophy (MD):** male children with family history

G. **Fibromyalgia:** more common in women; stress

H. **Bone tumors:** genetic link, exposure to chemotherapy or radiation (osteosarcomas), Paget's disease

I. **Systemic lupus erythematosus (SLE):** women of childbearing years, family history, ethnicity (African Americans, Asians, and Hispanics)

J. **Scleroderma:** women of childbearing years; African American women; coal miners; occupational exposure to polyvinyl chloride, epoxy resins, and aromatic hydrocarbons; genetic link probable

K. **Fractures:** trauma, active participation in sports, elderly clients at risk for falls, clients with bone disease

L. **Compartment syndrome:** more frequent in crushing injuries and fractures of forearm or lower leg

M. **Osteoporosis:** postmenopausal women; ethnicity (Caucasian and Asians); clients with endocrine disorders such as hyperparathyroidism, hyperthyroidism, Cushing's syndrome, and diabetes mellitus; use of the following substances: glucocorticoids, caffeine, nicotine, tetracycline, and aluminum-containing antacids; sedentary lifestyle; both genders over 80 years of age

II. OSTEOARTHRITIS (OA)

A. **Overview**

1. Defined as a form of arthritis with progressive destruction of cartilage in both synovial joints and vertebrae

2. Characteristics

a. Most common form of arthritis, also referred to as *degenerative arthritis*

b. Chronic, progressive, nonsystemic disease

c. Characterized by degeneration of **articular cartilage** (connective tissue covering the **epiphysis** [proximal and distal end of long bones] where joint surfaces meet) in hands: proximal interphalangeal (PIP) and distal interphalangeal (DIP) joints, feet (metatarsophalangeal [MTP] joints), shoulder, lumbar and cervical spine, hips, and knees

    3. Classifications and causes

        a. *Primary idiopathic:* unknown etiology, however, risk factors usually present

        b. *Secondary disorder:* OA resulting from conditions that predispose a client to degenerative changes in joints, such as rheumatoid arthritis, diabetes mellitus, congenital deformities, joint trauma, or repetitive movement of a joint related to participation in sports or work activities

B. Pathophysiology

    1. Primary idiopathic OA: articular cartilage decreases friction during joint movement and displaces force of workload onto subchondral bone, thereby decreasing stress within joint itself

        a. Type II collagen, normally present in healthy articular cartilage, contains proteoglycans; proteoglycans are macromolecules that provide elasticity and stiffness to articular cartilage allowing it to resist compression

        b. It is thought that clients with primary idiopathic OA have some type of malfunction in production of proteoglycans; body attempts to compensate by producing more proteoglycans and collagen; however, these substances are destroyed faster than they can be synthesized

        c. Type II collagen is eventually replaced with Type I collagen (normally present in skin and tendons); as Type I collagen continues to replace Type II collagen with disease progression, composition of articular cartilage is altered, and it is unable to perform its original function

        d. In response to changes in the articular cartilage, synovitis (inflammation of a synovial joint) often occurs within joint and subchondral bone responds to cartilage damage by producing **osteophytes** (outgrowth of bony tissue commonly referred to as spurs)

    2. Secondary OA

        a. Repetitive movements that apply excessive workloads to joints will result in breakdown of cartilage and changes in subchondral bone

        b. Ability of cartilage to lubricate joint becomes depleted and friction increases between joint surfaces during joint motion

        c. The outcome is similar to that of primary idiopathic OA; joint narrowing occurs with cartilage breakdown, and synovitis and formation of osteophytes occurs with disease progression

    3. Signs and symptoms

        a. Dull, aching pain in affected joint with movement and weight bearing and relieved with rest

        b. Numbness or tingling at night, associated with disease progression secondary to nerve damage

        c. Crepitus with joint movement

        d. Edema and stiffness in affected joint

        e. Decreased range of motion (ROM) and ability to participate in activities of daily living (ADLs)

        f. Joint deformities: **Heberden's nodes** (formation of hard nodules in DIP joints, resulting in joint deformity) and **Bouchard's nodes** (formation of hard nodules in PIP joints, resulting in joint deformity)

        g. Symptoms vary in severity and may range from mild intermittent discomfort to complete disability

C. Nursing assessment

1. Assessment includes baseline ROM, participation in ADLs and work/leisure activities, pain assessment, safety with ambulation, baseline weight and dietary habits, presence of Heberden's nodes and Bouchard's nodes

2. Diagnostic tests

   a. X-ray: loss of joint cartilage, narrowing of space between adjacent bones, and formation of osteophytes in progressive disease states

   b. Eosinophil sedimentation rate (ESR): normal, slight increase with synovitis, used to differentiate other forms of arthritis

D. Nursing management

1. Medications include acetaminophen (Tylenol) preferred or acetylsalicylic acid (aspirin), corticosteroids (intra-articular injection or other forms), nonsteroidal antiinflammatory drugs (NSAIDs)

2. Instruct on weight reduction

3. Collaborate with physical therapy (PT) regarding an aerobic exercise program to reduce and eliminate strain on joints: swimming, biking, walking, water aerobics

4. Collaborate with occupational therapy (OT) regarding assistive devices for ADLs

5. Implement and assess effectiveness of pain relief measures

   a. Teach action and side effects of medications used for pain control

   b. Application of heat before exercising and application of cold after exercising

   c. Splints designed to immobilize joint

   d. Cotton gloves at night

   e. Paraffin dips

   f. Warm water soaks

   g. Neck collar and lumbar corsets for OA of vertebrae

   h. Firm mattress for sleeping

6. Preoperative teaching as required for surgery:

   a. Arthroscopy (use of an arthroscope to examine interior of a joint)

   b. Total or partial joint replacements for OA of hip and knee

   c. Joint fusions for OA of cervical spine

7. Instruct on safety in home (see Box 5-1)

III. RHEUMATOID ARTHRITIS (RA)

A. Overview

1. Defined as a chronic, progressive, systemic, autoimmune disease with inflammation of joints and deformity

---

Box 5-1	➤ Eliminate throw rugs in home.
Home Safety Tips for Clients with Musculoskeletal Health Problems	➤ Use good body mechanics when performing ADLs and work/leisure activities.
	➤ Use a shower chair and hand rails when bathing.
	➤ Use cane and walker as directed to decrease workload on hips and knees.
	➤ Use well-fitting, supportive shoes when ambulating.

2. Characteristics

   a. Onset is insidious and characterized by periods of remissions and exacerbations

   b. Characterized by chronic inflammation of bilateral joints and surrounding structures; multiple joints are usually involved

3. Unknown etiology; however, evidence supports that disease progression is related to autoimmune processes in middle age

4. Systemic complications

   a. Extrasynovial rheumatoid nodules on heart, lungs, eyes, or spleen

   b. Vasculitis

   c. Anemia

B. Pathophysiology

1. Exposure to a viral pathogen may initiate inflammatory response; immunoglobulin G (IgG) is formed in response to antigen, but for some unknown reason the body begins to produce autoantibodies (called rheumatoid factors) against IgG

   a. Rheumatoid factors combine with IgG to form immune complexes

   b. Continued presence of immune complexes within joint cavity results in chronic inflammation and destruction of articular cartilage as well as surrounding joint structures

2. Synovial membrane (located within joint capsule and responsible for producing synovial fluid to lubricate joint structures) hypertrophies and thickens secondary to chronic inflammation

   a. Blood supply to area is occluded and cellular necrosis occurs

   b. These events lead to formation of **pannus** (vascular granulation tissue that forms in synovial membrane of clients with RA)

   c. Pannus gradually extends from synovial membrane and surface of articular cartilage into joint capsule and subchondral bone causing destruction of bone

3. Fibrous adhesions and bony **ankylosis** (joint immobility or fixation secondary to an underlying disease process) occurs as involved bone is destroyed; the inflammatory process extends to support structures of bone, tendons and ligaments, and joint instability and deformities occur

4. Signs and symptoms

   a. Initially may present with vague systemic symptoms such as anorexia, weight loss, fever, and loss of energy

   b. Early disease states will present with inflammation, swelling, and decreased movement of joints in hand (PIP and MCP), feet (MTP), wrists, and elbows; as RA progresses, joints of knees, hips, and cervical spine may also be involved

   c. The American Rheumatism Association has developed diagnostic criteria for rheumatoid arthritis; evidence of four out of seven criteria must be present to confirm diagnosis (see Box 5-2)

C. Nursing assessment

1. Assessment includes low-grade temperature; decreased ROM; signs and symptoms of inflammation (tenderness, swelling, redness) involving multiple joints bilaterally; morning stiffness lasting greater than one hour; change in energy level and ability to participation in ADLs as well as work/leisure activities; pain assessment; neurological assessment (complaints of headache,

numbness, or tingling with involvement of cervical vertebrae); baseline weight and history of recent weight loss; presence of:

  a. Joint deformities

    1) Swan neck (hyperextension of PIP joints with flexion of DIP joints)

    2) Ulnar drift (joint deformity characteristic of RA)

    3) Boutonnière deformities (flexion of PIP joint and hyperextension of DIP joint)

  b. Rheumatoid nodules (firm, nontender subcutaneous masses found on olecranon bursae or extension surface of forearm) over pressure areas

2. Diagnostic tests

  a. X-ray: may show minimal changes early in disease; however, as disease progression occurs, narrowing of joint space, bone erosion, and bone deformities are evident bilaterally

  b. Serum rheumatoid factor: not exclusive for RA but positive in majority of clients

  c. Evidence of anemia with complete blood count (CBC)

  d. Elevated ESR

  e. Synovial fluid analysis: increased white blood cells (WBCs), increased turbidity, decreased viscosity

D. Nursing management

  1. Medications

    a. NSAIDs, used early in disease

    b. Systemic corticosteroids: long-term use is associated with severe side effects; they are usually utilized when NSAIDs are no longer effective

    c. Disease-modifying drugs (DMARDs): once the last drugs of choice for treatment, these drugs are now being used earlier in treatment regimen because evidence suggests that they may play a role in arresting disease progression

      1) Most drugs in this category are contraindicated in clients with a history of kidney and liver disease

      2) Drugs included in this category are auranofin (Ridaura), sulfasalazine (Azulfidine), and hydroxychloroquine (Plaquenil)

Box 5-2

Diagnostic Criteria for Rheumatoid Arthritis

➤ Morning stiffness lasting for at least 1 hour and persisting over at least 6 weeks

➤ Arthritis with swelling or effusion of three or more joints persisting for at least 6 weeks

➤ Arthritis of wrist, MCP, or PIP joints persisting for at least 6 weeks

➤ Symmetric arthritis with simultaneous involvement of corresponding joints on both sides of the body

➤ Rheumatoid nodules

➤ Positive serum rheumatoid factor

➤ Characteristic radiologic changes (erosions or decalcifications) of rheumatoid arthritis noted in hands and wrists

Source: Lemone, R.E. Burke, K. (2008). *Medical surgical nursing: Critical thinking In client care* (4th ed.). Upper Saddle River, NJ: Prentice Hall, p. 1461.

2. Instruct on disease process and treatment regimen

3. Refer to support groups including Arthritis Foundation

4. Emphasize rest to decrease joint stress

   a. Pace activities

   b. Perform activities while sitting when possible

   c. Splints for hands and wrists

   d. Relaxation techniques

   e. Guided imagery

> **▶ Practice to Pass**
>
> When providing health maintenance teaching to the client with rheumatoid arthritis (RA), what information should the nurse include regarding the best methods to increase joint mobility and maintain joint function?

5. Collaborate with physical therapist (PT) regarding therapeutic exercise program, isotonic exercises, passive ROM and active ROM exercise to maintain muscle strength and joint ROM

6. Collaborate with occupational therapist (OT) regarding assistive devices for ADLs, tips for joint protection and work simplification

7. Teach action and side effects of medications used for pain control

8. Implement and assess effectiveness of pain relief measures

   a. Medications

   b. Application of heat or cold, depending on what works for client

   c. Paraffin dips

   d. Firm mattress for sleeping and proper positioning in bed for comfort

9. Pre-operative teaching as required following surgery:

   a. Synovectomy (removal of synovial membrane)

   b. Total joint replacements for OA of hip and knee

   c. Joint fusions for RA of cervical spine

10. Instruct on home safety (refer back to Box 5-1)

11. Instruct on hazards of immobility if bedridden and teach prevention

IV. GOUTY ARTHRITIS

A. Overview

1. Defined as a metabolic disease marked by increased serum uric acid levels (hyperuricemia) and joint inflammation

2. Characteristics

   a. Not all clients with hyperuricemia will develop gouty arthritis

   b. Acute, painful episodes of monoarticular joint inflammation lasting about 10 to 14 days

   c. Acute episodes vary in frequency and are often precipitated by some stress: surgery, joint trauma, and emotional stress; it is self-limiting with treatment

3. Classifications and causes

   a. *Primary:* genetic alteration in purine (end product of nucleoprotein digestion, breaks down from uric acid) metabolism resulting in increased production of uric acid or decreased excretion of uric acid

   b. *Secondary:* hyperuricemia secondary to disease state or medications

B. Pathophysiology

1. Increased levels of serum uric acid precipitate within joint and initiate inflammatory response; sodium urates are deposited around or within joints

2. Phagocytosis of urate crystals occurs, leading to cell death and release of lysosomal enzymes

3. If untreated, chronic inflammation will lead to involvement of multiple joints, destruction of cartilage, bone, and formation of tophi

4. Signs and symptoms

   a. Sudden onset of severe pain in one joint; the great toe is most commonly affected; however, it may occur in the instep, wrist, tarsal joints, knees, elbows, and ankles

   b. Joint appears red or dusky, swollen, edematous, and is extremely tender to touch

   c. Tophi: hard, movable, nodules with irregular surfaces occur in synovium, helix of ear, olecranon bursa, and Achilles' tendon (most common locations); associated with chronic untreated gout; can resolve with treatment

C. **Nursing assessment**

1. Assessment includes: complete health history, determination of risk factors; pain assessment; inspection of affected joint for signs and symptoms of inflammation; and mobility and safety with ADLs

2. Diagnostic tests

   a. Serum uric acid level greater than 7.5 mg/dL (normal: male 2.1 to 8.5 mg/dL; female 2.0 to 6.6 mg/dL)

   b. Increased WBC and ESR during acute episodes

   c. 24-hour urine to evaluate uric acid excretion

      1) Levels will correlate with increased serum uric acid levels if there is an overproduction of uric acid

      2) In cases where excretion of uric acid is a problem, serum uric acid will be increased; however, 24-hour urine levels will be decreased

   d. Synovial fluid analysis (positive for urate crystals)

D. **Nursing management**

1. Medication

   a. Uric acid inhibiting drugs: used in prophylactic treatment of gouty arthritis and chronic gouty arthritis; allopurinol (Zyloprim), probenecid (Benemid), colchicine (also used for acute attacks), and sulfinpyrazone (Anturane)

   b. Narcotic analgesics and NSAIDs effectively relieve pain associated with acute attacks; acetylsalicylic acid (aspirin) is contraindicated because it decreases excretion of uric acid and interferes with action of uricosuric drugs

2. Instruct client on disease process and treatment plan; emphasize that disease prognosis is good with treatment compliance

3. Administer medications as ordered and instruct client on medication regime; instruct clients to increase fluid intake to 3 liters/day to decrease incidence of kidney stones associated with use of uricosuric agents unless contraindicated by other conditions

4. Instruct on strict bedrest for first 24 hours of acute attack, activity may aggravate and prolong acute symptoms; provide a bedcradle to relieve pressure from linens at affected area

5. Assist with weight reduction

6. Instruct on limiting intake of alcohol to a moderate or lower level

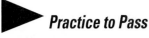

Practice to Pass

Explain how the results of a 24-hour urine for uric acid assists the health care provider in determining the etiology of gout.

V. OSTEOMYELITIS

A. Overview

1. Defined as an acute or chronic infection of bone
2. Characteristics
   a. Early diagnosis critical to prevent disease progression
   b. Most common causative agent: *Staphylococcus aureus*
3. Classifications and causes: osteomyelitis is classified by mode of entry as well as course of disease
   a. Entry
      1) Hematogenous: bloodborne infection localized in bone
      2) Direct entry: contamination through an open wound; most common form in adults
   b. Course
      1) Acute: less than 6 weeks
      2) Chronic: more than 6 to 8 weeks, can last years

B. Pathophysiology

1. Entry of pathogen occurs; organism lodges in bone, multiplies, and initiates inflammatory response
2. As pus accumulates, pressure within bone cavity increases and blood supply to area diminishes
3. If infection enters chronic stage, infection spreads through bone
4. Bone cells become necrotic and break off into segments called sequestra
5. Sequestra remain surrounded by pus and become a great medium for spread of bacteria to surrounding bone tissue
6. New bone formation, called involucrum, develops around necrotic bone cells and sinus tract formation often occurs
7. Signs and symptoms
   a. Hematogenous
      1) Acute onset of fever, chills, pain, and limited ROM at site of infection
      2) Involvement of **metaphysis** (growth plates located in area of flaring between epiphysis [proximal and distal end of long bones] and **diaphysis** [shaft or long portion of long bones]) of tibia, humerus, or femur in children
      3) Involvement of vertebrae in adults
   b. Direct entry
      1) A febrile or low-grade temperature
      2) Erythema, pain, tenderness at site of infection

C. Nursing assessment

1. Health history
   a. Recent episode of *Staphylococcus* infection in children younger than 10 years
   b. Illicit IV drug use
   c. Recent trauma, surgery, or puncture wound in adults
2. Assessment includes determining drug allergies; pain assessment (abrupt onset of pain, guarding of affected site); vital signs (VS); discomfort; decreased ROM at affected site; wound drainage; and decreased activity level

3. Diagnostic tests

   a. X-ray: no changes in early stages, elevation of **periosteum** (membrane covering bone that contains nerve, lymph, and blood vessels) and increased osteoclastic (bone cells responsible for resorption of bony tissue) activity with disease progression

   b. Bone scan (positive for active infection)

   c. Computed tomography (CT) scan or magnetic resonance imaging (MRI) (positive for sinus tracts, abscesses, and may assist in determining boundaries of infection)

   d. ESR and WBC (elevated)

   e. Blood and tissue cultures (positive)

D. Nursing management

   1. Medications include: antibiotics as ordered, over-the-counter (OTC) analgesics or narcotic analgesics for pain relief

   2. Administer medications as ordered, assess therapeutic/nontherapeutic effects

   3. Implement and assess effectiveness of pain relief measures; immobilize affected area

   4. Prevent spread of infection

      a. Implement aseptic technique

      b. Instruct on importance of proper handwashing

      c. Instruct on strict bedrest, mobility may mobilize bacteria

      d. Application of heat during acute infection is contraindicated; bacteria may spread as a result of vasodilation

   5. Splint foot to prevent foot drop

   6. Pre-operative teaching as required for incision and drainage (I&D) of wound

   7. Instruct on nutritious diet (increased protein, calcium, and vitamin C) for optimal wound healing

   8. Instruct on safety measures with use of assistive devices (crutches, walkers, wheelchair)

VI. PAGET'S DISEASE (OSTEITIS DEFORMANS)

A. Overview

   1. Defined as a chronic bone disease with inflammation of bone, hypertrophy of long bones, and deformity of flat bones

   2. Characteristics

      a. Early diagnosis is important to arrest disease progression

      b. Occurs most commonly in spine, cranium, hips, pelvis, thighs, and lower extremities

   3. Cause is unknown, may be viral

   4. Long-term complications

      a. Heart failure secondary to increased demand for blood to achieve **bone remodeling** (formation of new bone by osteoblasts and removal of old bone by osteoclasts)

      b. Lung disease if ribs are involved

      c. Neurological deficits secondary to pressure on brain from enlarged cranium

      d. Increased incidence of sarcoma

      e. Arthritis

      f. Renal calculi secondary to hypercalcemia

B. Pathophysiology

> **1.** Osteolytic phase: characterized by rapid growth of abnormal osteoclasts; formation of new bone cannot occur at same rate that bone resorption (destruction of bone) is taking place, and healthy bone is replaced with vascular, fibrous connective tissue

> **2.** Osteoblastic sclerotic phase: deformities occur as bone eventually becomes enlarged, rough, thicker, and weaker; the bone assumes a mosaic pattern called cement lines

   3. Signs and symptoms

      a. May remain asymptomatic for years

>   b. Bone pain is most common symptom

      c. Headache and hearing loss occur with involvement of cranium

      d. Increased head size

>   e. Bowing of legs

      f. Fatigue

C. Nursing assessment

   1. Assessment

      a. Pain assessment: increasing pain with weight bearing may indicate long bone involvement; headaches may indicate cranial bone involvement

      b. Waddling gait

      c. Bone deformities: kyphosis, enlarged skull, and bowing of legs

      d. Decrease in height

      e. Cardiac assessment: hypertension and arteriosclerosis

      f. Hearing or vision loss secondary to pressure on cranial nerves

      g. Pathological fractures

      h. Complaints of fatigue

   2. Diagnostic tests

      a. Serum alkaline phosphatase (elevated)

      b. Urine for hydroxyproline (elevated), an amino acid present in urine of clients with Paget's disease

      c. X-rays (reveal bone deformities, bone enlargement, widening of bone cortex)

      d. Bone scans (reveal active bone remodeling)

D. Nursing management

   1. Medications include NSAIDs; bone metabolism regulators such as calcitonin (Calcimar), and biphosphonates such as alendronate (Fosamax), pamidronate (Aredia) and tiludronate (Skelid)

   2. Implement and assess effectiveness of pain relief measures

      a. Medications

      b. Collaborate with PT or OT regarding proper fitting for a brace or corset

      c. Heat and massage therapy

▶ **Practice to Pass**

A client diagnosed with Paget's disease wants to know why physical therapy is needed. Relate the bone deformities common in clients with Paget's disease to the disease's pathophysiology.

3. Assess therapeutic/nontherapeutic effects of medication therapy

4. Encourage client to remain active

5. Assess for signs and symptoms of hypercalcemia caused by increased osteoclast activity (fatigue, depression, mental confusion, nausea, vomiting, increased urination, and electrocardiogram [ECG] changes)

6. Instruct on safety to prevent pathological fractures

7. Instruct client to increase fluid intake 2 to 3 liters/day to prevent renal calculi unless contraindicated because of other conditions

8. Assist with adaptation to hearing or vision loss

VII. MUSCULAR DYSTROPHY (MD)

A. Overview

1. Defined as a genetically transmitted disease that is progressive and involves specific muscles

2. Characteristics

   a. Condition includes several disease states characterized by progressive muscle wasting

   b. Has an insidious onset associated with progressive muscle weakness

3. Genetically transmitted by recessive gene on X-chromosome (mother to son) or spontaneous mutation form may occur in females

4. Classifications: there are several forms of the disease; characterized by age of onset, clinical manifestations, and disease progression

   a. Rapidly progressing: Duchenne's muscular dystrophy (DMD)

      1) X-linked recessive, onset usually by age 5

      2) Most common form

   b. Slower-progressing forms

      1) Becker's: onset 5 to 15 years of age; X-linked recessive

      2) Fascioscapulohumeral: onset 10 to 30 years; autosomal dominant

      3) Limb-girdle: onset 10 to 30 years; cause varies

B. Pathophysiology

1. Defect in gene that produces the protein dystrophin, which affects contraction of muscles and is normally found next to sarcolemma membrane

2. Muscle cells die, are phagocytized, and eventually replaced with fatty tissue

3. Muscle size increases causing pseudohypertrophy (false appearance of being enlarged), muscles become progressively weakened because of fatty deposits and connective tissue that enters muscle fibers

4. Signs and symptoms

   a. Duchenne's MD

      1) Symptoms present around 2 to 3 years of age with frequent falls

      2) Waddling gait and toe walking

      3) Pseudohypertrophy of muscles in lower extremities

      4) Kyphosis

      5) Progressive immobility, confined to wheelchair by teen years

      6) Death in early adulthood secondary to respiratory or cardiac failure

      7) Cardiac involvement in later stage of illness

      b. Becker's MD: generalized muscle involvement; normal life span

      c. Fascioscapulohumeral MD: face, neck, and shoulder muscles involved with muscle inflammation

      d. Limb-girdle MD: shoulder and pelvic muscle involvement; upper- and lower-extremity weakness in proximal muscles

C. Nursing assessment

  1. Assessment includes: family history; gait and walking in toddlers; kyphosis in preteen years; muscle strength; history of recurrent URIs with aging

  2. Diagnostic tests

      a. Serum creatinine phosphokinase (CPK), lactic dehydrogenase (LDH), glutamic transaminase, and glucose phosphate elevated

      b. Electromyograms (reveals decreased electrical signals within muscles)

      c. Muscle biopsy (muscle cell necrosis and scar tissue present)

      d. Prenatal testing for dystrophin gene for prevention

D. Nursing management

  1. No medications are recommended

  2. Access available resources and refer client and family to support groups

  3. Prevent upper respiratory infections

  4. Goal is to maintain mobility and prevent contractures

      a. Collaborate with PT regarding therapeutic exercise program

      b. Collaborate with OT regarding use of splints to prevent contractures

  5. Instruct on safe use of wheelchair

  6. Incorporate growth and developmental activities appropriate for age

VIII. FIBROMYALGIA

A. Overview

  1. Defined as a condition of muscles and joints resulting in chronic pain without evidence of arthritis

  2. Characteristics

      a. Condition may be precipitated or aggravated by stress or exertion

      b. Onset is usually gradual, but it can occur suddenly

  3. Cause: unknown etiology, may be associated with endocrine disorders, affective disorders, and disturbances in sleep; may be acute or chronic

B. Pathophysiology

  1. Unclear; inappropriate levels of neurotransmitters have been investigated

  2. Lacks characteristics of arthritis such as inflammation or structural changes in muscles or joints

  3. Signs and symptoms

      a. Muscle pain: local or generalized over entire body

      b. Most commonly occurs in neck, shoulders, lower back, and hips

      c. Fatigue

      d. Headache

      e. Sleep disturbances, particularly lack of non-REM sleep (stage 4)

        f. Irritable bowel syndrome

        g. Muscle spasms

C. Nursing assessment

    1. Assessment includes: pain, mobility, sleep patterns, sources of stress, bowel patterns, and psychosocial assessment

    2. Diagnostic tests: physical exam and the presence of 11 consistent tender points; tests to rule out other disorders such as OA or RA may be performed

D. Nursing management

    1. Medications include: NSAIDs for pain; antidepressants for sleep, benzodiazepine derivatives such as clonazepam (Klonopin), or mild analgesics

    2. Encourage activity and assist with exercise program

    3. Refer to support groups

    4. Instruct on importance of rest

    5. Stress management

    6. Nutritious diet

IX. BONE TUMORS

A. Overview

    1. Defined as a tumor or neoplasm involving skeletal tissue

    2. Characteristics

        a. *Primary bone tumors:* originate in bone; account for 1% of cancer in adults and 15% in children

            1) Commonly referred to as sarcomas

            2) Pathology may be malignant or benign

        b. *Metastatic bone tumors:* originate from a tumor elsewhere in body

            1) Occur more commonly than primary bone tumors

            2) Associated with primary cancer of breast, lung, prostate, and kidney

            3) Usually located in spine, pelvis, femur, humerus, or ribs

    3. Osteosarcoma

        a. Primary malignant bone tumor characterized by rapid growth, etiology unknown

        b. Occur more frequently in males between ages of 10 and 25 years, with greatest incidence during teenage years

        c. Tissue of origin: metaphysis of long bones

        d. Common sites: distal femur, proximal tibia, and proximal humerus

        e. Frequently discovered following an injury

    4. Chondrosarcoma

        a. Primary malignant bone tumor characterized by slow growth, etiology unknown

        b. Occurs more frequently in adult males

        c. Tissue origin: cartilage

        d. Common sites: pelvis, femur, and humerus

    5. Ewing's sarcoma

        a. Primary malignant bone tumor characterized by rapid metastasis to lung tissue, etiology unknown

  b. Occurs between ages of 10 and 25, with greatest incidence in teen years

  c. Tissue origin: nerve tissue within bone marrow

  d. Common sites: pelvis, humerus, femur, and ribs

B. Pathophysiology

  1. Growth of neoplastic cells in tissue of origin causes **osteolysis** (softening and breakdown of bone)

  2. Alteration in bone remodeling occurs, resulting in destruction of normal bone tissue

  3. Enlargement of bony surfaces occurs with tumor growth; bones become weak, leaving client at risk for pathological fractures

  4. Structures surrounding bone tissue are invaded as neoplastic cells continue to multiply

  5. Signs and symptoms vary based on size and location of tumor and include:

  a. Pain or tenderness and swelling at site of tumor

  b. Decreased ROM and function

  c. Neuralgia secondary to nerve compression

  d. Palpable mass

  e. Pathological fractures

  f. Temperature elevation

C. Nursing assessment

  1. Assessment includes symptom analysis of pain or swelling at affected site, activity level, complaints of weakness; conduct health history to determine risk factors; palpate for masses; and assess vital signs

  2. Diagnostic tests

  a. X-rays

   1) Benign tumors: well-defined tumor margins

   2) Malignant tumors: undefined tumor borders, extension of tumor beyond bone structure

  b. CT scan and MRI: can detect soft tissue sarcomas not detected on X-ray; also location of tumor, extent of tumor growth, as well as metastases

  c. Bone scans

  d. Bone biopsy

  e. Serum calcium and serum alkaline phosphatase: elevated

  f. Red blood count (RBC): elevated

D. Nursing management

  1. Medications include nonopioid and opioid analgesics and chemotherapy prior to surgery

  2. Implement and assess effectiveness of pain relief measures

  a. Proper positioning

  b. Use of assistive devices for ambulation

  3. Instruct on safety in home

  4. Provide rest periods between activities

  5. Instruct on chemotherapy and radiation therapies as treatment options

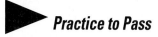

Practice to Pass

Identify the characteristics that differentiate osteosarcomas, chondrosarcomas, and Ewing's sarcomas.

6. Preoperative teaching as required for surgery: limb-salvage surgery (surgical removal of a bone tumor that prevents limb amputation) and limb amputation

7. Incorporate growth and developmental stage in nursing interventions

8. Collaborate with PT and/or OT regarding therapeutic exercise regime following surgery

9. Assist client and family in developing coping strategies in dealing with diagnosis and treatment plans and refer to cancer support groups

10. Place clients receiving opioids on a bowel monitoring and management regimen

X. SYSTEMIC LUPUS ERYTHEMATOSUS (SLE)

A. Overview

1. Defined as a chronic inflammatory, rheumatic, autoimmune disease, characterized by remissions and exacerbations

2. Characteristics

   a. Prognosis improves with early diagnosis and treatment

   b. May affect connective tissue of any body organ, disease progression varies from mild to severe depending on organ involvement

3. Classifications

   a. *Drug-induced lupus:* associated with use of procainamide (Procan SR), hydralazine (Apresoline), isoniazid (INH), and some antiepileptic drugs; symptoms usually subside after drugs are discontinued

   b. *Discoid lupus:* limited to involvement of skin

   c. *Systemic lupus:* involvement of one or more of these systems: musculoskeletal, lungs, kidneys, CNS, cardiovascular, hematological

4. Causes

   a. Infections from leukemia and renal failure are major causes of mortality

   b. Etiology is unknown but may be attributed to exposure to ultraviolet rays, genetic defect, or hormonal imbalance (which may explain increased incidence during pregnancy)

B. Pathophysiology

1. The body produces autoantibodies, specifically against DNA, secondary to hyperactivity of B-cells

2. These autoantibodies combine with antigens to form immune complexes; accumulation of immune complexes within connective tissue triggers an inflammatory response

3. Chronic inflammation destroys connective tissue; tissue damage varies with organ involvement

4. Signs and symptoms

   a. May be unpredictable and vary with organs involved

   b. General presenting symptoms include; fever, malaise, fatigue, weakness, and weight loss

   c. Musculoskeletal: polyarthralgia, symmetrical arthritis

   d. Integumentary: alopecia, butterfly rash, sclerosis of skin on fingers, discoid lesions

   e. Painless lesions in oral mucosa

  f. Cardiac: pericarditis

  g. Lungs: pleural effusions, pleuritis

  h. Kidney: glomerulonephritis, renal failure

  i. CNS: seizures, psychosis, cerebrovascular accident (CVA), senile dementias

  j. Hematological: anemia, leukopenia, and thrombocytopenia

  k. Infections

C. Nursing assessment

 1. Assessment includes identifying risk factors; complete drug history; nutrition (baseline weight and history of recent weight loss); skin assessment (rashes, hair loss, photosensitivity, ecchymosis, and petechiae may indicate hematologic involvement); respiratory assessment (pleural effusion and pleuritis); renal assessment: I & O; neurological assessment (seizure activity, changes in affect and/or cognitive abilities); cardiovascular assessment (VS, signs and symptoms of pericarditis); musculoskeletal assessment (symmetrical joint pain, assess ability to participate in ADLs, history of weakness)

 2. Diagnostic tests

  a. X-ray of affected joints (will not show degenerative changes or bone deformities characteristic of arthritis)

  b. Serum syphilis (false positive)

  c. Serum antinuclear antibody (ANA) (positive), but this is not exclusive to SLE

  d. Anti-DNA antibody (positive), which is definitive for SLE

  e. Serum complement levels (decreased)

  f. CBC (positive for anemia, leukopenia, and/or thrombocytopenia)

  g. Urinalysis (UA): positive for proteinuria and/or hematuria

  h. Blood urea nitrogen (BUN) and creatinine (Cr): elevated

  i. ESR (elevated)

D. Nursing management

 1. Medications

  a. NSAIDs: used for treatment of joint pain

  b. Antimalarials: used for treatment of joint pain and skin disorders

  c. Corticosteroids: used during acute exacerbations, may also use a low-maintenance dose during remissions

  d. Immunosuppressive drugs: toxic drugs used during acute life-threatening exacerbations only

 2. Instruct on disease process and treatment regimen

 3. Instruct on factors that may trigger exacerbations

  a. Pregnancy: provide counseling regarding family planning and alternatives to birth control pills

  b. Exposure to UV rays: use sunscreen with sun protection factor (SPF) of 15, wear sun hats, avoid sunbathing, and use a beach umbrella

  c. Medication: avoid use of birth control pills, sulfonamides, penicillin

 4. Refer to support groups

 5. Implement and assess effectiveness of joint pain relief measures

  a. Medications

      b. Application of heat

      c. Therapeutic exercise program

  6. Administer medications as directed and assess therapeutic and nontherapeutic responses

      a. Educate about side effects of corticosteroids (cushingoid effects, hypertension, weight gain)

      b. Advise regarding side effects of immunosuppressive drugs

      c. Blindness can occur with antimalarials; routine eye exams should be done

  7. Instruct on importance of good nutrition

  8. Instruct on handwashing and infection control at home to prevent infection

  9. Instruct on oral care

  10. If alopecia occurs from SLE, make referral for hair wig if appropriate to maintain positive body image

  11. Assist family and client in developing coping strategies to deal with cognitive changes

  12. Instruct family and client on appropriate safety interventions related to cognitive changes

XI. SCLERODERMA (SYSTEMIC SCLEROSIS)

A. Overview

  1. Defined as an uncommon, chronic, autoimmune connective tissue disorder involving skin and other organs, characterized by remissions and exacerbations

  2. Classifications are systemic sclerosis, CREST syndrome, and localized

  3. Unknown etiology; may include genetic, immune, or environmental factors

B. Pathophysiology

  1. Unknown etiology

  2. Overproduction of collagen leads to fibrosis and inflammation resulting in damage to affected area

  3. Types of scleroderma

      a. *Systemic sclerosis* (SS): involvement of skin of fingers, hands, face, and trunk as well as visceral organs

         1) Most common visceral organs affected are esophagus, intestines, lungs, heart, and kidney

         2) May progress quickly and be life-threatening depending on extent of organ involvement

      b. *CREST syndrome:* acronym representing

         1) Calcinosis (abnormal deposits of calcium salts on skin)

         2) Raynaud's syndrome

         3) Esophageal dysfunctions

         4) Sclerodactyly (scleroderma localized within fingers)

         5) Telangiectasis (small, dilated blood vessels with a bright-red center point and spikerlike branches)

         6) Prognosis is good and disability is limited

       c. Localized or limited: involvement of skin on fingers, hands, and face; self limiting with good prognosis

!   **4.** Signs and symptoms

    a. Skin

      1) Shiny, thick skin on fingers, hands progressing to arms, trunk, and face

      2) Pursed lips

      3) Nonpitting edema of affected areas

      4) Calcium deposits on skin

      5) Telangiectasis

      6) Hyperpigmentation

    b. Vascular: Raynaud's syndrome

    c. Musculoskeletal: polyarthralgia and joint stiffness

    d. Esophageal: heartburn and dysphagia

    e. Intestinal: constipation, diarrhea, malabsorption, abdominal distention

    f. Heart: ECG changes, signs and symptoms of pericarditis

    g. Lungs: shortness of breath (SOB) on exertion

    h. Kidneys: renal failure

C. Nursing assessment

  1. Assessment

    a. Skin assessment: for changes previously listed

    b. Baseline height and weight; recent weight loss

    c. Gastrointestinal: dietary intake, bowel patterns, abdominal assessment, complaints of heartburn and dysphagia

!   **d.** Musculoskeletal: decreased ROM in affected areas, complaints of polyarthralgia and joint stiffness, clawlike appearance of hands

    e. Respiratory assessment for exertional dyspnea

    f. Cardiac: heart rate and rhythm, hypertension

    g. Renal: I&O for fluid retention

  2. Diagnostic tests

    a. ESR (elevated)

    b. Urinalysis (proteinuria)

    c. BUN and creatinine (elevated with renal failure)

    d. ANA (elevated)

    e. Skin biopsy (results indicate dermal collagen thickening, confirms diagnosis)

    f. Pulmonary function tests (abnormal with decreased function)

D. Nursing management

  1. Medications

    a. NSAIDs or analgesics for joint pain

    b. H_2 antagonists and proton pump inhibitors for gastrointestinal (GI) symptoms

    c. Antibiotics if needed; may be used prophylactically as indicated

    d. Corticosteroids and immunosuppressive drugs are used in advanced life-threatening disease states

        e. Stool softeners to decrease constipation from analgesics, if appropriate

        f. Anticoagulants to prevent deep vein thrombasis

  2. Instruct on disease process and treatment regimen

  3. Refer to support groups

  4. Musculoskeletal symptoms

        a. Collaborate with PT regarding therapeutic exercises to maintain joint mobility

        b. Collaborate with OT regarding assistive devices and ADL training

  5. GI symptoms

        a. Consult dietitian for nutritional support

        b. Maintain high-Fowler's position during and following meals

        c. Small frequent meals

  6. Raynaud's syndrome

        a. Instruct to avoid cold temperatures

        b. Wear gloves and socks to warm hands and improve circulation

        c. Avoid smoking

  7. Skin care: instruct to inspect skin daily for breakdown and utilize skin moisturizers

XII. FRACTURES

A. Overview

  1. Defined as a break in a bone, which occurs secondary to trauma or bone disease

  2. Classifications: according to location of break, angle of break, and/or relationship with external environment

        a. Relationship to external environment

           1) Open or compound: penetration of skin, bone protrudes through

           2) Closed: no penetration of bone through the skin

        b. Type of break

           1) Complete: bone broken all the way through

           2) Incomplete: partially broken or splintered

        c. Name of fracture

           1) Comminuted: bone shatters into pieces

           2) Compression: bone is crushed

           3) Impacted: ends of broken pieces are jammed together

           4) Spiral: bone twists and causes jagged break

           5) Greenstick: incomplete break

           6) Transverse: complete break at right angle to long axis of bone

  3. A client may be able to move affected area even though a fracture exists

  4. Causes include accidents, trauma, motor vehicle accidents, abuse, neglect, and disease processes such as osteoporosis or metastatic disease

B. Pathophysiology

  1. Hematoma formation: bleeding occurs immediately following fracture secondary to ruptured blood vessels within bone and trauma to surrounding tissue; presence of clotting factors within hematoma leads to formation of a fibrin mesh around fracture site

    2. Granulation tissue: during first 48 to 72 hours, new capillary beds form and proliferation of osteoblasts (bone cell responsible for formation of new bone) and fibroblasts occurs within hematoma

      a. Granulation tissue replaces hematoma

      b. Phagocytosis also occurs and removes necrotic bone tissue

    3. Callus formation: within a week, granulation tissue changes and becomes callus (composed of new cartilage, calcium, phosphorus, and osteoblasts)

      a. Callus becomes interlaced among bony fragments and delicately links distal ends of fracture

      b. Eventually callus formation extends beyond fracture and serves as a temporary splint

      c. The process continues leading to increased strengthening of bone

      d. X-rays will confirm this stage of bone healing and help to determine treatment regimen

    4. Ossification: formation of mature bone replaces callus; the delicate link between distal ends of fracture solidifies and a strong connection is restored

    5. Remodeling: osteoclasts resorb excess callus and bone returns to pre-injury strength and shape

    6. Signs and symptoms

      a. Pain and muscle spasms

      b. Asymmetrical appearance of limb secondary to bone displacement

      c. Numbness and or tingling at affected site secondary to nerve compression

      d. Loss of function

      e. Edema secondary to tissue trauma

      f. Crepitus with movement

C. Nursing assessment

    1. Assessment includes

      a. Subjective data describing event

      b. Pain assessment including guarding of affected site

      c. Loss of function

      d. Crepitus

      e. Edema, ecchymosis, and tenderness at affected site

      f. Presence of pulses

      g. Asymmetrical appearance

    2. Diagnostic test: X-ray will confirm fracture

D. Nursing management

    1. Medications include analgesics to control pain, antibiotics for open fracture

    2. Emergency nursing care: immobilize fracture, control bleeding, and clean wound (unless an open fracture exists, which will be cleaned in surgery)

    3. Assess 5 Ps (see Figure 5-1)

    4. Teach action and side effects of medications; obtain consent for operation prior to medicating, if surgery is pending

    5. Preoperative teaching as required for surgery

      a. Closed reduction

      b. Open reduction

Practice to Pass

A 10-year-old client diagnosed with a fractured humerus is discharged from the Emergency Department after application of a cast. Develop a teaching plan for the child and caregivers regarding cast care.

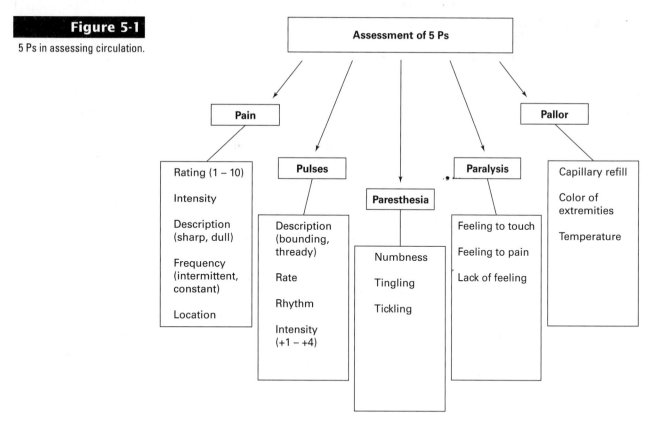

Figure 5-1

5 Ps in assessing circulation.

6. Instruct on safety and use of assistive devices
7. Elevate extremity and apply an ice pack to relieve edema
8. Assess and provide client teaching on prevention of hazards of immobility
9. Recognize and treat early complications
   a. Hypovolemic shock
   b. Fat emboli (petechial rash, tachycardia, tachypnea)
   c. Deep vein thrombosis
   d. Compartment syndrome (see below)
10. Instruct on cast care if applicable (see Box 5-3)
11. Provide traction care if applicable (see Box 5-4)
12. Maintain nutritional status

XIII. COMPARTMENT SYNDROME

A. Overview

1. Defined as muscle and nerve damage related to excessive swelling in area of a fracture
2. Classifications
   a. *Acute:* occurs following a crushing injury or bone fracture, when a cast has been applied
   b. *Chronic:* occurs most frequently in young adults who participate in activities that require repetitive motion, causing excessive strain on lower extremities; for example, long-distance running

Box 5-3	➤ During the first 24 hours after application of the cast, apply ice directly over the fracture, elevate the extremity, and promote drying of the cast by leaving it exposed to air and supporting it on pillows.
Teaching Tips for Clients with Casts	➤ Report any of the following symptoms to your health care provider: increased pain, change in color, coolness of extremity, lack of movement, or numbness and tingling.
	➤ Do not place any item in the cast; use a blowdryer on the cool setting to relieve itching.
	➤ Keep plaster casts dry at all times; cover with plastic during bathing.
	➤ Fiberglass casts may get wet; be sure to dry them completely with a blowdryer on cool setting.
	➤ Report drainage or cast odor to your health care provider.

B. Pathophysiology

1. Two factors leading to compartment syndrome

    a. Hemorrhage and edema occur following a fracture, causing a reduction in ability of **fascia** (fibrous connective tissue responsible for supporting and connecting structures of musculoskeletal system) to accommodate excessive edema

    b. A closed compartment may be created with application of a tightly fitting external dressing, splint, or cast, which causes increased pressure on limb

2. As pressure within compartment increases, both venous and arterial circulation become obstructed and tissue perfusion is diminished

3. Consequently, tissue ischemia, loss of function, and nerve damage occur; pressures of 30 mmHg or more can result in permanent muscle and nerve damage

4. Signs and symptoms

    a. Severe pain unrelieved by analgesics and aggravated by elevation

    b. Paresthesias

    c. Loss of function and decreased reflexes

    d. Pallor, extremity cool to touch

    e. Pulse is decreased in volume or may not be present

C. Nursing assessment

1. Assessment

    a. Symptom analysis of pain

    b. Neurovascular checks following fractures; pulses may be present during early stages of compartment syndrome

Box 5-4	➤ Maintain correct alignment at all times.
Nursing Implications for Clients Receiving Traction	➤ All weights should clear the floor at all times.
	➤ Inspect the skin at pressure points for skin breakdown.
	➤ Implement skin care measures that prevent skin breakdown.
	➤ Implement nursing interventions that prevent hazards of immobility.
	➤ Inspect pin sites for signs and symptoms of infection.
	➤ Provide pin care according to agency policy.

      c. Assess external dressings, splint, or cast for tightness

      d. Excessive edema at fracture site

    2. Diagnostic tests: no tests are recommended

D. Nursing management

    1. Medications include analgesics for pain

    2. Notify health care provider

    3. Elevate extremity and apply ice immediately to increase venous return and decrease edema as a means of *preventing* compartment syndrome

    4. Remove or loosen constrictive dressings and or splint, assist with bivalving cast if directed once it has occurred

    5. Conduct preoperative teaching as indicated for a fasciotomy (surgical procedure to cut and divide a fascia)

XIV. OSTEOPOROSIS

A. Overview

    1. Defined as a musculoskeletal disorder characterized by loss of bone mass

    2. Disease process predisposes clients to fractures

    3. Classifications

      a. *Type I:* associated with early postmenopausal estrogen deficiency

      b. *Type II:* senile osteoporosis associated with calcium deficiency

    4. Cause related to endocrine disorder, malignancy, or aging process

B. Pathophysiology

    1. The disease process is characterized by an increase in activity of osteoclasts and a decrease in activity of osteoblasts; this leads to rate of bone resorption that exceeds bone formation

    2. Outer cortex (outer surface of bone composed of hard, cortical bone) of the diaphysis and metaphysis becomes thinner secondary to enlargement of bone

    3. Advanced disease process leads to loss of trabeculae (spongy bone containing red bone marrow located in area of metaphysis of long bones) from cancellous (spongy bone located towards interior of bone containing red or yellow bone marrow) bone and thinning of cortex; these changes in bone structure increase risk of a client's experiencing a bone fracture

    4. Signs and symptoms: loss of height, kyphosis, low back pain, fractures of forearm, spine, and hip

C. Nursing assessment

    1. Assessment includes analysis of possible risk factors; height (pattern of decrease); pain assessment; and any recent fractures

    2. Diagnostic test: bone density studies; x-rays (will not show changes in bone mass until a loss greater than 30% exists)

D. Nursing management

    1. Medications include calcium supplements; calcitonin and fluoride; selective estrogen receptor modulators (SERMs) such as raloxifene hydrochloride (Evista); biphosphonates such as alendronate (Fosamax), etidronate (Didronel), and pamidronate (Aredia)

2. Instruct clients at risk and those diagnosed on the following:

   a. Implement an exercise regimen that incorporates weight bearing exercises; jogging, walking, rowing, and weight lifting

   b. Instruct on adequate calcium intake through diet or supplements

      1) Premenopausal women 1,000 mg/day

      2) Postmenopausal women 1,500 mg/day

   c. Instruct elderly clients at risk on safety with ambulation in home (see Box 5-1)

Case Study

A 45-year-old client sustains fractures of the right leg and arm because of a motor vehicle accident. The client is treated in the Emergency Department and then admitted to an orthopedic unit for observation.

1. What are the priorities of care at the scene of the accident?

2. Outline the nursing care of the client after casts are placed on the right arm and leg.

3. What discharge instructions should the nurse give to the client?

4. Forty-eight hours after the accident, the client complains of excruciating pain in his right arm unrelieved by analgesics. What complication should the nurse suspect?

5. What are the priorities of care in question 4 above?

For suggested responses, see page 534.

POSTTEST

1 A client has had a fracture reduced and immobilized. To determine if the client is experiencing compartment syndrome, which of the following is a priority area for assessment by the nurse?

1. Assessing for edema at the fracture site
2. Palpation of a pulse distal to the fracture site
3. Performing a pain assessment
4. Assessing for the presence of drainage on the cast

2 In reviewing the medication order sheet for a client with systemic sclerosis (scleroderma), the nurse concludes that the ordered calcium channel blocker and alpha-adrenergic blocker are being given to treat which of the following problems accompanying this disease?

1. Renal failure
2. Pericarditis
3. Bradycardia
4. Raynaud's phenomenon

3 Which of the following lab values is most significant to the nurse when assessing a client for complications associated with Paget's disease?

1. Calcium level of 15 mg/dL
2. Positive rheumatoid factor (RF)
3. Blood urea nitrogen (BUN) of 90 mg/dL
4. Eosinophil sedimentation rate (ESR) of 30 mm/hr

4 A female client has breast cancer that has metastasized to the bones. The nurse would develop which goals of nursing care for this client? Select all that apply.

1. Treat primary cancer and prevent further metastasis
2. Control pain to allow activities of daily living
3. Promote survival with maximal function
4. Prevent pathological fractures
5. Prevent complications from hypercalcemia

POSTTEST

5 An adult male limps into the ambulatory clinic reporting a red, hot, swollen joint in his great toe. The problem developed after a night of heavy alcohol use. He asks the nurse what caused his gout pain to return. The nurse formulates a response based on what underlying pathophysiology?

1. Increased immune complexes are deposited within the joint cavity
2. Alteration in purine metabolism results in hyperuricemia; alcohol consumption may trigger it
3. Excessive bone remodeling is secondary to increased levels of phosphorus, related to overeating
4. Presence of fibrous adhesions within bony cartilage causes pain and a limping gait

6 A client is diagnosed with osteomyelitis involving the foot. The wound is draining and dressing changes are being done daily or more often as needed. What is the nurse's highest priority at this time?

1. Maintaining adequate pain control
2. Implementing aseptic technique
3. Promoting adequate nutrition
4. Splinting the foot to prevent foot drop

7 The nurse is counseling the parents of a child diagnosed with muscular dystrophy. Which of the following statements by the nurse most accurately describes the disease progression?

1. "Prognosis is favorable with early detection."
2. "With aggressive physical therapy and the use of a walker, your child will remain ambulatory through adulthood."
3. "The muscles and the lungs may also become involved, and this can shorten your child's lifespan."
4. "Muscle weakness is progressive and rapid, and your child will most likely be confined to a wheelchair by the age of 5."

8 The nurse is explaining osteoarthritis (OA or degenerative joint disease) to a client. The nurse incorporates which of the following concepts about the underlying pathology in the discussion?

1. Changes in composition of the articular cartilage contribute to increased friction during joint movement
2. Joint inflammation occurs secondary to the presence of immune complexes within the joint cavity
3. Excessive bone necrosis within the joint occurs secondary to increased osteoclastic activity
4. Bone damage occurs secondary to osteolysis and excessive bone remodeling

9 An adult client is being treated in the early stages of rheumatoid arthritis (RA). Which of the following drugs would the nurse expect to be included in the client's drug regime? Select all that apply.

1. Nonsteroidal antiinflammatory drugs (NSAIDs) such as ibuprofen (Motrin) or aspirin
2. Systemic corticosteroids such as prednisone (Deltasone)
3. Disease-modifying anti-rheumatoidal drugs (DMARDs) such as methotrexate (Trexall)
4. Oral opioid analgesics such as oxycodone (Oxycontin)
5. Routine injections of an opioid such as morphine sulfate

10 The nurse is explaining the pathophysiology of osteoporosis to a female client. Which of the following statements should the nurse include in the discussion to best describe the disease process?

1. Increased amounts of estrogen in postmenopausal women contribute to bone loss
2. Imbalance is seen between the formation of new bone and the absorption of existing bone
3. Decrease in blood supply to the bone results in bony necrosis or death of bone cells
4. Invasion of a pathogen leads to infection and destruction of bone

➤ *See pages 183–185 for Answers & Rationales.*

ANSWERS & RATIONALES

Pretest

1 Answer: 3 The joints should not be further damaged so activities are chosen that allow range of motion (ROM) but do not further injure a joint. Aerobic exercises such as swimming help the client to maintain maximum ROM and mobility while minimizing strain on joints. Weight-bearing exercises such as tennis, jogging, and volleyball place excessive strain on diseased joints and should not be activities of choice.
Cognitive Level: Application **Client Need:** Health Promotion and Maintenance **Integrated Process:** Nursing Process: Evaluation **Content Area:** Adult Health: Musculoskeletal **Strategy:** Consider what activity is aerobic and yet does not abuse damaged joints. The correct option stands out from the others. **Reference:** Porth, C. M. (2005) *Pathophysiology: Concepts of altered health states* (7th ed.). Philadelphia, PA: Lippincott Williams & Wilkins, p. 1432.

2 Answers: 2, 4, 5 Swan neck deformities of the hand are classic deformities associated with rheumatoid arthritis secondary to the presence of fibrous connective tissue within the joint space. Clients with RA experience morning stiffness lasting from 30 minutes up to several hours. Systemic manifestations include weakness, fatigue, and weight loss. RA is characterized by symmetrical joint involvement. Heberden's nodes and morning stiffness lasting less than 30 minutes are characteristic of osteoarthritis.
Cognitive Level: Analysis **Client Need:** Physiological Integrity: Physiological Adaptation **Integrated Process:** Communication and Documentation **Content Area:** Adult Health: Musculoskeletal **Strategy:** The core issue of the question is the ability to distinguish between RA and OA. Use nursing knowledge and the process of elimination to make a selection. **Reference:** LeMone, P., & Burke, K. (2008). *Medical-surgical nursing: Critical thinking in client care* (4th ed.). Upper Saddle River, NJ: Pearson/Prentice Hall, pp. 1449–1460.

3 Answer: 2 A liberal fluid intake is recommended to reduce calculi formation and increase urate excretion. Alkalizing agents such as bicarbonate or citrate may also minimize uric acid stone formation. Bed rest is indicated during an acute attack to rest the joint but rest does not prevent renal problems.
Cognitive Level: Application **Client Need:** Physiological Integrity: Physiological Adaptation **Integrated Process:** Nursing Process: Implementation **Content Area:** Adult Health: Musculoskeletal **Strategy:** Utilize principles of fluid balance and renal excretion to answer the question. Critical words include *facilitate* and *excretion*. Identify options that are opposite in nature if the correct answer is unknown because one of these would have to be incorrect. **Reference:** LeMone, P., & Burke, K. (2008). *Medical-surgical nursing: Critical thinking in client care* (4th ed.). Upper Saddle River, NJ: Pearson/Prentice Hall, pp. 1443–1447.

4 Answers: 2, 3, 4, 5 Immobilizing the joint, providing analgesia, and maintaining asepsis are appropriate nursing interventions when caring for a client diagnosed with osteomyelitis to manage the pain and prevent the spread of infection. The application of heat is contraindicated because it can increase edema and pain in the affected area and spread bacteria through vasodilatation.
Cognitive Level: Application **Client Need:** Physiological Integrity: Physiological Adaptation **Integrated Process:** Nursing Process: Implementation **Content Area:** Adult Health: Musculoskeletal **Strategy:** Identify the actions that provide comfort and maintain function. These will be the correct options in the question. **Reference:** LeMone, P., & Burke, K. (2008). *Medical-surgical nursing: Critical thinking in client care* (4th ed.). Upper Saddle River, NJ: Pearson/Prentice Hall, pp. 1477–1481.

5 Answer: 4 Serum alkaline phosphatase is elevated because of increased activity of bone cells. Inflammation is in the bone and usually does not reveal an elevated serum WBC, ESR, or the presence of *Staphylococcus*.
Cognitive Level: Application **Client Need:** Physiological Integrity: Reduction of Risk Potential **Integrated Process:** Nursing Process: Analysis **Content Area:** Adult Health: Musculoskeletal **Strategy:** Choose the option that reflects loss of bone tissue. Eliminate the options related to infection. **Reference:** Porth, C. M. (2005). *Pathophysiology: Concepts of altered health states* (7th ed.). Philadelphia, PA: Lippincott Williams & Wilkins, pp. 1412–1413.

6 Answer: Osteosarcomas are most commonly seen in children and young adults. Middle-aged males (option 1), females age 50 to 60 (option 2), and females of child-bearing age (option 3) are less likely to develop osteosarcoma.
Cognitive Level: Application **Integrated Process:** Nursing Process: Assessment **Client Need:** Health Promotion and Maintenance **Content Area:** Adult Health: Musculoskeletal **Strategy:** If this question is difficult and you need to make an educated guess, note that one option stands

out as different from the others. **Reference:** Porth, C. M. (2005). *Pathophysiology: Concepts of altered health states* (7th ed.). Philadelphia, PA: Lippincott Williams & Wilkins, p. 1385.

7 **Answer: 1** Although the etiology of SLE is unknown, certain environmental factors have been associated with the onset of symptoms. The administration of procainamide (Procan SR) and hydralazine (Apresoline) have been associated with SLE symptoms, which usually subside after the drug is discontinued.
Cognitive Level: Application **Client Need:** Physiological Integrity: Pharmacological and Parenteral Therapies **Integrated Process:** Nursing Process: Analysis **Content Area:** Adult Health: Musculoskeletal **Strategy:** The core issue of the question is knowledge of which drugs have adverse effects resembling SLE. Use this knowledge and the process of elimination to make a selection. **Reference:** Porth, C. M. (2005). *Pathophysiology: Concepts of altered health states* (7th ed.). Philadelphia, PA: Lippincott Williams & Wilkins, p. 1423.

8 **Answer: 1** Raynaud's disease is characterized by spasms of the blood vessels within the fingers of the hands resulting in diminished circulation. Gloves protect the hands from cold temperatures and provide warmth, which promotes blood flow to the affected areas. Raynaud's phenomenon is seen in the CREST syndrome, a type of scleroderma.
Cognitive Level: Application **Client Need:** Physiological Integrity: Physiological Adaptation **Integrated Process:** Teaching/Learning **Content Area:** Adult Health: Musculoskeletal **Strategy:** Recall that treatment is supportive to prevent vascular spasms due to cold temperatures. Identify options that are opposite and consider whether one of them may be the correct option. **Reference:** Porth, C. M. (2005). *Pathophysiology: Concepts of altered health states* (7th ed.). Philadelphia, PA: Lippincott Williams & Wilkins, pp. 1424–1425.

9 **Answer: 3** During earlier stages of bone healing, overproduction of callus enlarges the bone and acts as a splint. Callus is eventually replaced with mature bone during the ossification phase of bone healing, and then the excess callus is resorbed during the remodeling phase to return the bone to its original shape.
Cognitive Level: Application **Client Need:** Physiological Integrity: Physiological Adaptation **Integrated Process:** Nursing Process: Analysis **Content Area:** Adult Health: Musculoskeletal **Strategy:** Apply principles of healing. Recall that remodeling is the last stage. **Reference:** LeMone, P., & Burke, K. (2008). *Medical-surgical nursing: Critical thinking in client care* (4th ed.). Upper Saddle River, NJ: Pearson/Prentice Hall, pp. 1402–1404.

10 **Answer: 1** Edema is expected immediately following a fracture, but because the fascia is non-elastic, excessive swelling will lead to increased capillary pressure within the area, resulting in nerve and muscle damage if left untreated. Damage is irreversible if the capillary pressure reaches 30 mmHg. A pulse may still be present during early stages of compartment syndrome. One factor that can differentiate pain associated with trauma from the fracture and that from compartment syndrome is the ineffectiveness of analgesics when compartment syndrome occurs.
Cognitive Level: Application **Client Need:** Physiological Integrity: Physiological Adaptation **Integrated Process:** Nursing Process: Analysis **Content Area:** Adult Health: Musculoskeletal **Strategy:** Consider the hemorrhage and edema that occur at a fracture site and use the process of elimination to make a selection. **Reference:** LeMone, P., & Burke, K. (2008). *Medical-surgical nursing: Critical thinking in client care* (4th ed.). Upper Saddle River, NJ: Pearson/Prentice Hall, pp. 1403, 1406.

Posttest

1 **Answer: 3** Although assessing for edema, pulses, and the presence of drainage is important in the care of a client with a fracture, pain unrelieved by analgesics is the symptom most indicative of compartment syndrome.
Cognitive Level: Analysis **Client Need:** Physiological Integrity: Physiological Adaptation **Integrated Process:** Nursing Process: Assessment **Content Area:** Adult Health: Musculoskeletal **Strategy:** Identify the critical word *priority* in the stem of the question. With this in mind, expect all options to be plausible. Select the best one after reading all the options. **Reference:** LeMone, P., & Burke, K. (2008). *Medical-surgical nursing: Critical thinking in client care* (4th ed.). Upper Saddle River, NJ: Pearson/Prentice Hall, pp. 1403, 1406.

2 **Answer: 4** When clients with scleroderma develop Raynaud's phenomenon, which is characterized by vasospasms of the arteries and veins of the hands, calcium channel blockers (such as nifedipine) or alpha-adrenergic blockers (such as prazosin) are the treatment of choice. ACE inhibitors would be used for renal involvement. Bradycardia is not specific to scleroderma. Clients may experience pericarditis, but this is not treated with calcium channel or alpha adrenergic blockers.
Cognitive Level: Application **Client Need:** Physiological Integrity: Pharmacological and Parenteral Therapies **Integrated Process:** Nursing Process: Analysis **Content Area:** Adult Health: Musculoskeletal **Strategy:** Recognize that all the options are possible concerns for a client with scleroderma. Consider which complication may be

ANSWERS & RATIONALES

treated with the drugs in the stem of the question. **Reference:** Porth, C. M. (2005). *Pathophysiology: Concepts of altered health states* (7th ed.). Philadelphia, PA: Lippincott Williams & Wilkins, pp. 1424–1425.

3 Answer: 1 Hypercalcemia (option 1) can occur as a complication of Paget's disease secondary to increased osteoclast activity. The other tests are not specific to Paget's disease although they are all abnormal values. **Cognitive Level:** Analysis **Client Need:** Physiological Integrity: Reduction of Risk Potential **Integrated Process:** Nursing Process: Analysis **Content Area:** Adult Health: Musculoskeletal **Strategy:** Find the laboratory test result that reflects the abnormal bone reabsorption and formation seen in Paget's disease. **Reference:** LeMone, P., & Burke, K. (2008). *Medical-surgical nursing: Critical thinking in client care* (4th ed.). Upper Saddle River, NJ: Pearson/Prentice Hall, pp. 1441–1443.

4 Answers: 2, 3, 4, 5 Metastatic bone disease weakens the bones, predisposing the client to pathological fractures. The major symptom is pain. The goal is to prevent pathological fractures and promote survival while maximizing function, maintaining mobility, and controlling pain as much as possible. Hypercalcemia occurs in 10% to 20% of clients with metastatic bone disease because of demineralization. **Cognitive Level:** Application **Client Need:** Physiological Integrity: Physiological Adaptation **Integrated Process:** Nursing Process: Planning **Content Area:** Adult Health: Musculoskeletal **Strategy:** Do not choose goals that are unrealistic. **Reference:** Porth, C. M. (2005). *Pathophysiology: Concepts of altered health states* (7th ed.). Philadelphia, PA: Lippincott Williams & Wilkins, pp. 1388–1389.

5 Answer: 2 The pathophysiology of gouty arthritis is related to overproduction or decreased excretion of uric acid in the primary form. The pathophysiology does not involve deposits of immune complexes, increased phosphorus, or fibrous adhesions. **Cognitive Level:** Application **Client Need:** Physiological Integrity: Physiological Adaptation **Integrated Process:** Nursing Process: Analysis **Content Area:** Adult Health: Musculoskeletal **Strategy:** The critical words in the question are *gout* and *alcohol*. Use nursing knowledge and the process of elimination to make a selection. **Reference:** LeMone, P., & Burke, K. (2008). Medical-surgical nursing: Critical thinking in client care (4th ed.). Upper Saddle River, NJ: Pearson/Prentice Hall, p. 1444.

6 Answer: 2 Although all the items listed are important in the plan of care for the client diagnosed with osteomyelitis, maintaining aseptic technique and preventing the spread of infection is crucial to resolving the

disease process. Maslow's hierarchy may identify option 1 as highest priority, but infection is the cause of the pain, making this the best option. **Cognitive Level:** Analysis **Client Need:** Physiological Integrity: Physiological Adaptation **Integrated Process:** Nursing Process: Planning **Content Area:** Adult Health: Musculoskeletal **Strategy:** Think of what causes the problem and deal with that first in a question such as this. **Reference:** Porth, C. M. (2005). *Pathophysiology: Concepts of altered health states* (7th ed.). Philadelphia, PA: Lippincott Williams & Wilkins, pp. 1380–1383.

7 Answer: 3 Symptoms of muscular dystrophy usually manifest themselves in early childhood. The child has a waddling gait and experiences frequent falls. There is no cure for the disease and muscles become progressively weaker. Most children are wheelchair confined by the teen years. As the disease progresses, heart and lung muscle are affected, resulting in cardiac and pulmonary failure. The child lives, on average, 15 years after onset. **Cognitive Level:** Application **Client Need:** Physiological Integrity: Physiological Adaptation **Integrated Process:** Communication and Documentation **Content Area:** Adult Health: Musculoskeletal **Strategy:** Recall that this is a progressive disease and the options are linear. Use this information and the process of elimination to make a selection. **Reference:** LeMone, P., & Burke, K. (2008). *Medical-surgical nursing: Critical thinking in client care* (4th ed.). Upper Saddle River, NJ: Pearson/Prentice Hall, pp. 1458–1459.

8 Answer: 1 Articular cartilage is responsible for decreasing friction during joint movement and displacing the force of the workload onto the subchondral bone. In OA, the composition of the articular cartilage is changed because of a malfunction in the release of cytokines and proteases. Consequently, the articular cartilage can no longer perform its original function. **Cognitive Level:** Application **Client Need:** Physiological Integrity: Physiological Adaptation **Integrated Process:** Nursing Process: Analysis **Content Area:** Adult Health: Musculoskeletal **Strategy:** Eliminate the options that describe other diseases. Another clue lies in the other name for the disease. **Reference:** Porth, C. M. (2005). *Pathophysiology: Concepts of altered health states* (7th ed.). Philadelphia, PA: Lippincott Williams & Wilkins, pp. 1430–1431.

9 Answers: 1, 3 DMARDs are now being used earlier in the treatment regime for RA because evidence suggests that they may play a role in arresting the disease process. NSAIDs are used in combination with this drug classification for pain management. Systemic corticosteroids are not used until NSAIDs are no longer effective because of the severe side effects associated with their use. Narcotics are not indicated in the early disease process. **Cognitive Level:** Application **Client Need:** Physiological Integrity: Pharmacological and Parenteral Therapies **Integrated Process:** Nursing Process: Implementation **Content Area:** Adult Health: Musculoskeletal **Strategy:** Note the clue words *early stages* in the stem. With this in mind, select agents that are useful to the disease process and analgesics that are milder in nature. **Reference:** Porth, C. M. (2005). *Pathophysiology: Concepts of altered health states* (7th ed.). Philadelphia, PA: Lippincott Williams & Wilkins, pp. 1420–1422.

10 **Answer: 2** Osteoporosis is characterized by excessive bone resorption that exceeds the body's ability to produce new bone. It is more prevalent in postmenopausal women with low levels of estrogen. There is a decrease in the number and activity of osteoblasts that form new bone and an increase in the number and activity of osteoclasts that absorb bone. The incorrect options describe other diseases. **Cognitive Level:** Application **Client Need:** Physiological Integrity: Physiological Adaptation **Integrated Process:** Teaching/Learning **Content Area:** Adult Health: Musculoskeletal **Strategy:** Eliminate the options that relate to other diseases. **Reference:** LeMone, P., & Burke, K. (2008). *Medical-surgical nursing: Critical thinking in client care* (4th ed.). Upper Saddle River, NJ: Pearson/Prentice Hall, pp. 1434–1435.

References

Adams, M., Holland, L. & Bostwick, P. (2005). *Pharmacology for nurses: A pathophysiologic approach* (2nd ed.). Upper Saddle River, NJ: Prentice Hall.

Arthritis Foundation (2001). DMARDs. Retrieved on November 24, 2005 from http://www.arthritis.org/answers/default.asp

Bush, M. (2004). Nursing management of arthritis and connective tissue diseases. In S. Lewis, M. Heitkemper, & S. Dirkson (Eds.), *Medical-surgical nursing: Assessment and management of clinical problems* (6th ed.). St. Louis, MO: Mosby.

Gunta, K. (2005). Disorders of skeletal function: Developmental and metabolic disorders. In C. Porth (Ed.), *Pathophysiology: Concepts of altered health states* (7th ed.). Philadelphia: Lippincott Williams & Wilkins, pp. 1393–1415.

Gunta, K. & Hightower, M. (2005). Alterations in skeletal function: Trauma, infections and neoplasms. In C. Porth (Ed.), *Pathophysiology: Concepts of altered health states* (7th ed.). Philadelphia: Lippincott Williams & Wilkins, pp. 1367–1391.

LeMone, P. & Burke, K. (2008). *Medical surgical nursing: Critical thinking in client care* (4th ed.). Upper Saddle River, NJ: Prentice Hall.

Porth, C. M. (2005). *Pathophysiology: Concepts of altered health states* (7th ed.). Philadelphia, PA: Lippincott Williams & Wilkins.

Rizzo, D. (2005). Alterations in skeletal function: rheumatic disorders. In C. Porth (Ed.), *Pathophysiology: Concepts of altered health states* (7th ed.). Philadelphia: Lippincott Williams & Wilkins, pp. 1417–1439.

Venes, C. & Thomas, C. L. (2006). *Taber's cyclopedic medical dictionary* (20th ed.). Philadelphia, PA: F. A. Davis.

Wilson, B. A., Shannon, M. T., & Stang, C. L. (2006). *Nursing drug guide: 2006.* Upper Saddle River, NJ: Prentice Hall.

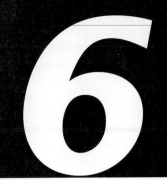

6

Eye, Ear, Nose, and Throat Health Problems

Chapter Outline

Risk Factors Associated with Eye, Ear, Nose, and Throat Health Problems

Glaucoma

Cataracts

Eye Injury

Macular Degeneration

Retinal Detachment

Sensorineural Hearing Impairment

Conductive Hearing Impairment

Otitis Media

External Otitis

Ménière's Disease

Epistaxis

Sinusitis

Laryngeal Cancer

NCLEX-RN® Test Prep

Use the CD-ROM enclosed with this book to access additional practice opportunities.

Objectives

➤ Define key terms associated with eye, ear, nose, and throat health problems.

➤ Identify risk factors associated with the development of eye, ear, nose, and throat health problems.

➤ Explain the common etiologies of eye, ear, nose, and throat health problems.

➤ Describe the pathophysiologic processes associated with specific eye, ear, nose, and throat health problems.

➤ Distinguish between normal and abnormal eye, ear, nose, and throat findings obtained from nursing assessment.

➤ Prioritize nursing interventions associated with specific eye, ear, nose, and throat health problems.

Review at a Glance

audiometry test used to evaluate ability to hear pure tones of varying intensity

Caldwell-Luc procedure procedure used to treat epistaxis and chronic sinusitis involving entry into maxillary sinus through an incision under upper lip; when used for epistaxis, involves ligating artery responsible for bleeding; when used for sinusitis, allows for creation of a window to increase aeration of sinus and promote drainage

cholesteatoma an inflamed cyst or mass filled with epithelial cells and debris that remains infected, enlarges, and may destroy ossicles, causing permanent hearing loss; results from chronic otitis media

endolymph pale, transparent fluid within membranous labyrinth of ear

gonioscopy test used to measure depth of anterior chamber of the eye; used to differentiate open-angle from narrow (angle-closure) glaucoma

intraocular pressure (IOP) pressure of aqueous humor within eye; normally ranges from 12 to 21 mmHg

labyrinth term used to describe inner ear; composed of two parts: bony labyrinth, a system of open channels that houses second part (membranous labyrinth); bony

labyrinth contains vestibule, semicircular canals, and cochlea

laryngectomy removal of all or part of larynx; partial laryngectomy is used for tumors confined to a specific portion of larynx; total laryngectomy involves removal of entire larynx and surrounding structures and is used for tumors extending beyond vocal cords; requires creation of permanent tracheostomy

miotic pharmacological agents that cause pupil constriction

mydriatic pharmacological agents that cause pupil dilation

myringotomy incision into tympanic membrane to relieve pressure; also known as tympanocentesis

nystagmus involuntary, rapid movements of eye

otosclerosis familial condition of stapes (ossicles of middle ear) characterized by resorption of bone followed by overgrowth of new, hard sclerotic bone; sclerotic changes impact the stapes and oval window and impair sound transmission into inner ear

presbycusis age-related loss of ability to hear high-frequency sounds; may impair ability to hear normal speech

Rinne test test done by alternately placing a tuning fork on mastoid bone and in front of ear canal to compare air and bone conduction; with conductive hearing loss, bone conduction is greater than air conduction; with sensorineural loss, the opposite results are noted

stapedectomy surgical removal and replacement of diseased stapes to restore hearing

tonometry indirect measure of intraocular pressure using contact or non-contact methods

tympanocentesis aspiration of fluid/pus from middle ear using a needle

tympanometry an indirect measurement of compliance of middle ear to sound transmission; an audiometer with a sealed probe tip is used to deliver a continuous tone to tympanic membrane; an instrument records energy reflected from surface of membrane; also known as impedance audiometry

tympanoplasty surgical reconstruction of ossicles and tympanic membrane of middle ear to help restore hearing

Weber test diagnostic test using a tuning fork held against midline of top of head to differentiate conductive hearing loss from sensorineural hearing loss

PRETEST

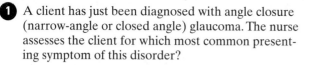

1 A client has just been diagnosed with angle closure (narrow-angle or closed angle) glaucoma. The nurse assesses the client for which most common presenting symptom of this disorder?

1. Halo vision
2. Dull eye pain
3. Severe eye and face pain
4. Impaired night vision

2 The nurse notes a cloudy appearance to the lens of an 80-year-old client's eye. Which of the following additional assessment findings would help confirm the diagnosis of cataracts?

1. Sense of a curtain falling over the visual field
2. Persistent, dull eye pain
3. Loss of red reflex
4. Double vision

3 The nurse would take which of the following as a priority action for the client with a penetrating eye injury from a visible foreign body?

1. Patch both eyes
2. Immobilize the foreign body and cover the eye
3. Irrigate the eye with copious amounts of water
4. Administer carbonic anhydrase inhibitors as prescribed

4 A client is diagnosed with conductive hearing loss and asks how this occurred. The nurse should respond by stating that conductive hearing loss:

1. Has an unknown etiology.
2. Occurs as a result of damage to the hair cells of the inner ear.
3. Usually results from chronic exposure to loud noise.
4. Occurs as a result of damage to the middle ear structures.

5 The nurse should assess a client with sensorineural hearing loss using which of the following?

1. Tympanocentesis
2. Transillumination of the sinuses
3. Electronystagmography
4. Weber and Rinne tests

6 The nurse should include which of the following information in a teaching plan for the parents of an infant with acute otitis media? Select all that apply.

1. Antibiotics can be discontinued when infant is afebrile
2. When bottle-feeding, infant should be maintained in an upright position
3. Orange juice and other fruit juices should be eliminated from the diet
4. Cigarette smoke in the home is a significant risk factor in acute otitis media
5. Infant should be fed in a horizontal position, not upright

7 The nurse developing a teaching plan for a client with atrophic macular degeneration should include information about which of the following?

1. Surgical treatment options
2. Availability of aids to enhance vision and promote safety
3. Risks associated with the loss of peripheral vision
4. Antibiotic therapy

8 The nurse anticipates that which of the following ophthalmic medications would be ordered for the client who has open-angle glaucoma? Select all that apply.

1. Cholinergic such as pilocarpine (Pilocar)
2. Beta blocker such as timolol (Timoptic)
3. Anticholinergic such as atropine sulfate
4. Prostaglandin analog such as latanoprost (Xalatan)
5. Warm compresses instead of medications as this is the less severe form of glaucoma

9 A 60-year-old male presents to the clinic complaining of hoarseness and a cough for at least two months. His spouse states his voice has changed in the last few months. The nurse interprets that the client's symptoms are consistent with which of the following disorders?

1. Gastroesophageal reflux disease (GERD)
2. Coronary artery disease (CAD)
3. Laryngeal cancer
4. Chronic sinusitis

10 The nurse is caring for a client immediately after surgery. The client has nasal packing. What is the most important action that the nurse should take to provide safe care to this client?

1. Provide frequent oral care
2. Ensure adequate intake of oral fluids
3. Monitor respiratory function and oxygen saturation
4. Administer analgesics as prescribed

➤ *See pages 211–213 for Answers and Rationales.*

I. RISK FACTORS ASSOCIATED WITH EYE, EAR, NOSE, AND THROAT HEALTH PROBLEMS

   A. **Glaucoma:** advancing age, ethnicity, diabetes, and family history

   B. **Cataracts:** advancing age, tobacco smoking associated with alcohol consumption, exposure to ultraviolet light, ocular trauma, and family history

   C. **Eye injury:** environmental and workplace hazards, motor vehicle accidents, sports injuries, and physical assault

   D. **Macular degeneration:** advancing age, family history, and nutritional factors have been implicated

   E. **Retinal detachment:** advancing age, myopia, and trauma (i.e., sudden blows to head)

   F. **Sensorineural hearing impairment:** advancing age, ototoxic medications, and persistent exposure to loud noise

   G. **Conductive hearing impairment:** otosclerosis, infections of external or middle ear, trauma to tympanic membrane and middle ear

   H. **Otitis media:** age (i.e., common in infants and children), upper respiratory infections, and allergies

   I. **Ménière's disease:** age (i.e., increased incidence in middle-age) and family history

   J. **Epistaxis:** nasal trauma (i.e., blunt trauma or mild irritation from manipulation), nasal allergies, substance abuse (i.e., cocaine) sinusitis, upper respiratory infections (URI), tobacco smoking, use of oxygen, certain climates or altitudes, prescription medications, and anatomic variations (i.e., deviated nasal septum, nasal polyps)

   K. **Laryngeal cancer:** tobacco smoking, alcohol consumption associated with tobacco smoking, occupational exposure to chemicals and toxins, and family history

II. GLAUCOMA

   A. **Overview**

   1. Defined as a group of conditions characterized by increased **intraocular pressure (IOP);** if untreated, it results in ischemia and degeneration of retina and optic nerve, loss of vision, and complete blindness

   2. Normal intraocular pressure ranges from 12 to 21 mmHg

   3. Caused by alterations in circulation and resorption of aqueous humor

   4. Classified as *open-angle* (wide-angle) or *closed-angle* (narrow-angle or acute-angle closure)

   5. Manifests as a *primary* or *secondary* disorder and may be congenital or acquired

   a. Primary glaucoma occurs without evidence of preexisting eye or systemic disease

   b. Secondary glaucoma results from inflammatory processes, tumors, long-term steroid use, or ocular trauma

   B. **Pathophysiology**

   1. Aqueous humor serves to maintain IOP and support metabolism of lens and posterior cornea

   2. Formation/secretion of aqueous humor is an active process that begins at ciliary body (ciliary epithelium) in posterior chamber; aqueous humor flows through pupil into anterior chamber; resorption into venous system occurs through trabecular meshwork of anterior chamber into Canal of Schlemm (Figure 6-1)

Figure 6-1

Internal structures of the eye.

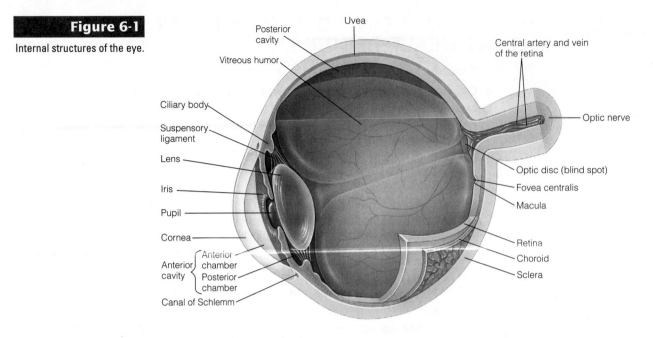

3. Open-angle (wide-angle) glaucoma
   a. Etiology is unclear; there is no obstruction between trabecular meshwork and anterior chamber
   b. May occur because of an abnormality of trabecular meshwork (network) that impairs flow of aqueous humor into Canal of Schlemm; the resulting increased pressure in anterior chamber causes increased pressure in posterior chamber
   c. Usually affects both eyes, has a genetic component, and is frequently seen in adults over 60 years of age
   d. Onset is insidious with no symptoms in early stages
   e. Signs and symptoms include tunnel vision (an initial symptom) from loss of peripheral vision, pain (persistent, dull eye pain, lasting over 20 minutes), halo and/or blurred vision, inability to detect colors, and mild headaches

4. Closed-angle (narrow-angle or acute-angle closure) glaucoma
   a. An *acute medical emergency* resulting in narrowing of angle between pupil and lateral cornea resulting in impaired outflow of aqueous humor
   b. Symptoms relate to sudden, intermittent increases in IOP and may occur following prolonged sitting in a darkened room, during emotional upset or stress, or any condition causing prolonged pupil dilation
   c. Often unilateral; other eye may be affected at a later time and accounts for only 5 to 10% of cases
   d. Signs and symptoms include sudden, severe eye and face pain, severe headache accompanied by nausea and vomiting (may be confused with migraine), blurred vision and/or complaints of halos around lights, redness of eye, haziness (steaminess) of cornea, and fixed dilated pupil at midpoint that is nonreactive to light

C. Nursing assessment

1. Open-angle (wide-angle) glaucoma

    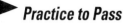

    a. Assessment includes eye examination for loss of peripheral vision, tunnel vision, or complaints of seeing halos around lights; ability to focus on near objects or differentiate colors, symptom analysis of headaches and eye or face pain, and family history of glaucoma

    b. Diagnostic tests: intraocular pressure measurement (**tonometry**), examination of optic disk, visual field testing, **gonioscopy** (visualization and measurement of angle of anterior chamber) to differentiate open-angle from closed-angle glaucoma

2. Closed-angle (narrow-angle or acute-angle closure) glaucoma

    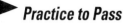

    a. Assessment includes symptom analysis of acute onset of severe eye pain, headaches associated with nausea and vomiting, assessment of eye for color and clarity as well as pupil response, and recent history of prolonged exposure to darkened room, high stress, or emotional distress

    b. Diagnostic tests: same as those used for open-angle glaucoma; blindness can occur if increased IOP persists for 24 to 48 hours

D. Nursing management

1. Medications

    a. Beta-adrenergic blocking eyedrops such as timolol maleate (Timoptic) or betaxolol are (Betaoptic) used to decrease production of aqueous humor; watch for systemic effects

    b. **Miotics** (drugs that constrict pupil); constriction of pupil stimulates ciliary muscle to pull on trabecular meshwork surrounding Canal of Schlemm, which facilitates flow of aqueous humor; pilocarpine hydrochloride (Pilocar) is a typical drug in anticholinergic drug class

    c. Carbonic anhydrase inhibitors (CAIs) such as acetazolamide (Diamox) and dichlorphenamide (Daranide) are used in closed-angle glaucoma to reduce secretion/formation of aqueous humor by ciliary body

    d. Sympathomimetics, prostaglandins, and osmotic diuretics may be used

2. For closed-angle glaucoma, surgical procedures to facilitate drainage of aqueous humor can include trabeculectomy, laser traberculoplasty, iridectomy, or laser iridotomy

3. Teach importance of early detection; urge clients to begin regular eye examinations at age 40 and continue annually

4. Avoid **mydriatrics** (drugs that dilate pupils) such as atropine sulfate (Isopto Atropine); memory trick: "d" is in both mydriatic and dilate

5. Obtain Medic-alert card or bracelet

6. Use safety precautions (i.e., lights, handrails) to compensate for reduced vision

7. Client teaching

    a. Importance of daily compliance with medication; stress that noncompliance may lead to permanent loss of vision

    b. Actions and side effects of specific medications (i.e., systemic effects of ophthalmic beta blockers)

    c. Procedures for correct and safe self-administration of eye drops

    d. Postoperative home care

Practice to Pass

A client who has just been diagnosed with open-angle glaucoma states that her mother "went blind" from glaucoma and that she fears the same will happen to her. How should the nurse respond?

e. Importance of reading over-the-counter (OTC) labels since many of these drugs can increase IOP

III. CATARACTS

A. Overview

1. Defined as a progressive clouding or opacity of lens of eye that interferes with transmission of light to retina, leading to painless loss of vision

2. Cataracts due to aging (senile cataracts) are most common; other causes are foreign body ocular trauma causing lens swelling and rupture, congenital factors (i.e., Down syndrome, intrauterine rubella infection, and fetal exposure to radiation), metabolic disorders (i.e., diabetes mellitus, hypoparathryoidism), certain medications such as systemic corticosteroids, chlorpromazine (Thorazine) and busulfan (Mylcran), exposure to ultraviolet light (UV-B)

B. Pathophysiology

1. As a result of aging or injury, cells in lens degenerate beginning at periphery and moving to center; with progression, entire lens becomes involved

2. Cellular debris from deteriorating lens escapes through degenerating lens capsule into aqueous humor and may contribute to obstruction of outflow of aqueous humor resulting in increased IOP

3. Partial opacity is termed "immature cataract"; opacity of entire lens is termed "mature cataract"

4. Age-related (senile) cataracts are usually bilateral but may be asymmetrical in development

5. Signs and symptoms include blurred vision, visual distortion, decreased night vision, glare and/or abnormal presence of light in visual field, decline in near and distant vision, white or gray opacity filling pupil opening (aperture); as cataract matures, retina becomes impossible to visualize; loss of red reflex occurs

C. Nursing assessment

1. Assessment includes an eye examination, determining client's understanding of cause, symptoms, and treatment options related to cataracts, and assessing client's fears of blindness and/or permanent disability related to cataracts and proposed cataract surgery

2. Diagnostic tests: direct examination of eye using an ophthalmoscope or slit-lamp (lens opacity and absence of red reflex) and Snellen vision testing to assess loss of visual acuity

D. Nursing management

1. Medications include postoperative management with analgesics, anti-inflammatories, and antibiotics to decrease discomfort and prevent infection; no effective medicine is available to remove a cataract

2. Surgical interventions: lens extraction and intraocular lens implantation or use of convex corrective lens (rare); methods utilized include:

   a. Extracapsular extraction: involves removal of lens nucleus and cortex; posterior lens capsule remains intact to help support lens implant; currently is most popular method

   b. Phacoemulsification (use of sound waves to break up lens) has enhanced success of extracapsular extraction

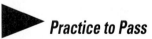

Practice to Pass

Following cataract surgery with lens implantation, the client asks the nurse to explain at-home activity restrictions. What specific instructions should be given to the client?

      c. Cryoextraction involves use of forceps or a supercooled probe to extract lens through a small incision in cornea

      d. Intracapsular extraction involves removal of entire lens and surrounding capsule

      e. Newest technology involves laser removal of lens opacities

  3. Surgical procedures are done on outpatient basis using local anesthesia; usually they are performed on one eye at a time with the second procedure completed within several weeks or months

  4. Identify safety concerns in environment related to loss of visual acuity and propose adaptive measures; if a lens implant is not performed, safety measures must be reinforced related to the loss of accommodation

  5. Caution clients to avoid night driving prior to surgical correction

  6. Client teaching related to surgery (see Box 6-1)

IV. EYE INJURY

A. Overview

  1. Defined as any injury to a part of eye; since even minor injuries can threaten vision, all should be considered emergencies and immediate evaluation and care should be obtained

  2. Major causes of eye injury include corneal abrasion, blunt trauma, penetrating trauma, and burns

B. Pathophysiology

  1. Corneal abrasion

      a. Characterized by a disruption of superficial epithelium of cornea

      b. Common causative agents include contact lenses, foreign bodies (i.e., dust, dirt, fingernails, eyelashes), and chemical irritants

      c. Drying of surface of eye contributes to corneal abrasion

---

Box 6-1	The following should be included when teaching clients undergoing cataract surgery:
Teaching Clients Undergoing Cataract Surgery	➤ Anticipated pre- and postoperative procedures
	➤ Importance of leaving eye patch in place until changed or removed by surgeon at postoperative visit, usually within 24 to 48 hours
	➤ Importance and procedure for administering eye drops and/or ointments during the postoperative period
	➤ Need for eye protection such as sunglasses during the day and eye shields at night; photophobia is common after eye surgery
	➤ Need to avoid sleeping on operative side and bending over
	➤ Insertion and care of postoperative contact lenses if prescribed
	➤ If convex corrective lens are prescribed, explain the loss of peripheral visual fields and need for *turning* the head from side to side to prevent accidents; measures to compensate for loss of depth perception should be emphasized
	➤ Teach symptoms to report to health care provider: eye pain or pressure, redness, cloudiness, drainage, decreased vision, floaters, halos around objects

    d. Superficial cornea abrasions are extremely painful but generally heal without scarring; deeper abrasions may lead to infection and scar formation

    e. Signs and symptoms include pain, tearing, photophobia, and visual impairment (usually temporary)

  2. Blunt trauma

    a. Common causes include sports injuries from baseballs, tennis rackets, handballs as well as from contact sports such as basketball, football, boxing, and wrestling; motor vehicle accidents, physical assault, and falls

    b. Signs and symptoms include lid ecchymosis (black eye), subconjunctival hemorrhage, hyphema, and orbital blowout fracture

      1) Subconjunctival hemorrhage is caused by blood vessel rupture under conjunctiva, (membrane that lines inner surface of eye); manifests as a well-defined, red, painless area; usually requires no treatment; blood reabsorbs within 2 to 3 weeks

      2) Hyphema is characterized by bleeding into anterior chamber of eye; symptoms include pain, decreased visual acuity and reddish tint in visual field; blood is visible to examiner when visualized at an angle

      3) Orbital blowout fracture is caused by fracture of any part of orbit; ethmoid bone on orbital floor is most common site; with fracture, orbital contents including fat, muscles, and eye can herniate into maxillary sinus; symptoms include diplopia, pain with upward movement, decreased sensation on affected cheek, limited eye movement with upward movement, and enophthalmos (sunken appearance to eye)

  3. Penetrating trauma

    a. Common causes include shards of glass, pieces of metal produced from high-speed drilling, gunshot wounds (including BBs), arrows, and knives

    b. In penetrating injuries, layers of eye reapproximate immediately after injury, and injury may not be readily apparent

    c. In perforating injuries, layers of eye do not reapproximate and rupture of globe and loss of ocular contents may occur

    d. Symptoms include pain, loss of vision, bleeding, and possible loss of eye contents

  4. Burns

    a. Chemical burns are most common; other causes include heat, radiation, and explosions

    b. Sources of chemical burns include both acid substances (i.e., acid from car batteries) and alkaline substances (i.e., ammonia, lye from oven cleaners)

    c. Alkaline burns are generally more serious because of progressive damage from particles of offending agent remaining in contact with conjunctival sac; acid burns are generally less serious

    d. Symptoms include eye pain, decreased vision, swollen eyelids, conjunctival reddening, and edema and cloudiness of cornea; ulcerations of cornea and sloughing of conjunctival tissue may occur with chemical burns

C. Nursing assessment

  1. Assessment includes presence of other injuries (i.e., nasal fractures, skin abrasions, facial and scalp lacerations/burns), eye movement, and visual acuity

  2. Diagnostic tests: examination of eye under magnification using topical anesthetics to facilitate examination, fluorescein staining to identify abrasions, and facial x-rays or computed tomography (CT) scanning to identify orbital fractures and/or to evaluate foreign bodies

D. Nursing management

1. Corneal abrasions

   a. Medications include application of ophthalmic antibiotics and eye pad to reduce pain and photophobia

   b. If foreign body present, removal with sterile applicator and/or irrigate with sterile solution

   c. Client education to prevent reinjury

2. Blunt trauma

   a. Medications include carbonic anhydrase inhibitors to reduce IOP as ordered

   b. Place client on bedrest in semi-Fowler's position

   c. Patch affected eye; unaffected eye may also be patched to decrease eye movement

   d. Client education about importance of using protective eyewear during sports activities

3. Penetrating trauma

   a. Medications include opioid analgesics, sedatives and/or antiemetics for vomiting, topical and/or intravenous antibiotics to prevent infection

   b. Do not attempt to remove embedded foreign body

   c. Immobilize foreign body and cover eye to protect from further injury with metal eye shields; paper cups may be substituted for metal shield if foreign body is too large

   d. Patching unaffected eye decreases movement of affected eye

   e. Institute bed rest to prevent further injury

   f. Client education to avoid future injuries

4. Burns

   a. Medications include topical anesthetics to decrease pain during irrigation; following irrigation, apply topical antibiotics as ordered

   b. For chemical burns, immediately flush with copious amounts of normal saline or water

   c. Following irrigation, evaluate vision with and without any corrective eyeglasses

   d. During irrigation, evert eyelid to ensure thorough irrigation of conjunctival sac

   e. Client education on importance of protective eyewear

V. MACULAR DEGENERATION

A. Overview

1. Defined as degeneration of macular area of retina in eye; most common cause of blindness; most common type is termed age-related macular degeneration (ARMD)

2. Macula (located in center of retina) receives light from center of visual field and has greatest visual acuity

3. Causes of age-related macular degeneration are unknown; injury, inflammation, nutritional and hereditary factors have been implicated; males and females are affected equally

B. Pathophysiology

1. In ARMD, gradual failure of outer layer of retina (pigmented epithelium) occurs; pigmented epithelium attaches retina to choroid layer and functions to remove cellular wastes; as outer layer fails, photoreceptor cells are lost, waste products and toxins accumulate in subretinal space, and cell death occurs

2. Types

   a. Atrophic ("dry") form: characterized by gradual, progressive bilateral loss of vision caused by atrophy and degeneration of outer pigmented layer of retina that is attached to choroid

   b. Exudative ("wet") form: characterized by more rapid, severe loss of vision because of accumulation of serous or hemorrhagic fluid in subretinal space; accumulated fluid leads to separation of retina from choroids; scar formation leads to death of retinal cells and loss of vision

3. Signs and symptoms include loss of central vision (peripheral vision remains intact), pale yellow spots called "drusen" appear on macula, visual distortion of images (i.e., straight lines may appear wavy), and difficulty with activities requiring close central vision (i.e., reading and sewing)

C. Nursing assessment

1. Assessment includes eye examination and symptom analysis of appearance of wavy lines and changes in ability to perform close-up work

2. Diagnostic tests: ophthalmologic examination, visual acuity, visual field and color vision tests, and electroretinography (ERG) to measure retinal responses to light

D. Nursing management

1. No medications are required for macular degeneration; treatment modalities include:

   a. Laser photocoagulation for exudative macular degeneration

   b. No current therapy for atrophic macular degeneration

2. Early referral for ophthalmologic examination and early intervention may preserve vision and slow progression of disease

3. Reassurance that loss of central vision does not progress to loss of peripheral vision

4. Assessment of home environment to prevent injuries related to loss of vision

5. Client education

   a. Availability of aids to enhance vision and promote safety (i.e., magnification devices, enhanced lighting)

   b. Availability of large-print books and newspapers as well as audio books

   c. Importance of home safety evaluation to minimize risk of injuries and falls

VI. RETINAL DETACHMENT

A. Overview

1. Defined as separation of sensory layer of retina from choroid

2. Usually occurs spontaneously but may result from trauma such as sudden blows to head

3. Spontaneous retinal detachment occurs most frequently in clients older than 50 years

Practice to Pass

A client is admitted to the outpatient surgery unit for scleral buckling of a detached retina. How should the nurse explain retinal detachment and respond to the client's fears about permanent loss of vision?

4. Causes include eye tumors, inflammatory disorders, myopia, and cataract extraction

B. **Pathophysiology**

1. Retina may tear and fold back onto itself or remain intact and be pulled away from choroid as vitreous humor shrinks because of aging

2. Breaks in retina allow fluid from vitreous cavity to seep into defect; additionally, fluids from choroid vessels, the pull of gravity, and traction imposed by the vitreous enhance separation

3. Separation of retina from choroid causes ischemia, death of retinal neurons, and permanent loss of vision

4. Retinal damage can progress slowly or can enlarge quickly resulting in complete detachment

5. It is considered a medical emergency requiring immediate intervention

6. Signs and symptoms include sudden appearance of floaters, irregular lines and/or flashes of light in visual field, sensation of having a curtain drawn across field of vision, progressive deterioration of vision, blurred vision, weeping of eye (when trauma occurs), loss of central vision if macula is involved, and hemorrhage into vitreous; ophthalmic examination may reveal gray opaque appearance of retina and/or evidence of tears, holes, or folds in retina; detachment is usually painless

C. **Nursing assessment**

1. Assessment includes symptom analysis of visual changes such as floating spots and/or flashing lights, loss of visual acuity, blurred vision, and/or sense of curtain or veil coming down into visual field, any history of trauma to eye, and physical examination for weeping and visual redness

2. Diagnosis based on ophthalmoscope examination

D. **Nursing management**

1. Medications include antibiotics, anti-inflammatory agents, and analgesics as ordered

2. Treatment modalities include the following surgical interventions:

   a. Scleral buckling utilizes laser photocoagulation or cryothermy to produce adhesions that seal retinal layers; silicone is used to indent or "buckle" sclera to enhance contact between layers

   b. Pneumatic retinopexy involves injecting air/gas into vitreous to force detached retina to come into contact with choroid

   c. Laser photocoagulation or cryothermy can also be used without scleral buckling to create areas of inflammation and adhesions, which fuse separated layers together

   d. Surgical instrumentation is used to manipulate detached retina into place

3. Provide for emergency care with an ophthalmologist

4. Ensure that client's head is positioned with detached area in a dependent position to assist gravity to pull retina back closer to choroid

5. Instruct client to avoid bending forward or making sudden head movements

6. Cover both eyes with patches to limit ocular movement

7. Protect client from injury (i.e., bed in low position, side rails up, call bell within reach)

8. Provide pre- and postoperative instructions

9. Offer psychological support to alleviate anxiety related to sudden loss of vision and fear of permanent blindness

10. Provide diversional activities for distraction such as books on tape or mirror to view television while lying in head-dependent position

VII. SENSORINEURAL HEARING IMPAIRMENT

A. Overview

1. Defined as abnormalities of cochlear apparatus or auditory nerve decreasing and/or distorting transfer of sounds to brain, resulting in loss of hearing; sound transmission to inner ear is normal

2. Occurs with disorders affecting inner ear, auditory nerve, or auditory pathways to brain

3. Characterized by loss of perception of high-frequency tones, making speech recognition difficult in noisy environments

4. Causes of sensorineural hearing loss include persistent exposure to loud noise, trauma to head or inner ear, vascular lesions, ototoxicity from medications (i.e., aminoglycosides, salicylates, diuretics, vancomycin, antineoplastic agents); infections (i.e., bacterial meningitis), Ménière's disease, **presbycusis** (degenerative changes resulting from aging), endocrine disorders (i.e., diabetes mellitus, hypothyroidism), intrauterine infections (i.e., maternal rubella), developmental malformations, and tumors (i.e., acoustic neuroma, meningioma, metastatic brain tumors)

5. In presbycusis, degenerative changes may begin in early adulthood but not be clinically significant until later in life; men are affected earlier and experience greater hearing loss than women

6. Hearing loss is usually permanent

7. May occur along with conductive hearing loss; termed mixed hearing loss

B. Pathophysiology

1. Inner ear (**labyrinth**) contains vestibule, semicircular canals, and cochlea; the cochlea houses the organ of Corti (see Figure 6-2)

2. Exposure to high levels of noise on an intermittent or constant basis damages hair cells of organ of Corti

3. With presbycusis, hair cells of organ of Corti degenerate; gradual, progressive hearing loss results in difficulty hearing high-pitched tones and conversational speech; eventually, ability to hear middle and lower tones is lost

4. Signs and symptoms of sensorineural hearing loss include deafness (usually bilateral), inability to hear low, middle and/or high-pitched sounds, tinnitus (ringing in ear), dizziness, and pain

C. Nursing assessment

1. Nursing assessment includes signs of hearing loss (i.e., increased voice volume, requests for information to be repeated, inappropriate responses to questions, lack of response, and turning head to direction of a speaker)

2. Diagnostic tests: **audiometry** to assess hearing, **Weber** and **Rinne tests** (tuning fork tests) to differentiate sensorineural hearing loss from conductive hearing

Figure 6-2

Structures of the external ear, middle ear, and inner ear.

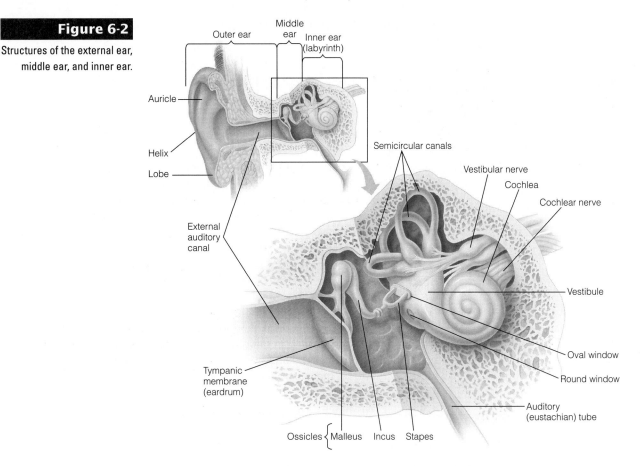

loss, brainstem auditory evoked response (BAER), and brain imaging studies to rule out intracranial lesions

D. Nursing management

1. Medications are not recommended; treatment modalities are limited but include:
   a. Cochlear implants: provide clients with perception of sound but not normal hearing; allow clients to recognize warning sounds of telephones, sirens, and automobiles; alert clients to incoming communication; and provide some help for clients even if no auditory nerve function exists
   b. Hearing aids not generally helpful; serve only to intensify distorted sounds
   c. Use of devices that provide "white noise" to mask unpleasant or distressing sounds associated with tinnitus (such as tinnitus marker)
2. Avoid shouting; address clients in normal, low-pitched voice
3. Provide adequate visual contact and lighting when communicating with clients to foster speech lip-reading; face client directly
4. Provide alternative means of communication (i.e., use sign language, provide written instructions)
5. Reduce background noises when communicating with clients
6. Use short sentences and gestures (i.e., pointing) when appropriate
7. Educate family about social isolation associated with sensorineural hearing loss, including apparent inattention, withdrawal, and/or disinterest

8. Evaluate safety of home environment (i.e., ability to hear smoke detectors, telephones)

VIII. CONDUCTIVE HEARING IMPAIRMENT

A. Overview

1. Defined as an interruption in sound transmission from external auditory canal to inner ear

2. Causes include obstruction of external auditory canal by impacted cerumen; edema of canal lining, foreign objects, and neoplasms; rupture or scarring of tympanic membrane; disruption or fixation of bones in middle ear secondary to trauma or **otosclerosis** (a familial disorder of hearing loss); otitis externa or otitis media, presence of fluid in middle ear; and congenital malformations of external or middle ear

3. Termed mixed hearing loss if occurs in conjunction with sensorineural hearing loss

B. Pathophysiology

1. Changes in hearing may be sudden or gradual depending upon cause

2. With otosclerosis, bone resorption is followed by overgrowth of new, hard sclerotic bone; stapes (ossicle in middle ear) becomes immobilized against oval window thus decreasing transmission of sound to inner ear; pressure of otosclerotic bone on inner ear structures or 8th cranial nerve may also result in sensorineural hearing loss

3. Often unilateral; may be bilateral if caused by otosclerosis

4. Signs and symptoms include loss of sound at all frequencies and tinnitus with otosclerosis

C. Nursing assessment

1. Assessment includes presence of foreign bodies, infection and/or cerumen in external auditory canal, integrity of tympanic membrane and presence of otitis media

2. Diagnostic tests: Weber and Rinne tests, audiometry, **tympanometry** (an indirect measurement of compliance of middle ear to sound transmission), and otoscopic examination

D. Nursing management

1. No medications are recommended; treatment modalities include:

   a. Removal of cerumen or foreign body by health care provider; medications such as carbamide peroxide (Debrox) help with dry cerumen

   b. Hearing aids to amplify sound

   c. Assistive listening devices ("pocket talker")

   d. Reconstructive procedures to restore hearing: **stapedectomy** (making an incision in stapes to improve hearing) for otosclerosis and **tympanoplasty** (surgical procedure to restore function of middle ear to transmit sound more efficiently)

2. Client teaching related to conductive hearing loss (see Box 6-2)

3. Utilize techniques appropriate for hearing impaired as noted in section on nursing management of sensorineural hearing loss

4. Provide appropriate pre- and postoperative care

IX. OTITIS MEDIA

A. Overview

1. Defined as inflammation and/or infection of middle ear

2. Primarily affects infants and young children; may occur in adults

3. Major cause of conductive hearing loss

4. Two common forms of otitis media include *serous otitis media* and *acute otitis media*

5. Causes

    a. Serous otitis media: upper respiratory infections, allergies, and narrow or edematous Eustachian tubes

    b. Acute otitis media: *Streptococcus pneumoniae, Haemophilus influenzae,* and *Streptococcus pyogenes*

B. Pathophysiology

1. Tympanic membrane protects middle ear from external auditory canal; Eustachian tube (auditory tube) connects middle ear with nasopharynx and serves to equalize pressure in middle ear with atmospheric pressure

2. *Serous otitis media*

    a. Occurs when Eustachian tube is obstructed for a prolonged period of time, causing impaired equalization of air pressure within middle ear

    b. Air in middle ear is absorbed; continued obstruction of Eustachian tube prevents more air from entering, and negative pressure in middle ear results; serous fluid moves into middle ear forming a sterile effusion

    c. Signs and symptoms of serous otitis media include: decreased hearing in affected ear, complaints of "snapping" or "popping," decreased mobility of tympanic membrane, retracted or bulging of tympanic membrane indicating presence of fluid or air bubbles, pain, bleeding and/or rupture of tympanic membrane, rupture of round window with sensory hearing loss, and vertigo

3. *Acute otitis media*

    a. Results from entry of pathogens from oronasopharynx via Eustachian tube into normally sterile environment of middle ear

    b. Typically follows upper respiratory infections

Box 6-2	The following points should be included in a teaching plan for clients with conductive hearing loss:
Teaching Clients with Conductive Hearing Loss	➤ Technique for proper insertion and cleaning of hearing aids
	➤ Proper insertion of hearing aid batteries; need for extra batteries
	➤ Availability of assistive listening devices (i.e., "pocket talkers")
	➤ Postoperative and home care following stapedectomy or tympanoplasty
	➤ Methods to protect ears from injury; use of ear plugs while swimming and diving
	➤ Care of ears and ear canal, including cleaning and removal of cerumen
	➤ Signs of middle ear infection and the importance of early and complete treatment

c. Common in infants and children because of short, straight Eustachian tubes; higher incidence noted in bottle-fed infants/toddlers who maintain a more horizontal position during feeding and in those living with smokers

d. Invasion and colonization by bacteria along with white blood cell invasion leads to pus formation; pus increases middle ear pressure and may lead to rupture of tympanic membrane

e. Signs and symptoms of acute otitis media include: pain, often severe, in affected ear; infants and young children may pull at affected ear; fever; impaired hearing; dizziness and vertigo; red, inflamed or dull, bulging tympanic membrane; decreased movement of membrane; tenderness over mastoid area indicating development of mastoiditis

4. Chronic, recurring otitis media may result in permanent perforation of tympanic membrane, permanent hearing loss, and/or the formation of a benign epithelial-cell tumor, called **cholesteatoma**

5. Complications of untreated acute otitis media include meningitis, osteomyelitis of skull, and facial paralysis

C. **Nursing assessment**

1. Assessment includes visualization of tympanic membrane using otoscope, pain (intensity, description, and location); note that pain associated with otitis media, unlike that of external otitis, is not aggravated by ear movement; history for recurrent otitis media

2. Diagnostic tests: visualization of tympanic membrane with pneumatic otoscope, tympanometry, complete blood count (CBC) to assess for an elevated white blood cell count, and culture of middle ear effusion if membrane has ruptured or **myringotomy** (incision into tympanic membrane) has been done

D. **Nursing management**

1. Serous otitis media

a. Medications include systemic or intranasal decongestants to reduce edema of Eustachian tube and maintain patency, analgesics, and antipyretics

b. Treatment includes autoinflation of middle ear by forcefully exhaling against closed nostrils

c. Avoidance of air travel and underwater diving

2. Acute otitis media

a. Medications include antibiotic therapy with or without decongestants; therapy often continued for 10 to 12 days; analgesics, and antipyretics

b. **Tympanocentesis:** aspiration of fluid from middle ear

c. Myringotomy with or without insertion of tympanostomy tubes (ventilation tubes)

3. Stress importance of completing full course of antibiotic therapy

4. Stress importance of increasing fluid intake and consuming nutritious diet to enhance immune system and hasten resolution of infection

5. Alert clients or parents of possibility of superinfections due to antibiotic therapy, such as diarrhea or thrush

6. If tympanostomy tubes are present, caution clients to avoid swimming, diving, or allowing water to enter ear

7. Provide appropriate pre- and postoperative care for myringotomy and/or insertion of tympanostomy tubes

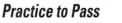

Practice to Pass

A young mother brings her 12-month-old child in with recurrent acute otitis media. What should the nurse suggest to help prevent recurrence of these middle ear infections?

X. EXTERNAL OTITIS

A. Overview

1. Defined as an inflammation of outer ear canal; known as swimmer's ear

2. Caused by excess moisture in ear canal, fungi or bacteria, trauma, or local hypersensitivity; common organisms include *Pseudomonas aeruginosa*

B. Pathophysiology

1. Removal of cerumen, which has water-repellant and antimicrobial properties, leaves ear canal susceptible to infection; excess moisture, vigorous cleaning, or excess drying of ear canal can assist in removing cerumen

2. Signs and symptoms include severe pain, fullness in ear, and decreased hearing; pain with application of pressure on tragus is a hallmark sign; visual examination shows clusters of white particles on side of canals and edema; tympanic membrane may be difficult to see but will appear normal and pearly gray

C. Nursing assessment

1. Assessment includes a symptom analysis of when pain began (frequency, description), occupation or frequency in swimming, physical palpation of tragus

2. Diagnostic tests: ear examination with otoscope

D. Nursing management

1. Medications include topical antibiotics, topical corticosteroids such as polymixin B-neomycin hydrocortisone (Cortisporin otic), benzocaine and antipyrine (Auralgan), pain medication as needed, and aluminum sulfate and calcium acetate (Dome Burrow) solution to irrigate ear

2. Instruct client to use topical antibiotic for prescribed time in order to completely eliminate organism and avoid swimming for 7 to 10 days

3. Educate client to use drying agents before and after swimming (such as Swimmer's Ear™ or a 2% acetic acid solution with alcohol), earplugs should be used for clients with ear tubes

XI. MÉNIÈRE'S DISEASE

A. Overview

1. Defined as a chronic inner ear disorder characterized by a triad of symptoms including vertigo, tinnitus, and sensorineural hearing loss, known as *endolymphatic hydrops*

2. Usually unilateral, affecting men and women equally; high-risk group includes adults between ages of 35 and 60

3. Causes include trauma, infection, allergies, adrenal-pituitary insufficiency, hypothyroidism, immune system dysfunction, increased sodium intake, stress, and premenstrual fluid retention; a genetic predisposition may exist

B. Pathophysiology

1. Most common form is idiopathic

2. An overaccumulation of fluid (**endolymph**) in membranous labyrinth of inner ear results in dilation of lymphatic channels and labyrinth dysfunction; autonomic nervous system control of labyrinthine circulation may be impaired, also contributing to labyrinth dysfunction

3. Excess fluid is thought to be caused by an impaired absorption of endolymph

4. Onset of symptoms may be gradual or sudden

5. Signs and symptoms include severe rotary vertigo (lasting from minutes to hours, may be associated with nausea and vomiting and may cause immobility), tinnitus, sensorineural hearing loss, sense of fullness in ears, hypotension, diaphoresis, and **nystagmus** (irregular eye movements) during acute attacks

C. Nursing assessment

1. Assessment includes subjective reports of dizziness, nausea, vomiting, sweating, tinnitus, incapacitating vertigo, blurred vision, sensitivity to light, and roaring sensation in ears; objective assessment should include heart rate (HR) (bradycardia), diarrhea, and disequilibrium; history often includes past otitis media, allergies, and arteriosclerosis

2. Diagnostic tests

    a. Electronystagmography (ENG): a series of tests used to evaluate vestibular-ocular reflexes by identifying nystagmus as a response to specific stimuli; caloric ice water test is one part of ENG

    b. Caloric ice water testing involves instillation of cold water into external auditory canal; in clients with impaired inner ear function, normal nystagmus response is blunted or absent; this test is not recommended if tympanic membrane is perforated

    c. X-rays and CT scans are used to evaluate anatomic changes of central portion of inner ear known as the vestibule

    d. Rinne and Weber tests utilize a tuning fork to test hearing

    e. Auditory dehydration test involves administration of fast-acting diuretics or hyperosmolar substances (i.e., glycerin) orally to decrease fluid pressure in inner ear; acute, temporary improvement is considered diagnostic

    f. Audiometry testing

D. Nursing management

1. Medications for *acute attacks*

    a. Anticholinergics: atropine sulfate (Isopto Atropine) and scopolamine (Isopto Hyoscine) to decrease response peripheral nervous system

    b. Central nervous system (CNS) depressants: diazepam (Valium), lorazepam (Ativan) as an alternative to anticholinergics

    c. Antiemetics: prochlorperazine (Compazine), meclizine (Antivert)

    d. Sedatives/antiemetics: droperidol (Inapsine)

    e. Antihistamines: diphenhydramine (Benadryl)

    f. Antibiotics in large doses for bacterial labyrinthitis

2. Medications *between attacks* include oral diuretics (such as furosemide [Lasix] or hydrochlorothiazide/triamterene [Dyazide] to decrease pressure in labyrinth, as well as vasodilators

3. Ensure client safety *during attacks* (i.e., assist with ambulation, side rails up, bed in low position, call bell within reach), limit movement, and replace fluid and electrolytes

4. Medical treatment options *between* acute attacks focus on prevention; interventions include a sodium-restricted diet and avoidance of substances causing vasoconstriction (i.e., tobacco, alcohol, and caffeine)

5. Surgical interventions

   a. Endolymphatic sac decompression and shunting, which releases pressure in labyrinth and shunts endolymph from membranous labyrinth to subarachnoid space

   b. Vestibular nerve resection: removal of part of 8th cranial nerve

   c. Labyrinthectomy: complete removal of labyrinth

6. When administering diuretics, monitor for electrolyte imbalance

7. Ensure adequate hydration and nutrition if attacks are frequent

8. Client teaching

   a. Signs of impending attack (i.e., feeling of ear fullness, increasing tinnitus, vertigo, nausea and vomiting)

   b. Avoidance of attack triggers (i.e., stress, fatigue, blinking lights, loud noises, quick or jerky body movements)

   c. Safety measures if attack occurs while driving (i.e., pull off to side of road, need for car phone and "HELP POLICE" sign)

   d. Need for adequate rest and sleep; avoid tobacco

   e. Relaxation techniques

   f. Availability of organizations offering information and support (i.e., Vestibular Disorders Association and Ménière's Network)

   g. Need for Medic-alert bracelet, card, or necklace

   h. Salt-restricted or salt-free diet

XII. EPISTAXIS

A. Overview

1. Defined as a nosebleed; the nose is highly vascular, receiving blood from major arterial vessels originating from both internal and external carotid arteries

2. Men are affected by nosebleeds more often than women

3. Bleeding may originate in anterior or posterior nose

4. Identified by area where bleeding originates: *anterior epistaxis* or *posterior epistaxis*

5. Causes include medications, particularly antiplatelets or anticoagulants, and the following:

   a. Anterior epistaxis: drying, infection, blunt trauma or trauma from manipulation, cocaine use, and local infection

   b. Posterior epistaxis: blood dyscrasias, hypertension, diabetes, and trauma

B. Pathophysiology

1. Ninety percent of all nosebleeds arise from Kiesselbach's area, a rich vascular plexus in anterior nasal spectum or from rupture of vessels caused by trauma

2. Posterior epistaxis tends to be more severe; occurs more often in older adults

C. Nursing assessment

1. Assessment includes identifying amount of blood lost and source of bleeding by examining both nares and back of throat to rule out posterior bleeding, client's health history, medication history including use of herbal products, and vital signs

    2. There are no diagnostic tests; a CBC may be obtained if severe blood loss has been experienced

    3. Drying of nasal passages can trigger nosebleeds

D. Nursing management

    1. Medications include topical application of vasoconstrictors such as phenylephrine (Neo-Synephrine), oxymetazoline hydrochloride (Afrin), or adrenaline; chemical cauterization using silver nitrate or Gelfoam, topical antibacterial ointment to inner nares, and analgesics (particularly if packing has been placed)

    2. Treatment options

        a. First aid measures

            1) Assess for respiratory distress; administer supplemental oxygen as indicated

            2) Instruct client to sit upright with head tilted forward

            3) Apply pressure, by pinching nose toward septum, for 5 to 10 minutes

            4) Apply ice packs to nose and/or forehead to promote vasoconstriction

            5) Encourage client to expectorate blood to prevent nausea and vomiting resulting from swallowed blood

            6) Estimate blood loss when possible

            7) Maintain an attitude of calm reassurance

        b. Nasal packing

        c. Surgery including cauterization and ligation of vessels (i.e., **Caldwell-Luc procedure**)

    3. Following nasal packing

        a. Monitor respiratory function and oxygen saturation

        b. Assess packing for odor, color, and amount of drainage

        c. Administer analgesics as needed

        d. Monitor vital signs to assess for cardiovascular complications and infection

        e. Monitor position of catheter (i.e., rubber or inflatable type) if used to provide hemostasis

        f. Provide frequent oral care; use bedside humidifier or high humidity face mask to reduce drying of oral mucous membranes

    4. Provide pre- and postoperative teaching and care as indicated

XIII. SINUSITIS

A. Overview

    1. Defined as inflammation with resulting infection of mucous membranes of one or more of paranasal sinuses

    2. Commonly follows upper respiratory tract infections or viral rhinitis

    3. Classified as *acute, subacute,* or *chronic*

        a. Acute sinusitis lasts from 1 day to 3 weeks

        b. Subacute sinusitis persists from 3 weeks to 3 months

        c. Chronic sinusitis lasts longer than 3 months

    4. Immunocompromised clients may be at greater risk for sinusitis and may be more difficult to treat

5. Causes include: upper respiratory infections, viral rhinitis, nasal polyps, deviated nasal septum, tooth abscess, prolonged nasotracheal or nasogastric intubation in hospitalized client, abuse of nasal decongestants, swimming and diving, exposure to frequent changes in barometric pressure (i.e., pilots, flight attendants), smoking, nasal packing (epistaxis), and allergies

B. Pathophysiology

1. Paranasal sinuses are air cells that connect with nasal cavity and are named for the bone in which they are located (i.e., frontal, sphenoid, ethmoid, and maxillary)

2. Sinuses are lined with cilia; cilia facilitate movement of fluids and microorganisms into nasal cavity for exit from body

3. Viral illness produces inflammation of sinus mucosa causing obstruction of normal ciliary action, creating an ideal environment for bacterial growth

4. Following invasion of microorganisms into sinuses, the inflammatory response increases swelling and congestion, further compromising normal ciliary action; bacterial growth continues

5. Common organisms associated with sinusitis include *Streptococcus pyogenes, Staphylococcus aureus, Streptococcus pneumoniae,* and *Haemophilus influenzae;* gram-negative species and fungi may also be causative

6. Signs and symptoms

   a. Acute sinusitis: constant, often severe pain and tenderness over infected sinuses, pain in teeth may indicate maxillary sinusitis, headache, fever, malaise, and fatigue, nasal congestion, purulent nasal discharge, halitosis, sore and inflamed throat because of swallowed secretions (postnasal drip)

   b. Subacute or chronic sinusitis: dull, intermittent or constant pain, purulent nasal discharge, chronic cough, and loss of sense of smell

7. Local and intracranial complications of sinusitis

   a. Periorbital abscesses and/or cellulitis

   b. Osteomyelitis of the facial bones

   c. Cavernous sinus thrombosis

   d. Meningitis

   e. Brain abscess

   f. Sepsis

C. Nursing assessment

1. Assessment includes frequency of sinusitis, precipitating factors, pain, and need for analgesics

2. Diagnostic tests: physical examination including inspection of nose and throat, cultures of nasal discharge, transillumination of sinuses, x-rays and CT scans to detect opacity of sinuses, and nasal endoscopy to visualize anterior nasal cavity and sinus openings

D. Nursing management

1. Medications include antibiotic therapy, oral or intranasal decongestants, intranasal corticosteroids, expectorants such as guaifenesin (Robitussin) to liquefy secretions, saline nasal sprays and/or steam inhalation, saline irrigation of maxillary sinus (i.e., antral irrigation) using needle access to sinus, and

analgesics; clients with allergies may use medications to decrease allergic response, such as desloratidine (Clarinex), loratidine (Claritin), budesonide (Rhinocort) or fexofenadine (Allegra)

2. Surgical interventions

   a. Endoscopic sinus surgery

   b. Caldwell-Luc procedure

   c. External sphenoethmoidectomy: removal of diseased tissue from sphenoid or ethmoid sinuses via a surgical incision along side of nose

   d. Administer analgesics as necessary; institute comfort measures (i.e., application of ice packs, elevate head of bed)

   e. Provide teaching

      1) Importance of completing full course of antibiotic therapy

      2) Uses and hazards of nasal decongestants, such as rebound effect

      3) Signs and symptoms of recurrent infection

      4) Importance of adequate hydration

      5) Postoperative management including avoidance of strenuous activity and blowing the nose

XIV. LARYNGEAL CANCER

A. Overview

1. Defined as cancer of glottis (true vocal cords), supraglottis, or subglottis

2. Causes are prolonged use of tobacco and alcohol, chronic laryngitis, occupational exposure to chemicals and toxins, exposure to selected types of human papilloma virus, and genetic predisposition

3. Squamous cell carcinoma is most common type of laryngeal malignancy

4. With early diagnosis and treatment, 80 to 90% of small lesions can be cured

B. Pathophysiology

1. Exposure to irritants (i.e., tobacco smoke, chemicals, toxins) result in changes to laryngeal mucosa

2. Precancerous leukoplakia (white, patchy lesions) and erythroplakia (red, velvet-like patches) appear on laryngeal mucosa

3. Lesions may occur in any of three areas of larynx (i.e., glottis, supraglottis, or subglottis); lesions along edges of glottis (true vocal cords) are most common (see Figure 6-3)

4. Lesions of glottis are usually well-differentiated and slow-growing

5. Structures in supraglottis include epiglottis, arytenoid muscles and cartilage, and false vocal cords; subglottis is located below vocal cords and terminates at tracheal ring; tumors of supraglottis are often large before symptoms are noted and very rare

6. Laryngeal tumors initially metastasize to regional lymph nodes; metastasis to lungs may follow

7. Signs and symptoms include hoarseness, change in voice, dyspnea, pain and burning in throat when drinking hot liquids or citrus juices, dysphagia, foul-smelling breath, pain radiating to ear, persistent cough, and palpable lump in neck

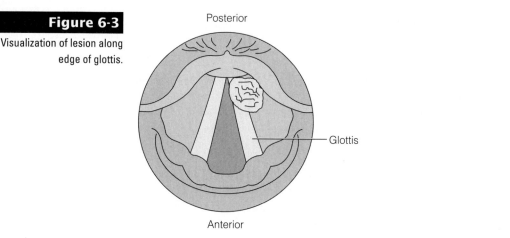

Figure 6-3

Visualization of lesion along edge of glottis.

Posterior

Glottis

Anterior

C. Nursing assessment

1. Assessment includes early recognition of signs and symptoms, signs of respiratory distress, nutritional status, and psychosocial needs; prompt assessment and early referral of clients presenting with symptoms of laryngeal cancer; early diagnosis is critical to survival

2. Diagnostic tests

   a. Laryngoscopy with biopsy of leukoplakia (precancerous lesions) and erythroplakia (precancerous patches)

   b. X-ray studies of head, neck, and chest; CT or MRI scans

   c. Barium swallow to evaluate swallowing and/or presence of tumor in esophagus

D. Nursing management

1. Medications include adjunctive chemotherapy

2. Treatment options

   a. Surgical interventions: partial, supraglottic, or total **laryngectomy** (removal of part or all of larynx) depending upon tumor location; radical neck dissection with cervical lymph node involvement

   b. External beam radiation or implants for early tumors

3. Monitor respiratory status

4. Provide supplemental nutrition

5. Assess emotional status and possible grieving, encourage client to ventilate feelings and concerns

6. Provide postoperative care as indicated and client teaching as follows:

   a. Postoperative and home care following partial or total laryngectomy (i.e., tracheotomy care, enteral nutrition)

   b. Need for radiation treatments and/or chemotherapy

   c. Options available for restoration of speech (i.e., esophageal speech, battery-operated speech generator)

   d. Availability of support services (i.e., American Cancer Society, support groups, pastoral care)

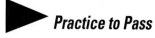

Practice to Pass

The client asks the nurse about the methods available to restore speech following total laryngectomy. How should the nurse respond?

Case Study

R. M., a 48-year-old female client, has been admitted to the Emergency Department with severe vertigo accompanied by nausea and vomiting. She also complains of tinnitus and a sense of fullness in the left ear. She is diagnosed with acute Ménière's disease.

1. What other assessment findings can be expected?

2. What medical interventions can be anticipated during the acute phase of this illness?

3. What diagnostic tests can be anticipated for this client?

4. How should the nurse explain Ménière's disease to the client?

5. What discharge instructions should be given to the client?

For suggested responses, see pages 534–535.

POSTTEST

1 A client reports sudden onset of continuous eye pain and impaired vision. Pupil dilation is noted. The nurse concludes that this assessment data is consistent with which of the following disorders?

1. Closed-angle (narrow-angle) glaucoma
2. Open-angle glaucoma
3. Cataracts
4. Retinal detachment

2 The nurse is assessing a client with Ménière's disease. What subjective assessment data does the nurse expect to obtain?

1. Bilateral hearing impairment
2. Vertigo and nausea
3. Pain when the tragus is touched
4. Tenderness over the mastoid area

3 A male client has just had a cataract operation with a lens implant. In discharge teaching, the nurse will instruct the client's wife to:

1. Prepare only soft foods for several days to prevent facial movement.
2. Encourage sleeping on the affected side for greater comfort.
3. Have her husband resume all normal activities starting the next day.
4. Instill eye drops correctly.

4 An adult client presents to the Emergency Department after having a large rock hit his eye while weeding along a ditch near a busy highway. The event occurred several hours earlier. The nurse assesses the eye and finds redness and weeping, but the client denies any pain. Which of the following early symptoms would help confirm retinal detachment? Select all that apply.

1. Pain
2. Floaters
3. Subconjunctival hemorrhage
4. Sensation of curtain drawn across the vision
5. Dark lines or spots in the field of vision

5 A young child has had a recent upper respiratory infection. The child now reports severe pain in the right ear and says, "I can't hear." The nurse concludes that the pathology that led to this problem is most likely which of the following?

1. Tympanic membrane has ruptured causing hearing loss
2. Child has been exposed to secondhand smoke, which caused an acute allergic response
3. Narrowed auditory tube impaired equalization of pressure in the middle ear, stopping air from entering
4. Edema of the auditory tube followed the respiratory infection impairing drainage of the middle ear

6 The community health nurse interprets that which of the following clients is at highest risk for macular degeneration?

1. Biochemist exposed to various toxins
2. Elderly client
3. Youth hit in the eye with a baseball
4. Young adult with multiple allergies

7 A client presents to the clinic with reports of pain in the cheekbones that is worse when bending forward. What other symptoms should the nurse expect if the diagnosis is acute sinusitis? Select all that apply.

1. Nausea and food intolerances
2. Nasal congestion and purulent discharge
3. Bad breath
4. Nuchal rigidity
5. Pain in the upper teeth

8 Which of the following is a priority nursing diagnosis that the nurse would address for a client with epistaxis?

1. Anxiety with risk for aspiration
2. Risk for infection
3. Pain
4. Impaired verbal communication

9 The community health nurse interprets that which of the following clients is at highest risk for laryngeal cancer? A client who:

1. Has an injury to the larynx.
2. Is 85 years old.
3. Has chewed tobacco and smoked for 20 years.
4. Suffers from chronic sinusitis and seasonal allergies.

10 The nurse would include which interventions in the plan of care for a client with sensorineural hearing loss?

1. Provide information about availability of hearing aids to amplify sound
2. Educate family members about social isolation and depression
3. Administer antibiotics as prescribed
4. Prepare client for tympanoplasty

➤ *See pages 213–214 for Answers & Rationales.*

ANSWERS & RATIONALES

Pretest

1 **Answer: 3** Angle closure or narrow-angle glaucoma develops abruptly and manifests with acute face and eye pain and is a medical emergency. Halo vision, dull eye pain, and impaired night vision are symptoms commonly associated with open-angle glaucoma. **Cognitive Level:** Application **Client Need:** Physiological Integrity: Physiological Adaptation **Integrated Process:** Nursing Process: Assessment **Content Area:** Adult Health: Eye and Ear **Strategy:** Use nursing knowledge to answer the question. If none of the options are recognizable,

keep in mind that when options are opposite, one of them is more likely to be correct. **Reference:** Lemone, P., & Burke, K. (2008). *Medical-surgical nursing: Critical thinking in client care* (4th ed.). Upper Saddle River, NJ: Pearson/Prentice Hall, p. 1707.

2 **Answer: 3** A cloudy-appearing lens is symptomatic of cataract development. As the cataract matures, the red reflex is lost. A sense of a curtain falling over the visual field is associated with detached retina. Eye pain and double vision are not associated with cataracts. **Cognitive Level:** Application **Integrated Process:** Nursing Process: Assessment **Client Need:** Physiological Integrity:

Physiological Adaptation **Content Area:** Adult Health: Eye and Ear **Strategy:** Recall normal assessment findings related to the eye. Consider what other assessment changes would occur if the lens is clouding. **Reference:** Lemone, P., & Burke, K. (2008). *Medical-surgical nursing: Critical thinking in client care* (4th ed.). Upper Saddle River, NJ: Pearson/Prentice Hall, p. 1704.

3 **Answer: 2** The foreign body should not be removed or manipulated. It should be immobilized if possible and the eye covered to protect from further injury. A paper cup can be used in place of an eye patch. Patching both eyes is an appropriate intervention to prevent ocular movement but follows immobilization of the foreign body. Irrigation with water is an intervention for chemical burns to the eyes. Carbonic anhydrase inhibitors are used to decrease intraocular pressure following blunt trauma.
Cognitive Level: Analysis **Client Need:** Physiological Integrity: Physiological Adaptation **Integrated Process:** Nursing Process: Implementation **Content Area:** Adult Health: Eye and Ear **Strategy:** For emergency actions, choose the option that stabilizes the client and prevents further injury. **Reference:** Lemone, P., & Burke, K. (2008). *Medical-surgical nursing: Critical thinking in client care* (4th ed.). Upper Saddle River, NJ: Pearson/Prentice Hall, pp. 1702–1703.

4 **Answer: 4** Conductive hearing loss results from changes that occur in the external or middle ear. Hearing aids, assistive listening devices (i.e., "pocket talkers"), and reconstructive surgeries can improve or correct hearing loss. Exposure to high levels of noise on an intermittent or constant basis damages the hair cells of the Organ of Corti, resulting in sensorineural hearing loss.
Cognitive Level: Application **Client Need:** Physiological Integrity: Physiological Adaptation **Integrated Process:** Teaching/Learning **Content Area:** Adult Health: Eye and Ear **Strategy:** Note the clarifying word *conductive* in the stem of the question that identifies the type of hearing loss. Read the question carefully and choose the option that is consistent with this form of hearing loss.
Reference: Lemone, P., & Burke, K. (2008). *Medical-surgical nursing: Critical thinking in client care* (4th ed.). Upper Saddle River, NJ: Pearson/Prentice Hall, pp. 1729–1733.

5 **Answer: 4** Weber and Rinne tests are used to differentiate conductive hearing loss from sensorineural. The Weber and Rinne tests are physical examination techniques that are within the nurse's role to complete. Tympanocentesis is the aspiration of fluid/pus from the middle ear to identify the causative organism of acute otitis media. Transillumination of the sinuses is a diagnostic tool used to assess for sinusitis. The diagnosis of Mé-

nière's disease is confirmed by electronystagmography, a series of tests to evaluate vestibular-ocular reflexes.
Cognitive Level: Application **Client Need:** Physiological Integrity: Reduction of Risk Potential **Integrated Process:** Nursing Process: Assessment **Content Area:** Adult Health: Eye and Ear **Strategy:** Decode unfamiliar terms by finding the root word and prefixes or suffixes. Be careful to select a test that the nurse can perform. **Reference:** Porth, C. M. (2005). *Pathophysiology: Concepts of altered health states* (7th ed.). Philadelphia, PA: Lippincott Williams & Wilkins, pp. 1339–1343.

6 **Answers: 2, 4** A higher incidence of acute otitis media is noted in infants who are bottle-fed in a horizontal position and who live in homes with smokers. The full 10- to 12-day course of antibiotic therapy must be administered. There is no relationship between the ingestion of fruit juices and acute otitis media.
Cognitive Level: Application **Client Need:** Physiological Integrity: Physiological Adaptation **Integrated Process:** Teaching/Learning **Content Area:** Adult Health: Eye and Ear **Strategy:** The wording of the question indicates the correct options contain true information. Use nursing knowledge and the process of elimination to make selections. **Reference:** Porth, C. M. (2005). *Pathophysiology: Concepts of altered health states* (7th ed.). Philadelphia, PA: Lippincott Williams & Wilkins, p. 1333.

7 **Answer: 2** Atrophic macular degeneration causes loss of central vision. Magnification devices and enhanced lighting help to promote safety. Peripheral vision remains intact. Although laser photocoagulation is effective for exudative macular degeneration, there is no treatment for the atrophic form. Since macular degeneration is not an infectious process, antibiotic therapy is not indicated.
Cognitive Level: Application **Client Need:** Physiological Integrity: Physiological Adaptation **Integrated Process:** Teaching/Learning **Content Area:** Adult Health: Eye and Ear **Strategy:** Apply knowledge of anatomy and physiology and determine what the macula does. Choose the option that can assist with the lost function. **Reference:** Lemone, P., & Burke, K. (2008). *Medical-surgical nursing: Critical thinking in client care* (4th ed.). Upper Saddle River, NJ: Pearson/Prentice Hall, pp. 1713–1714.

8 **Answers: 1, 2, 4** Ophthalmic cholinergics, beta blockers, and prostaglandin analogs are used to manage open-angle glaucoma. Atropine and other anticholinergics are contraindicated in angle-closure glaucoma and not usually used with any glaucoma because of the mydriatic effect.
Cognitive Level: Application **Client Need:** Physiological Integrity: Pharmacological and Parenteral Therapies **Integrated Process:** Nursing Process: Planning **Content Area:**

Adult Health: Eye and Ear **Strategy:** The core issue of the question asks for anticipated medications, so eliminate option 5 first. Since option 1 and 3 are opposites, one of them cannot be correct. Keep in mind which drug blocks pupil dilation to choose correctly between them. **Reference:** Lemone, P., & Burke, K. (2008). *Medical-surgical nursing: Critical thinking in client care* (4th ed.). Upper Saddle River, NJ: Pearson/Prentice Hall, pp. 1709–1710.

9 **Answer: 3** These symptoms, along with dysphagia, foul-smelling breath, and pain when drinking hot or acidic fluids, are common signs of laryngeal cancer. Chronic sinusitis can produce foul breath and pain or burning in the throat. GERD and CAD may produce epigastric and/or chest pain, but hoarseness and change of voice do not occur.

Cognitive Level: Application **Client Need:** Physiological Integrity: Physiological Adaptation **Integrated Process:** Nursing Process: Analysis **Content Area:** Adult Health: Eye and Ear **Strategy:** Recall that these are classic warning signs of cancer. **Reference:** Lemone, P., & Burke, K. (2008). *Medical-surgical nursing: Critical thinking in client care* (4th ed.). Upper Saddle River, NJ: Pearson/Prentice Hall, p. 1253.

10 **Answer: 3** All of the nursing actions listed are appropriate for the client following nasal packing for epistaxis or surgery; however, the risk of aspiration is high, and monitoring respiratory function essential.

Cognitive Level: Analysis **Client Need:** Physiological Integrity: Physiological Adaptation **Integrated Process:** Nursing Process: Implementation **Content Area:** Adult Health: Eye and Ear **Strategy:** Notice the question asks for the priority intervention. Use the process of elimination and physiological priorities in making a selection. **Reference:** Lemone, P., & Burke, K. (2008). *Medical-surgical nursing: Critical thinking in client care* (4th ed.). Upper Saddle River, NJ: Pearson/Prentice Hall, pp. 1243–1244.

Postest

1 **Answer: 1** Closed or narrow-angle glaucoma has an abrupt onset and is characterized by severe pain of sudden onset. The pain usually lasts longer than 20 minutes with closed-angle glaucoma. Eye pain that comes and goes quickly can be indicative of allergies. Open-angle glaucoma occurs gradually with no initial manifestations. Pain is not associated with cataracts or retinal detachment.

Cognitive Level: Application **Client Need:** Physiological Integrity: Physiological Adaptation **Integrated Process:** Nursing Process: Analysis **Content Area:** Adult Health: Eye and Ear **Strategy:** Eliminate the diseases that do not

cause pain. **Reference:** Lemone, P., & Burke, K. (2008). *Medical-surgical nursing: Critical thinking in client care* (4th ed.). Upper Saddle River, NJ: Pearson/Prentice Hall, pp. 1707–1708.

2 **Answer: 2** Ménière's disease is associated with vertigo that may last for hours as well as fluctuating hearing loss, nausea, and vomiting. The disorder is unilateral, but because hearing is bilateral, the client often does not realize the extent of the hearing loss. Option 3 is indicative of swimmer's ear, and option 4 is indicative of acute otitis media.

Cognitive Level: Application **Client Need:** Physiological Integrity: Physiological Adaptation **Integrated Process:** Nursing Process: Assessment **Content Area:** Adult Health: Eye and Ear **Strategy:** Note that the incorrect options are found with other ear disorders. **Reference:** LeMone, P., & Burke, K. (2008*). Medical-surgical nursing: Critical thinking in client care* (4th ed.). Upper Saddle River, NJ: Pearson/Prentice Hall, pp. 1726–1727.

3 **Answer: 4** Postoperative information includes limitations on reading, lifting, strenuous activity, and sleeping on the affected side. A family member needs to be taught to instill eye drops. There are no dietary restrictions.

Cognitive Level: Application **Client Need:** Physiological Integrity: Physiological Adaptation **Integrated Process:** Teaching/Learning **Content Area:** Adult Health: Eye and Ear **Strategy:** What implementations are needed for safety and home care after eye surgery? **Reference:** Lemone, P., & Burke, K. (2008). *Medical-surgical nursing: Critical thinking in client care* (4th ed.). Upper Saddle River, NJ: Pearson/Prentice Hall, p. 1705.

4 **Answers: 2, 4, 5** Retinal detachment is painless, but eventually floaters, lines or spots, and visual loss will be manifested, especially if hemorrhage has occurred. Dark lines, spots, or sensation of a curtain drawn across the field of vision is a common manifestation. Subconjunctival hemorrhage is a manifestation of blunt trauma to the eye and not of retinal detachment.

Cognitive Level: Analysis **Client Need:** Physiological Integrity: Physiological Adaptation **Integrated Process:** Nursing Process: Assessment **Content Area:** Adult Health: Eye and Ear **Strategy:** Consider the consequences of damage to the retina, which receives visual stimuli. **Reference:** Lemone, P., & Burke, K. (2008). Medical-surgical nursing: Critical thinking in client care (4th ed.). Upper Saddle River, NJ: Pearson/Prentice Hall, p. 1716.

5 **Answer: 4** In acute otitis media, the auditory tube provides entry of pathogens. This infection typically follows an upper respiratory infection. Edema of the tube causes mucus and fluid to accumulate and the pathogens to grow. Hearing loss is common in otitis media and is a conductive loss due to the exudate. There is no evidence in the question to indicate rupture of the tympanic membrane or exposure to secondhand smoke. Sterile fluid in the middle ear occurs in serous otitis media. **Cognitive Level:** Analysis **Client Need:** Physiological Integrity: Physiological Adaptation **Integrated Process:** Nursing Process: Analysis **Content Area:** Adult Health: Eye and Ear **Strategy:** Consider the history of URI and apply knowledge of complications. Also remember that the client is a child. **Reference:** Lemone, P., & Burke, K. (2008). *Medical-surgical nursing: Critical thinking in client care* (4th ed.). Upper Saddle River, NJ: Pearson/Prentice Hall, pp. 1721–1723.

6 **Answer: 2** Age-related macular degeneration is the leading cause of loss of vision in clients over 50 years of age. Blunt trauma, exposure to toxins, and allergies are not known causes of macular degeneration.

Cognitive Level: Application **Client Need:** Health Promotion and Maintenance **Integrated Process:** Nursing Process: Analysis **Content Area:** Adult Health: Eye and Ear **Strategy:** Consider the factors associated with macular degeneration. Note that three of the options include the age of the client. **Reference:** LeMone, P., & Burke, K. (2008). *Medical-surgical nursing: Critical thinking in client care* (4th ed.). Upper Saddle River, NJ: Pearson/Prentice Hall, pp. 1713–1714.

7 **Answers: 2, 3, 5** Manifestations of acute sinusitis include nasal congestion with postnasal drip, and purulent discharge. Bad breath is a frequent finding. With involvement of the maxillary sinuses, pain and pressure may be felt in the upper teeth. Food intolerances are not related. Nuchal rigidity would indicate a more serious problem.

Cognitive Level: Application **Client Need:** Physiological Integrity: Physiological Adaptation **Integrated Process:** Nursing Process: Assessment **Content Area:** Adult Health: Eye and Ear **Strategy:** Consider upper respiratory symptoms of infection. **Reference:** LeMone, P., & Burke, K. (2008). *Medical-surgical nursing: Critical thinking in client care* (4th ed.). Upper Saddle River, NJ: Pearson/Prentice Hall, pp. 1235–1238.

8 **Answer: 1** Since the amount of blood lost in a nosebleed can be frightening to clients, anxiety is a priority nursing diagnosis. Blood draining into the nasopharynx poses a risk of aspiration. Risk for infection and pain are appro-

priate nursing diagnoses related to nasal packing but are not the priorities. Impaired verbal communication is unlikely.

Cognitive Level: Analysis **Client Need:** Physiological Integrity: Physiological Adaptation **Integrated Process:** Nursing Process: Analysis **Content Area:** Adult Health: Eye and Ear **Strategy:** Which diagnosis poses the most immediate threat? **Reference:** LeMone, P., & Burke, K. (2008). *Medical-surgical nursing: Critical thinking in client care* (4th ed.). Upper Saddle River, NJ: Pearson/Prentice Hall, pp. 1243–1244.

9 **Answer: 3** The two major risk factors for laryngeal cancer are prolonged smoking along with concomitant use of alcohol. Although the majority of cases occur in men ages 50 to 75, advancing age does not significantly increase risk. Injury to the larynx, seasonal allergies, and chronic sinusitis are not risk factors.

Cognitive Level: Application **Client Need:** Health Promotion and Maintenance **Integrated Process:** Nursing Process: Analysis **Content Area:** Adult Health: Eye and Ear **Strategy:** Consider unhealthy lifestyle as etiology for many disorders. **Reference:** Lemone, P., & Burke, K. (2008). *Medical-surgical nursing: Critical thinking in client care* (4th ed.). Upper Saddle River, NJ: Pearson/Prentice Hall, p. 1253.

10 **Answer: 2** The client with sensorineural hearing loss experiences social isolation and depression and may appear withdrawn. Amplification devices such as hearing aids are helpful for clients with conductive hearing loss but only amplify noxious sounds for the client with sensorineural hearing loss. Antibiotics are not helpful for sensorineural hearing loss, and tympanoplasty is used to correct damage to structures in the middle ear.

Cognitive Level: Application **Client Need:** Psychosocial Integrity **Integrated Process:** Nursing Process: Implementation **Content Area:** Adult Health: Eye and Ear **Strategy:** The critical word *sensorineural* in the stem of the question tells what type of hearing loss is being tested. Consider the psychological as well as physical problems and then determine the nursing actions needed. **Reference:** LeMone, P., & Burke, K. (2008). *Medical-surgical nursing: Critical thinking in client care* (4th ed.). Upper Saddle River, NJ: Pearson/Prentice Hall, pp. 1730–1733.

References

Adams, S., & Holland, L. & Bostwick, P. (2008). *Pharmacology for nurses: A pathophysiologic approach* (2nd ed.). Upper Saddle River, NJ: Prentice Hall.

Carroll, E., Porth, C.M. Captis R. (2005). Disorder of visual function. In C. Porth (Ed.), *Pathophysiology: Concepts of altered health states* (7th ed.). Philadelphia, PA: Lippincott Williams & Wilkins, pp. 1237–1308.

LeMone, P., & Burke, K. (2008). *Medical surgical nursing: Critical thinking in client care* (4th ed.). Upper Saddle River, NJ: Prentice Hall.

Nelsen-Marsh, J. (2005). Alterations in special sensory function. In L. E. Copstead & J. Banasik (Eds.), *Pathophysiology: Biological and behavioral perspectives* (3rd ed.). Philadelphia, PA: W. B. Saunders, pp. 1151–1169.

Porth, C. M. (2005). Alterations in respiratory function: Respiratory tract infections, neoplasms, and childhood disorders. In C. Porth (Ed.), *Pathophysiology: Concepts of altered health states* (7th ed.). Philadelphia, PA: Lippincott Williams & Wilkins, pp. 659–687.

Porth, C. M. (2005). *Pathophysiology: Concepts of altered health states* (7th ed.). Philadelphia, PA: Lippincott Williams & Wilkins.

Porth, C., & Curtis, R. (2005). Disorders of hearing and vestibular function. In C. Porth (Ed.), *Pathophysiology: Concepts of altered health states* (7th ed.). Philadelphia, PA: Lippincott Williams & Wilkins, pp. 1329–1353.

Wilson, B., Shannon, M., & Stang, C. (2006). *Nurse's drug guide 2006.* Upper Saddle River, NJ: Prentice Hall.

7 Gastrointestinal Health Problems

Chapter Outline

Risk Factors Associated with Gastrointestinal Health Problems

Gastroesophageal Reflux Disease (GERD)

Peptic Ulcer Disease (PUD)

Hiatal Hernia

Crohn's Disease (Regional Enteritis)

Ulcerative Colitis

Diverticular Disease

Intestinal Obstruction

Appendicitis

Peritonitis

Neoplasms of the Gastrointestinal Tract

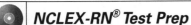

NCLEX-RN® Test Prep

Use the CD-ROM enclosed with this book to access additional practice opportunities.

Objectives

➤ Define key terms associated with gastrointestinal health problems.

➤ Identify risk factors associated with the development of gastrointestinal health problems.

➤ Explain the common etiologies of gastrointestinal health problems.

➤ Describe the pathophysiologic processes associated with specific gastrointestinal health problems.

➤ Distinguish between normal and abnormal gastrointestinal findings obtained from the nursing assessment.

➤ Prioritize nursing interventions associated with specific gastrointestinal health problems.

Review at a Glance

borborygmus rumbling sounds in gastrointestinal (GI) tract

Crohn's disease an inflammatory bowel condition in which there are patchy areas of inflammation anywhere along entire GI tract; also known as regional enteritis

dumping syndrome rapid emptying of stomach contents into small intestine, causing sweating and weakness after a meal; usually occurs after a gastric resection

dyspepsia burning, epigastric pain

erythroplakia red patches in mouth

fecalith a hard piece of stool that is stone-like and may cause bleeding

gastroparesis delayed gastric emptying time

hematemesis vomiting up blood

Helicobacter pylori Gram-negative bacteria that play a role in development of peptic ulcers

intussusception intrusion of one part of intestine into another part that is distal to it

leukoplakia white patches on mouth

McBurney's point point halfway between umbilicus and right iliac crest

melena black, tarry feces caused by presence of blood

peptic ulcer disease (PUD) an ulcer that may be located in lower end of esophagus, stomach, or duodenum

peritonitis infection of membrane that lines peritoneum or abdominal cavity

pyrosis severe epigastric pain or heartburn

rebound tenderness severe pain over an area of tenderness when pressure is applied to that area by examiner and quickly released

volvulus obstruction a twisting of bowel resulting in a large bowel obstruction

Zollinger-Ellison syndrome a condition in which a pancreatic tumor causes secretion of excess amounts of gastrin, which stimulates secretion of hydrochloric acid and pepsin; these events can lead to formation of a peptic ulcer

PRETEST

1 A client being admitted to the hospital with reports of severe lower abdominal pain is lying on the bed with the knees flexed. Admission vital signs reveal an oral temperature of 101.2° F. The nurse would conclude that which of the following additional findings is consistent with a diagnosis of appendicitis?

1. Localized pain at a position halfway between umbilicus and right iliac crest
2. Client describes pain as occurring two hours after eating
3. Pain subsides after eating
4. Pain is in left lower quadrant

2 An elderly client presents with fever, leukocytosis, left lower quadrant pain, and diarrhea alternating with constipation. The nurse concludes that these are frequently seen in clients with which health problem?

1. Appendicitis
2. Diverticulitis
3. Peptic ulcer disease
4. Irritable bowel syndrome

3 A client says to the nurse, "My doctor told me my ulcer may have been caused by bacteria. I thought ulcers were caused by diet and too much stress." Which of the following responses by the nurse is the best?

1. "If it was caused by bacteria, you would have a fever as a result of the inflammatory process."
2. "We know that ulcers are communicable. They can be spread easily. Be careful you don't spread them to your children."
3. "Diet and stress have nothing to do with developing an ulcer."
4. "Even though the bacteria *Helicobacter pylori* causes inflammation, other factors may cause increased acid in the stomach."

4 The nurse is caring for a client with a hiatal hernia. The client asks what could have prevented the problem. The nurse's response will be based on what knowledge of the etiology of the disorder?

1. Heavy lifting may have been a factor
2. "Junk" foods with a high fat content irritated the stomach
3. Commonly seen in younger adults
4. Fair-skinned females over 40 are more at risk

PRETEST

5 An elderly male client is worried about red blood in his stool along with feeling tired and worn out. The nurse considers that these symptoms may be caused by which of the following? Select all that apply.

1. Ascending (right-sided) colon cancer
2. Descending (left-sided) colon cancer
3. Sigmoid colon cancer
4. Gastric ulcers
5. Hemorrhoids

6 A client states, "My doctor told me to stop taking aspirin since I've developed this ulcer. I have to take aspirin to keep my arthritis from hurting. I don't know what to do." Which response on the part of the nurse is best?

1. "Let's worry about treating your ulcer. Your arthritis will have to wait."
2. "Aspirin is one of the medications that makes an ulcer worse. Your primary care provider can determine which drug is best for you."
3. "Go ahead and take the aspirin if it helps, but watch closely for bleeding."
4. "The doctor knows what is best for you, and you should follow those instructions."

7 The nurse is caring for a female client during recuperation following development of a duodenal ulcer. The client suddenly experiences severe abdominal pain, increased heart rate, increased respiratory rate, and diaphoresis. On palpation, the abdomen is rigid; bowel sounds are faint and diminished. Which nursing action is most appropriate?

1. Immediately place her in high Fowler's position to facilitate breathing
2. Help her walk to the bathroom to get rid of any flatus
3. Check to see if she has food allergies and see if she ate anything to which she might be allergic
4. Establish IV access and call the doctor to report the assessment data

8 A female client complains of a burning, cramping pain in the top part of the abdomen that worsens in the middle of the afternoon and sometimes awakens her at night. She reports that eating something usually helps the pain go away but that the pain is now becoming more intense. Which of the following is the best conclusion for the nurse to draw?

1. Symptoms are consistent with peptic ulcer disease
2. Client is probably developing cholelithiasis
3. Client probably has indigestion and needs to watch what she eats
4. Snack before bed should be recommended

9 The nurse considers that which of the following clients would be most at risk for an intestinal obstruction?

1. Jewish client who smokes and consumes large amounts of caffeine
2. Elderly client who is on bed rest because of postoperative abdominal surgery
3. Individual eating a low-fiber, high-fat diet
4. Adult diagnosed with cirrhosis of the liver

10 A client is complaining of dyspepsia, frequent belching, and increased salivation. The nurse suspects which of the following?

1. Peptic ulcer disease (PUD)
2. Ulcerative colitis
3. Paraesophageal hiatal hernia
4. Gastroesophageal reflux disease (GERD)

➤ *See pages 234–235 for Answers & Rationales.*

I. RISK FACTORS ASSOCIATED WITH GASTROINTESTINAL HEALTH PROBLEMS

A. Gastroesophageal reflux disease (GERD): prolonged gastric intubation, infections, systemic diseases, systemic lupus erythematosus (SLE), ingestion of corrosive substances, acidic foods, obesity, smoking, and alcohol intake

B. ***Peptic ulcer disease (PUD):*** chronic diseases such as COPD, rheumatoid arthritis (RA), or cirrhosis; stress; smoking; continued or excessive use of nonsteroidal antiinflammatory drugs (NSAIDs) or aspirin products; ***Helicobacter pylori*** infection; duodenal ulcers are more prominent with type O blood and may be genetically transmitted

C. **Hiatal hernia:** aging, trauma, surgery, hereditary, obesity

D. ***Crohn's disease:*** genetic and familial predisposition, race (Jewish highest), stress

E. **Ulcerative colitis:** race, genetic predisposition, stress, autoimmune disease

F. **Diverticular disease:** diseases such as ulcerative colitis and Crohn's disease; obesity; poor dietary habits (high intake of refined foods), especially in elderly

G. **Intestinal obstruction:** clients having abdominal surgeries; elderly; trauma

H. **Appendicitis:** fecal impactions, kinking of bowel, parasites, infections

I. ***Peritonitis:*** diseases such as Laënnec's cirrhosis, tuberculosis, PUD, inflammatory conditions, trauma or perforation of abdominal viscus, surgery

J. **Neoplasms of gastrointestinal (GI) tract:** tobacco use (oral cancer); excessive alcohol and tobacco consumption; diet lacking fruits and vegetables; esophageal disorders (esophageal cancer); genetic predisposition; diet high in gastric irritants; conditions such as chronic gastritis or achlorhydria (stomach cancer); low-fiber, high-fat diet and diseases such as Crohn's disease, polyps, ulcerative colitis (intestinal cancer)

II. GASTROESOPHAGEAL REFLUX DISEASE (GERD)

A. **Overview**

1. Defined as a backflow of gastric contents into esophagus; also known as heartburn or esophagitis

2. Etiologies include high-fat diet; hiatal hernia; pregnancy, obesity; conditions that reduce lower esophageal sphincter (LES) tone (such as excess caffeine intake); congenital defects; **gastroparesis** (delayed gastric emptying time); activities such as vomiting, coughing, lifting, or bending

B. **Pathophysiology**

1. Gastric contents that are regurgitated into esophagus are acidic and irritate esophageal lining; LES should completely close when food is consumed into stomach; when LES is weakened or incompetent, higher pressure within stomach forces contents into esophagus where pressure is less; this same concept of a higher pressure area emptying into a lower pressure area accounts for incidence of GERD in conditions such as pregnancy, obesity, and overindulgence of food

2. Esophagus has mucus-producing cells to protect its lining, but in less quantity than the stomach, where a high acid environment is normal

3. Severe GERD can cause epithelial cell damage and erosion of muscularis

4. Complications include strictures, bleeding, reflux-induced asthma, laryngitis

5. Signs and symptoms include **dyspepsia** (burning, epigastric pain); frequent belching with a sour taste; pain after eating, when lying down, and after straining or lifting; increased salivation; flatulence; history of high stress level

C. **Nursing assessment**

1. Assessment includes symptom analysis of pain (1–2 hours after eating), nutritional assessment, analysis of any other symptoms, and evidence of complications

2. Diagnostic tests: pH probe test is used to determine number and length of declines in pH of stomach contents (less than 4.0); barium swallow; otherwise history determines diagnosis

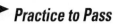 **D. Nursing management**

1. Medications include antacids, H_2-receptor blockers, proton pump inhibitors, antihistamines; separate all antacids from meals by 1 hour and from other medications by 1 to 2 hours

2. Teach client about possible surgery (fundoplication)

3. Offer several small meals rather than three large ones; suggest weight loss if necessary; limit or eliminate caffeine, heavy spices, and smoking

4. Elevate head of the bed while sleeping

5. Instruct client to avoid eating in a supine position and to drink extra fluids unless contraindicated

6. Instruct client to keep a diary of foods that seem to increase symptoms and avoid these when determined

7. Discuss stress reduction methods and resources, as well as weight reduction

Practice to Pass

A 42-year-old male client is diagnosed with GERD after being admitted with severe pains in his chest, frequent indigestion, and pain after meals. Since he thought he was having a heart attack, how should the nurse explain the difference in the symptoms between the two diagnoses?

III. PEPTIC ULCER DISEASE (PUD)

A. Overview

1. Defined as an ulcer, which may be located in lower end of esophagus, stomach, or duodenum

2. Occurs equally between males and females; mortality increases with age over 75

3. Causes include: excessive stress, *H. pylori* infection (a gram-negative bacteria), excessive use of NSAIDs and aspirin products; any situation where there is damage to mucosa; and **Zollinger-Ellison syndrome** (a pancreatic tumor that causes excess amounts of gastrin to be excreted)

4. Three main types are gastric, duodenal, and stress; may be acute or chronic

    a. Gastric ulcers: etiologies include ingestion of medications, tobacco, caffeine, alcohol; *H. pylori* infection; chronic bile reflux and increased serum gastrin

    b. Duodenal ulcers: etiologies include hypersecretion of pepsinogen, autosomal dominant trait, *H. pylori* infection (95–100% of cases)

B. Pathophysiology

1. Three main factors contribute to ulcer development

    a. *Excess acid* can lead to a break or ulceration in mucosa of stomach or duodenum; the break allows mucosa to be subjected to an acid environment and thus autodigestion occurs

    b. *Decreased mucus production* can leave mucosal cells unprotected from acid environment; hypoxia, shock, severe burns, etc., can lead to injury of mucus-producing cells

    c. *Increased delivery of acid* can cause protective mucus layer to be irritated because of rapid movement of stomach contents, such as in **dumping syndrome** (rapid emptying of stomach contents into small intestine causing sweating, weakness, etc., after a meal)

2. Ulcers can be superficial or deep

   a. Superficial ulcers are also called erosions

   b. Deep lesions extend through musculature and penetrate blood vessels causing hemorrhage; can also cause perforation of wall of stomach or intestines

3. Infection with bacteria *H. pylori* is a major factor in gastric and duodenal ulcers, causing death of mucosal epithelial cells; it also releases toxins and enzymes that produce inflammation and ulcer development; increased levels of gastrin and/or pepsinogen have been attributed to presence of bacteria

4. Rapid gastric emptying (such as in dumping syndrome) may cause increased acid in duodenum and aid ulcer development (Figure 7-1)

5. Stress, caffeine, cigarette smoking, and alcohol consumption increase acid production; aspirin and NSAID medications inhibit prostaglandin, which helps protect lining of stomach

6. Gastric ulcers are usually small and singular, located at lesser curvature of stomach; duodenal ulcers are usually deep and occur at beginning area of duodenum near to pyloric sphincter

7. A Curling's ulcer is an acute stress ulcer that usually follows a severe illness (especially burns, trauma, surgery, shock, renal failure); tends to be multiple, superficial, and tends to erode several areas of gastric mucosa

8. Signs and symptoms

   a. Gastric ulcers: severe **pyrosis** (epigastric pain or heartburn); may radiate to back or flank; usually occurs immediately after or during a meal; food usually does not relieve pain

   b. Duodenal ulcers: right epigastric pain; radiates to back or thorax; often occurs when stomach is empty; food and antacids relieve pain

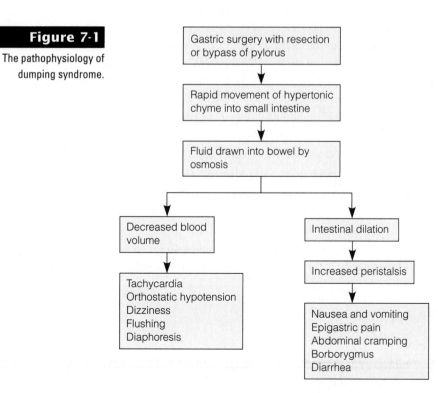

Figure 7-1

The pathophysiology of dumping syndrome.

  c. Other: fullness after eating, nausea, vomiting, bloating, anorexia, gnawing type of pain; weight loss or weight gain (with duodenal ulcers because eating relieves pain); pain may come and go; **hematemesis** (vomiting up blood), **melena** (black, tarry feces because of presence of blood) or hematochezia (blood in stool)

C. Nursing assessment

  1. Assessment includes symptom analysis of pain; relationship of pain to food intake; any hematemesis or melena; use of NSAID medications, list of all medications taken at home; intake of alcohol or use of cigarettes; history of stress level

  2. Diagnostic tests: blood serum for presence of *H. pylori* antibodies; endoscopy, barium studies and upper GI (ulcer craters present); CBC (decreased RBC, hemoglobin, hematocrit); stool specimen (positive for occult blood), electrolytes

D. Nursing management

  1. Medications

    a. H$_2$ blockers such as cimetidine (Tagamet), ranitidine (Zantac), famotidine (Pepcid) or nizatidine (Axid)

    b. Proton pump inhibitor such as omeprazole (Prilosec), lansoprazole (Prevacid), esomeprazole (Nexium), pantoprazole (Protonix), or rabeprazole (Aciphex)

    c. Mucosal barrier such as sucralfate (Carafate)

    d. Antacids to neutralize gastric acid (with exception of bicarbonate of soda)

    e. Cytoprotective agent such as synthetic *E. prostaglandin* (Cytotec) to promote mucus production for healing

    f. Antibiotics to destroy *H. pylori*

      1) Frequently this disorder can be treated by giving two antibiotics such as tetracycline hydrochloride (Achromycin) or clarithromycin (Biaxin) and metronidazole (Flagyl)

      2) Often recommended to give bismuth compound (Pepto-Bismol) with the antibiotics (but may make stools appear as melena)

  2. Individualize diet by determining which foods cause pain and eliminate them; suggest six small meals daily rather than three large ones; limit food intake, caffeine, and alcohol late at night

  3. Limit milk to one glass per meal

  4. Avoid caffeine, cigarettes, and alcohol

  5. Encourage rest and stress reduction

  6. Monitor for indications of perforation such as severe abdominal pain, rigidity in abdomen, distention, absent bowel sounds, and signs of shock

  7. Monitor weight periodically

  8. Avoid use of NSAIDs and acetylsalicylic acid (aspirin) products; instruct client that many pain medications and most arthritis medications contain these agents and should be avoided

IV. HIATAL HERNIA

A. Overview

  1. Defined as a protruding of stomach into mediastinal cavity by way of diaphragm (see Figure 7-2)

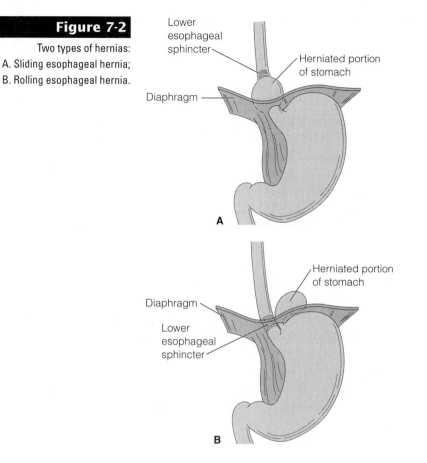

Figure 7-2

Two types of hernias:
A. Sliding esophageal hernia;
B. Rolling esophageal hernia.

2. Types

    a. Sliding esophageal hernia (most common, 90%): herniated section of stomach slides back and forth through hiatus with position changes and increased peristalsis

    b. Paraesophageal hiatal hernia: fundus and greater curvature of stomach roll into thorax next to esophagus; can have serious complications

3. Causes include weakening of esophageal muscles due to aging, trauma, surgery or an anatomic defect; heavy straining or lifting

B. Pathophysiology

    1. In a sliding esophageal hernia, there is gastroesophageal reflux caused by weakened esophageal hiatus muscles; this accounts for symptoms experienced

    2. In a paraesophageal hernia, increased intrathoracic pressure occurs because of protrusion of thoracic contents by hernia

    3. It may be asymptomatic, or signs and symptoms may vary according to type of hernia

        a. Sliding: dysphagia, pyrosis, regurgitation, bloating, and heartburn

        b. Rolling: shortness of breath, chest pain (similar to anginal pain), and tachycardia

C. Nursing assessment

    1. Assessment includes symptom analysis of pain, vital signs (VS), complaints of shortness of breath, analysis of symptoms that would suggest angina versus GI pain (description of pain)

   2. Diagnostic tests: upper GI, arterial blood gases (ABGs) if shortness of breath is experienced, CXR shows stomach in thorax

D. Nursing management

   1. Medications include antacids, H$_2$-receptor blockers, analgesics
   2. Monitor and educate about proper diet and taking six small meals rather than three large ones; begin on weight reduction program if necessary
   3. Educate client about head elevation for sleep and eating
   4. Explain surgery if indicated
   5. Discourage intake of alcohol, high amounts of caffeine, and cigarettes

V. CROHN'S DISEASE (REGIONAL ENTERITIS)

A. Overview

   1. Defined as a chronic inflammatory condition of bowel in which there are patchy areas of inflammation anywhere in entire GI tract; most common in ileum or colon; referred to as a chronic inflammatory bowel disease (IBD) and grouped with ulcerative colitis because symptoms are similar
   2. Incidence is higher among young adults and teenagers; occurs equally in both genders; more often seen in clients of Jewish and Caucasian backgrounds
   3. Develops slowly, with remissions and exacerbations; emotional factors related to family matters or work aggravate the illness
   4. Cause is unknown but thought to be multifactoral, probably involving an infectious process (bacteria, viruses, mycobacteria), allergy or immune disorder, psychosomatic, dietary, hormonal, and environmental factors

B. Pathophysiology

   1. Inflammatory lesions may occur anywhere from mouth to anus; more often lesions occur in ascending colon and terminal ileum
   2. Lesions are local and involve all layers of intestinal wall; wall contains shallow long ulcers with long or short areas of stricture
   3. Lesions involve some areas of bowel but not all areas (called skip lesions)
   4. Because of involvement of submucosal layers, mucosa has a granuloma (tumor-like growth) that gives tissue a cobblestone appearance
   5. Bowel wall becomes congested, thickened, and may develop abscesses; fistulas may develop between infected area and bladder or other areas of intestine, resulting in malabsorption of nutrients (see Figure 7–3)
   6. Scar tissue may interfere with movement of chyme and perforation or obstruction may occur
   7. Complications caused by excessive diarrhea include fluid and electrolyte imbalance as well as dehydration; deficiency in absorption of folic acid, calcium, and vitamin D; anal fissures, perianal abscesses, fistula, and obstruction
   8. Signs and symptoms include nausea, vomiting, flatulence, malaise, weight loss cause by anorexia, three to five semisolid foul-smelling stools/day; intermittent, localized pain in right lower quadrant (worsening as disease progresses); mucus in stools with possible pus (blood may also be present); urgency at night to defecate; fluid and electrolyte imbalance, dehydration, fever, elevated WBC, iron-deficiency anemia, perianal abscesses and fistulas, and hypoalbuminemia

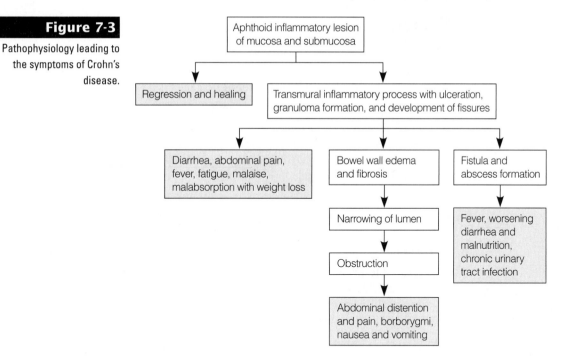

Figure 7-3

Pathophysiology leading to the symptoms of Crohn's disease.

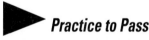

C. Nursing assessment

1. Assessment includes nutritional and fluid status, symptom analysis of symptoms and pain, bowel pattern assessment, daily weight, activity tolerance, visual examination of stool, history of risk factors/stress level and emotional factors, VS, skin/nail color changes secondary to anemia

2. Diagnostic tests: CBC (elevated WBC, low RBC, Hgb, and Hct), barium enema (reveals characteristic "string sign," or skip lesions) colonoscopy, albumin level (low), high erythrocyte sedimentation rate (ESR), electrolytes (hypocalcemia), folic acid level, possibly serum levels of vitamins

D. Nursing management

1. Medications include sulfasalazine (Azulfidine), mesalamine (Asacol, Rowasa), or olsalazine (Dipentum) to control infection; corticosteroids to decrease inflammation; analgesics to control abdominal pain; anticholinergics to control diarrhea; vitamin and mineral replacements; electrolyte replacements as needed; antipyretics if fever occurs; immunosuppressant drugs; many of the electrolytes (especially potassium and calcium) should be given with food to decrease GI irritation

2. Attempt to control diarrhea since distended intestinal wall may lead to perforation; monitor temperature

3. Fluid replacement may be given to correct dehydration; monitor for symptoms of dehydration; TPN may be added if necessary to provide for nutritional needs while allowing GI tract to rest

4. Give low-residue, low-fat, high-protein, high-calorie diet

5. Instruct about lifestyle management to reduce stress

▶ *Practice to Pass*

How should the nurse determine whether a client with Crohn's disease is becoming dehydrated?

VI. ULCERATIVE COLITIS

A. Overview

1. Defined as an inflammatory disease affecting mucous membranes of colon; affects part of or all of colon and rectum

2. Occurs between ages 10 to 40; more common in those of Caucasian and Jewish backgrounds

3. Considered under general heading of chronic inflammatory bowel disease (IBD) along with Crohn's disease; disease has stages of exacerbations and remissions

4. Disease is labeled as mild, moderate, or fulminating

5. Disease is of unknown etiology; suggested causes include a genetic basis, viruses, bacteria, autoimmunity, and stress

B. Pathophysiology

1. Ulcerated lesions form small erosions in mucosal layer; there are no skip lesions as in Crohn's disease; affects large bowel in a continuous pattern progressing from distal to proximal

2. These cavities may feature small hemorrhages and abscesses

3. Wall of bowel thickens and ulcerations are fibrotic in later stages of illness

4. Complications can include intestinal obstruction, dehydration, fluid and electrolyte imbalances, malabsorption and iron-deficiency anemia

5. Signs and symptoms include chronic, bloody diarrhea mixed with mucus (worsens as disease increases in severity); fever; weight loss; abdominal cramping and pain; nausea and vomiting; urge to defecate

C. Nursing assessment

1. Assessment includes bowel habits, visual inspection of stool, VS, recent or progressive weight loss, symptom analysis of pain, activity tolerance, bowel sounds, and nutritional status

2. Diagnostic tests: CBC (low RBC, Hgb, Hct), electrolytes (low potassium), colonascopy, stool for occult blood

D. Nursing management

1. Medications include antipyretics; antiinflammatory drugs such as sulfasalazine (Azulfidine); antibiotics; corticosteroids; antimicrobial agents, metronidazole (Flagyl); antidiarrheals; antispasmodics

2. Offer bulk-free diet and nutritional supplements as necessary; weigh client weekly, individualizing plan of care as needed

3. Offer psychological support and counseling

4. Monitor bowel sounds and bowel movements

5. Assess for signs of dehydration; monitor intake and output; administer IV fluids as ordered

VII. DIVERTICULAR DISEASE

A. Overview

1. Defined as *diverticula* or *diverticulum:* an outpouching of walls of colon; *diverticulitis:* inflammation of a diverticulum within intestinal tract;

diverticulosis: condition of having diverticula within colon without any inflammation or symptoms

2. More common in clients over 60 years of age who eat a low-residue diet

3. May be *acute* (similar to appendicitis) or *chronic* (characterized by severe constipation and pain, distention, and flatulence)

4. Causes include severe constipation, obesity, lack of dietary fiber or roughage

B. Pathophysiology

1. An increase in intraluminal pressure causes outpouching of colon wall; there is usually a weakness in intestinal wall from effects of diet

2. Bacteria from food that becomes trapped in pouches then causes diverticulitis

3. A lack of adequate blood supply or nutrients from diet may also contribute to development of this disease

4. Chronic diverticulitis may cause thickening of intestinal walls and possibly obstruction

5. Complications include rupture of intestinal wall leading to peritonitis; obstruction, and abscesses (rare)

6. Signs and symptoms include constipation, lower left-sided abdominal pain, signs of peritonitis (fever, guarding, abdominal rigidity); occasional rectal bleeding; diarrhea (not as common as constipation); elevated WBC; may be asymptomatic

C. Nursing assessment

1. Assessment includes: symptom analysis of complaints and any pain, VS, palpation of abdomen, auscultation of bowel sounds, bowel habits, any posturing

2. Diagnostic tests: ultrasound, colonoscopy, guaiac stool, barium enema, CT scan, flexible sigmoidoscopy

D. Nursing management

1. Medications include antidiarrheals and antispasmodics (occasionally), stool softeners, analgesics, antipyretics if fever occurs, broad-spectrum antibiotics for acute stage: metronidazole (Flagyl), ciprofloxacin (Cipro), or trimethoprim/sulfamethoxazole (Septra, Bactrim)

2. Monitor vital signs and treat fever as necessary

3. Encourage 2 to 3 liters of fluid per day unless contraindicated by another condition

4. Assess stools for color, consistency, frequency, presence of blood

5. Encourage rest periods and discourage lifting, straining, or bending

6. Offer high dietary roughage (fruit, vegetables, fiber)

7. Educate client about symptoms of disease and a lifestyle that can decrease these symptoms

8. Encourage cessation of smoking and alcohol use for general GI health

VIII. INTESTINAL OBSTRUCTION

A. Overview

1. Defined as inability of intestinal contents to progress through bowel in a normal manner; sites of blockage may be located in small intestine (high blockage) or colon (low blockage)

    2. Classified as mechanical or paralytic obstructions

        a. *Mechanical* is caused by any condition that hinders patency of bowel lumen (tumors, adhesions); most common type overall

            1) A **volvulus obstruction** refers to a twisting of bowel and results in a large bowel obstruction; most common in elderly clients

            2) **Intussusception** is intrusion of a part of intestine into another part that lies distal to it; most common in infants 10–15 months

        b. *Functional* or *paralytic* (adynamic) is caused by neurogenic or muscular impairment that hinders peristalsis (postsurgery, prolonged bedrest)

    3. Children most commonly have mechanical obstructions (especially younger than 2 years) rather than paralytic obstructions

    4. Causes include intestinal adhesions, hernias, tumors, severe constipation, surgery, debilitated state with prolonged bedrest

B. Pathophysiology

    1. Blockage of intestine (regardless of cause) leads to intestinal distention by gas and air, pooling of gastric and biliary secretions, and loss of fluids, electrolytes, and proteins

    2. Distention caused by pooling of secretions leads to decreased absorption of water and electrolytes through bowel wall; vomiting and pooling lead to hypovolemia, dehydration, and ultimately hypovolemic shock

    3. Impaired blood supply leads to increased peristalsis initially, ischemia and acidosis, bacterial invasion, and possibly subsequent necrosis and peritonitis

    4. Cellular disruption and tissue hypoxia, along with stasis of secretions, provide an excellent medium for bacteria growth

    5. Complications include fluid and electrolyte imbalances, gangrene of bowel, strangulation of a bowel segment, and perforation

    6. Signs and symptoms include colicky pain, distention of bowel; bowel sounds may be **borborygmus** (rumbling sounds) initially, then change to hypoactive or absent; nausea and vomiting (bilious, feculent); anorexia; diarrhea or lack of bowel movement; abdominal tenderness, rigidity, fever; restlessness; electrolyte abnormalities; hypovolemic or septic shock may occur

C. Nursing assessment

    1. Assessment includes bowel habits and patterns, symptom analysis of pain, bowel sounds, palpation of abdomen, visual inspection of stool, intake and output (I&O), nutritional status, VS and oxygen (O_2) saturation, abdominal girth

    2. Diagnostic tests: CBC, electrolytes, abdominal x-ray, amylase level, barium enema, CT scan (use gastrografin if obstruction suspected; check for allergies), ultrasound of abdomen, ABGs

D. Nursing management

    1. Medications include laxatives (oral or suppository), enemas, electrolyte replacements as needed

    2. Monitor bowel sounds and bowel movements; check for a fecal impaction and remove if possible

    3. Measure I&O; weight, and amount of food consumed each meal

    4. Provide privacy to have a bowel movement; offer air freshener

    5. Decompression of bowel through a nasogastric or nasoenteric tube or surgical intervention may be needed

▶ *Practice to Pass*

An elderly female client presents with a distended abdomen, hypoactive bowel sounds, tenderness and pain upon palpation and states her last bowel movement was 7 days ago. What changes could occur within the next few hours that would warrant immediate attention if the obstruction is not treated?

6. Postsurgery, encourage early ambulation and increased fluid intake

7. Monitor VS; provide IV fluids as ordered

8. Educate client about need to prevent constipation (use of natural laxatives, stool softeners, increased fluid intake, and increased activity)

9. Monitor use and frequency of opioid analgesics that decrease motility

IX. APPENDICITIS

A. Overview

1. Defined as an inflammation of vermiform appendix

2. Occurs often in children and young adults ages 10 to 30 years; males are affected more often than females

3. May be acute (sudden, severe), chronic (follows an acute attack), or gangrenous (extreme inflammation); an appendix may rupture

4. Symptoms in females must be differentiated from ovarian cysts, ectopic pregnancy, and pelvic inflammatory disease

5. Causes include unknown etiology, obstruction of appendix from stool, or necrosis of organ

B. Pathophysiology

1. Appendix is attached to cecum just below ileocecal valve and in normal individuals is small, serving no known purpose

2. Obstruction of lumen can occur due to stool (**fecalith**—a hard piece of stool that is stone-like), tumors, parasites, or foreign bodies

3. Obstruction can lead to inflammation and bacterial invasion can occur

4. Occlusion of capillaries and venules causes increased intraluminal pressure, leading to decreased blood flow to mucosa and hypoxic tissue

5. Gangrene can develop from thrombosis of luminal blood vessels, which may lead to perforation and possibly resultant peritonitis (infection of membrane that lines peritoneum or abdominal cavity)

6. Signs and symptoms include pain in right lower quadrant of abdomen that may localize at **McBurney's point** (halfway between umbilicus and right iliac crest); GI disturbances (anorexia, nausea, vomiting, diarrhea, or sometimes constipation); **rebound tenderness** (severe pain over area of tenderness when pressure is applied to appendix area and quickly released); posturing by lying on side or back with knees flexed; fever, elevated BP and/or heart rate caused by pain and fever; malaise

7. If a confirmed diagnosis of appendicitis is made and the pain suddenly stops without any intervention, appendix may have ruptured; pain is lessened because appendix is no longer distended; surgery is still needed and is an emergency to reduce risk of peritonitis

C. Nursing assessment

1. Assessment includes VS, symptom analysis of pain, palpation of abdomen (rebound tenderness) until diagnosis is made, history of bowel movements, history of menses in women, and activity tolerance

2. Diagnostic tests: CBC (elevated WBC [note differential] with rupture), ultrasound, CT scan

▶ Practice to Pass

A 15-year-old is brought to the Emergency Department complaining of right lower quadrant pain and diarrhea. There are no other signs and symptoms present. What assessment and nursing intervention would help to rule out appendicitis?

D. Nursing management

1. Medications include IV antibiotics, analgesics for pain, and antipyretics for fever

2. Comfort measures until a diagnosis is confirmed; surgery is recommended treatment

3. Administer IV fluids in preparation for surgery if diagnosis is confirmed; in absence of rebound tenderness, IV fluids are given to confirm a possible GI virus (pain improves after fluids are given with a virus)

4. Avoid enemas, cathartics, heating pads, or abdominal palpation with a confirmed diagnosis to prevent a rupture

5. Monitor vital signs, especially temperature

6. Administer standard postoperative care: turn, cough, deep-breathing; early ambulation, assess bowel sounds, monitor urinary output, and provide wound care

X. PERITONITIS

A. Overview

1. Defined as local or generalized inflammation of peritoneum (lining that covers abdominal viscera)

2. May be primary (bacterial infection), secondary (trauma, surgical injury, chemical irritation), or as a complication of GI accessory organ disease

3. Caused by a ruptured appendix or peptic ulcer, diverticulitis, bowel obstruction, ruptured urinary bladder, infection from reproductive tract, or as a postoperative complication resulting in leakage from an intestinal anastomosis

B. Pathophysiology

1. Peritoneum is a semipermeable membrane; as an attempt to maintain homeostasis, fluid shifts may occur with third-spacing into peritoneal cavity; dehydration, decreased urinary output, hypovolemia, electrolyte imbalance, and even shock may occur

2. If secretions or chemical irritants leaking into peritoneum are sterile, irritation is primarily chemical; if they are infected, an intense inflammatory response is generated

3. Generalized peritonitis progresses to septicemia, which leads to septic shock and multiple organ failure; symptoms may be overlooked in an elderly client until condition is severe

4. Signs and symptoms include abdominal pain that is intense, often localized at site of involvement; chills and fever; anorexia, nausea, and vomiting; guarding and rigidity of abdomen; abdominal distention; diminished or absent bowel sounds; sweating, tachycardia, tachypnea; oliguria; restlessness, disorientation; elevated WBC; pallor; reduced urine output from dehydration

C. Nursing assessment

1. Assessment includes symptom analysis of pain and other complaints, VS, auscultation of bowel sounds, palpation of abdomen, urinary output, mental status, skin color, and nutritional assessment

2. Diagnostic tests: CBC, electrolytes, abdominal ultrasound, BUN, creatinine, peritoneal aspiration with cultures, blood cultures, flat plate x-ray (supine and standing)

D. Nursing management

1. Medications include antibiotic therapy (after cultures are obtained); analgesics for pain control; potassium replacement if kidney function is adequate

2. Replacement of fluid and electrolytes

3. Monitor urine output and venous pressure

4. Mechanical ventilation or monitoring of pulmonary artery pressure by a Swan-Ganz catheter may be necessary for severely ill clients

5. Total parenteral nutrition (TPN) may be used for nutritional needs

6. NG tube is often necessary for abdominal distention and reduced peristalsis; postoperative feeding may be done by jejunostomy tube if client is unable to take an oral diet

7. Emotional support for both client and family is important

8. Routine postoperative care, discharge planning, and referrals are essential

XI. NEOPLASMS OF THE GASTROINTESTINAL TRACT

A. Overview

1. Defined as oral cancer (lips, pharynx, tongue, soft palate, and uvula); esophageal, stomach, or colon and rectum (colorectal) cancer

2. **Leukoplakia** (white patches on mouth) and **erythroplakia** (red patches in mouth) are precancerous lesions that should be reported; ulcers on lips or in mouth that don't heal, as well as enlarged lymph nodes, should be investigated as possible harmful lesions

3. Early diagnosis is essential in both oral and colorectal cancer for higher survival rates to be achieved

4. Causes include tobacco and alcohol use; diet low in fiber, high in fat, and low in fruits and vegetables; genetic disposition

B. Pathophysiology

1. Squamous cells in mouth are susceptible to developing squamous cell carcinoma; oral cancer spreads very rapidly because of rich vascular supply in mouth

2. Esophageal tumors encircle esophagus and invade lymphatic system

3. Stomach cancer includes adenocarcinoma occurring within pyloric region of stomach; spreads through lymphatic system and into other organs

4. Most colorectal cancers are moderately differentiated adenocarcinomas; colorectal cancers tend to grow slowly; start in mucosa and most extend over a considerable amount of tissue before reaching lymph channel and metastasizing

5. Signs and symptoms

    a. Oral: difficulty or pain in chewing, swallowing, or speaking; presence of a precancerous lesion or an ulcer in the tissue

    b. Esophageal: dysphagia, pulmonary complications, regurgitation, aspiration, or fistula formation

    c. Stomach: loss of appetite, weight loss, gastric discomfort, weakness, pain

    d. Colorectal

        1) Right-sided (ascending): mild bleeding; weakness, fatigue, lack of energy; anorexia and weight loss

        2) Left-sided (descending): change in bowel habits such as going from diarrhea to constipation; small or pencil-shaped stools, gas or bloating, dark blood in stool or rectal bleeding; another complaint is a feeling of incomplete emptying on defecation

    e. Anorexia, weakness, and weight loss are indications of any tumor growth; in advanced stages, tumor mass would be palpable

C. Nursing assessment

    1. Assessment includes changes in bowel habits, nutritional status, weight loss or gain, palpation of abdomen, activity tolerance, symptom analysis of any pain, visual inspection of any oral lesions (oral lesions frequently can be palpated with a gloved finger before they are visible, any firm, asymmetric enlargement should be suspect and reported); visual inspection of stool specimen

    2. Diagnostic tests: guaiac test for occult blood, biopsy, colonoscopy or sigmoidoscopy, barium enema, CBC, liver function tests, CT scan/MRI, bronchoscopy, endoscopy, carcinoembryonic antigen (CEA), upper and lower GI series, coagulation panel

D. Nursing management

    1. Medications and other treatment

        a. Radiation and/or surgery is often the treatment recommended

        b. Chemotherapy may be given alone or in combination with radiation therapy and surgery

        c. Other: analgesics, antiemetics, stool softeners, antibiotic therapy if indicated

    2. Client teaching is important regarding detection of any GI cancer and includes use of sunscreens, necessity for annual physical examinations, and avoidance of potential risk factors such as smoking, tobacco, or snuff

    3. Over age 40, a colonoscopy is recommended and then every 10 years, especially if a family history exists or a client has rectal polyps or diverticulosis; an annual guaiac test is recommended for clients over age of 5

    4. If surgery is performed, provide standard postoperative care

    5. Provide pain management

    6. Maintain patent airway after oral surgery

    7. Monitor nutritional status; provide good oral care; hydrate well after an endoscopy or GI series

    8. Provide emotional support and referral as needed for client and family

    9. After surgery for colorectal cancer, monitor bowel patterns closely (frequency, volume, and consistency) or provide ostomy care if created

Case Study

A 34-year-old female is admitted who reports abdominal pain and diarrhea. She is very pale and emaciated. Her admitting diagnosis is rule out Crohn's disease.

1. What specific questions should the nurse ask her as part of the admission history?

2. What objective data should the nurse collect?

3. What information will be helpful regarding the client's social history? Why?

4. What nursing measures are important to prevent the complication of dehydration?

5. What other nursing interventions should the nurse anticipate providing?

For suggested responses, see page 535.

POSTTEST

1 A client presents to the clinic with "bad pain" in the middle of the abdomen, vomiting, and "not knowing what is wrong." Palpation reveals rebound tenderness with increased pain halfway between the umbilicus and the top of the pelvis. The client seems to have less pain when lying on the left side and flexing the knees. What is the best conclusion for the nurse to draw?

1. To make sure client does not have an impaction, an enema should be given
2. Since client is vomiting, the problem is probably gastroenteritis
3. Client should be checked for possible appendicitis
4. Since client has been vomiting, nourishment may help

2 A client with Zollinger-Ellison syndrome thinks she has a rare form of cancer. The nurse explains that this syndrome is characterized by which of the following?

1. Destruction of mucus-protecting cells of the stomach that could lead to an ulcer
2. Condition that causes increased secretion of pepsin and hydrochloric acid
3. Twisting of bowel that leads to intestinal obstruction
4. Crohn's disease, which is an inflammatory bowel disorder

3 A client who is exhibiting borborygmi, cramping pain, vomiting, and diarrhea has a diagnosis of peptic ulcer disease (PUD) with recent surgical treatment. The nurse considers that the client is probably experiencing which of the following?

1. Dumping syndrome
2. Complications of the PUD
3. Perforation of the stomach
4. Peritonitis

4 A client diagnosed with peptic ulcer disease (PUD) wants to know why antibiotics are being given. The nurse's best answer would be:

1. "Antibiotics help calm the stomach and decrease the symptoms."
2. "Antibiotics decrease dumping syndrome, which can lead to PUD."
3. "*H. pylori* is a bacterial cause for PUD, and antibiotics will treat the cause."
4. "The excess acid can be decreased when the stomach is sterile."

5 A client is being treated for peptic ulcer disease. The nurse anticipates orders for which medications that might be used to decrease gastric acid content or protect the stomach? Select all that apply.

1. Proton pump inhibitors such as omeprazole (Prilosec) or lansoprazole (Prevacid)
2. Bismuth compounds (Pepto-Bismol) to stimulate mucosal bicarbonate
3. NSAIDS such as ibuprofen (Motrin) to reduce the inflammation
4. Laxatives such as bisacodyl (Dulcolax) to prevent constipation
5. Sucralfate (Carafate) to form a barrier against acid and pepsin in the ulcer base

6 The nurse explains to a family that the main physiological reason for weight loss in a client with Crohn's disease is which of the following?

1. Symptoms of anorexia prevent client from eating
2. Inflammation of the disease decreases the appetite
3. Thickening and congestion of bowel wall results in malabsorption
4. "Skip lesions" interfere with food passage through the bowel

7 The nurse explains to a certified nursing assistant (CNA) who is also a nursing student that the reason elderly clients are more prone to diverticulitis is because of:

1. Poor, deficient diet and constipation.
2. Chronic diarrhea with resulting infection.
3. Frequent use of stimulating laxatives.
4. Sedentary lifestyle.

8 The nurse should caution a client who has Crohn's disease and is noncompliant about the risk for which of the following?

1. Perforation of the bowel
2. Cancer of the small intestine or colon
3. Peptic ulcer disease (PUD)
4. Ulcerative colitis

9 Prior to giving an analgesic for pain to a postoperative client who has a history of peptic ulcer disease (PUD), the nurse should check to see that the medication does not contain which of the following?

1. Opioid product
2. Acetaminophen (Tylenol)
3. Acetylsalicylic acid (aspirin)
4. Hydrocodone

10 A client is admitted to the unit with a large, distended bowel, acute tenderness upon palpation of the abdomen, fever, rigidity, and absent bowel sounds. After being on the unit, the client's level of consciousness decreases, and he begins to have feculent vomit. The nurse anticipates the need for what therapeutic interventions? Select all that apply.

1. Reduce fever through oral antipyretics
2. Insert NG tube to suction and monitor the output
3. Administer narcotic pain medications to relax client
4. Begin to prepare client for surgery
5. Insert IV line to begin fluid administration

➤ *See pages 236–237 for Answers & Rationales.*

ANSWERS & RATIONALES

Pretest

1 **Answer: 1** Pain over McBurney's point, the point halfway between the umbilicus and the iliac crest, is diagnostic for appendicitis. Assessment for rebound tenderness would also assist in the diagnosis. Options 2 and 3 are common with ulcers; option 4 may suggest ulcerative colitis or diverticulitis.
Cognitive Level: Application **Integrated Process:** Nursing Process: Assessment **Client Need:** Physiological Integrity: Physiological Adaptation **Content Area:** Adult Health: Gastrointestinal **Strategy:** Consider the anatomical location of the appendix and determine where the pain should be felt. **Reference:** LeMone, P., & Burke, K. (2008). *Medical-surgical nursing: Critical thinking in client care* (4th ed.). Upper Saddle River, NJ: Pearson/Prentice Hall, pp. 766–767.

2 **Answer: 2** Fever indicates an infection, ruling out options 3 and 4. Appendicitis typically causes pain in the umbilical area or right lower quadrant and is not usually accompanied by diarrhea. Fever and diarrhea accompany diverticulitis.
Cognitive Level: Application **Client Need:** Physiological Integrity: Physiological Adaptation **Integrated Process:** Nursing Process: Analysis **Content Area:** Adult Health:

Gastrointestinal **Strategy:** Eliminate the wrong options considering the fever, elevated white blood cells, and pain. **Reference:** LeMone, P., & Burke, K. (2008). *Medical-surgical nursing: Critical thinking in client care* (4th ed.). Upper Saddle River, NJ: Pearson/Prentice Hall, p. 815.

3 **Answer: 4** *H. pylori* causes release of toxins and enzymes that promote inflammation and ulceration. It is not spread from one person to another. Contributing factors are those that increase secretion of acid and pepsin such as NSAIDs and cigarette smoking.
Cognitive Level: Application **Client Need:** Physiological Integrity: Physiological Adaptation **Integrated Process:** Communication and Documentation **Content Area:** Adult Health: Gastrointestinal **Strategy:** Apply current knowledge of the pathophysiology of peptic ulcers. Look for the broadest answer. **Reference:** LeMone, P., & Burke, K. (2008). *Medical-surgical nursing: Critical thinking in client care* (4th ed.). Upper Saddle River, NJ: Pearson/Prentice Hall, pp. 681–685.

4 **Answer: 1** Heavy lifting is one factor that may lead to development of a hiatal hernia if it increases the intra-abdominal pressure. Dietary management may involve limiting fat intake or spicy foods, but "junk" food did not cause the problem. The incidence increases with age. Fair-skinned individuals are not more prone to this condition.

Cognitive Level: Application **Client Need:** Physiological Integrity: Physiological Adaptation **Integrated Process:** Nursing Process: Planning **Content Are:** Adult Health: Gastrointestinal **Strategy:** Recall that a hiatal hernia occurs when part of the stomach protrudes into the thorax. Consider the etiology to be primarily mechanical. **Reference:** LeMone, P., & Burke, K. (2008). *Medical-surgical nursing: Critical thinking in client care* (4th ed.). Upper Saddle River, NJ: Pearson/Prentice Hall, pp. 667–668.

5 **Answers: 2, 3, 5** Red blood in the stool is more characteristic of left-sided colon cancer. If blood occurs in the stool in right-sided colon cancer or gastric ulcers, it will be black and tarry. Bright red blood can also occur with hemorrhoids.

Cognitive Level: Application **Client Need:** Physiological Integrity: Physiological Adaptation **Integrated Process:** Nursing Process: Analysis **Content Area:** Adult Health: Gastrointestinal **Strategy:** Consider the appearance of digested heme or older blood. Where must bleeding be to be seen as red in the stool? **Reference:** Porth, C. M. (2005). *Pathophysiology: Concepts of altered health states* (7th ed.). Philadelphia, PA: Lippincott Williams & Wilkins, p. 912.

6 **Answer: 2** Aspirin is one of the nonsteroidal anti-inflammatory drugs (NSAIDs). These drugs are predisposing or contributing factors in the development of a peptic ulcer, because of the effect on prostaglandins. Many of the medications used for arthritis may also irritate an ulcer; therefore, a physician or the primary health care provider should be consulted.

Cognitive Level: Application **Client Need:** Physiological Integrity: Pharmacological and Parenteral Therapies **Integrated Process:** Communication and Documentation **Content Area:** Adult Health: Gastrointestinal **Strategy:** The treatment for one health problem may aggravate another condition. Comorbidities must be managed. **Reference:** LeMone, P., & Burke, K. (2008). *Medical-surgical nursing: Critical thinking in client care* (4th ed.). Upper Saddle River, NJ: Pearson/Prentice Hall, pp. 681–685.

7 **Answer: 4** These are all signs of perforation. If the client is going into shock, it is important to establish IV access before the veins collapse. The doctor will probably schedule emergency surgery. If a client has a possible perforation, she should be in low Fowler's position (option 1) to contain the secretions in the abdomen. Walking (option 2) is not recommended, and food allergies (option 3) are not as likely to be the problem.

Cognitive Level: Analysis **Client Need:** Physiological Integrity: Physiological Adaptation **Integrated Process:** Nursing Process: Implementation **Content Area:** Adult Health: Gastrointestinal **Strategy:** This is an emergency situation. What is needed most to support the anticipated emergency care? **Reference:** LeMone, P., & Burke, K. (2008). *Medical-surgical nursing: Critical thinking in client care* (4th ed.). Upper Saddle River, NJ: Pearson/Prentice Hall, pp. 681–685.

8 **Answer: 1** This description of pain is consistent with ulcer pain. The pain is epigastric and is worse when the stomach is empty and is relieved by food. These symptoms are not common with cholelithiasis. Ordinary indigestion does not present with this clinical scenario.

Cognitive Level: Application **Client Need:** Physiological Integrity: Physiological Adaptation **Integrated Process:** Nursing Process: Analysis **Content Area:** Adult Health: Gastrointestinal **Strategy:** Consider the factors related to the timing of the pain, such as an empty stomach. **Reference:** LeMone, P., & Burke, K. (2008). *Medical-surgical nursing: Critical thinking in client care* (4th ed.). Upper Saddle River, NJ: Pearson/Prentice Hall, p. 684.

9 **Answer: 2** One form of intestinal obstruction is paralysis, caused by decreased movement of the intestinal contents by normal peristalsis. The client in option 1 is at high risk for Crohn's disease and ulcerative colitis. Option 3 enhances the risk of cancer of the colon and diverticular disease; option 4 is consistent with peritonitis.

Cognitive Level: Application **Client Need:** Physiological Integrity: Physiological Adaptation **Integrated Process:** Nursing Process: Assessment **Content Area:** Adult Health: Gastrointestinal **Strategy:** Intestinal obstruction may be mechanical or functional—that is, from problems outside the intestine or from failure of peristalsis. What clients are at risk for either of these? **Reference:** Lemone, P., & Burke, K. (2008). *Medical-surgical nursing: Critical thinking in client care* (4th ed.). Upper Saddle River, NJ: Pearson/Prentice Hall, pp. 812–813.

10 **Answer: 4** Gastroesophageal reflux disease causes epigastric pain usually described as burning; it is accompanied by belching with a sour taste, pain after eating, increased salivation, and flatulence. The symptoms of a sliding hiatal hernia are similar to GERD, but not those of a paraesophageal hiatal hernia. Symptoms of PUD are more pronounced and reflective of a full or empty stomach. Ulcerative colitis symptoms are related to pain and bowel movements.

Cognitive Level: Application **Client Need:** Physiological Integrity: Physiological Adaptation **Integrated Process:** Nursing Process: Analysis **Content Area:** Adult Health: Gastrointestinal **Strategy:** Eliminate options that present with different symptoms. **Reference:** LeMone, P., & Burke, K. (2008). *Medical-surgical nursing: Critical thinking in client care* (4th ed.). Upper Saddle River, NJ: Pearson/Prentice Hall, pp. 663–667.

Posttest

1 Answer: 3 Lying on the side with legs flexed, pain over McBurney's point, and rebound tenderness are characteristic symptoms of appendicitis. Vomiting frequently accompanies the pain. The client definitely should not have an enema if appendicitis is suspected. If surgery is needed for appendicitis, the client needs to be NPO. **Cognitive Level:** Analysis **Client Need:** Physiological Integrity: Physiological Adaptation **Integrated Process:** Nursing Process: Analysis **Content Area:** Adult Health: Gastrointestinal **Strategy:** The findings described in the question are common characteristics of a problem. What organ is in the anatomical area where the pain is located? **Reference:** LeMone, P., & Burke, K. (2008). *Medical-surgical nursing: Critical thinking in client care* (4th ed.). Upper Saddle River, NJ: Pearson/Prentice Hall, pp. 766–767.

2 Answer: 2 Zollinger-Ellison syndrome is a condition usually caused by a gastrin-secreting tumor of the pancreas, stomach, or intestines that leads to the increased secretion of pepsin and hydrochloric acid. This often leads to peptic ulcer disease. Option 1 explains one of the pathologic reasons for peptic ulcer disease; option 3 explains a volvulus obstruction, and another name for Crohn's disease is regional enteritis. **Cognitive Level:** Application **Client Need:** Physiological Integrity: Physiological Adaptation **Integrated Process:** Nursing Process: Analysis **Content Area:** Adult Health: Gastrointestinal **Strategy:** The nurse must identify the description of Zollinger-Ellison syndrome. If the disease is unfamiliar, eliminate the options that describe diseases that are known. **Reference:** LeMone, P., & Burke, K. (2008). *Medical-surgical nursing: Critical thinking in client care* (4th ed.). Upper Saddle River, NJ: Pearson/Prentice Hall, p. 684.

3 Answer: 1 Dumping syndrome is the rapid influx of stomach contents into the duodenum or jejunum, causing increased peristalsis and dilation of the intestines. Although this occurs primarily after a gastrectomy, the condition can cause an ulcer. **Cognitive Level:** Application **Client Need:** Physiological Integrity: Physiological Adaptation **Integrated Process:** Nursing Process: Analysis **Content Area:** Adult Health: Gastrointestinal **Strategy:** The clue event is the recent surgery. Review complications following gastric surgery. **Reference:** Porth, C. M. (2005). *Pathophysiology: Concepts of altered health states* (7th ed.). Philadelphia, PA: Lippincott Williams & Wilkins, p. 877.

4 Answer: 3 The bacteria *H. pylori* has been discovered to be the leading cause of many ulcers and can be treated with success by antibiotics. Options 1, 2, and 4 are unrealistic answers for the action of antibiotics.

Cognitive Level: Application **Client Need:** Physiological Integrity: Physiological Adaptation **Integrated Process:** Communication and Documentation **Content Area:** Adult Health: Gastrointestinal **Strategy:** Review the actions of antibiotics if this question was difficult. **Reference:** LeMone, P., & Burke, K. (2008). *Medical-surgical nursing: Critical thinking in client care* (4th ed.). Upper Saddle River, NJ: Pearson/Prentice Hall, pp. 681–685.

5 Answers: 1, 2, 5 Proton pump inhibitors, histamine receptor blockers, sucralfate (Carafate), and bismuth compounds are all used to treat PUD. NSAIDs are contraindicated. Some drugs cause constipation, but laxatives are not routinely given to treat PUD. **Cognitive Level:** Application **Client Need:** Physiological Integrity: Pharmacological and Parenteral Therapies **Integrated Process:** Nursing Process: Planning **Content Area:** Adult Health: Gastrointestinal **Strategy:** Choose the drugs that reduce gastric acid content or protect the gastric mucosa. **Reference:** LeMone, P., & Burke, K. (2008). *Medical-surgical nursing: Critical thinking in client care* (4th ed.). Upper Saddle River, NJ: Pearson/Prentice Hall, pp. 684–685.

6 Answer: 3 The bowel wall becomes congested, thickens, and sometimes develops fistulas, which can become infected. This leads to malabsorption and deficiency in absorption of folic acid, calcium, and vitamin D. The anorexia can play a role in weight loss, but most clients eat and cannot explain why they have weight loss. **Cognitive Level:** Application **Client Need:** Physiological Integrity: Physiological Adaptation **Integrated Process:** Teaching/Learning **Content Area:** Adult Health: Gastrointestinal **Strategy:** Systemic manifestations are common responses to inflammatory diseases. Edematous bowel does not function properly. **Reference:** LeMone, P., & Burke, K. (2008). *Medical-surgical nursing: Critical thinking in client care* (4th ed.). Upper Saddle River, NJ: Pearson/Prentice Hall, pp. 782–786.

7 Answer: 1 A high-fiber diet reduces the risk of complications with diverticulosis such as development of diverticulitis. Elderly clients often eat less food with less roughage and fiber and therefore do not obtain the proper nutrients from their diet, which can aid in the development of the disease. Most often chronic constipation, not diarrhea, is a cause. Sedentary lifestyle may contribute to the constipation but is not a direct etiology. **Cognitive Level:** Application **Client Need:** Physiological Integrity: Physiological Adaptation **Integrated Process:** Teaching/Learning **Content Area:** Adult Health: Gastrointestinal **Strategy:** Consider the relationship of diet and disease. Identify the opposite options. **Reference:** LeMone, P., & Burke, K. (2008). *Medical-surgical nursing: Critical thinking in client care* (4th ed.). Upper Saddle River, NJ: Pearson/Prentice Hall, pp. 814–818.

ANSWERS & RATIONALES

8 **Answer: 2** Clients with long-standing Crohn's disease have 4 to 5 times the risk of developing cancer of the small intestine or colon. A noncompliant client increases that risk and should be educated that Crohn's can be successfully kept under control. Fistulas are common but perforation of the bowel is not.
Cognitive Level: Application **Client Need:** Health Promotion and Maintenance **Integrated Process:** Nursing Process: Analysis **Content Area:** Adult Health: Gastrointestinal **Strategy:** Consider the cell changes that result from chronic inflammation such as Crohn's disease. **Reference:** LeMone, P., & Burke, K. (2008). *Medical-surgical nursing: Critical thinking in client care* (4th ed.). Upper Saddle River, NJ: Pearson/Prentice Hall, pp. 782–786.

9 **Answer: 3** A client with any GI disorder, especially a peptic ulcer, should never receive any aspirin product or NSAID. Many pain medications contain aspirin or ibuprofen and are combined with an opioid analgesic. The nurse administering the pain medication should know what ingredients are in it. Hydrocodone is a schedule III opioid analgesic and if combined with acetaminophen is acceptable to use with clients who have PUD.
Cognitive Level: Analysis **Client Need:** Physiological Integrity: Pharmacological and Parenteral Therapies **Integrated Process:** Nursing Process: Implementation **Content Area:** Adult Health: Gastrointestinal **Strategy:**

What classification of analgesic is contraindicated in PUD? That is the correct answer. **Reference:** LeMone, P., & Burke, K. (2008). *Medical-surgical nursing: Critical thinking in client care* (4th ed.). Upper Saddle River, NJ: Pearson/Prentice Hall, pp. 681–685.

10 **Answers: 2, 4, 5** This is an urgent situation. The client probably has an obstructed or ruptured bowel. NPO must be maintained because of the nonfunctioning GI system and preparation for surgery. Narcotics may mask worsening level of consciousness and are not indicated at his time. Inserting an NG tube will decompress the bowel, which will relieve the vomiting and pain and hopefully prevent the client from going into shock. This may be a measure to institute only until surgery can be performed. Vomiting fecal matter can be dangerous (as well as unpleasant) because of the possibility of aspiration, especially with a decreasing level of consciousness. An IV line is needed if not already present.
Cognitive Level: Analysis **Client Need:** Physiological Integrity: Physiological Adaptation **Integrated Process:** Nursing Process: Implementation **Content Area:** Adult Health: Gastrointestinal **Strategy:** What actions are needed to manage this emergency situation? What is contraindicated? **Reference:** LeMone, P., & Burke, K. (2008). *Medical-surgical nursing: Critical thinking in client care* (4th ed.). Upper Saddle River, NJ: Pearson/Prentice Hall, pp. 811–814.

References

Adams, M., Holland, L. & Bostwick, P. (2008.) *Pharmacology for nurses: A pathophysiologic approach* (2nd ed.). Upper Saddle River, NJ: Prentice Hall.

Ignatavicius, D., Workman, M., & Mishler, M. (2006). *Medical surgical nursing: Critical thinking for colloborative care* (5th ed.). Philadelphia, PA: W. B. Saunders, pp. 1159–1297.

LeMone, P., & Burke, K. (2008). *Medical surgical nursing: Critical thinking in client care* (4th ed.). Upper Saddle River, NJ: Prentice Hall.

McCance, K., & Huether, S. (2006). *Pathophysiology: The biologic basis for disease in adults and children* (5th ed.). St. Louis, MO: Mosby.

Porth, C. M. (2005). *Pathophysiology: Concepts of altered health states* (7th ed.). Philadelphia, PA: Lippincott Williams & Wilkins, pp. 885–913.

Sands, J. (2006). Management of persons with problems of the stomach and duodenum. In W. Phipps, J. Sands, & J. Marek. (Eds.), *Medical-surgical nursing: Health and illness perspectives.* (8th ed.). St. Louis: Mosby.

Venes, C., Thomas, C. L. (2006). *Taber's cyclopedic medical dictionary.* (20th ed.). Philadelphia, PA: F. A. Davis.

Wilson, B. A., Shannon, M. T., & Stang, C. L. (2006). *Nursing drug guide: 2006.* Upper Saddle River, NJ: Prentice Hall.

ANSWERS & RATIONALES

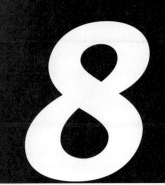

8 Hepatobiliary Health Problems

Chapter Outline

Risk Factors Associated with Hepatobiliary Health Problems

Cirrhosis

Hepatitis

Cancer of the Liver

Cholelithiasis

Cholecystitis

Pancreatitis

Cancer of the Pancreas

 NCLEX-RN® Test Prep

Use the CD-ROM enclosed with this book
to access additional practice opportunities.

Objectives

➤ Define key terms associated with hepatobiliary health problems.

➤ Identify risk factors associated with the development of hepatobiliary health problems.

➤ Explain the common etiologies of hepatobiliary health problems.

➤ Describe the pathophysiologic processes associated with specific hepatobiliary health problems.

➤ Distinguish between normal and abnormal hepatobiliary findings obtained from nursing assessment.

➤ Prioritize nursing interventions associated with specific hepatobiliary health problems.

Review at a Glance

ascites increased amount of fluid in abdominal cavity

bile a thick, yellow-green fluid secreted from biliary tract and duodenum; responsible for digestion of food, absorption of fats and fat-soluble vitamins, and stimulation of peristalsis

biliary cirrhosis cirrhosis characterized by a prolonged state of jaundice because of retention of bile and bile duct inflammation

cholecystitis inflammation of gallbladder

cholelithiasis condition in which there are stones present in gallbladder

cirrhosis scarring of liver tissue, which interferes with normal liver function and results in structural changes within liver

fulminant hepatitis necrosis and shrinking of liver, possibly resulting in liver failure; a complication of viral hepatitis

hemochromatosis a genetically transmitted disease where iron is excessively absorbed and accumulated

hepatic encephalopathy damage to brain tissue, which occurs as a complication of cirrhosis of liver caused by ammonia in brain tissue

hepatitis an inflammation of liver

jaundice yellow-tinged color of skin, body organs, or body fluids caused by abnormally high accumulation of bile pigment (bilirubin) in blood

Laënnec's cirrhosis development of cirrhosis associated with chronic alcoholism

melena black tarry-colored feces as a result of secretions from intestines on free blood

pancreatitis inflammation of pancreas

portal hypertension increase in pressure in portal vein caused by obstruction or congestion; a complication of cirrhosis of liver

splenomegaly an enlarged spleen

steatorrhea excessive elimination of fat; fatty stools

thrombocytopenia a decrease in number of platelets

varices dilation of a vein that is usually tortuous

Wilson's disease an autosomal recessive disorder where ceruloplasmin is decreased, which leads to increased copper in several organs (liver, brain, kidney, and cornea)

PRETEST

1 The nurse is reviewing a client's liver biopsy report, which confirmed a fatty liver and the diagnosis of cirrhosis. The nurse interprets that hepatic fat accumulation in a 55-year-old male is usually a result of which type of cirrhosis?

1. Biliary
2. Metabolic
3. Postnecrotic
4. Laënnec's

2 A concerned mother doesn't understand how her child acquired hepatitis A, when the child was perfectly healthy up to a week ago. The nurse considers that one characteristic of hepatitis A that may help her to understand is that hepatitis A has:

1. An incubation period of 60 to 180 days.
2. A fecal-oral mode of transmission.
3. A positive carrier state.
4. A sexual mode of transmission.

3 The nurse is analyzing the physical assessment findings of spider angiomas, palmar erythema, peripheral edema, ascites, and change in mental status of the client. These findings are consistent with which of the following disorders?

1. Cholelithiasis
2. Cholecystitis
3. Cirrhosis
4. Pancreatitis

4 A 45-year-old female hospitalized with acute pancreatitis has orders for morphine sulfate 8 mg IM every three hours as needed for pain. The nurse explains that morphine has been ordered because:

1. It has a slower onset of action than oxycodone (Percocet).
2. It is less addictive than meperidine (Demerol).
3. The pain of acute pancreatitis is severe.
4. It has fewer cognitive side effects.

5 A 65-year-old female with a history of hepatic encephalopathy is hospitalized for pneumonia and dehydration. When she complains to the nurse about the small portions of meat ordered by the dietitian, the best response would be:

1. "Ask your doctor about it in the morning."
2. "I will call and order larger portions for you."
3. "The amount of meat on your tray is dictated by certain blood test results."
4. "Your protein is being limited, but you can have more food that is not meat or protein."

6 The physical assessment of a 55-year-old female with end-stage cirrhosis reveals a protuberant abdomen with bulging flanks and dullness to the dependent side while lying laterally. The appropriate terminology for that the nurse uses to document this assessment is:

1. Fluid overload.
2. Malnutrition.
3. Ascites.
4. Distention.

7 The nurse is teaching a client who has been diagnosed with advanced pancreatic cancer. The client asks the nurse why it was not diagnosed earlier. Which of the following statements by the nurse would be correct to teach this client? Select all that apply.

1. "The onset of pancreatic cancer is usually insidious."
2. "Pancreatic cancer causes black tarry stools."
3. "Pancreatic cancer presents with slow weight loss and jaundice."
4. "Pancreatic cancer often is diagnosed early and rarely metastasizes."
5. "The pain with pancreatic cancer is a dull epigastric pain that may not be reported right away."

8 When providing discharge teaching to the client with chronic cirrhosis, the spouse asks the nurse to explain why there is so much emphasis on bleeding precautions. Which of the following provides the most appropriate response?

1. "The liver affected by cirrhosis is unable to produce clotting factors."
2. "The low protein diet will result in reduced clotting factors."
3. "The increased production of bile decreases clotting factors."
4. "The required medications reduce clotting factors."

9 A nurse sustained a needle stick injury with a client's used intramuscular needle. The nurse has previously had the three doses of hepatitis B vaccine but requests postexposure prophylaxis for hepatitis B. What advice should the occupational health nurse give to this nurse?

1. Nurse needs a booster vaccination to provide protection for this new exposure
2. If nurse's hepatitis B titer is positive, nurse does not need prophylactic treatment
3. Real risk is hepatitis A, which requires an immune globulin injection for prophylaxis
4. Antiviral drug is needed for six months to prevent development of any type of hepatitis

10 A male client with a history of alcoholism and long time intravenous drug use has been diagnosed with primary liver cancer. He asks the nurse to explain the cause of his cancer. Which of the following are risk factors that might fit this client's history? Select all that apply.

1. Chronic hepatitis C infection
2. Chronic hepatitis B infection
3. Drinking from the city's treated water supply
4. Alcoholic cirrhosis of the liver
5. Taking folic acid and vitamins as a dietary supplement

➤ *See pages 258–259 for Answers & Rationales.*

I. RISK FACTORS ASSOCIATED WITH HEPATOBILIARY HEALTH PROBLEMS

A. *Cirrhosis:* alcoholism (primary); viral hepatitis, toxic reactions to drugs and chemicals, biliary obstruction, cardiac disease; **hemochromatosis** (a genetically transmitted disease where iron is excessively absorbed and accumulated); **Wilson's disease** (an autosomal recessive disorder where ceruloplasmin is decreased, leading to increased copper in several organs [liver, brain, kidney, and cornea])

B. *Hepatitis*

1. Hepatitis A: drinking contaminated milk or water and consumption of shellfish from contaminated waters; children in day care centers and institutionalized adults are at increased risk

2. Hepatitis B: contact with blood or serum and oral or sexual contact

3. Hepatitis C: intravenous (IV) drug abusers, persons receiving blood transfusions, health care workers, persons on hemodialysis, those with high-risk sexual behavior, and organ transplant recipients

4. Hepatitis D: IV drug users and those receiving clotting factor concentrates

5. Hepatitis E: pregnant women in developing countries

C. **Cancer of liver:** persons with chronic hepatitis B infection, hepatitis C, or cirrhosis, and consumption of hepatocarcinogens in food such as aflatoxin in moldy peanuts

D. *Cholecystitis:* diet high in fat content, cholelithiasis

E. *Cholelithiasis:* aging process, family history, cirrhosis, Crohn's disease, sickle-cell anemia, hyperlipidemia, congenital malformation of biliary ducts, obesity and rapid weight loss, diabetes mellitus, drugs that reduce cholesterol, and hyperalimentation; other risk factors include: Native American, Caucasian or Mexican American ethnicity and female gender (pregnancy or use of oral contraceptives)

F. *Pancreatitis:* alcohol in men, gallstones in women, hyperlipidemia, hyperparathyroidism, viral infections, and abdominal trauma

G. **Cancer of pancreas:** smoking (major risk); industrial chemicals, environmental toxin exposure, high-fat diet, pancreatitis, age, and diabetes mellitus

II. CIRRHOSIS

A. Overview

1. Cirrhosis is defined as scarring of liver tissue, which interferes with normal liver function and results in structural changes within lobes of liver

2. Characterized by structural and functional disorganization as a result of diffuse fibrosis and nodules of regenerated tissue

3. Three types

a. Laënnec's or alcoholic cirrhosis

b. Biliary cirrhosis

c. Posthepatic cirrhosis

4. Causes

a. Laënnec's (or alcoholic) cirrhosis: consumption of a pint or more of alcohol per day

        b. Biliary cirrhosis: hepatotoxins, any obstruction of common bile duct, severe congestive heart failure (CHF)

        c. Posthepatic cirrhosis: results from chronic hepatitis B or C

B. Pathophysiology

    1. Laënnec's (or alcoholic) cirrhosis: development of cirrhosis associated with chronic alcoholism

        a. Alcohol is transformed to acetaldehyde, which begins to alter hepatocyte function

        b. Acetaldehyde inhibits removal of proteins from liver and alters metabolism of vitamins and minerals

        c. As large amounts of alcohol are consumed, fat accumulates in liver, known as "fatty liver"

    2. Biliary cirrhosis is cirrhosis characterized by a prolonged state of bile duct inflammation and jaundice (late manifestation) because of retention of **bile** (a thick yellow-green fluid secreted from biliary tract to duodenum; responsible for digestion of food, absorption of fat and fat-soluble vitamins, and stimulation of peristalsis)

        a. *Primary:* inflammation, destruction, fibrosis, and obstruction of intrahepatic bile ducts results in nodular regeneration and cirrhosis; women are more commonly affected than men and this type of cirrhosis does not usually begin before age 30 years

        b. *Secondary:* inflammation and scarring of bile ducts occurs proximal to an obstruction caused by neoplasms, strictures, or gallstones

    3. Posthepatic cirrhosis: fibrous, nodular scar tissue replaces necrotic tissue because of viral hepatitis B or C, drugs, toxins, or autoimmune disease

    4. Metabolic cirrhosis: inflammation and scarring, which is a result of defects or storage diseases; examples are antitrypsin deficiency, glycogen storage disease, Wilson's disease, and galactosemia

    5. Progression of disease

        a. Fatty infiltration results in inflammation, which in turn results in necrosis and fibrosis of liver, followed by regeneration and scarring

        b. Damage is increased if client has a poor nutritional state

        c. Normal structure of liver is lost and replaced by disorganized arrangement of scars and nodules

        d. Widespread scarring puts pressure on and obstructs blood vessels and biliary ducts

        e. Increased capillary pressure causes increased fluid in abdomen and development of **portal hypertension** (increase in pressure in portal vein caused by obstruction or congestion; a complication of cirrhosis of liver)

        f. Decreased production of albumin results in decreased colloidal osmotic pressure; fluid leaves blood vessels and enters abdomen (third spacing)

        g. Decreased metabolism of aldosterone results in sodium retention and increased fluid retention

        h. Portal hypertension causes collateral circulation to develop in stomach, rectum, and esophagus; these vessels become distended and cause **varices** (tortous dilation of a vein); in the esophagus varices are irritated by alcohol and food causing rupture and excessive bleeding, **melena** (black tarry-colored feces as a result of secretions of free blood from intestines), hematemesis; this is also aggravated by coughing, vomiting, lifting, or straining

    i. Portal hypertension causes stasis of blood into the splenic vein, which results in **splenomegaly** (enlarged spleen), and increased breakdown of white blood cells (WBCs) (leukopenia), red blood cells (RBCs) (anemia), and platelets (**thrombocytopenia**), and thus decreased defense against infection

    j. Decreased liver function results in inability to inactivate adrenocortical hormones, estrogen, testosterone, and aldosterone

    k. Normally, ammonia is produced by bacteria and enzymes, which break down amino acids

      1) Ammonia goes to liver to be converted to urea and eliminated

      2) If liver is not functioning, ammonia is not broken down; it accumulates in bloodstream, crosses blood-brain barrier and goes into brain tissue, leading to **hepatic encephalopathy** (damage to brain tissue as a complication of cirrhosis of liver caused by to ammonia in brain tissue); precipitated by any major hemodynamic insult to body such as bleeding, shock, toxins to body, hypovolemia, or anything that can increase metabolic needs on liver

  6. Signs and symptoms of cirrhosis include weakness, fatigue, fever, anorexia, weight loss, nausea, vomiting, indigestion, increased flatulence, change in memory or level of consciousness (LOC), sexual dysfunction (loss of libido, change in menstrual pattern), edema, ascites, change in secondary sex characteristics (gynecomastia), bruising or hematoma, spider angiomas (a telangiectasis with a red, elevated center and small radiating blood vessels), palmar erythema (redness of palm), jaundice, dark urine, light-colored feces, enlarged liver and spleen, muscle wasting, decreased strength, insomnia

  7. Signs and symptoms of hepatic encephalopathy include restlessness, change in LOC, inability to concentrate, altered sleep, forgetfulness, confusion, asterixis (flapping tremor of hands when extending arms), muscle twitching, and coma

C. Nursing assessment

  1. Assessment includes fluid and electolyte balance (sodium and water retention), vital signs (VS), bowel sounds, abdominal girth, dilation of abdominal wall veins, pulse quality, **ascites** (increased amount of fluid in abdominal cavity), peripheral edema, color, mental status, reproductive history, urine and stool color, palpate abdominal muscle strength, weight, gastrointestinal (GI) complaints

  2. Diagnostic tests: electrocardiogram (ECG), electrolytes, blood urea nitrogen (BUN), creatinine (CR), stool for occult blood, ultrasound (US) of abdomen, complete blood count (CBC), clotting studies, prothrombin time (PT), partial thromboplastin time (PTT), international normalized ratio (INR), urine specific gravity, arterial blood gases (ABGs), liver function tests: alanine aminotransferase (ALT), aspartate aminotransferase (AST), alkaline phosphatase, gamma-glutamyl transpeptidase (GGT), bilirubin levels, liver biopsy (to verify cirrhosis and only if necessary), protein, albumin, ammonia levels, glucose, cholesterol, esophagascopy

D. Nursing management

  1. Medications

    a. Diuretics for ascites: spironolactone (Aldactone) is drug of choice and furosemide (Lasix)

  b. Lactulose (Chronulac) and neomycin (Mycifradin) to reduce high ammonia levels by metabolism of lactulose to organic acids by intestinal bacteria and decreasing pH of colon; a more acid pH converts ammonia to a nonabsorbable food so it is expelled in feces

  c. Ferrous sulfate and folic acid

  d. Vitamin K (Aquamephyton) to enhance clotting

  e. Antacids if gastritis is present

  f. Beta blockers such as nadolol (Corgard) with isosorbide mononitrate (Imdur)

2. Avoid medications highly metabolized by liver such as barbiturates, sedatives, acetaminophen (Tylenol), and alcohol-containing products

3. Monitor weight, abdominal girth, and peripheral edema daily

4. Administer low-sodium, low-protein diet of 500 to 2,000 mg of sodium with restricted fluids; protein is controlled to reduce ammonia; sodium is controlled to limit fluid accumulation

5. Inspect skin integrity every 8 hours

6. Be cautious about amount and frequency of medications administered (especially acetaminophen, barbiturates, sedatives, and hypnotics)

7. Monitor neurologic functioning for early signs of encephalopathy

8. Check VS every 8 hours

9. Institute bleeding precautions

  a. Avoid manipulation of rectum, including prevention of constipation

  b. Avoid injections

  c. Assess and report ecchymosis and purpura

  d. Apply extra pressure for areas that begin to bleed

  e. Use a soft toothbrush and assess gums for bleeding

  f. Avoid harsh blowing of nose

  g. Try to coordinate timing of lab work to prevent excess venipunctures

10. Position in high Fowler's with feet elevated, avoid supine position

11. Monitor respiratory status and administer O_2 as indicated

12. Use warm — not hot — water for bathing to reduce pruritus

13. Institute skin protocols to prevent breakdown

14. Be cautious in administering antihistamines for itching because of liver disease and impaired metabolism

15. Priority nursing diagnoses are Excess fluid volume; Impaired tissue perfusion; Risk for injury: bleeding; Risk for impaired gas exchange; Impaired skin integrity

E. Complications

1. Portal hypertension

  a. Overview

  1) Defined as an abnormally high blood pressure in portal venous system

  2) Occurs when blood flow through portal system is obstructed or impeded due to thrombosis, inflammation, or fibrous changes in hepatic sinuses with cirrhosis or hepatitis; parasitic diseases and right-sided congestive heart failure can also cause portal hypertension

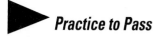

Practice to Pass

How should the nurse determine if a client is developing ascites? What lab data are important?

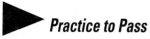

Practice to Pass

A known client with alcoholism is admitted with a BP of 210/110, strong ammonia odor, tenderness in the abdomen, anorexic look, and reports eating only one meal per day containing less than nutritional foods. The client develops a GI hemorrhage and is treated for a GI bleed. Relate the signs and symptoms to Laënnec's cirrhosis.

b. Pathophysiology

   1) Portal veins carry blood from GI tract, pancreas, and spleen to liver

   2) Blood then flows through liver, empties into inferior vena cava, and is delivered to right atrium

   3) Normal pressure in this system is 3 mmHg; with portal hypertension, pressure reaches 10 mmHg

   4) Obstruction causes blood to back up into portal circulation and increase pressure; high pressure in portal veins causes collateral circulation to develop between portal veins and systemic veins

   5) Decreased protein synthesis results in a decrease in albumin, which leads to edema and ascites

   6) Long-term portal hypertension causes distended, twisted collateral veins; gradually these become transformed to varicosities

   7) Major complication is hemorrhage

c. Nursing assessment

   1) Assess abdomen for distention of collateral veins radiating over abdomen; hematemesis, melena; signs of shock (cool, pale skin, drop in blood pressure [BP], increase in heart rate [HR] and respirations) review history for jaundice, hepatitis, or alcoholism

   2) Diagnostic tests: CBC, clotting factors

d. Nursing management

   1) There is no effective medical treatment for portal hypertension, and nursing care is same as treatment of cirrhosis

   2) Nursing diagnoses are: Risk for injury: bleeding; Risk for impaired gas exchange; Risk for impaired skin integrity; and Imbalanced nutrition: less than body requirements

2. Esophageal varices

a. Overview

   1) Defined as distended, tortuous collateral veins that occur from prolonged elevation of pressure

   2) Most commonly located in stomach and lower esophagus but varices may also be found in rectum

   3) Mortality from ruptured esophageal varices ranges from 30 to 60%, and many individuals die within 1 year

b. Pathophysiology

   1) Increased pressure in portal veins causes development of collateral vessels to occur between portal veins and systemic veins, where blood pressure is lower

   2) Blood then bypasses obstructed portal vessels and is carried via collateral veins in esophagus, anterior abdominal wall, and rectum

   3) First sign of esophageal varices is usually vomiting of copious amounts of dark-colored blood; ruptured varices do not cause pain and the rupture is usually precipitated by increased venous pressure and gastric acid

c. Nursing assessment

   1) Assessment includes: hematemesis and melena

   2) Diagnostic tests: CBC, clotting studies, type and cross-match

    d. Nursing management

!▷   **1)** Medications include: vasopressin (Pitressin) to lower portal BP; beta blockers to lower BP; antacids; lactulose (Chronulac) or neomycin (Mycifradin) to decrease production of ammonia if caused by cirrhosis; vitamin K (Aquamephyton) for clotting

!▷   **2)** Ruptured esophageal varices are a medical emergency, and management includes compression with insertion of a Sengstaken-Blakemore tube; varices may be managed by injection of a sclerosing agent (sclerotherapy) or surgical construction of a portacaval shunt

      3) Replace blood loss with administration of blood and IV fluids

      4) Maintain patent airway

      5) Monitor VS every 30 minutes

      6) Use gastric lavage with cool saline to control bleeding

      7) Monitor for signs of shock

III. HEPATITIS

A. Overview

    1. Hepatitis is defined as an inflammation of liver, usually viral in nature

    2. Known hepatitis viruses are (see Table 8-1)

!▷   **a.** Hepatitis A (HAV)

!▷   **b.** Hepatitis B (HBV): causes high amount of liver damage

    c. Hepatitis B–associated delta virus (HDV)

!▷   **d.** Hepatitis C virus (HCV): causes high amount of liver damage

Table 8-1	**Classification and Characteristics of Viral Hepatitis**				
	Hepatitis A HAV	**Hepatitis B HBV**	**Hepatitis C HCV**	**Hepatitis D HDV**	**Hepatitis E HEV**
Onset	Abrupt	Insidious	Insidious	Abrupt	Abrupt
Transmission	Fecal-oral	Blood and body fluids	Blood and body fluids	Blood and body fluids; perinatal	Fecal-oral
Incubation Period	2–6 weeks	6 weeks to 4 months	2–12 weeks	1–6 months	3 weeks to 2 months
Antibody-Antigens	Anti-HAV*	Anti-HBs, HBsAg+	Anti-HCV (indicates infection, no confirmation of immunity +HCV RNA	Anti-HDV*, HDVAg+	Anti-HEV*
Carrier State	No	Yes	Yes	Yes	No
Post-Exposure Treatment	Gamma globulin	Hepatitis B immune globulin	None available	Immune globulin	Gamma globulin does not offer protection
Vaccination	Immune globulin HAV vaccine	HBV vaccine	None	HBV vaccine	None

*Demonstrates immunity

+Presence of this antigen signifies acute infection or carrier state

     e. Hepatitis E (HEV)

     f. Hepatitis F

     g. Hepatitis G

  3. Each virus differs in mode of transmission, incubation period, degree of liver damage, and ability to create a carrier state

     a. HAV and HEV are both spread by fecal-oral contamination; major sources of infection are inadequate handwashing, infected food handlers, contaminated food or water, and improper cleaning of utensils

     b. HBV, HCV, and HDV are all spread by bloodborne organisms; control of contaminated needles, standard precautions for health care workers, and control of blood administration are primary means to control infection

     c. Hepatitis F and G, little is known yet of transmission and mechanism of hepatic injury; hepatitis F is an enteric virus isolated from human stool, and hepatitis G is associated with acute and chronic non-ABCDE hepatitis; hepatitis G is transmitted parenterally

     d. Depending upon cause, hepatitis can exist in either an acute or chronic form; chronic form results in cirrhosis

     e. Causes other than viruses include hepatobiliary obstruction from gallstones or from toxic effects of alcohol, drugs, toxins, or infectious agents

B. Pathophysiology

  1. Viral infections of liver create same pathologic lesions as viral infections in other parts of body; hepatic cell necrosis, scarring, Kupffer cell hyperplasia, and infiltration by mononuclear phagocytes occur in varying amounts and severity

  2. Cytotoxic T-cells and natural killer cells become activated by immune response and promote cellular injury; hepatic cells begin to regenerate within 48 hours of injury

  3. Distortion of normal structure of liver interferes with flow of blood and bile

  4. Obstruction of portal and hepatic blood flow increases portal pressure causing engorgement, hepatomegaly, and splenomegaly

  5. Cholestasis and obstructive **jaundice** (yellow-tinged color of skin, body organs, or body fluids caused by abnormally high accumulation of bile [bilirubin] in blood) are a result of inflammatory effect on bile canaliculi

  6. Signs and symptoms are specific to stages

     a. Preicteric stage (before jaundice occurs): malaise, fatigue, nausea, vomiting, diarrhea, anorexia (and aversion to food, especially protein and fat), enlarged liver and lymph nodes, electrolyte imbalances; conjunctivitis; skin rash; pain (headache, muscle aches, painful joints, fever, and sore throat)

     b. Icteric stage (onset of jaundice): jaundice, pruritus, light-colored stools, brown urine, malaise, preicteric symptoms improve or subside

     c. Posticteric stage (convalescent phase): decrease in fatigue, appetite returns to normal, laboratory work improves, and pain subsides

  7. A complication of hepatitis is **fulminant hepatitis** (necrosis and shrinking of liver, possibly resulting in liver failure): develops 6 to 8 weeks after initial symptoms, anorexia, and vomiting, abdominal pain, progressive jaundice followed by ascites, GI bleeding, lethargy, disorientation, and coma develop; mortality rate is high

C. Nursing assessment

1. Assessment

   a. Preicteric: assess for energy level; nutritional status; GI complaints; genitourinary (GU) patterns; presence of any pain; palpate liver and lymph nodes; VS

   b. Icteric phase: assess skin for color and integrity; stools and urine characteristics, VS, GI symptoms; nutritional status

   c. Posticteric: assess for improvement in all laboratory results and symptoms

2. Diagnostic tests

   a. Preicteric stage

      1) Electrolytes: abnormal

      2) Liver function tests (AST, ALT, alkaline phosphatase [ALP]): elevated

      3) Virus and antibodies present in serum

   b. Icteric stage

      1) Total, conjugated, and unconjugated serum bilirubin: elevated

      2) Urinalysis: bilirubinuria

   c. Posticteric stage

      1) Serum bilirubin and enzymes: normal or returning to normal

      2) Serum antibodies: elevated

   d. Other diagnostic tests

      1) Hepatitis A: anti-HAV (antibody to HAV demonstrates immunity); IgM anti-HAV (antibody to HAV in recent infections to 6 months)

      2) Hepatitis B: HBsAG (Hepatitis B surface-antigen indicating active disease); HBeAg (antigen in chronic carriers of hepatitis B); anti-HBs (immunity following hepatitis B vaccine); anti-HBc-IgM (indicates core infection in hepatitis B)

      3) Hepatitis C: anti-HCV (antibody found in hepatitis C clients that indicates an infection but not necessarily immunity)

      4) Hepatitis D: HDAg (antigen in acute infection); anti-HDV (antibody found in hepatitis D)

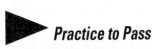

Practice to Pass

A client asks, "How can I keep from developing hepatitis B?" What should the nurse tell him?

D. Nursing management

1. Medications are for symptom control and include antiemetics to control nausea; use of antihistamines such as diphenhydramine (Benadryl), dimenhydrinate (Dramamine) or trimethobenzamide hydrochloride (Tigan); and emollient creams and lotions on skin

2. Avoid acetaminophen (Tylenol), prochlorperazine (Compazine), or other drugs detoxified in liver

3. Eliminate risk for infection (transmission): standard precautions and meticulous handwashing are essential to prevent transmission of hepatitis A and E

4. Diet should consist of 16 carbohydrate kcalories per kilogram of ideal body weight; calories should be consumed in morning hours since most clients are nauseated by afternoon and evening; decrease fat content as fat is generally not appetizing

5. Monitor fluid and electrolytes

6. Prevent skin breakdown and avoid use of hot water for bathing

7. In fulminant hepatitis, protein is restricted

8. Supportive care with rest and gradual return to normal activities
9. Prevention for health care workers
   a. Use of standard precautions
   b. Meticulous handwashing or hand hygiene (hand rubs)
   c. Hepatitis A and B vaccines

IV. CANCER OF THE LIVER

A. Overview

1. Defined as metastatic carcinoma or primary neoplasm of liver
2. Liver cancer as a primary site is not common in United States, but frequently metastasis occurs from pulmonary, breast, and GI primary sites
3. Primary cancers arise from bile duct in 10% of cases; alcohol-induced cirrhosis and hepatitis A or B account for most primary liver cancers in United States
4. Causes include chronic cirrhosis, vinyl chloride exposure, inorganic arsenic, aflatoxins, nitrosamines, pesticides, prolonged androgen therapy, and contraceptive steroids

B. Pathophysiology

1. Major types
   a. Hepatocellular carcinoma, arising from liver cells
   b. Cholangiocarcinoma, primary cancer of cells of bile duct
2. Hepatocellular carcinoma is classified as nodular, massive, or diffuse
3. Metastasis to heart, lung, brain, kidney, and spleen is rapid because of invasion of hepatic and portal veins
4. Benign tumors of liver are adenomas often affecting women and related to oral contraceptives
5. Manifestations are usually related to effects of tumor or functional changes in liver
   a. Bile products are secreted because of secretion of substances by tumors
   b. Tumor secretes hormones that lead to polycythemia, hypoglycemia, and hypercalcemia
   c. Obstruction of biliary system leads to jaundice, portal hypertension, ascites
   d. Impairment of hepatocytes results in metabolic disturbances
   e. Invasion of tumor into liver, which is often inoperable, causes hepatomegaly, hemorrhage, and liver failure
   f. Other signs and symptoms
      1) GI: nausea, vomiting, fullness, pressure, and dull ache in right upper abdomen, anorexia, malaise, fever of unknown origin (FUO)
      2) Pain, as a result of enlargement of tumor
      3) Debilitation, weight loss, cachexia
      4) Symptoms of cirrhosis

C. Nursing assessment

1. Assessment includes presence of GI symptoms, pain, weight, nutritional status, fluid status (I&O), measurement of abdominal girth, and presence of bleeding
2. Diagnostic tests: magnetic resonance imagery (MRI), computed tomography (CT) scans, ultrasound, and alpha-fetoprotein serum markers (specific to detecting hepatocellular carcinoma)

D. Nursing management

1. Medications include narcotics and analgesics for pain; chemotherapeutic agents [5-fluorouracil (5-FU), methotrexate (MTX), doxorubicin (Adriamycin)]
2. There is no cure; palliative care is the goal
3. Monitor for and prevent infection
4. Inspect skin and prevent breakdown
5. Manage pain and instruct client to ask for pain medication prior to onset of severe pain
6. Offer support for client and family for grief and coping

V. CHOLELITHIASIS

A. Overview

1. Cholelithiasis is defined as a formation of stones in biliary duct system or gallbladder
2. Approximately 10 to 20% of men and 20 to 40% of women are affected
3. Causes include obesity, oral contraceptives and estrogen therapy, family history, diseases (cirrhosis, Crohn's disease, hyperlipidemia, diabetes mellitus), hyperalimentation (total parenteral nutrition or TPN)

B. Pathophysiology

1. Gallstones form when cholesterol and calcium precipitate as solid crystals within mucous lining of gallbladder
2. This process is enhanced by delayed emptying of gallbladder
3. If gallstone obstructs cystic duct, acute cholecystitis occurs
4. Manifestations result from presence and location of stone (see Figure 8-1)
   a. Stones lodged in cystic duct cause distention of gallbladder and colicky pain (severe, cramplike)
   b. Pain may radiate to subscapular area
   c. Obstruction of common bile duct causes reflux of bile into liver and jaundice
   d. Other signs and symptoms include nausea, vomiting, epigastric pain, heartburn, and intolerance to fat-containing foods

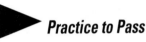

Practice to Pass

A client with cholelithiasis is admitted to the medical-surgical unit. What nursing diagnoses are appropriate for the plan of care and what specific interventions would be necessary to institute?

Figure 8-1

Common location of gallstones.

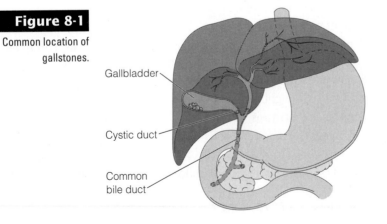

Gallbladder

Cystic duct

Common bile duct

C. Nursing assessment

1. Assessment includes pain, color, stool characteristics, nutritional status, GI symptoms (epigastric pain, heartburn, nausea, vomiting, right upper abdominal pain)

2. Diagnostic tests: serum bilirubin (direct bilirubin elevated if biliary ducts involved, indirect bilirubin elevated if liver damage occurs), alkaline phosphatase (elevated), cholangiography or radioactive scan, ultrasound of gallbladder, gallbladder scans

D. Nursing management

1. Medications include: oral bile acids or dissolvers: ursodiol(Actigall) and chenodiol (Chenix); analgesics such as morphine sulfate; cholestyramine (Questran) for pruritis

2. Clients should be taught to avoid high-fat foods because these stimulate gallbladder contractions: avoid whole-milk products, fried foods, nuts, gravies, cooking oils, hot dogs, chocolate, and cheese

3. Obese or overweight clients should be instructed in weight loss

4. Goal is to reduce inflammation and blockage

VI. CHOLECYSTITIS

A. Overview

1. Cholecystitis is defined as an inflammation of cystic duct caused by lodging of a gallstone in duct

2. May be acute or chronic

3. Causes

   a. Cholelithiasis

   b. Without cholelithiasis: trauma, fasting, TPN, surgery

B. Pathophysiology

1. A lodged gallstone in cystic duct exerts pressure against wall of gallbladder, decreasing blood flow

2. Ischemia follows with possibility of necrosis and perforation of gallbladder

3. Chemical irritation from obstruction or presence of a bacterial infection prevents outflow of bile from gallbladder

4. Signs and symptoms include pain that suddenly or gradually develops (classically in back or right shoulder), fever, nausea, vomiting, jaundice, clay-colored stools, intolerance to fat-containing foods, epigastric pain, heartburn

C. Nursing assessment

1. Assessment includes rebound tenderness, VS, abdominal muscle guarding, GI distress (epigastric pain, heartburn, nausea, vomiting, right upper quadrant abdominal pain), skin color, stool characteristics, and nutritional status

2. Diagnostics tests: serum bilirubin (direct bilirubin elevated if biliary ducts involved, indirect bilirubin elevated if liver damage), alkaline phosphatase (elevated), serum amylase (normal unless pancreas involved), CBC (elevated WBC), electrolytes, cholangiography or radioactive scan, ultrasound of the gallbladder, gallbladder scans

D. Nursing management

1. Medications include: oral bile acids or dissolvers: ursodiol (Actigall) and chenodiol (Chenix); antibiotics, antipyretics; analgesics such as morphine sulfate; cholestyramine (Questran) for pruritis

2. Clients should be taught to avoid whole-milk products, fried foods, nuts, gravies, cooking oils, hot dogs, chocolate, and cheese

3. Obese or overweight clients should be instructed in weight loss

4. For clients with surgical interventions, focus on Deficient knowledge, both pre- and postoperatively; other nursing diagnoses include: Pain, Risk for impaired gas exchange, and Risk for infection

5. Teaching for home care

   a. Focus of nonsurgical interventions is diet management and instructions for stone-dissolving medications; include information about function of gallbladder and purpose of bile

   b. Teaching for postoperative client is focused upon pain control, monitoring for infection, eating low-fat foods, and managing a T-tube by:

      1) Ensuring patency of tube

      2) Monitoring amount of drainage: as much as 500 mL within first 24 hours, 200 mL the next 2 to 3 days, and minimal after that

      3) Maintaining a Fowler's position to promote drainage

      4) Assessing skin around tube for integrity

      5) Assisting and teaching client to ambulate with tube

      6) Monitoring for signs of infection

VII. PANCREATITIS

A. Overview

1. Pancreatitis is defined as an inflammation of pancreas

2. Classification

   a. Acute: necrosis, suppuration (abscesses), gangrene, and hemorrhage occurs

   b. Chronic: formation of scar tissue that interferes with organ function

3. Causes

   a. Alcoholism (excessive intake of liquor or wine for 6 years or more)

   b. Biliary (obstruction of pancreatic duct by a gallstone)

   c. Other: high triglyceride levels, hypercalcemia, or infections

B. Pathophysiology

1. Acute

   a. When pancreas is injured and/or function is disrupted, pancreatic enzymes (phosopholipase A, lipase, and elastase) leak into pancreatic tissue and initiate autodigestion

   b. Trypsin and elastase are activated proteolases and along with lipases, break down tissue and cell membranes, resulting in edema, vascular damage, hemorrhage and necrosis

c. Replacement of pancreatic tissue by fibrous changes causes exocrine and endocrine changes with loss of function of islets of Langerhans, which secrete insulin, resulting in diabetes mellitus

d. Multiple-organ failure and mortality occurs when toxic enzymes are released into bloodstream and distributed by vessels into major organs

1) Activation of kinin occurs, resulting in vasodilation

2) Increased stickiness of leukocytes occurs, causing emboli

3) Coagulopathy occurs, which causes disseminated intravascular coagulopathy (DIC)

4) Increased permeability causes movement of fluid and circulatory insufficiency

5) Myocardial depressant factor (MDF) is released, which decreases cardiac function

6) Activation of renin-angiotensin system decreases kidney function as a result of decreased renal perfusion

e. Types

1) Acute interstitial: pancreas and surrounding tissue are engorged with interstitial fluid; this form may progress to hemorrhagic

2) Acute hemorrhagic: bleeding into gland and other structures occurs

2. *Chronic:* a structural or functional impairment of pancreas, most commonly associated with chronic alcohol abuse

a. Chronic form is irreversible and leaves connective tissue in place of pancreatic tissue

b. Pancreatic cysts are common lesions found in chronic pancreatitis, which are walled-off pockets of pancreatic juice, necrotic debris, or blood

c. Types

1) Chronic calcifying pancreatitis is associated with alcoholism; alcohol causes a spasm of sphincter of Oddi leading to blockage of passage of secretions out of pancreas; enzymes then pass into pancreas, resulting in autodigestion of pancreatic tissue

2) Chronic obstructive pancreatitis is associated with gallstones in women

3. Signs and symptoms

a. Acute pancreatitis

1) Sudden onset of severe epigastric and abdominal tenderness and pain that radiates to back; may be relieved by sitting up and leaning forward, flexing left leg or by walking; may be initiated by fatty meal or excessive alcohol intake

2) GI: nausea, vomiting, and distention

3) Cardiac: tachycardia, hypotension

4) Other: fever, decreased bowel sounds, and cold, clammy skin; mild jaundice may occur within 24 hours of acute symptoms, retroperitoneal bleeding after 3 to 6 days, weakness, anxiety, pallor

b. Chronic pancreatitis

1) Left upper abdominal pain radiating to back

2) GI: nausea, vomiting, weight loss, flatulence, constipation, **steatorrhea** (excessive elimination of fat, fatty stools), malabsorption

C. Nursing Assessment

1. Assessment includes symptom analysis of pain, GI complaints, nutritional status, energy level, stool characteristics, VS, skin color, bleeding—positive Turner's sign (flank bruising) or Cullen's sign (umbilical bruising)

2. Diagnostic tests

   a. Acute
      1) Serum amylase: elevated
      2) Serum lipase: elevated
      3) Serum calcium: decreased
      4) ABGs

   b. Chronic
      1) Serum and urinary amylase levels: elevated
      2) Serum bilirubin: elevated

D. Nursing management

1. Medications

   a. Pancreatic enzyme replacement such as pancrelipase (Lipancreatin)
   b. Opioid analgesics such as morphine sulfate
   c. Antibiotics
   d. Antacids
   e. H$_2$-blockers such as rantidine (Zantac) or famotidine (Pepcid)
   f. Proton pump inhibitors such as omeprazole (Prilosec)
   g. Carbonic anhydrase inhibitors: acetazolamide (Diamox)
   h. Antispasmodics: dicyclomine (Bentyl)
   i. Antiemetics
   j. Antipyretics

2. Assess and reassess pain at regular intervals for location, radiation, duration, character, and intensity

3. Maintain nothing by mouth (NPO) status (3 to 7 days) in order to reduce gastric secretions and aggravation of pancreatic pain; gastric suction may be ordered to minimize secretions

4. Decrease physical movement and mental stimulation to minimize gastric secretions and pain

5. Provide moisture to dry mucous membranes, which result from NPO status

6. Prevent visualization of food since gastric secretions are stimulated by sight of food

7. Encourage a position of comfort, which is elevation of head at 45 degrees, side lying with knees flexed

8. Daily weight

9. Assess bowel sounds

10. Assess cardiovascular status at regular intervals, monitor VS

11. Assess respiratory function at regular intervals because abdominal pain causes shallow respirations; pleural effusion is also a complication of pancreatitis

Practice to Pass

In trying to determine the etiology of a client's abdominal pain, various laboratory tests are ordered. What specific symptoms and lab work would differentiate cholecystitis, pancreatitis, and cirrhosis?

12. IV fluid replacement with electrolytes and possibly total parenteral nutrition (TPN)
13. IV albumin may be needed to combat third-spacing
14. Monitor O_2 saturation

VIII. CANCER OF THE PANCREAS

A. Overview

1. Defined as tumors of pancreas that are ductal adenocarcinomas; nearly all cases are fatal

2. Seventy percent of tumors are located in pancreatic head, 20% in body of pancreas, and 10% in tail

3. Causes include longstanding diabetes, chronic pancreatitis, and smoking; it is not associated with coffee drinking, alcoholism, and cholelithiasis

B. Pathophysiology

1. Pancreatic cancer has a slow onset and is usually not detected until tumor has spread

2. Cancer of head of pancreas obstructs bile flow while tumors in body of pancreas press on celiac ganglion

3. Cancer cells often invade the stomach, duodenum, bile duct, colon, spleen, kidney, and major blood vessels

4. Signs and symptoms

   a. Common symptoms: weight loss, anorexia, nausea, vomiting, flatulence, epigastric pain, malaise, diarrhea and constipation, palpable abdominal mass, hematemesis, melena

   b. Cancer of head of pancreas specifically causes jaundice (from biliary obstruction), clay-colored stools, dark urine, and pruritus

   c. Cancer in tail of pancreas may cause no symptoms until metastasis has occurred

   d. Tumors in body of pancreas may cause pain and nausea during eating or when lying supine

C. Nursing assessment

1. Assessment includes weight, GI symptoms, symptom analysis of pain, stool and urine characteristics, skin color, fluid and electrolyte status, nutritional status, energy level

2. Diagnostic tests: carcinoembryonic antigen (elevated), bilirubin levels (increased), urine urobilinogen (decreased), alkaline phosphatase (elevated), ultrasonography

D. Nursing management

1. Medications

   a. Opioid narcotic analgesics

   b. Antiemetics

2. Client may be a candidate for resection called a Whipple's procedure (removal of head of pancreas, entire duodenum, one-third of stomach, part of jejunum, and lower-half of common bile duct with restructuring of pancreas, stomach, and

common bile duct); postoperative care is consistent with that of any abdominal surgery and demands special attention to:

   a. Pain management

   b. Respiratory expansion

   c. Monitoring of complications related to oxygenation

   d. Renal function

   e. Level of consciousness

   f. Blood chemistries

3. Have dietitian evaluate client's needs, especially during NPO status

4. Palliative care if appropriate (terminally ill client)

Case Study

M. S. is a 55-year-old female presenting as a hospital admission for surgery in the morning. She is a divorced mother of three adult children and has smoked one pack of cigarettes daily for 30 years. In the past month, she has lost 20 pounds, cannot sleep lying on her back, and is unable to tolerate solid foods. The client became jaundiced in the past 48 hours and computed tomography (CT) scan confirmed a mass in the pancreas.

1. What are the primary risk factors present for pancreatic cancer?

2. Where is the likely location of the tumor based upon the client's symptoms?

3. What are the primary preoperative nursing interventions?

4. What are the primary postoperative nursing interventions?

5. What is the likely prognosis for this client?

For suggested responses, see pages 535–536.

POSTTEST

1 The nurse is asked about the risk factors for pancreatitis. The nurse responds that which of the following clients is more likely to develop pancreatitis?

   1. 59-year-old male with a history of occasional alcohol use

   2. Client with renal problems and hypocalcemia

   3. Client recovering from a myocardial infarction with hypercholesterolemia

   4. Client with a stone lodged in the pancreatic duct

2 What is the best explanation for the nurse to give a client who asks how pancreatic enzymes caused the damage leading to pancreatitis?

   1. Pancreatic enzymes are used in the intestine for digestion of food

   2. Pancreas self-destructs by autodigestion with its own enzymes

   3. Intestinal enzymes go into the pancreas and cause inflammation

   4. Bile duct can become clogged if stones pass out of the gallbladder

3 The following laboratory results were returned on a client who is suspected of having pancreatitis. The nurse concludes that which result gives positive evidence of pancreatitis?

1. Lipase 230 IU/liter
2. Calcium 9.3 mg/dL
3. Blood glucose 75 mg/dL
4. White blood cell count 5,000/mm^3

4 An adult female is diagnosed with cholecystitis and is being treated conservatively at home. The nurse visits her at home and begins teaching diet for healthy weight loss and reducing the pain episodes. What diet should the nurse recommend?

1. Very low calorie diet to promote faster weight loss
2. Higher fat diet to stimulate the gallbladder to empty
3. Low carbohydrate, low fat, higher protein diet
4. Low protein diet with adequate carbohydrate and no fat at all

5 The nurse is assessing an older male client. Which of the following findings would strongly indicate the possibility of cirrhosis?

1. Dry skin
2. Hepatomegaly
3. Peripheral edema
4. Pruritus

6 The nurse is reviewing the laboratory reports for a female client with cirrhosis of the liver. What abnormal results does the nurse note that are consistent with severe cirrhosis? Select all that apply.

1. Arterial PCO$_2$ of 34 mmHg
2. Arterial pH of 7.48
3. Prothrombin time (PT) 20 seconds; INR 1.8
4. White blood cell count (WBC) 3,000 mm^3
5. Red blood cell (RBC) count 3.2 × 10^{12}/liter; hemoglobin 10.4 grams/dL

7 The nurse considers that which of the following clients is most likely to acquire hepatitis A?

1. Child who is immunosuppressed
2. Health care worker after a puncture with a used needle
3. Adult who uses recreational intravenous drugs
4. Person who drinks water that is contaminated with fecal material

8 In reviewing the possible causes of hepatitis A in a 22-year-old male, the nurse concludes that which of the following would be the most likely factor?

1. Contact with blood in his profession as a policeman
2. Receiving a blood transfusion during surgery
3. Eating shrimp at the local pub
4. Admitting to being sexually active

9 A client is admitted to the unit with reports of malaise, nausea, vomiting, anorexia, and headaches. The laboratory results show abnormal electrolytes and elevated aspartate aminotransferase (AST), alanine aminotransferase (ALT), and alkaline phosphatase (ALP). Hepatitis B surface antigen (HbsAG) is also present. The nurse would conclude that the client has:

1. Hepatitis A.
2. Hepatitis B.
3. Cirrhosis.
4. Pancreatitis.

10 A client is admitted with possible liver cancer. The nurse interprets that which test would be the most confirming of this diagnosis and tumor type?

1. Abdominal ultrasound (US)
2. Liver biopsy
3. Alpha-fetoprotein markers
4. Computed tomography (CT) scan

➤ *See pages 259–260 for Answers & Rationales.*

POSTTEST

ANSWERS & RATIONALES

Pretest

1 **Answer: 4** A fatty liver is one of the main effects of alcohol consumption, known as Laënnec's cirrhosis. Other factors such as dietary intake of fat, body stores of fat, and hormonal status can also contribute to fatty liver. The liver is fibrotic in other types of cirrhosis.
Cognitive Level: Application **Client Need:** Physiological Integrity: Physiological Adaptation **Integrated Process:** Nursing Process: Analysis **Content Area:** Adult Health Gastrointestinal **Strategy:** If the answer is not known, eliminate the options known to be incorrect and select the option that is most familiar. **Reference:** LeMone, P., & Burke, K. (2008). *Medical-surgical nursing: Critical thinking in client care* (4th ed.). Upper Saddle River, NJ: Pearson/Prentice Hall, p. 710.

2 **Answer: 2** Hepatitis A has an acute onset, and accounts for about 25 percent of hepatitis cases in the United States. The usual incubation period is 15 to 40 days. The disease is spread where there is fecal contamination of water supplies and from oral contamination (such as in day care or contaminated food).
Cognitive Level: Application **Client Need:** Physiological Integrity: Physiological Adaptation **Integrated Process:** Nursing Process: Analysis **Content Area:** Adult Health: Gastrointestinal **Strategy:** Relate the answer to hepatitis type A and eliminate the options that refer to other types of hepatitis. **Reference:** LeMone, P., & Burke, K. (2008). *Medical-surgical nursing: Critical thinking in client care* (4th ed.). Upper Saddle River, NJ: Pearson/Prentice Hall, pp. 705–707.

3 **Answer: 3** Portal hypertension and liver cell failure contribute to the late manifestations of cirrhosis. Cholelithiasis and cholecystitis will be accompanied by pain, food intolerances, and/or vomiting. Pancreatitis presents with pain radiating to the back, mild cardiovascular changes, and hypocalcemia.
Cognitive Level: Application **Client Need:** Physiological Integrity: Physiological Adaptation **Integrated Process:** Nursing Process: Analysis **Content Area:** Adult Health: Gastrointestinal **Strategy:** Recognize that two options relate to gallbladder disease, which is not manifested with the findings in the question. Eliminate those options. **Reference:** LeMone, P., & Burke, K. (2008). *Medical-surgical nursing: Critical thinking in client care* (4th ed.). Upper Saddle River, NJ: Pearson/Prentice Hall, p. 784.

4 **Answer: 3** The pain of acute pancreatitis is severe and requires early intervention and narcotic analgesics. Both morphine and Demerol have the potential for addiction. Percocet is an oral preparation with a slower onset of action. All narcotic analgesics have side effects.
Cognitive Level: Application **Client Need:** Physiological Integrity: Pharmacological and Parenteral Therapies **Integrated Process:** Nursing Process: Planning **Content Area:** Adult Health: Gastrointestinal **Strategy:** One option stands out as different from the others. This option answers what is asked. **Reference:** LeMone, P., & Burke, K. (2008). *Medical-surgical nursing: Critical thinking in client care* (4th ed.). Upper Saddle River, NJ: Pearson/Prentice Hall, pp. 727–728.

5 **Answer: 4** Ammonia is a by-product of protein metabolism and is not converted to urea by a damaged liver. The client is at increased risk for a return of the encephalopathy because of the diagnosis of pneumonia and dehydration. Dietary protein intake must be controlled (or eliminated) in order to minimize the ammonia levels in the bloodstream.
Cognitive Level: Analysis **Client Need:** Physiological Integrity: Physiological Adaptation **Integrated Process:** Communication and Documentation **Content Area:** Adult Health: Gastrointestinal **Strategy:** Usually options that defer to the physician are incorrect if the nurse can implement the care. Look for the option that is client-centered. **Reference:** LeMone, P., & Burke, K. (2008). *Medical-surgical nursing: Critical thinking in client care* (4th ed.). Upper Saddle River, NJ: Pearson/Prentice Hall, p. 715.

6 **Answer: 3** Decreased serum proteins and increased aldosterone, along with portal hypertension, causes ascites, an accumulation of fluid in the abdominal cavity. Gravity causes the fluid to sink, creating the shifting dullness during assessment. This is different than distention and not related to nutrition or fluid overload.
Cognitive Level: Analysis **Client Need:** Physiological Integrity: Physiological Adaptation **Integrated Process:** Communication and Documentation **Content Area:** Adult Health: Gastrointestinal **Strategy:** Only one option fits the percussion findings. Associate dullness that shifts with position changes to indicate ascites. **Reference:** LeMone, P., & Burke, K. (2008). *Medical-surgical nursing: Critical thinking in client care* (4th ed.). Upper Saddle River, NJ: Pearson/Prentice Hall, p. 568.

7 **Answers: 1, 3, 5** Most cancers of the pancreas have already metastasized by the time of diagnosis. The onset is insidious with pain, jaundice, and weight loss as the classic symptoms. Black tarry stools are caused by GI bleeding such as from gastric or intestinal cancers. **Cognitive Level:** Application **Client Need:** Physiological Integrity: Physiological Adaptation **Integrated Process:** Teaching/Learning **Content Area:** Adult Health: Gastrointestinal **Strategy:** Select options that are general and fit for any area of the pancreas. **Reference:** Porth, C. M. (2005). *Pathophysiology: Concepts of altered health states* (7th ed.). Philadelphia, PA: Lippincott Williams & Wilkins, p. 946.

8 **Answer: 1** Clotting is altered by vitamin K deficiency and impaired liver production of clotting factors II, VII, IX, and X. Increased platelet destruction secondary to splenomegaly is also a factor. **Cognitive Level:** Application **Client Need:** Physiological Integrity: Physiological Adaptation **Integrated Process:** Communication and Documentation **Content Area:** Adult Health: Gastrointestinal **Strategy:** Consider the role of the liver in the coagulation process. In chronic cirrhosis the liver function is impaired. **Reference:** LeMone, P., & Burke, K. (2008). *Medical-surgical nursing: Critical thinking in client care* (4th ed.). Upper Saddle River, NJ: Pearson/Prentice Hall, p. 722.

9 **Answer: 2** Hepatitis B prophylaxis is not needed if the exposed person has been vaccinated and is known to be immune—that is, with a positive titer. Hepatitis immune globulin is given for short-term immunity to persons who are not already immune. Hepatitis A is transmitted by the fecal-oral route. **Cognitive Level:** Application **Client Need:** Safe, Effective Care Environment: Safety and Infection Control **Integrated Process:** Nursing Process: Planning **Content Area:** Adult Health: Gastrointestinal **Strategy:** How can the immune status be determined? Consider the epidemiology of hepatitis A and B. **Reference:** LeMone, P., & Burke, K. (2008). *Medical-surgical nursing: Critical thinking in client care* (4th ed.). Upper Saddle River, NJ: Pearson/Prentice Hall, pp. 705–710.

10 **Answers: 1, 2, 4** With the history of IV drug use, it is likely that he has either chronic hepatitis B or C, which are risk factors for liver cancer. His alcoholism predisposes him to cirrhosis, which is another risk factor for liver cancer. Although arsenic-containing water and carcinogens in food are risk factors, food supplements and municipal water are considered safe. **Cognitive Level:** Analysis **Client Need:** Physiological Integrity: Physiological Adaptation **Integrated Process:** Nursing Process: Implementation **Content Area:** Adult Health: Gastrointestinal **Strategy:** Look at his lifestyle and determine what liver disorders he may have as a consequence. Which of these are risk factors for liver

cancer? **Reference:** LeMone, P., & Burke, K. (2008). *Medical-surgical nursing: Critical thinking in client care* (4th ed.). Upper Saddle River, NJ: Pearson/Prentice Hall, p. 723.

Posttest

1 **Answer: 4** Causes of pancreatitis include alcohol abuse of excessive intake of liquor or wine for six years or more; high triglyceride levels, and hypercalcemia. Stones lodged in the pancreatic duct can cause obstruction and lead to inflammation of the pancreas. **Cognitive Level:** Analysis **Client Need:** Physiological Integrity: Physiological Adaptation **Integrated Process:** Nursing Process: Analysis **Content Area:** Adult Health: Gastrointestinal **Strategy:** Eliminate options that do not represent a primary risk factor. **Reference:** LeMone, P., & Burke, K. (2008). *Medical-surgical nursing: Critical thinking in client care* (4th ed.). Upper Saddle River, NJ: Pearson/Prentice Hall, p. 726.

2 **Answer: 2** When the pancreas is injured and/or has an impaired or disrupted function, pancreatic enzymes leak into pancreatic tissue and initiate autodigestion. Option 1 is a normal function; option 3 is false; option 4 describes gallbladder disease. **Cognitive Level:** Application **Client Need:** Physiological Integrity: Physiological Adaptation **Integrated Process:** Teaching/Learning **Content Area:** Adult Health: Gastrointestinal **Strategy:** Which option describes an autoimmune process? **Reference:** LeMone, P., & Burke, K. (2008). *Medical-surgical nursing: Critical thinking in client care* (4th ed.). Upper Saddle River, NJ: Pearson/Prentice Hall, p. 726.

3 **Answer: 1** In pancreatitis, the lipase, amylase, glucose, and white blood count (WBC) are all elevated. The calcium is low for 7 to 10 days and is a sign of severe pancreatitis. Options 2, 3, and 4 contain normal values. **Cognitive Level:** Analysis **Client Need:** Physiological Integrity: Reduction of Risk Potential **Integrated Process:** Nursing Process: Assessment **Content Area:** Adult Health: Gastrointestinal **Strategy:** This question draws on knowledge of laboratory results and what is normal and abnormal. If this question was problematic, review normal lab values for each of these tests. **Reference:** LeMone, P., & Burke, K. (2008). *Medical-surgical nursing: Critical thinking in client care* (4th ed.). Upper Saddle River, NJ: Pearson/Prentice Hall, p. 728.

4 **Answer: 3** A low carbohydrate, low fat, higher protein diet will reduce symptoms of cholecystitis. The goal is a healthy rate of weight loss and reduced pain episodes. Fasting and very low carbohydrate diets are contraindicated. Fat is an essential nutrient and is needed in a

balanced diet. A fat-soluble vitamin supplement may be needed if obstructed bile flow has reduced the absorption of fats.
Cognitive Level: Application **Client Need:** Health Promotion and Maintenance **Integrated Process;** Nursing Process: Planning **Content Area:** Adult Health: Gastrointestinal **Strategy:** Consider a moderate, healthy diet for gradual weight loss while controlling the fat. **Reference:** LeMone, P., & Burke, K. (2008). *Medical-surgical nursing: Critical thinking in client care* (4th ed.). Upper Saddle River, NJ: Pearson/Prentice Hall, p. 698.

5 **Answer: 2** Although option 4 is correct, it is not a strong indicator of cirrhosis. Pruritus can occur for many reasons. Options 1 and 3 are incorrect, fluid accumulation is usually in the form of ascites in the abdomen. Hepatomegaly is an enlarged liver, which is correct. The spleen may also be enlarged.
Cognitive Level: Application **Client Need:** Physiological Integrity: Physiological Adaptation **Integrated Process:** Nursing Process: Analysis **Content Area:** Adult Health: Gastrointestinal **Strategy:** Read carefully. One word may change the meaning and make an option wrong. **Reference:** LeMone, P., & Burke, K. (2008). *Medical-surgical nursing: Critical thinking in client care* (4th ed.). Upper Saddle River, NJ: Pearson/Prentice Hall, pp. 714–715.

6 **Answers: 3, 4, 5** Clients with cirrhosis have used their clotting factors, and the liver is unable to provide enough clotting factors. A prothrombin time is an indication of the time needed for blood to clot; the high PT/INR indicates slow clotting. Low WBC and anemia also are seen with cirrhosis. The other abnormal laboratory results are not related to the liver function.
Cognitive Level: Analysis **Client Need:** Physiological Integrity: Reduction of Risk Potential **Integrated Process:** Nursing Process: Analysis **Content Area:** Adult Health: Gastrointestinal **Strategy:** Although all these results are abnormal, only two are influenced by impaired liver function. Continue to review normal and abnormal labs. **Reference:** LeMone, P., & Burke, K. (2008). *Medical-surgical nursing: Critical thinking in client care* (4th ed.). Upper Saddle River, NJ: Pearson/Prentice Hall, p. 715.

7 **Answer: 4** Hepatitis A (HAV) and E (HEV) are spread by the fecal-oral route. Types B, C, and D are spread by blood and body fluids. The contaminated water could contain the virus causing the infection.
Cognitive Level: Analysis **Client Need:** Physiological Integrity: Physiological Adaptation **Integrated Process:** Nursing Process: Assessment **Content Area:** Adult Health: Gastrointestinal **Strategy:** Eliminate the two equally plausible options (IV exposure). Focus on the other op-

tions for the correct answer. **Reference:** LeMone, P., & Burke, K. (2008). *Medical-surgical nursing: Critical thinking in client care* (4th ed.). Upper Saddle River, NJ: Pearson/Prentice Hall, p. 706.

8 **Answer: 3** Hepatitis A is transmitted by fecal-oral route. The virus is excreted in oropharyngeal secretions (nose and throat) and transmitted by direct contact person to person, or by fecal contamination of food or water. A worker could have hepatitis A and transfer it to food. Options 1, 2, and 4 are classic of hepatitis B, C, and D.
Cognitive Level: Application **Client Need:** Physiological Integrity: Physiological Adaptation **Integrated Process:** Nursing Process: Analysis **Content Area:** Adult Health: Gastrointestinal **Strategy:** This question is similar to the last one but it focuses on an action causing a problem for a specific client. NCLEX may test material in either format. **Reference:** Lemone, P., & Burke, K. (2008). *Medical-surgical nursing: Critical thinking in client care* (4th ed.). Upper Saddle River, NJ: Pearson/Prentice Hall, p. 706.

9 **Answer: 2** The symptoms in preicteric hepatitis are vague and more flulike as described above. The physician usually needs laboratory work to verify a diagnosis. In this case, the presence of the antigen HBsAG concludes that the client has an active form of the disease since hepatitis B surface antigen is present.
Cognitive Level: Analysis **Client Need:** Physiological Integrity: Reduction of Risk Potential **Integrated Process:** Nursing Process: Assessment **Content Area:** Adult Health: Gastrointestinal **Strategy:** Evaluate the laboratory findings in the question along with vague symptoms. The options are all hepatobiliary problems—which one fits the description? A clue is the surface antigen result. **Reference:** LeMone, P., & Burke, K. (2008). *Medical-surgical nursing: Critical thinking in client care* (4th ed.). Upper Saddle River, NJ: Pearson/Prentice Hall, p. 705.

10 **Answer: 2** Abdominal ultrasound, x-ray, and CT scans are useful in the diagnosis of cancer of the liver. The alpha-fetoprotein serum markers are specific to detecting primary hepatocellular carcinoma. To confirm the diagnosis and identify the tumor type or origin, a biopsy is done.
Cognitive Level: Application **Client Need:** Physiological Integrity: Reduction of Risk Potential **Integrated Process:** Nursing Process: Assessment **Content Area:** Adult Health: Gastrointestinal **Strategy:** What is the best diagnostic test to confirm almost any cancer type? **Reference:** LeMone, P., & Burke, K. (2008). *Medical-surgical nursing: Critical thinking in client care* (4th ed.). Upper Saddle River, NJ: Pearson/Prentice Hall, p. 724.

References

Adams, M., Holland, L. & Bostwick, P. (2005). *Pharmacology for nurses: A pathophysiologic approach* (2nd ed.). Upper Saddle River, NJ: Prentice Hall.

Bickley, L. (2004). *Bates' guide to physical examination and history taking* (8th ed.). Philadelphia, PA: Lippincott.

Johnson, A. (2006). Disorder of the liver. In D. Ignatavicius, M. Workman, & M. Mishler, (Eds.). *Medical-surgical nursing: Critical thinking for collaborative care* (5th ed.). Philadelphia, PA: W. B. Saunders.

Karch, A. (2005). *Focus on nursing pharmacology* (3rd ed.). Philadelphia, PA: Lippincott.

LeMone, P., & Burke, K. (2008). *Medical-surgical nursing: Critical thinking in client care* (4th ed.). Upper Saddle River, NJ: Prentice Hall.

McCance, K., & Huether, S. (2006). *Pathophysiology: The biologic basis for disease in adults and children* (5th ed.). St. Louis, MO: Mosby.

Porth, C. M. (Ed.). (2005). *Pathophysiology: Concepts of altered health status* (7th ed.). Philadelphia, PA: Lippincott Williams & Wilkins.

Ralph, S., & Taylor, C. (2005). *Sports and Taylor's nursing diagnosis reference manual* (6th ed.). Philadelphia, PA: Lippincott Williams & Wilkins.

Sands, J. (2006). Management of persons with problems of the stomach and duodenum. In W. Phipps, J. Sands, & J. Marek (Eds.), *Medical-surgical nursing: Health and illness perspectives* (8th ed.). St. Louis: Mosby.

9

Endocrine and Metabolic Health Problems

Chapter Outline

Risk Factors Associated with Endocrine and Metabolic Health Problems

Thyroid Hyperfunction Disorders

Thyroid Hypofunction Disorders

Parathyroid Disorders

Adrenal Cortex Hyperfunction Disorders

Adrenal Cortex Hypofunction Disorder: Addison's Disease

Adrenal Medulla Hyperfunction Disorder: Pheochromocytoma

Anterior Pituitary Disorders

Posterior Pituitary Disorders

Diabetes Mellitus

NCLEX-RN® Test Prep

Use the CD-ROM enclosed with this book to access additional practice opportunities.

Objectives

➤ Define key terms associated with endocrine and metabolic health problems.

➤ Identify risk factors associated with the development of endocrine and metabolic health problems.

➤ Explain the common etiologies of endocrine and metabolic health problems.

➤ Describe the pathophysiologic processes associated with specific endocrine and metabolic health problems.

➤ Distinguish between normal and abnormal endocrine and metabolic findings obtained from nursing assessment.

➤ Prioritize nursing interventions associated with specific endocrine and metabolic health problems.

Review at a Glance

Addison's disease chronic adrenocortical insufficiency as a result of destruction of adrenal glands

Addisonian crisis acute adrenocortical insufficiency precipitated by stress or abrupt withdrawal of glucocorticoids; signs and symptoms include hypotension and shock

antidiuretic hormone (ADH) hormone secreted by posterior pituitary gland; purpose is to control serum osmolality

Conn's syndrome (hyperaldosteronism) primary hyperaldosteronism; hypersecretion of aldosterone in which hypertension is a major complication

Cushing's syndrome symptoms produced by excess cortisol from adrenal cortex; classic signs and symptoms are moon face, truncal obesity, and "buffalo hump"

diabetes insipidus (DI) disorder caused by antidiuretic hormone (ADH) insufficiency, results in excess fluid excretion

diabetes mellitus (DM) a pancreatic disorder caused by lack of secretion or inadequate secretion of insulin, or insulin resistance, resulting in hyperglycemia, and leading to multisystem effects

diabetic ketoacidosis (DKA) life-threatening state of hyperglycemia and metabolic acidosis

exophthalmos abnormal protrusion of eyeballs; seen in hyperthyroidism; may affect one or both eyes

goiter enlargement of thyroid gland, most often seen in hyperthyroidism, but also may occur in hypothyroidism or euthyroidism

Graves' disease hyperthyroidism leading to a hypermetabolic state

hyperparathyroidism increase in secretion of parathyroid hormone (PTH)

hyperthyroidism increase in secretion of thyroid hormone (TH)

hypoparathyroidism decrease in secretion of parathyroid hormone (PTH)

hypothyroidism decrease in secretion of thyroid hormone (TH)

insulin hormone produced by pancreas, responsible for controlling serum glucose level

myxedema form of hypothyroidism characterized by non-pitting edema that is generally found in periorbital and pretibial areas

myxedema coma life-threatening state of hypothyroidism

pheochromocytoma tumor (usually benign) of adrenal medulla resulting in excessive secretion of catecholamines, which leads to severe hypertension

syndrome of inappropriate antidiuretic hormone (SIADH) excessive secretion of antidiuretic hormone (ADH) from pituitary gland; results in excessive water retention

thyroid storm life-threatening form of hyperthyroidism, characterized by extreme state of hypermetabolism

PRETEST

1 The nurse is obtaining a health history on a 36-year-old female who reports an increase in appetite, weight loss, intolerance to heat, and nervousness. On physical assessment, the client is noted to have thin hair and moist skin. Based on this information, the nurse would suspect which of the following?

1. Hypothyroidism
2. Hyperthyroidism
3. Hypoparathyroidism
4. Hyperparathyroidism

2 A client is returning from a subtotal thyroidectomy for the treatment of hyperthyroidism. The immediate priority of the nurse who is assigned to this client is to assess for which of the following?

1. Respiratory distress
2. Fluid volume status
3. Neurological status
4. Incisional pain

3 The nurse has given medication instructions to a client newly diagnosed with hypothyroidism who will be taking levothyroxine sodium (Synthroid). Which statement made by the client would indicate additional teaching is required?

1. "I know I will be on this medication for the rest of my life."
2. "I won't eat excessive amounts of cabbage or spinach."
3. "I'll take my Synthroid with food."
4. "I'll take my Synthroid in the morning."

4 In providing care for a client being admitted for severe hyperparathyroidism, the nurse anticipates implementing which of the following actions?

1. Administering intravenous (IV) calcium gluconate
2. Administering large amounts of IV saline
3. Maintaining strict fluid restriction
4. Monitoring for tetany

5 A client is receiving supplemental calcium as treatment for hypoparathyroidism. The nurse concludes that the client has achieved therapeutic results of drug therapy when the serum calcium level has reached at least _____ mg/dL. Provide a numeric answer.

Answer: _____

6 A client with Cushing's syndrome is admitted with the symptoms of hypertension, fatigue, and edema. The priority nursing diagnosis for this client would be which of the following?

1. Deficient fluid volume
2. Excess fluid volume
3. Anxiety
4. Deficient knowledge

7 A client with Conn's syndrome (hyperaldosteronism) who will not be treated surgically is receiving spironolactone (Aldactone). The nurse explains to the client that the purpose of this drug is to do which of the following?

1. Reverse the hyperaldosteronism
2. Decrease the serum potassium level
3. Promote fluid retention
4. Treat hypertension and hypokalemia

8 A client with Addison's disease is being discharged home and will be taking hydrocortisone (Cortisol). Which of the following statements by the client indicates that the teaching about the disease and its management was successful? Select all that apply.

1. "I will monitor closely for any signs of infection."
2. "I will wear a Medic-Alert bracelet indicating disease and treatment."
3. "I will report any rapid weight gain or fluid in my legs if it persists for over two weeks."
4. "I will take safety measures at home to prevent injuries."
5. "I will have to take this medicine for the rest of my life."

9 The nurse is establishing a plan of care for a client newly admitted with syndrome of inappropriate antidiuretic hormone secretion (SIADH). The priority nursing diagnosis for this client would be which of the following?

1. Deficient fluid volume
2. Anxiety
3. Excess fluid volume
4. Risk for injury

10 The nurse is discussing the treatment regimen for a client newly diagnosed with Type 1 diabetes mellitus. While discussing insulin administration, the client asks, "Why can't I just take a pill like my friend does?" Which of the following statements indicates the client understands the nurse's explanation?

1. "Because my body does not produce insulin, I must receive the injections."
2. "I will be on insulin for a short while, then I can take the pills."
3. "The pills are not as effective as the insulin injections."
4. "When my body starts making insulin again, I can stop taking the injections."

➤ *See pages 291–293 for Answers & Rationales.*

I. RISK FACTORS ASSOCIATED WITH ENDOCRINE AND METABOLIC HEALTH PROBLEMS

A. Thyroid hyperfunction disorders

1. Graves' disease: immunological factors, genetic predisposition, infection, stress, excessive intake of thyroid medications; occurs 8 times more frequently in females
2. Goiter: inadequate intake of iodine, increase in thyroid hormone demand
3. Thyroid storm: stress, injury, infection, surgery

B. Thyroid hypofunction disorders

1. Hypothyroidism: congenital defect, immunological factors, elderly, infection, iodine deficiency, antithyroid drugs
2. Myxedema: undiagnosed or untreated hypothyroidism

C. **Parathyroid disorders**

1. Hyperparathyroidism: elderly, female, thyroid adenoma

2. Hypoparathyroidism: accidental removal or damage to parathyroid during thyroidectomy

D. **Adrenal cortex hyperfunction disorders**

1. Cushing's syndrome: tumor of pituitary gland, excess administration of corticosteroids or adrenocorticotropic hormone (ACTH), although exogenous hormone may also suppress endogenous function

2. Conn's disease: tumors of adrenal gland

E. **Adrenal cortex hypofunction disorder (Addison's disease):** immunological factors, surgical removal of adrenal glands, infection of adrenal glands, tumor of adrenal gland, head trauma (affects pituitary gland), withdrawal of exogenous glucocorticoids or ACTH

F. **Adrenal medulla hyperfunction disorder (pheochromocytoma):** genetic predisposition, middle age

G. **Anterior pituitary disorders**

1. Gigantism: pituitary adenoma (hyperfunction)

2. Acromegaly: pituitary adenoma (hyperfunction)

3. Dwarfism: pituitary adenoma, congenital inheritance, trauma, and radiation (hypofunction)

H. **Posterior pituitary disorders**

1. Diabetes insipidus (hypofunction of ADH secretion): head trauma, brain tumor, removal of pituitary gland, irradiation of pituitary gland, genetic predisposition, renal disease

2. Syndrome of inappropriate antidiuretic hormone (SIADH; hyperfunction of ADH): head trauma, brain tumor, infection, brain surgery, some pharmacologic agents

I. **Diabetes mellitus (DM)**

1. Type 1 diabetes mellitus: genetic predisposition, immunological factors, environmental factors, age < 30, increased in African Americans and Native Americans; hypertension, and elevated cholesterol are common associated conditions

2. Type 2 diabetes mellitus: age > 30 years, obesity, genetic predisposition

3. Diabetic ketoacidosis: increased insulin requirements, insufficient exogenous insulin

4. Hyperosmolar hyperglycemic non-ketotic coma (HHNK): stressors such as infection, trauma, surgery coupled with underlying (and perhaps unknown) hyperglycemia, and type 2 DM; also called hyperosmolar coma (HOC)

II. THYROID HYPERFUNCTION DISORDERS

A. **Overview**

1. Thyroid gland is located in lower neck anterior to trachea; its primary function is to produce, store, and secrete hormones:

   a. Thyroxine (T_4)—responsible for cellular metabolism

   b. Triiodothyronine (T_3)—responsible for regulating cellular metabolism

   c. Thyrocalcitonin (calcitonin)—role is calcium regulation

   d. T_3 and T_4 are known collectively as thyroid hormone

2. Iodine is necessary for thyroid gland to synthesize and secrete hormones

3. Thyroid hormone (T_3 and T_4) stimulates body growth, increases metabolic rate, heart rate, and glucose; overall role is to maintain metabolism and regulate growth and development

4. Calcitonin acts on kidneys and bones to decrease serum calcium levels

5. Causes of thyroid hyperfunction disorders include autoimmune responses, neoplasms, excessive intake of thyroid medications, and excess secretion of thyroid-stimulating hormone (TSH) from anterior pituitary gland

B. Pathophysiology

1. Thyroid hormone (TH) production depends on adequate secretion of TSH from anterior pituitary; the hypothalamus regulates pituitary secretion of TSH by negative feedback

2. **Hyperthyroidism** (hyperfunction of thyroid gland) leads to an excess of TH in body

   a. The presence of excess TH leads to a hypermetabolic state, which causes an increase in metabolic function, O_2 consumption by tissues, and heat production

   b. Thyroid hyperfunction disorders

      1) Graves' disease

      2) Toxic goiter

      3) Thyroid storm: leads to increased protein, lipid, carbohydrate, and vitamin metabolism

3. **Graves' disease** (most common cause of hyperthyroidism) is seen most often in women under age 40

   a. Exact cause is unknown, but it is considered an autoimmune disorder in response to stimulation of thyroid gland from a long-acting thyroid stimulator (LATS)

   b. An excess production of TH results, which leads to a *hypermetabolic state*

4. **Goiter** describes an enlargement or hypertrophy of thyroid gland in an attempt to compensate for inadequate TH, and may be present in hyperthyroidism or hypothyroidism

   a. Goiter may result from response to excess TSH stimulation, excess growth-stimulating immunoglobulins, or presence of substances that inhibit TH synthesis

   b. A goiter may become so large that respiratory complications arise as a result of compression to neck and chest

5. *Toxic multinodular goiter* exists when small, independently functioning nodules in thyroid gland tissue are present and secrete TH

   a. Nodules may be benign or malignant

   b. Manifestations develop more slowly than Grave's disease

   c. Toxic goiter is most often seen in women age 60 or older, who have had goiter for several years

6. **Thyroid storm** (also known as thyroid crisis or thyrotoxicosis) is a *life-threatening condition*, which describes an extreme state of hyperthyroidism

   a. Excessive thyroid hormone causes a rapid increase in metabolic rate

   b. Immediate treatment is necessary to avoid death

7. Signs and symptoms

   a. Hyperthyroidism (see Figure 9-1): note all symptoms are elevated or high except weight loss, sex drive, and fluid volume

   b. Symptoms are caused by excessive stimulation of:

   1) Sympathetic (adrenergic) branch of central nervous system (CNS): cardiac activity, reflexes

   2) Thyroxine: increased metabolism, weight loss, and psychological symptoms

   c. Thyroid storm: leads to extreme hyperthermia (102°F to 106°F), tachycardia, agitation, seizures

   d. Classic symptoms are weight loss, nervousness, **exophthalmos** (protrusion of eyeballs), increased appetite, palpitations, and heat intolerance

C. Nursing assessment

   1. Assessment for hyperthyroidism includes assessment of eyes, vital signs (VS), cardiac monitor for rhythm changes, signs of congestive heart failure (CHF), nutritional assessment, complaints of GI distress, muscle strength and appearance, presence of goiter, reproductive history, integument assessment, weight, and fluid status

   2. Assessment findings for thyroid storm include elevated temperature, symptom analysis of pain, bowel/GI complaints, neurological, development of seizures, changes in VS, respiratory status

   3. Diagnostic tests

   a. Serum thyroid antibodies (Serum TA): elevated

   b. Thyroid-stimulating hormone (TSH): decreased

   c. Serum thyroxine (T_4): increased; decreased in primary hyperthyroidism

   d. Serum triiodothyronine (T_3): increased

   e. T_3 uptake test (T_3RU): increased

   f. Radioactive iodine (RAI) uptake with thyroid suppression test: increased

D. Nursing management (see Table 9–1)

   1. Medications

   a. Antithyroid medications to reduce TH production

   1) Methimazole (Tapazole)

   2) Propylthiouracil (PTU, Propyl-Thracil)

   b. Propranolol (Inderal) to treat cardiac dysrhythmias

   c. Glucocorticoids: interfere with conversion of T_4 to T_3

   d. Lugol's solution (iodine) to decrease vascularity and size of thyroid prior to surgery

   e. Antipyretics if needed

   2. Educate client that it may take several weeks before therapeutic effects of antithyroid medications are noticed

   a. Instruct to take medication as prescribed and to not abruptly discontinue medication

   b. Educate about signs of hypothyroidism, which may occur if too much medicine is taken or dose needs adjusting

   3. Monitor for cardiac dysrhythmias, tachycardia

   4. Implement antipyretic measures

Figure 9-1 Body system effects of hyperthyroidism.

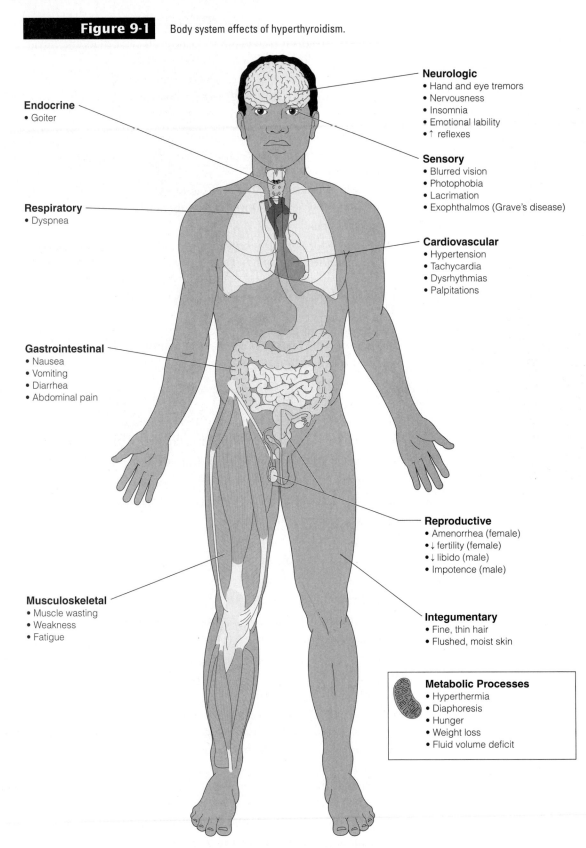

Endocrine
• Goiter

Respiratory
• Dyspnea

Gastrointestinal
• Nausea
• Vomiting
• Diarrhea
• Abdominal pain

Musculoskeletal
• Muscle wasting
• Weakness
• Fatigue

Neurologic
• Hand and eye tremors
• Nervousness
• Insomnia
• Emotional lability
• ↑ reflexes

Sensory
• Blurred vision
• Photophobia
• Lacrimation
• Exophthalmos (Grave's disease)

Cardiovascular
• Hypertension
• Tachycardia
• Dysrhythmias
• Palpitations

Reproductive
• Amenorrhea (female)
• ↓ fertility (female)
• ↓ libido (male)
• Impotence (male)

Integumentary
• Fine, thin hair
• Flushed, moist skin

Metabolic Processes
• Hyperthermia
• Diaphoresis
• Hunger
• Weight loss
• Fluid volume deficit

Table 9-1	Comparison of Symptoms and Treatment of Hyperthyroidism and Hypothyroidism	
	Hyperthyroidism	**Hypothyroidism**
Etiology	Autoimmune responses, excess secretion of thyroid-stimulating hormone (TSH), neoplasms, excessive intake of thyroid medications	Congenital defects, antithyroid medications, iodine deficiency, damage to thyroid from surgery or radiation
Clinical Manifestations	Emotional lability, agitation, exophthalmos, increased reflexes, tachycardia, diarrhea, muscle weakness, fatigue, flushed skin, goiter, hyperthermia, weight loss, heat intolerance, diaphoresis *Hint:* Everything is elevated except weight	Memory impairment, confusion, decreased reflexes, periorbital edema, hypotension, bradycardia, constipation, muscle weakness, goiter, edema, weight gain, hypothermia, cold intolerance *Hint:* Everything is decreased except weight
Laboratory Values	• Elevated serum thyroid antibodies (Serum TA) • Decreased thyroid-stimulating hormone (TSH) in primary hyperthyroidism • Increased serum triiodothyronine (T_3) • Increased T_3 uptake	• Increased thyroid-stimulating hormone (TSH) in primary hyperthyroidism • Decreased serum thyroxine (T_4) • Decreased serum triiodothyronine (T_3) • Decreased T_3 uptake • Hyponatremia
Treatment	Pharmacologic agents: methimazole (Tapazole), propylthiouracil (PTU), propranolol (Inderal), glucocorticoids Lugol's Solution Radioactive therapy Thyroidectomy	Pharmacologic agents Levothyroxine sodium (Levothroid, Synthroid) Liothyronine sodium (Cytomel) Liotrix (Euthroid) Vasopressor agents

5. Elevate head of bed to decrease eye pressure

6. Teach eye care and monitor for vision changes if exophthalmos occurs, since it will not change even after medications have been started

7. Monitor dietary intake: client may require up to 4,000 to 5,000 calories a day during hypermetabolic state

8. Monitor intake and output

9. Monitor weight

10. Keep environment cool and quiet because of symptoms

11. Radioactive therapy may be recommended to destroy thyroid cells in order to reduce production of TH

   a. Give radioactive iodine orally; results are expected in 6 to 8 weeks

   b. Does not require hospitalization or radiation precautions

   c. Contraindicated in pregnant women

   d. Monitor for signs of *hypothyroidism*

12. Preoperative and postoperative care for surgical intervention to remove all or part of thyroid (thyroidectomy)

   a. Subtotal thyroidectomy leaves part of thyroid gland intact in order to produce adequate amounts of TH

   b. If a total thyroidectomy is performed (usually for treatment of cancer), *lifelong* thyroid hormone replacement is necessary; educate client about importance of compliance with medication regime

   c. Preoperative care includes administering antithyroid medications to promote an euthyroid state, and iodine preparations to decrease vascularity of gland;

teach client how to support neck with both hands while sitting up, moving, or coughing following surgery to reduce strain on suture line

   d. Postoperative care includes monitoring for complications such as hemorrhage, respiratory distress, laryngeal nerve damage, and tetany (positive Chvostek's and Trousseau's signs); assess for pain and treat accordingly

13. Priority nursing diagnoses for thyroid hyperfunction disorders: Activity intolerance; Imbalanced nutrition: Less than body requirements; Hyperthermia; Risk for injury

III. THYROID HYPOFUNCTION DISORDERS

A. Overview

1. Hypofunction of thyroid leads to an insufficient amount of thyroid hormone (TH), a condition known as **hypothyroidism**

2. Decreased TH results in a *hypometabolic state* manifested by a decrease in metabolic function, a decrease in O_2 consumption by tissue, and a decrease in heat production

3. Thyroid hypofunction disorders

    a. Hypothyroidism

    b. Myxedema

    c. Myxedema coma

4. Classified as primary or secondary

5. Causes of primary and secondary hypothyroidism

    a. Causes of primary hypothyroidism include congenital defects, loss of thyroid tissue from surgery or radiation, antithyroid medications, endemic iodine deficiency, or thyroiditis

    b. Causes of secondary hypothyroidism include peripheral resistance to thyroid hormones or pituitary TSH deficiency

B. Pathophysiology

1. *Hypothyroidism* describes an insufficient amount of thyroid hormone (TH), which leads to a decrease in metabolic rate; manifestations develop slowly over months to years

2. **Myxedema** describes a generalized hypometabolic state occurring with untreated hypothyroidism

    a. Accumulation of proteins in interstitial spaces results in an increase in interstitial fluids, causing mucinous edema (myxedema)

    b. This non-pitting edema is most commonly found in pretibial and facial areas

3. **Myxedema coma** (also known as *hypothyroid crisis*) results from extreme or prolonged hypothyroidism; though rare, it is a life-threatening condition

    a. Characterized by a severe hypometabolic state: lactic acidosis, hypoglycemia, hyponatremia, hypotension, bradycardia, cardiovascular collapse, hypothermia, hypoventilation, and coma

    b. Precipitated by inadequate thyroid replacement, infection, trauma, exposure to cold temperatures, central nervous system depressants

4. *Iodine deficiency:* iodine is necessary for TH synthesis and secretion

    a. Iodine deficiency occurs as a result of antithyroid drugs, lithium intake or inadequate iodine intake

b. In the United States, thyroid deficiency because of inadequate iodine intake is rare because of use of iodized salt

5. *Hashimoto's thyroiditis* is an autoimmune disorder generally affecting women age 30 to 50, in which antibodies develop and destroy thyroid tissue

  a. TH levels decrease as a result of fibrous tissue replacing functional thyroid tissue

  b. Goiter develops as thyroid enlarges to compensate for decreasing TH levels

6. Signs and symptoms

  a. Hypothyroidism (see Figure 9-2): notice that most symptoms are decreased except weight and fluid volume

  b. Myxedema coma: hypothermia, cardiovascular collapse, coma, hyponatremia, hypoglycemia, lactic acidosis

C. Nursing assessment

1. Assessment of hypothyroidism includes neurological assessment, presence of periorbital edema, VS, cardiac rhythm, bowel habits, muscle strength, integument assessment, presence of goiter, reproductive history, fluid status, weight, activity tolerance, respiratory status

2. Assessment in myxedema coma includes VS, cardiac assessment, neurological assessment, and other assessments performed for hypothyroidism

3. Diagnostic tests

  a. Serum thyroid antibodies (serum TA): normal; elevated in Hashimoto's thyroiditis

  b. Thyroid stimulating hormone (TSH) in primary hypothyroidism: increased

  c. Serum thyroxine (T_4): decreased (normal 5 to 12 ng/dL)

  d. Serum triiodothyronine (T_3): decreased (normal 80 to 200 ng/dL)

  e. T_3 uptake test (T_3RU): decreased

  f. Radioactive iodine (RAI) uptake test (thyroid scan) with thyroid suppression test: no change or decreased

  g. Hyponatremia (dilutional)

  h. Increased cholesterol and triglyceride levels

  i. Myxedema coma: glucose decreased, ABGs show metabolic acidosis

D. Nursing management (see Table 9-1 again, p. 269)

1. Medications

  a. Thyroid replacement medications

    1) Levothyroxine sodium (T_4) (Levoxyl, Levoid, Levothroid, Synthroid, Synthrox)

    2) Liothyronine sodium (T_3) (Cytomel)

    3) Liotrix (Euthroid, Thyrolar)

  b. Vasopressor agents to maintain adequate perfusion

2. Intravenous glucose

3. Monitor for signs of digitalis toxicity if receiving digoxin (Lanoxin)

4. Monitor for hyperthyroidism with excess medication; teach signs and symptoms of both hyper- and hypothyroidism

5. Monitor for hyperglycemia and also for hypoglycemia (since myxedema can lead to this)

Figure 9-2 Body system effects of hypothyroidism.

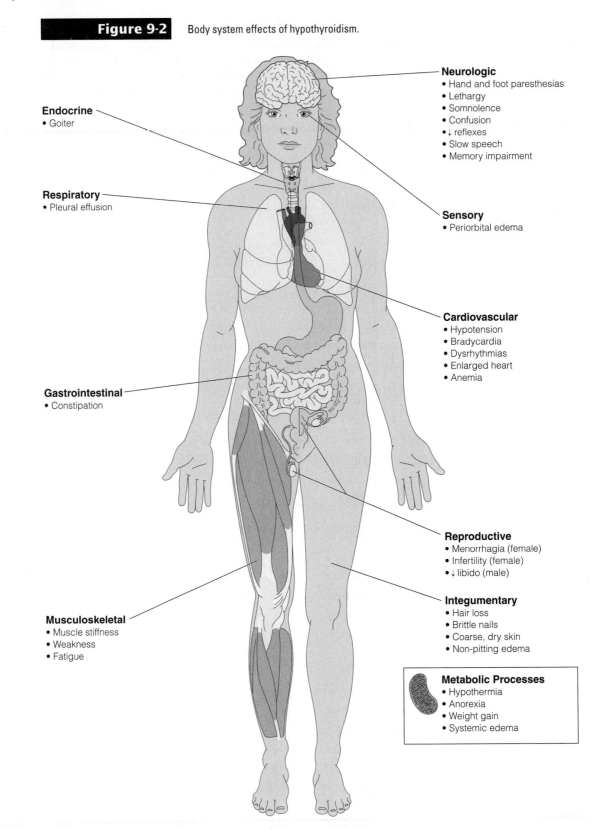

Neurologic
• Hand and foot paresthesias
• Lethargy
• Somnolence
• Confusion
• ↓ reflexes
• Slow speech
• Memory impairment

Endocrine
• Goiter

Respiratory
• Pleural effusion

Sensory
• Periorbital edema

Cardiovascular
• Hypotension
• Bradycardia
• Dysrhythmias
• Enlarged heart
• Anemia

Gastrointestinal
• Constipation

Reproductive
• Menorrhagia (female)
• Infertility (female)
• ↓ libido (male)

Integumentary
• Hair loss
• Brittle nails
• Coarse, dry skin
• Non-pitting edema

Musculoskeletal
• Muscle stiffness
• Weakness
• Fatigue

Metabolic Processes
• Hypothermia
• Anorexia
• Weight gain
• Systemic edema

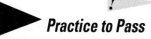

6. Monitor VS, daily weight
7. Client education

   a. Educate client to take medications 1 hour before or 2 hours after meals for optimal absorption and to take medication in morning

   b. Medication replacement is *lifelong*

   c. Do not substitute drug brands or use generic equivalents without prior approval from health care provider as dosing may be different

   d. Avoid excessive intake of foods such as cabbage, carrots, spinach, turnips, and peaches, which inhibit TH utilization

   e. Report nervousness, insomnia, palpitations, excess weight loss or leg cramps to primary health care provider (possible excess medication)

8. Priority nursing diagnoses for thyroid hypofunction disorders: Activity intolerance; Imbalanced nutrition: More than body requirements; Decreased cardiac output; Hypothermia; Risk for impaired skin integrity; Risk for injury

▶ *Practice to Pass*

The nurse is providing teaching to a client newly diagnosed with hypothyroidism. Her family is also included in the teaching process. What instructions should the nurse provide to the client and the client's family?

IV. PARATHYROID DISORDERS

A. Overview

1. Parathyroid glands are located posterior to thyroid glands

   a. Their major function is to maintain normal serum calcium levels by secreting parathyroid hormone (PTH), which increases bone resorption of calcium

   b. PTH responds to decreased calcium levels by increasing calcium absorption from bone, kidneys, and intestines

2. **Hyperparathyroidism** is an *increase* in PTH, which leads to hypercalcemia, hypophosphatemia, bone damage, and renal damage

3. **Hypoparathyroidism** is a *decrease* in PTH, which leads to hypocalcemia, hyperphosphatemia, hyperreflexia, and an altered sensorium

4. Most common cause of hypoparathyroidism is dàmage to or removal of parathyroid glands during thyroidectomy

5. Causes of hyperparathyroidism

   a. *Primary hyperparathyroidism* results from an adenoma or hyperplasia of one of parathyroid glands

   b. *Secondary hyperparathyroidism* occurs as a response of parathyroid glands to chronic hypocalcemia (usually caused by renal failure)

   c. *Tertiary hyperparathyroidism* results from hyperplasia of parathyroid glands and a resulting loss of response to serum calcium levels

B. Pathophysiology

1. Hyperparathyroidism

   a. Increased PTH causes an increased resorption of calcium by kidneys, leading to *hypercalcemia,* and an increased excretion of phosphate by kidneys, leading to hypophosphatemia

   b. Increased PTH causes an increased release of phosphorus and calcium by the bones, leading to bone decalcification and formation of renal calculi

   c. Increased PTH causes an increased bicarbonate excretion and decreased acid excretion, leading to hypokalemia and metabolic acidosis

2. Hypoparathyroidism

    a. Decreased PTH causes a decrease in bone and renal resorption of calcium, leading to *hypocalcemia,* and a decrease in renal excretion of phosphate, elevating serum phosphate levels (hyperphosphatemia)

    b. Calcifications may form on eyes, causing cataracts, and on basal ganglia, causing brain calcifications

    c. Decreased serum calcium levels cause muscular excitability, tetany, and laryngeal spasms

3. Signs and symptoms

    a. Hyperparathyroidism

        1) Neurological: depression, psychosis, paresthesias, decreased neuromuscular irritability, impaired vision, altered level of consciousness (LOC)

        2) Cardiovascular: hypertension, dysrhythmias

        3) Gastrointestinal: nausea, abdominal pain, constipation, peptic ulcers, gastric bleeding, thirst, anorexia, pancreatitis

        4) Renal: renal calculi, hypercalciuria, hyperphosphaturia

        5) Musculoskeletal: muscle atrophy and weakness, bone pain, pathologic fractures, back pain, osteoporosis, demineralization of bone

        6) Metabolic: metabolic acidosis, weight loss, polyuria, polydipsia, dehydration

    b. Hypoparathyroidism

        1) Neurological: hyperactive reflexes; increased intracranial pressure; irritability; anxiety; depression; paresthesias of lips, hands, and feet; laryngeal spasms; seizure activity

        2) Cardiovascular: dysrythmias

        3) Gastrointestinal: malabsorption syndromes, abdominal cramps

        4) Musculoskeletal: carpopedal spasms, facial grimacing, muscle spasms, tetany, seizures, positive Chvostek's and Trousseau's signs, hyperactive deep tendon reflexes, calcification of bones

        5) Renal: renal colic

        6) Integumentary: dry and scaly skin, hair loss, brittle nails

C. Nursing assessment

1. Assessment of hyperparathyroidism includes neurological assessment including LOC, VS, heart rhythm, GI assessment, complaints of pain, muscle strength, weight, I&O

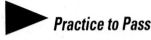

Practice to Pass

The nurse is providing care to a client who has recently had a thyroidectomy. What clinical manifestations and abnormal laboratory values should the nurse expect to observe if the client was experiencing symptoms related to damage of the parathyroid gland?

2. Diagnostic tests for hyperparathyroidism

    a. Serum calcium level: hypercalcemia: normal 9 to 11 mg/dL

    b. Serum phosphorus level: hypophosphatemia; normal 2.5 to 4.5 mg/dL

    c. ABGs: metabolic acidosis

    d. Serum potassium level: hypokalemia

    e. Urine calcium (leads to stones): increased

    f. Urine phosphates: increased

    g. Parathyroid hormone (PTH): increased

    h. Alkaline phosphate: increased

    i. Radiological examinations reveal deposits of calcium in soft tissues and renal structures, osteoporotic changes, demineralization of bone

3. Nursing assessment of hypoparathyroidism includes reflexes and other neurological assessments, VS, cardiac rhythm, GI complaints, Chvostek's and Trousseau's signs, signs of tetany, any integumentary or renal complaints

4. Diagnostic tests for hypoparathyroidism

   a. Serum calcium levels (hypocalcemia)

   b. Serum phosphate levels (hyperphosphatemia)

   c. Parathyroid hormone (PTH): decreased

   d. Urine calcium: decreased

   e. Radiologic examination reveals calcification of skull

D. Nursing management

1. Hyperparathyroidism

   a. Medications

      1) Biophosphate regulator: alendronate sodium (Fosamax) or pamidronate disodium (Aredia)

      2) Furosemide (Lasix) (oral or intravenous [IV]) to promote diuresis

      3) Phosphates (oral or IV) for replacement

      4) Calcitonin (Calcimar): IV to decrease release of calcium by bones

      5) Plicamycin (Mithracin) to inhibit bone resorption of calcium

      6) Gallium nitrate (Gallium) to inhibit bone resorption of calcium

      7) Glucocorticoids to decrease GI absorption of calcium

   b. Educate client to consume diet low in calcium and vitamin D, and increase oral intake of fluids as prescribed

   c. Intravenous saline fluids to increase excretion of calcium

   d. Preoperative and postoperative care for surgical removal of parathyroid gland (parathyroidectomy) for primary hyperparathyroidism

   e. Strain urine for stones, monitor I&O

   f. Monitor EKG rhythm, VS

2. Hypoparathyroidism

   a. Medications

      1) Calcium gluconate (Kalcinate) IV initially, then supplemental oral calcium replacement

      2) Oral vitamin D

      3) Administer parathyroid hormone (PTH)

   b. Educate client to consume a diet high in calcium and low in phosphate

   c. Monitor for seizure activity and laryngeal spasms; provide protective environment if seizures occur

   d. Perform Chvostek's and Trousseau's signs for hypocalcemia

   e. Keep tracheostomy set at bedside for respiratory emergencies caused by laryngeal spasm

   f. Monitor neuromuscular function

3. Priority nursing diagnoses for parathyroid disorders: Impaired physical mobility; Risk for injury; Pain

V. ADRENAL CORTEX HYPERFUNCTION DISORDERS

A. Overview

1. Adrenal glands are located superior to each kidney and composed of adrenal medulla (inner layer of adrenal gland) and adrenal cortex (outer layer of adrenal gland)

   a. Adrenal medulla secretes catecholamines: epinephrine, norepinephrine, and dopamine

   b. Adrenal cortex secretes mineralocorticoids (aldosterone), glucocorticoids (cortisol), androgens and estrogens (sex hormones)

2. Epinephrine and norepinephrine (catecholamines) increase metabolic rate, increase alertness, increase insulin levels, and are responsible for "fight-or-flight" response

3. Glucocorticoids (cortisol) assist body's response to stress; suppress inflammation; increase serum glucose by acting as an insulin antagonist; regulate metabolism of carbohydrates; fat; and protein; enhance protein synthesis; increase breakdown of protein and fatty acids, and decrease pain

4. Adrenocorticotropic hormone (ACTH) functions as an aid to growth and development

5. Mineralocorticoids (aldosterone) aid in sodium (Na$^+$) and water retention, and potassium (K$^+$) excretion

6. Androgens and estrogens contribute to growth and development

7. Adrenal cortex hyperfunction disorders result in excess production of

   a. Cortisol: **Cushing's syndrome**—or hypercortisolism

   b. Aldosterone: **Conn's syndrome**—hyperaldosteronism

8. Causes of hypercortisolism include adrenal tumors, adrenal hyperplasia, or exogenous glucocorticoids

9. Causes of hyperaldosteronism include an adrenal lesion or any condition that stimulates overproduction of aldosterone: heart failure, cirrhosis of liver, dehydration, renal disease

B. Pathophysiology

1. Cushing's syndrome (also known as hypercortisolism)

   a. Functions of glucocorticoids (cortisol, ACTH) include promoting gluconeogenesis, maintaining serum glucose levels, adaptation to stress, and augmenting release of catecholamines to increase blood pressure (BP)

   b. *Primary Cushing's syndrome* is caused by a benign or malignant adrenal tumor, which stimulates an increased production of cortisol

   c. *Secondary Cushing's syndrome* results from disorders of pituitary or hypothalamus, which causes an increased release of ACTH, or from an ectopic disorder that produces ACTH

   d. *Iatrogenic Cushing's syndrome* (most common cause of Cushing's syndrome) results from use of long-term glucocorticoid therapy, which results in excess cortisol levels

   e. Signs and symptoms of hypersecretion of cortisol include

      1) Neurological: psychosis, emotional liability, loss of memory, depression, poor concentration

      2) Cardiovascular: hypertension, dysrhythmias

3) Gastrointestinal: peptic ulcers

4) Musculoskeletal: muscle weakness, muscle wasting, osteoporosis, "buffalo" hump, truncal obesity

5) Integumentary: ecchymosis, hirsutism, purple striae on abdomen, poor wound healing, skin infections, thin skin, acne

6) Renal: glycosuria, polyuria, polydipsia, renal calculi

7) Reproductive: decreased libido, impotence, amenorrhea, masculine characteristics in females

8) Metabolic: hypokalemia, hypernatremia, edema, "moon face," weight gain

9) Classic symptoms of Cushing's syndrome: moon face, "buffalo" hump, purple striae, truncal obesity

2. Conn's syndrome (primary hyperaldosteronism)

a. Role of aldosterone (a mineralocorticoid) is sodium and water retention

b. Aldosterone affects tubular resorption of sodium (Na^+) and water; also has role in excretion of potassium (K^+) and hydrogen ions (H^+)

c. In *primary hyperaldosteronism* the effects of excessive secretion of aldosterone cause an increase in Na^+ retention, an increase in water retention, and an increase in K^+ excretion

1) As BP increases, renin production is suppressed

2) BP continues to rise to dangerous levels, potentially leading to renal damage and cerebral infarcts

3) Despite water and Na^+ retention, edema is *rarely* a complication because water is generally excreted with K^+ ions in urine

d. In *secondary hyperaldosteronism* hypertension is uncommon

e. Signs and symptoms include visual disturbances, paresthesias, hypertension, dysrhythmias, fluid retention, renal damage or failure, polyuria, muscle weakness, tetany, and electrolyte and acid–base imbalance

C. Nursing assessment

1. Assessment of Cushing's syndrome includes VS; cardiac rhythm; neurological assessment; history of GI, renal, and reproductive problems; muscle strength; integument assessment; weight; presence of edema; I&O

2. Diagnostic tests for Cushing's syndrome

a. Serum cortisol levels: increased

b. Serum Na^+ levels: increased (hypernatremia)

c. Serum K^+ levels: decreased (hypokalemia)

d. Serum glucose levels: increased (hyperglycemia)

e. Serum ACTH levels in secondary Cushing's syndrome: increased

f. Serum ACTH levels in primary Cushing's syndrome: decreased

g. 24-hour urine collection for 17-ketosteroids and 17-hydroxycorticosteroids: increased

h. ACTH suppression test is performed in order to identify cause; dexamethasone suppression test is done to determine if cause is pituitary or adrenal

i. White blood cell count (WBC) >10,000/mm³

j. Radiological examinations reveal pituitary tumor or adrenal tumor

3. Assessment of Conn's syndrome includes neurological assessment, eye exam, VS, cardiac rhythm, fluid status, I&O, muscle strength, electrolytes, and renal status

4. Diagnostic tests for Conn's syndrome
   a. Serum Na^+ levels: increased (hypernatremia)
   b. Serum K^+ levels: decreased (hypokalemia)
   c. ABGs: metabolic alkalosis (elevated HCO_3^-)
   d. Serum aldosterone levels: elevated
   e. Urine aldosterone levels: elevated
   f. Serum renin levels (primary hyperaldosteronism): decreased
   g. Serum renin levels (secondary hyperaldosteronism): increased
   h. Radiological examinations reveal tumor

D. **Nursing management**
   1. Cushing's syndrome
      a. Medications
         1) Mitotane (Lysodren): cytotoxic antihormonal agent that inhibits corticosteroid synthesis without destroying cortical cells
         2) Trilostane (Modrastane) or aminoglutethimide (Cytadren): block synthesis of glucocorticoids and adrenal steroids
         3) Antiinfective ketoconazole (Fluconazole) or metyrapone to inhibit corticosteroid synthesis
         4) Cyproheptadine (Periactin), somatostatin (Octreotide), or bromocriptine (Parlodel): interferes with ACTH production
         5) Lifelong steroid replacement if bilateral adrenalectomy is performed
         6) Somatostatin analog (Octreotide) to suppress ACTH
      b. Preoperative and postoperative care for adrenalectomy if performed
      c. Assist in monitoring effects of radiation therapy if performed
      d. Monitor for Addisonian crisis caused by drug therapy
      e. Priority nursing diagnoses for Cushing's syndrome: Excess fluid volume; Risk for infection; Risk for injury; Activity intolerance; Anxiety; Deficient knowledge; Risk for impaired skin integrity

   2. Conn's syndrome
      a. Medications
         1) Spironolactone (Aldactone) to treat hypertension and hypokalemia for those clients who will not be treated surgically
         2) Amiloride (Midamor) for those clients unable to tolerate spironolactone
         3) Administer glucocorticoids preoperatively as prescribed to prevent adrenal hypofunction
      b. Preoperative and postoperative care for unilateral or bilateral adrenalectomy
      c. Educate client that if bilateral adrenalectomy is performed, lifetime replacement of glucocorticoids is necessary; unilateral surgery may require temporary replacement until remaining gland adjusts hormonal output
      d. Monitor BP, urine output, electrolytes
      e. Educate client about low-Na^+ diet
      f. Teach side effects of medications
      g. Priority nursing diagnoses for Conn's syndrome: Excess fluid volume; Risk for injury

Practice to Pass

The nurse is providing care to a client with Cushing's syndrome. What nursing interventions should be implemented for a diagnosis of Fluid volume excess?

VI. ADRENAL CORTEX HYPOFUNCTION DISORDER: ADDISON'S DISEASE

A. Overview

1. **Addison's disease** is defined as a chronic adrenocortical insufficiency because of destruction of adrenal glands; also known as adrenal insufficiency

2. Adrenal cortex hypofunction results in a decreased production of cortisone and aldosterone

3. Causes include destruction of adrenal gland because of trauma, infection, hemorrhage into gland, or sudden stress

B. Pathophysiology

1. Gradual destruction of adrenal cortical tissue leads to hypofunction of adrenal glands

2. Insufficient hormonal secretion of mineralocorticoids and glucocorticoids results in deficient aldosterone, cortisol, and androgens

3. Insufficient levels of aldosterone lead to a reduction in Na^+ absorption and increased Na^+ excretion

4. Water follows Na^+, leading to increased water excretion and hypovolemia

5. Hypotension occurs as a result of hypovolemia

6. K^+ is retained (moves opposite direction of Na^+), resulting in hyperkalemia

7. **Addisonian crisis** can occur, which is an acute insufficiency of adrenocortical hormone from a lack of cortisol during stress, such as surgery or pregnancy, or when exogenous corticosteroid therapy is abruptly discontinued

   a. If not treated immediately, circulatory collapse, shock, and death may occur

   b. Signs and symptoms include severe nausea and vomiting, diarrhea, dehydration, sudden pain in lower back, abdomen and legs, hypotension, tachycardia, confusion, restlessness, fatigue, shock, headache

8. Signs and symptoms of Addison's disease include

   a. Neurological: neurosis, depression

   b. Cardiovascular: hypotension, EKG changes such as tall, peaked T waves because of hyperkalemia

   c. Musculoskeletal: muscle weakness, fatigue

   d. Integumentary: skin hyperpigmentation (bronzing)

   e. Gastrointestinal: diarrhea, nausea, vomiting, anorexia

   f. Reproductive: decreased libido, scant pubic hair

   g. Metabolic: hyperkalemia, hyponatremia, hypoglycemia, weight loss

C. Nursing assessment

1. Assessment includes neurological assessment, VS, cardiac monitoring, activity tolerance, muscle strength, GI symptoms, libido, electrolyte balance, weight

2. Diagnostic tests

   a. Serum cortisol levels: low

   b. Serum ACTH levels: high

   c. Serum Na^+ levels: low (hyponatremia)

   d. Serum K^+ levels: high (hyperkalemia)

   e. Serum aldosterone levels: decreased

Practice to Pass

The nurse is educating a client with Addison's disease about nutritional requirements for the management of this disease. What instructions should be provided?

     f. Urinary cortisol levels: decreased

     g. ABGs: metabolic acidosis (decreased HCO_3^-)

     h. Electrocardiogram

D. Nursing management

    1. Medications include mineralocorticoid and glucocorticoid replacement

     a. Addison's disease: administer cortisone, prednisone, or fludrocortisone acetate (Florinef) as prescribed

     b. Addisonian crisis: immediate IV glucocorticoid replacement and fluids with Na^+

    2. Monitor for signs of dehydration

    3. Maintain high-Na^+, low-K^+ diet

    4. Prepare client for surgical intervention if tumor is causative factor

    5. Priority nursing diagnoses for Addison's disease: Deficient fluid volume; Risk for injury

    6. Teach client about need to carry medical alert identification

VII. ADRENAL MEDULLA HYPERFUNCTION DISORDER: PHEOCHROMOCYTOMA

A. Overview

    1. **Pheochromocytoma** is a catecholamine-secreting tumor (usually benign) of adrenal medulla

    2. It is a rare disorder that causes severe hypertension in addition to hyperglycemia and hypermetabolism

    3. Cause is usually linked to individual with other multiple endocrine neoplasia syndromes

B. Pathophysiology

    1. A tumor in chromaffin cells of sympathetic nervous system arises, in most cases, in adrenal medulla

    2. Tumor causes secretion of excessive amounts of catecholamines (epinephrine and norepinephrine)

    3. The effects of excessive amounts of epinephrine and norepinephrine can lead to a risk of cerebral hemorrhage, cardiac failure, and death if left untreated

    4. Signs and symptoms

     a. Neurological: agitation, emotional outbursts, emotional instability, dilated pupils, severe headache, nervousness

     b. Cardiovascular: hypertension (may be persistent, intermittent, or fluctuating; may occur rapidly and abruptly cease), tachycardia, palpitations

     c. Gastrointestinal: nausea, vomiting, diarrhea

     d. Renal: glucosuria, polyuria

     e. Musculoskeletal: tremors

     f. Metabolic: hyperglycemia, cold extremities, excessive perspiration

C. Nursing assessment

    1. Nursing assessment includes VS, emotional stability, reports of neurological symptoms or headache, GI distress, I&O, skin temperature

    2. Diagnostic tests

       a. Urine catecholamines (metanephrines and vanillylmandelic acid [VMA]): positive

       b. Serum catecholamines: elevated

       c. Urine for glucose (glycosuria): elevated

       d. Serum glucose: elevated (hyperglycemia)

       e. Radiologic examinations reveal tumor

D. Nursing management

    1. Medications

       a. Phenoxybenzamine (Dibenzyline) preoperatively for hypertension control

       b. Metyrosine (Demser) to inhibit synthesis of norepinephrine

       c. IV antihypertensive agents for hypertensive crisis

    2. Preoperative and postoperative care for unilateral or bilateral adrenalectomy

    3. Monitor for heart failure, cerebrovascular accident, myocardial infarction, shock, renal failure

    4. Monitor BP, urinary output, neurological status

    5. Maintain seizure precautions

    6. Priority nursing diagnoses: Risk for injury; Pain

VIII. ANTERIOR PITUITARY DISORDERS

A. Overview

    1. Pituitary gland, referred to as "master gland," is located at base of brain adjacent to hypothalamus; it is responsible for regulating endocrine function by producing hormones that affect body systems and stimulate other endocrine glands to secrete hormones

    2. Hormones produced by anterior pituitary gland

       a. Growth hormone (GH)

       b. Thyroid-stimulating hormone (TSH)

       c. Adrenocorticotropic hormone (ACTH)

       d. Follicle-stimulating hormone (FSH)

       e. Leutinizing hormone (LH)

       f. Prolactin (PRL)

    3. Disorders of anterior pituitary gland result in excessive or insufficient pituitary hormones; disorders of pituitary gland are not as common as other endocrine gland disorders

    4. *Growth hormone* (GH) is a hormone necessary for growth that regulates cell division and synthesis of protein; exerts other metabolic effects on endocrine organs, skin, skeletal muscle, cardiac muscle, and connective tissue

    5. *Hyperfunction* of anterior pituitary (hyperpituitarism) results in excess production and secretion of one or more hormones: GH, prolactin (PRL), or ACTH, leading to manifestations such as tissue overgrowth seen in hyperpituitarism

    6. The most common cause of hyperpituitarism is benign adenoma

    7. *Hypofunction* of anterior pituitary (hypopituitarism) results in a deficiency of one or more of pituitary hormones: GH, FSH, TSH, LH, and ACTH

8. Causes of hypopituitarism include surgical removal of pituitary gland, pituitary tumors, pituitary infection, pituitary trauma, congenital defects, and radiation

9. Common disorders

    a. Hyperpituitarism: gigantism and acromegaly

    b. Hypopituitarism: dwarfism

B. Pathophysiology

1. Gigantism

    a. Gigantism results from GH hypersecretion that begins *before closure of epiphyseal plate*

        1) This hypersecretion leads person to become abnormally tall, often reaching 7 to 8 ft in height

        2) Body proportions are generally normal

    b. Most common cause of gigantism is tumor of pituitary gland

    c. Early detection, diagnosis, and treatment has made this disorder rare in occurrence

    d. Signs and symptoms include excessive height and acromegaly as an adult

2. Acromegaly

    a. Acromegaly is a result of GH hypersecretion beginning *during adulthood;* bone and connective tissue continue to grow, leading to *disproportionate* enlargement of tissues

    b. Most common cause of acromegaly is a tumor of pituitary gland

    c. Signs and symptoms include large hands and feet; protrusion of lower jaw; coarse facial features; signs of osteoporosis; change in hand, shoe, and glove size that slowly progresses; systemic symptoms: hypertension; coronary artery disease; congestive heart failure; enlarged adrenal, thyroid, and parathyroid glands; amenorrhea; headache; sweating; weakness

3. Dwarfism

    a. Dwarfism results from deficient secretion of anterior pituitary hormones

    b. Inadequate secretion of these hormones leads to growth retardation and accompanying metabolic disorders

    c. Signs and symptoms include short stature, obesity, high-pitched voice, slow-maturing skeletal system, hyperlipidemia, hypercholesterolemia

C. Nursing assessment

1. Assessment of gigantism includes growth chart for height and weight by age and visual exam

2. Assessment of acromegaly includes VS, visual disturbances, signs and symptoms of congestive heart failure or diabetes mellitus, growth and development, symptom analysis of any pain

3. Assessment of dwarfism includes growth chart for height and weight by age, development of sex organs

4. Diagnostic tests: bone scan, cholesterol, lipid panel, and hormone levels

D. Nursing management

1. Medications include cortisol and thyroid replacement drugs; growth hormone for dwarfism

2. Assist client in obtaining proper counseling to facilitate psychosocial adjustment to altered body image

3. Monitor for diabetes insipidus since posterior pituitary gland may be affected simultaneously

4. Priority nursing diagnoses for anterior pituitary disorders: Activity intolerance; Anxiety; Disturbed body image; Sexual dysfunction; Anticipatory grieving; Ineffective coping; Risk for disproportionate growth and development

IX. POSTERIOR PITUITARY DISORDERS

A. Overview

1. Posterior pituitary gland secretes hormones oxytocin and **antidiuretic hormone (ADH),** also known as vasopressin; purpose of ADH is to control serum osmolality

2. Disorders of posterior pituitary gland primarily result from excessive or deficient ADH secretion

   a. **Diabetes insipidus (DI)** results from ADH insufficiency, leading to excess fluid excretion

   b. **Syndrome of inappropriate antidiuretic hormone (SIADH)** results from excessive excretion of ADH and excessive water retention

3. Causes

   a. DI: unknown etiology in most cases; tumor or head trauma with damage to pituitary

   b. SIADH: occurs most often because of ectopic production of ADH by malignant tumors, but may also occur as a result of pituitary surgery, head injury, or certain medications such as diuretics, anesthetics, and barbiturates

B. Pathophysiology

1. Diabetes insipidus

   a. Normally, fluid balance is maintained by actions of hypothalamus, kidneys, and pituitary gland

      1) Hypothalamus detects dehydration, sends a message to pituitary, which in turn releases ADH and sends it to kidney

      2) In kidney it acts on collecting and distal tubules to reabsorb water, promoting *retention* to restore fluid balance

      3) When excess fluid volume occurs, hypothalamus sends a message to pituitary to inhibit secretion of ADH, promoting *excretion* to restore fluid balance

   b. In DI, ADH *insufficiency* leads to excretion of large amounts of urine (polyuria), up to 12 liters a day

   c. Classifications

      1) *Neurogenic DI* occurs when there is a decrease in synthesis and excretion of ADH; may be idiopathic, or may result from trauma or dysfunction of hypothalamus and pituitary gland

      2) *Nephrogenic DI* occurs when renal tubules are not sensitive to ADH

   d. If DI results from cerebral injury or other trauma, it may resolve without further incident, however, if disorder is chronic, lifelong treatment is required

   e. Signs and symptoms include polyuria, excess thirst, polydipsia, dehydration if client is unable to replace fluid loss, weakness

2. Syndrome of inappropriate antidiuretic hormone (SIADH)

   a. Normal feedback mechanisms (as previously described) from hypothalamus, pituitary gland, and kidney fail despite low serum osmolality and increased fluid volume, resulting in *excessive secretion* of ADH, which leads to excessive water retention

   b. Excessive water retention results in dilute plasma, decreased serum Na⁺ (dilutional hyponatremia), and water intoxication

   c. Signs and symptoms include lethargy, confusion, and/or other changes in neurological status, cerebral edema, muscle cramps, weakness, decreased urine output, fluid retention, and weight gain

C. Nursing assessment

1. Assessment of DI includes I&O, reports of thirst, signs of dehydration (poor skin turgor, dry skin, sunken eyeballs, weakness, decreased urinary output, complaints of thirst, dry mucous membranes)

2. Diagnostic tests for DI
   a. Serum Na⁺ level (hypernatremia)
   b. Urine specific gravity: low
   c. Serum osmolality: high
   d. Urine osmolality: decreased
   e. Serum ADH levels: decreased
   f. Vasopressin test and water deprivation test: increased (hyperosmolality); diagnostic for DI

3. Assessment of SIADH includes: LOC and other neurological indicators, I&O, weight

4. Diagnostic tests for SIADH
   a. Serum Na⁺ levels: low (hyponatremia)
   b. Serum osmolality: low
   c. Urine specific gravity: increased

D. Nursing management

1. Diabetes insipidus

   a. Medications include vasopressin (Pitressin, Pressyn) for treatment of neurogenic DI; desmopressin acetate (DDAVP) to reduce urine volume
   b. Administration of hypotonic IV fluids
   c. Increase oral fluid intake

   d. Treatment is lifelong for chronic DI
   e. Monitor I&O
   f. Monitor daily weight at same time on same scale in same amount of clothing

   g. Provide dietary instructions for low-Na⁺ diet and teach to avoid caffeine, since this increases urine output
   h. Educate client about need for Medic-Alert bracelet

2. Syndrome of inappropriate antidiuretic hormone
   a. Medications include diuretics, antibiotics such as demeclocycline hydrochloride (Declomycin)
   b. Administration of hypertonic saline IV fluids

   c. Oral fluid restriction
   d. Monitor I&O
   e. Monitor daily weight at same time on same scale in same amount of clothing

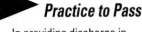

Practice to Pass

In providing discharge instructions to a client with chronic diabetes insipidus, what information should be included?

      f. Monitor for neurological changes and other signs of water intoxication

      g. Educate client about need for Medic-Alert bracelet

   3. Priority nursing diagnoses for posterior pituitary disorders: Excess fluid volume; Deficient fluid volume; Altered urinary elimination; Risk for injury; Deficient knowledge

X. DIABETES MELLITUS

A. Overview

   1. **Diabetes mellitus (DM)** is defined as a lack of or inadequate secretion of insulin, or insulin resistance resulting in hyperglycemia

      a. Is the most common chronic disorder of endocrine system

      b. Pancreas (beta cells of islets of Langerhans) fails to secrete an adequate amount of **insulin** (hormone responsible for glucose metabolism)

      c. Lack of adequate insulin secretion results in inappropriate *hyperglycemia*

      d. Obesity, especially when centralized in abdomen, may lead to insulin resistance

   2. Types

      a. *Type 1 diabetes* results from destruction of pancreatic beta cells, which leads to insulin dependence (no insulin is produced from beta cells of pancreas); insulin *must* be received exogenously

      b. *Type 2 diabetes* results from a decrease in beta cell weight and number or insulin resistance; may be managed with diet and exercise, and/or oral antidiabetic agents; situations increasing stress on body (surgery, illness, trauma) may create a need for supplemental insulin temporarily because of rise in glucose levels because of adrenal cortex response to stress

      c. Gestational DM: results from glucose intolerance during pregnancy

   3. Causes

      a. Type 1 DM: occurs as a result of genetic, environmental, or immunological factors that damage the pancreatic beta cells (the insulin-secreting cells)

      b. Type 2 DM: etiology is unknown; however, obesity is the single most important risk factor

      c. Other types may be caused by genetic defects, drugs or chemicals, infections or pancreatic disorders, or stress of pregnancy

B. Pathophysiology

   1. Type 1 DM

      a. Damage to pancreatic beta cells leads to uncontrolled glucose production by liver and subsequently results in hyperglycemia (elevated serum glucose)

      b. Renal threshold for glucose is approximately 180 to 200 mg/dL, therefore glucose spills into urine once it exceeds renal threshold

         1) Because glucose is highly osmotic, fluids "follow" glucose and are excreted from body in large amounts of urine (called *osmotic diuresis*), causing an excessive loss of fluids and electrolytes (*polyuria*)

         2) Loss of fluids leads to *polydipsia* (excessive thirst)

      c. Because of lack of insulin, body is unable to utilize carbohydrates, its primary source of energy; therefore, it must use proteins and fats for energy, leading to unexplained weight loss

         1) This use of fat results in *ketones,* which are acid end-products of fat metabolism

2) As ketones build in body, *acidosis* occurs

3) Breakdown of nutritional stores leads to excessive hunger, known as *polyphagia*

d. Polyuria, polydipsia, and polyphagia are classic signs of diabetes and are known as the "3 Ps"

e. Failure to receive adequate amounts of insulin results in continued fat metabolism, which produces ketone bodies leading to acidosis

f. Diabetic ketoacidosis (DKA) results in severe metabolic, fluid, and electrolyte disturbances, and is a life-threatening condition of hyperglycemia and metabolic acidosis requiring immediate action

2. Type 2 DM

a. Results from a decrease in beta cell weight and number or from insulin resistance

b. There is an *inadequate secretion of insulin* or an *insensitivity* (resistance) to insulin, which leads to hyperglycemia

c. Symptoms are generally same as for type 1 diabetes, but type 2 has a gradual onset and may be undetected for years (later adulthood); additionally, ketones are not usually present and excess weight rather than weight loss is noted

3. Signs and symptoms

a. Early manifestations of type 1 DM: polyuria, polydipsia, polyphagia, glucosuria, fatigue, weight loss, nausea, vomiting, abdominal pain

b. Early manifestations in type 2 DM: polyuria, polydipsia, blurred vision, weight gain

c. General multisystem findings (see Figure 9-3)

1) Sensory/neurological: diabetic retinopathy, cataracts, glaucoma, paresthesias, loss of sensation, peripheral neuropathy

2) Cardiovascular assessment: coronary artery disease, peripheral vascular disease, hypertension

3) Gastrointestinal assessment: constipation or diarrhea

4) Musculoskeletal assessment: contractures

5) Integumentary assessment: atrophy, foot ulcers, poor wound healing, chronic skin infections

6) Renal assessment: edema, chronic renal failure, albuminuria, urinary tract infections

7) Reproductive assessment: sexual dysfunction, vaginitis

8) Metabolic: hyperglycemia, hypokalemia, metabolic acidosis

d. Symptoms of diabetic ketoacidosis (DKA): abdominal pain, nausea and vomiting, metabolic acidosis, fruity breath odor, Kussmaul's respirations, altered level of consciousness, coma, and death if untreated

4. Complications include DKA, hypoglycemia, atherosclerosis, CVA, PVD, diabetic retinopathy, paresthesias (especially feet), diabetic neuropathy, renal failure, carpal tunnel syndrome, periodontal disease, gangrene, amputation, and inability to heal

C. Nursing assessment

1. Assessment includes symptom analysis, fluid status, I&O, nutritional status, weight, energy level, GI symptoms, neurological assessment, history of recent infections with difficulty healing

Figure 9-3 Body system effects of diabetes mellitus.

Early Manifestations
- Type 1 DM
  - Polyuria
  - Polydipsia
  - Polyphagia
  - Weight loss
  - Glycosuria
  - Fatigue
- Type 2 DM
  - Polyuria
  - Polydipsia
  - Blurred vision

Progressive Complications
- Hyperglycemia
  - Diabetic ketoacidosis
  - Hyperglycemic hyperosmolar nonketotic coma
- Hypoglycemia

Late Complications
Neurologic
- Somatic neuropathies
  - Paresthesias
  - Pain
  - Loss of cutaneous sensation
  - Loss of fine motor control
- Visceral neuropathies
  - Sweating dysfunction
  - Pupillary constriction
  - Fixed heart rate
  - Constipation
  - Diarrhea
  - Incomplete bladder emptying
  - Sexual dysfunction

Sensory
- Diabetic retinopathy
- Cataracts
- Glaucoma

Cardiovascular
- Orthostatic hypotension
- Accelerated atherosclerosis
- Cerebrovascular disease (stroke)
- Coronary artery disease (MI)
- Peripheral vascular disease
- Blood viscosity and platelet disorders

Renal
- Hypertension
- Albuminuria
- Edema
- Chronic renal failure

Musculoskeletal
- Joint contractures

Integumentary
- Foot ulcers
- Gangrene of the feet
- Atrophic changes

Immune System
- Impaired healing
- Chronic skin infections
- Periodontal disease
- Urinary tract infections
- Lung infections
- Vaginitis

2. Diagnostic tests

    a. Serum fasting glucose: increased (hyperglycemia > 126 mg/dL)

    b. Serum glycosylated hemoglobin levels: increased > 7%

    c. Urine for glucose and ketones: positive

    d. Urine for protein: positive

    e. Serum K^+: decreased (hypokalemia)

    f. 2-hour-plasma glucose (after meal) > 200 mg/dL

    g. Cholesterol and triglyceride levels: elevated

D. Nursing management

    1. Medications include insulin or oral antidiabetic agents

        a. Type 1 diabetes: short-acting (regular) insulin, intermediate-acting (NPH) insulin, long-acting (Lantus) insulin, or combination insulins such as Novolin 70/30; insulins are usually "U 100" with 100 units of insulin per mL; but may be U 500

        b. Type 2 diabetes: oral agents

            1) Sulfonylureas: glimepiride (Amaryl), glipizide (Glucotrol), glyburide (Micronase or DiaBeta), tolazamide (Tolinase), tolbutamide (Orinase)

            2) Meglitinides: repaglinide (Prandin)

            3) Biguanides: metformin (Glucophage)

            4) Alpha-glucosidase inhibitors: acarbose (Precose), miglitol (Glyet)

            5) Thiazolidinediones: rosiglitazone (Avandia), pioglitazone (Actos)

            6) D-phenylalanine derivative: netaglinide (Starlix)

    2. Monitor I&O, serum glucose, electrolytes

    3. Client education

        a. Teach signs and symptoms of hypoglycemia (irritability, fatigue, weakness, tremors, headache. possible coma) and hyperglycemia with appropriate interventions for each

        b. Teach self-administration of insulin or oral antidiabetic agents

        c. Teach onset and peak actions of insulin (see Table 9–2)

Table 9-2		Onset (hours)	Peak (hours)
Reaction Time of the Most Common Insulin Preparations	**Rapid-acting insulin** Regular (R) Regular Humulin	0.5–1	2–3
	Intermediate-acting NPH (N) Lente (L)	1–2	6–8
	Long-acting Lantus Ultralente	not defined 2	not defined 16–20
	Combinations Humulin 70/30 Novolin 70/30	0.5	4–8

      d. Teach self-monitoring of glucose

      e. Teach proper dietary management of diabetes (will need nutritionist consult): include need for balanced meal plan, food groups, food exchanges and need to correlate diet with serum glucose levels

      f. Teach proper diabetic foot care, need for proper shoe fit, and wound care

      g. Teach sick day rules: maintain or increase insulin when a common sickness occurs (virus, colds, etc.), and monitor glucose more often (every 2 to 4 hours) and maintain fluid intake

      h. Teach proper exercise to aid in management of diabetes

    4. Priority nursing diagnoses for diabetes mellitus: Imbalanced nutrition; Risk for self-care deficit; Risk for deficient fluid volume; Risk for impaired skin integrity; Risk for deficient knowledge

Case Study

A 16-year-old female is admitted for a workup because of symptoms of excessive weight loss, fatigue, inability to maintain her grades in school, and complaints of constant hunger. These symptoms began rather suddenly, and her mother did not recognize how severe her weight loss had become until she tried on bathing suits. Her admitting lab work was all within normal limits except glucose 425 mg/dL, and her urine test was positive for glucose and ketones. There is no family history of diabetes mellitus (DM). The doctor orders glucose monitoring before meals and at bedtime with regular insulin according to sliding scale along with NPH 30 units subcutaneous every morning.

1. When the physician confirms the diagnosis of DM, how should the nurse explain the disease so she can understand?

2. What are the most important symptoms she should be taught?

3. The mother is frantic and doubts the diagnosis because no one in the family has DM. How should the nurse handle this situation?

4. What should the client be taught about the possible problems associated with administration of both NPH and regular insulin?

5. What instructions should the client and her mother be given about hypoglycemia and hyperglycemia and why does she need instructions on both?

For suggested responses, see page 536.

For suggested responses, see page 536.

POSTTEST

1 A client with exophthalmos as a result of Graves' disease has expressed a desire for the medications to "hurry up and work so that my eyes will go down." The nurse's response to the client will be based on which of the following?

1. Reversal of exophthalmos will occur after therapeutic antithyroid medication has achieved a therapeutic level
2. Reversal of exophthalmos occurs after treatment with ophthalmic medications
3. Changes in the eyes as a result of Graves' disease are not reversible, even after treatment of the disease
4. Exophthalmos as a result of Graves' disease is only a temporary symptom and should resolve spontaneously

POSTTEST

❷ The nurse is providing care to a client with myxedema coma. Priority nursing care would include which of the following measures?

1. Reducing fever to achieve normal body temperature
2. Decreasing heart rate from tachycardic state
3. Maintaining circulating volume with intravenous fluids
4. Decreasing blood pressure to prevent hypertensive crisis

❸ A client diagnosed with primary hyperparathyroidism demonstrates to the nurse an understanding of the teaching plan by making which of the following statements?

1. "I know I must have surgery to remove my parathyroid gland."
2. "I must take diuretics the rest of my life."
3. "I must eat a diet low in potassium."
4. "I must limit my daily fluid intake."

❹ The nurse would select which of the following as the priority nursing diagnosis for a client with hypoparathyroidism?

1. Risk for excess fluid volume
2. Risk for injury
3. Anxiety
4. Knowledge deficit

❺ A client with Cushing's syndrome is receiving mitotane (Lysodren). When assessing the client's response to the medication, the nurse would expect therapeutic effects to be the result of which of the following?

1. Blocking utilization of glucocorticoids in the tissues
2. Suppression of adrenocorticotropic hormone (ACTH)
3. Direct suppression of activity of the adrenal cortex
4. Destruction of the pituitary gland

❻ The nurse has provided preoperative teaching for a client with Conn's syndrome who is scheduled for a bilateral adrenalectomy. The nurse concludes that the client understands the information presented after the client makes which statement?

1. "I will need to be on lifetime replacement of glucocorticoids."
2. "I will need to increase my salt intake."
3. "I need to avoid salt the rest of my life."
4. "I will need temporary replacements of glucocorticoids."

❼ A client with a history of Addison's disease is admitted to the unit with Addisonian crisis manifested by severe hypotension and unresponsiveness. Which statements provided by the client's spouse provide information to the nurse as to possible precipitating factors to the crisis? Select all that apply.

1. Client stopped taking prescribed hydrocortisone several days ago
2. Client began eating a very low salt diet
3. Client is taking fludrocortisone (Florinef)
4. Client has type 1 diabetes mellitus
5. Client has recently experienced several major stressors including an infection and an accident

❽ The nurse administering desmopressin (DDAVP) to a client with diabetes insipidus anticipates implementing which of the following actions for this client? Select all that apply.

1. Maintaining fluid restriction
2. Monitoring urine output and specific gravity
3. Administering oral fluids or hypotonic intravenous fluids
4. Monitoring blood glucose levels
5. Administering drug by route ordered, which may be oral, nasal, or parenteral

❾ The nurse would monitor which of the following as the highest priority for a client with pheochromocytoma?

1. Blood pressure
2. Urine output
3. Neurological status
4. Serum glucose levels

10 The nurse concludes that a client newly diagnosed with type 1 diabetes mellitus requires further teaching after the client makes which statement?

1. "I will notify my health care provider if my glucose levels run higher or lower than the target range."
2. "I will take my insulin as prescribed, and I will not miss a dose."
3. "I will check my glucose level 30 minutes before I eat and at bedtime."
4. "I will not take my insulin if I am sick and cannot eat."

➤ *See pages 293–294 for Answers & Rationales.*

ANSWERS & RATIONALES

Pretest

1 **Answer: 2** Hyperthyroidism is an excess of thyroid hormone (TH), which places the body in a hypermetabolic state manifested by increases in appetite, body temperature, and oxygen consumption. Hypothyroidism manifestations are the opposite of those seen in hyperthyroidism. The manifestations of parathyroidism are related to disturbances in calcium levels. **Cognitive Level:** Analysis **Client Need:** Physiological Integrity: Physiological Adaptation **Integrated Process:** Nursing Process: Analysis **Content Area:** Adult Health: Endocrine and Metabolic **Strategy:** Note that the options contain two pairs of opposites. To choose between the pairs, recall that the symptoms listed relate to metabolism, which is a function of the thyroid gland. Next consider that the signs are consistent with hyperthyroidism to choose this over the hypothyroid option. **Reference:** Lemone, P., & Burke, K. (2008). *Medical-surgical nursing: Critical thinking in client care* (4th ed.). Upper Saddle River, NJ: Pearson/Prentice Hall, pp. 534–536.

2 **Answer: 1** Though fluid volume status, neurological status, and pain are all important assessments, the immediate priority for postoperative thyroidectomy is airway management. Respiratory distress may result from hemorrhage, edema, laryngeal damage, or tetany. Assessment of respiratory status should include rate, depth, rhythm, and effort. **Cognitive Level:** Analysis **Client Need:** Physiological Integrity: Physiological Adaptation **Integrated Process:** Nursing Process: Assessment **Content Area:** Adult Health: Endocrine and Metabolic **Strategy:** The critical words in the question are *immediate priority*. This indicates that more than one option or all are correct but that one is better than the others. Use the ABCs—airway, breathing, and circulation—to make the correct selection. **Reference:** Lemone, P., & Burke, K. (2008). *Medical-surgical nursing: Critical thinking in client care* (4th ed.). Upper Saddle River, NJ: Pearson/Prentice Hall, p. 539.

3 **Answer: 3** For best absorption, thyroid medications should be taken one hour before meals or two hours after meals. Lifelong treatment of hypothyroidism is necessary. Foods that inhibit thyroid hormone (TH) synthesis, such as cabbage, spinach, and carrots, should not be consumed in excessive amounts. Thyroid medications should be taken in the morning to reduce the possibility of insomnia. **Cognitive Level:** Application **Client Need:** Physiological Integrity: Pharmacological and Parenteral Therapies **Integrated Process:** Nursing Process: Evaluation **Content Area:** Adult Health: Endocrine and Metabolic **Strategy:** The wording of the question indicates the correct option is an incorrect statement by the client. Eliminate options 1 and 4 first recalling that this is a lifelong condition and that the drug will aid metabolism (making morning the time of choice for administration). Use specific medication knowledge and the process of elimination to make a final selection. **Reference:** Lemone, P., & Burke, K. (2008). *Medical-surgical nursing: Critical thinking in client care* (4th ed.). Upper Saddle River, NJ: Pearson/Prentice Hall, p. 544.

4 **Answer: 2** Hypercalcemia is the primary complication of hyperparathyroidism, and the manifestations of the disorder are directly related to the effects of hypercalcemia. Administering large amounts of IV saline promotes renal excretion of calcium. Calcium gluconate would increase serum calcium levels, and tetany is a symptom of hypocalcemia. **Cognitive Level:** Application **Client Need:** Physiological Integrity: Physiological Adaptation **Integrated Process:** Nursing Process: Implementation **Content Area:** Adult Health: Endocrine and Metabolic **Strategy:** First recall that the calcium level is high in hyperparathyroidism. Next note that two options are opposites, making it more likely that one of them is correct. Consider that if the calcium level is high then increased fluid therapy will be needed to dilute the electrolyte, making option 2 correct. **Reference:** Lemone, P., & Burke, K. (2008).

POSTTEST

ANSWERS & RATIONALES

Medical-surgical nursing: Critical thinking in client care (4th ed.). Upper Saddle River, NJ: Pearson/Prentice Hall, pp. 524, 527.

5 Answer: 9 The normal serum calcium level is 9 to 11 mg/dL. The therapeutic response of supplemental calcium is demonstrated by normal calcium levels. **Cognitive Level:** Analysis **Client Need:** Physiological Integrity: Reduction of Risk Potential **Integrated Process:** Nursing Process: Evaluation **Content Area:** Adult Health: Endocrine and Metabolic **Strategy:** Specific knowledge of normal serum electrolyte levels (specifically calcium) is needed to answer the question. If needed, review the upper and lower limits of the normal reference range for calcium. **Reference:** Kee, J. (2006). *Laboratory and diagnostic tests with nursing implications* (7th ed.). Upper Saddle River, NJ: Pearson/Prentice Hall, p. 93.

6 Answer: 2 Cushing's syndrome is manifested by sodium retention, which leads to edema and hypertension. Excess fluid volume is the appropriate diagnosis. Treatment is aimed at restoring normal body fluid balance. If present, anxiety and knowledge deficit should be addressed after fluid volume excess. **Cognitive Level:** Application **Client Need:** Physiological Integrity: Physiological Adaptation **Integrated Process:** Nursing Process: Analysis **Content Area:** Adult Health: Endocrine and Metabolic **Strategy:** Use Maslow's hierarchy to determine that physiological needs take priority over psychosocial needs. Also note that two options are opposites, and link the term *edema* in the stem with *excess* in the correct option to make the correct selection. **Reference:** Lemone, P., & Burke, K. (2008). *Medical-surgical nursing: Critical thinking in client care* (4th ed.). Upper Saddle River, NJ: Pearson/Prentice Hall, p. 548.

7 Answer: 4 Hypertension and hypokalemia are the most common signs and symptoms of hyperaldosteronism. Surgical removal of the adrenal gland(s) is the treatment of choice; however, if that is not possible, the client is treated with Aldactone, a potassium-sparing diuretic, to treat the hypertension and correct the hypokalemia. **Cognitive Level:** Application **Client Need:** Physiological Integrity: Physiological Adaptation **Integrated Process:** Nursing Process: Implementation **Content Area:** Adult Health: Endocrine and Metabolic **Strategy:** Consider the function of aldosterone and what problems would come with an excess of the hormone. What does the drug do to reverse the response? **Reference:** Porth, C. M. (2005). *Pathophysiology: Concepts of altered health states* (7th ed.). Philadelphia, PA: Lippincott Williams & Wilkins, p. 521.

8 Answers: 1, 2, 4, 5 Weight must be monitored *daily;* any increase indicates fluid retention and should be re-

ported immediately. Waiting two weeks to report a problem is too long! Corticosteroids are immunosuppressants; therefore, careful monitoring for infection is necessary. Additionally, an increase in the medication may be required for stressors such as infection. A Medic-Alert bracelet is recommended to inform health care providers of Addison's disease and cortisol treatment. Safety measures are encouraged to prevent injuries. The treatment is lifelong. **Cognitive Level:** Analysis **Client Need:** Physiological Integrity: Physiological Adaptation **Integrated Process:** Nursing Process: Evaluation **Content Area:** Adult Health: Endocrine and Metabolic **Strategy:** First recall that Addison's disease is hypofunction of the adrenal gland, and therefore medication therapy must replace corticosteroids and mineralocorticoids. With this in mind, use the process of elimination to and knowledge of the possible adverse medication effects to make a selection. **Reference:** Lemone, P., & Burke, K. (2008). *Medical-surgical nursing: Critical thinking in client care* (4th ed.). Upper Saddle River, NJ: Pearson/Prentice Hall, p. 555.

9 Answer: 3 SIADH results in fluid retention and hyponatremia. Correction is aimed at restoring fluid and electrolyte balance. Anxiety and risk for injury should be addressed following excess fluid volume. **Cognitive Level:** Analysis **Client Need:** Physiological Integrity: Physiological Adaptation **Integrated Process:** Nursing Process: Analysis **Content Area:** Adult Health: Endocrine and Metabolic **Strategy:** Consider that fluid status is part of the circulation part of ABCs. With this in mind, consider fluid imbalance to be a higher priority using Maslow's hierarchy, followed by injury, and then anxiety. Use specific knowledge of SIADH to make a final selection, perhaps thinking of the "I" in SIADH as meaning *increased* instead of *inappropriate* will help to recall the direction of change. **Reference:** Lemone, P., & Burke, K. (2008). *Medical-surgical nursing: Critical thinking in client care* (4th ed.). Upper Saddle River, NJ: Pearson/Prentice Hall, pp. 558–559.

10 Answer: 1 Type 1, formerly called insulin-dependent diabetes, requires lifelong exogenous replacement of insulin, because no insulin is produced from the beta cells of the pancreas. Options 2, 3, and 4 are incorrect for Type 1 diabetes for the reason just explained. **Cognitive Level:** Application **Client Need:** Physiological Integrity: Physiological Adaptation **Integrated Process:** Teaching/Learning **Content Area:** Adult Health: Endocrine and Metabolic **Strategy:** Eliminate options 2 and 4 first because they are similar. Compare the differences between drug therapy for type 1 diabetes to type 2 diabetes mellitus. Which type does the client have? **Reference:** Lemone, P., & Burke, K. (2008). *Medical-surgi-

cal nursing: Critical thinking in client care (4th ed.). Upper Saddle River, NJ: Pearson/Prentice Hall, pp. 565–567.

Posttest

1 Answer: 3 Exophthalmos occurs as a result of accumulation of fat deposits and by-products in the retro-orbital tissues. Even with treatment of Graves' disease, these changes are not reversible. The client should receive instructions on proper eye care to prevent drying and injury.
Cognitive Level: Analysis **Client Need:** Physiological Integrity: Physiological Adaptation **Integrated Process:** Nursing Process: Analysis **Content Area:** Adult Health: Endocrine and Metabolic Strategy: Recall that exophthalmos is permanent. With this in mind, you will be able to eliminate many of the options. **Reference:** Lemone, P., & Burke, K. (2008). *Medical-surgical nursing: Critical thinking in client care* (4th ed.). Upper Saddle River, NJ: Pearson/Prentice Hall, p. 536.

2 Answer: 3 Myxedema coma is a life-threatening hypothyroid crisis manifested by hypothermia (not hyperthermia as implied by option 1), hyponatremia, hypoglycemia, lactic acidosis, cardiovascular collapse (not elevated pulse and BP as in options 2 and 4), and coma. Maintaining airway and circulation (with fluid volume) are the priority interventions along with replacement hormone because they are life-sustaining.
Cognitive Level: Application **Client Need:** Physiological Integrity: Physiological Adaptation **Integrated Process:** Nursing Process: Implementation **Content Area:** Adult Health: Endocrine and Metabolic **Strategy:** One option stands out as different from the others. Use Maslow's hierarchy helps in prioritizing. **Reference:** Lemone, P., & Burke, K. (2008). *Medical-surgical nursing: Critical thinking in client care* (4th ed.). Upper Saddle River, NJ: Pearson/Prentice Hall, pp. 541, 543.

3 Answer: 1 The treatment for primary hyperparathyroidism is a parathyroidectomy (surgical removal of parathyroid glands). Diuretic therapy, low potassium diet, and fluid restriction (options 2, 3, and 4, respectively) are incorrect treatments for primary hyperparathyroidism.
Cognitive Level: Application **Client Need:** Physiological Integrity: Physiological Adaptation **Integrated Process:** Teaching/Learning **Content Area:** Adult Health: Endocrine and Metabolic **Strategy:** Review the normal function of the parathyroid gland. Then eliminate the options that relate to other endocrine problems. **Reference:** Lemone, P., & Burke, K. (2008). *Medical-surgical nursing: Critical thinking in client care* (4th ed.). Upper Saddle River, NJ: Pearson/Prentice Hall, p. 547.

4 Answer: 2 Risk for injury related to hypocalcemia is the priority diagnosis as injury may occur as a result of low calcium levels and tetany. The client is at risk for fluid volume deficit, not excess, and anxiety and knowledge deficit would not take priority over injury.
Cognitive Level: Application **Client Need:** Physiological Integrity: Physiological Adaptation **Integrated Process:** Nursing Process: Analysis **Content Area:** Adult Health: Endocrine and Metabolic **Strategy:** First determine the pathophysiology and risks for a client with hypoparathyroidism. Next choose the nursing diagnosis that focuses on a physiological need and addresses the problem. **Reference:** Lemone, P., & Burke, K. (2008). *Medical-surgical nursing: Critical thinking in client care* (4th ed.). Upper Saddle River, NJ: Pearson/Prentice Hall, p. 548.

5 Answer: 3 The therapeutic effects of mitotane are the results of direct suppression of activity of the adrenal cortex to block hormone synthesis. Octreotide suppresses ACTH (option 2), and radiation destroys the pituitary gland (option 4).
Cognitive Level: Application **Client Need:** Physiological Integrity: Physiological and Parenteral Therapies **Integrated Process:** Nursing Process: Evaluation **Content Area:** Adult Health: Endocrine and Metabolic **Strategy:** Consider what the action of an "antiadrenal" agent might be. Find clues in the stem to help select an answer if guessing. **Reference:** Lemone, P., & Burke, K. (2008). *Medical-surgical nursing: Critical thinking in client care* (4th ed.). Upper Saddle River, NJ: Pearson/Prentice Hall, p. 550.

6 Answer: 1 Since the client will have a bilateral adrenalectomy, lifetime corticosteroid replacement is necessary. The surgery creates a state of permanent hypofunction of the gland because there is no hormone production. After the adrenalectomy, the client's aldosterone levels should return to normal; therefore, no dietary restrictions will be necessary.
Cognitive Level: Analysis **Client Need:** Physiological Integrity: Physiological Adaptation **Integrated Process:** Teaching/Learning **Content Area:** Adult Health: Endocrine and Metabolic **Strategy:** Note that two sets of opposites appear as options. Ask if salt or hormone is used to manage the problem to help make the appropriate distinctions among the various options. **Reference:** Lemone, P., & Burke, K. (2008). *Medical-surgical nursing: Critical thinking in client care* (4th ed.). Upper Saddle River, NJ: Pearson/Prentice Hall, p. 550.

7 Answer: 1, 2, 5 Hydrocortisone is given to replace cortisol in the client with adrenal insufficiency. Abrupt withdrawal of the hormone can precipitate Addisonian crisis. Hyponatremia is caused by aldosterone deficiency, which affects the renal tubules' ability to con-

serve sodium; therefore adding salt to the diet is recommended. Major stressors are a common precipitating factor in Addisonian crisis. Diabetes mellitus requiring insulin therapy is a complication of Addison's disease; however, there is no indication that diabetes precipitated the crisis.
Cognitive Level: Analysis **Client Need:** Physiological Integrity: Physiological Adaptation **Integrated Process:** Nursing Process: Analysis **Content Area:** Adult Health: Endocrine and Metabolic **Strategy:** Choose the events or behaviors that contribute to electrolyte imbalance or require corticosteroids for homeostasis. Remember which hormone is deficient in Addison's disease. (Think of the "d" in *Addison's* and the "d" in *down* to recall this is a hypofunction of the adrenal gland.) **Reference:** Lemone, P., & Burke, K. (2008). *Medical-surgical nursing: Critical thinking in client care* (4th ed.). Upper Saddle River, NJ: Pearson/Prentice Hall, pp. 555–557.

8 Answers: 2, 3, 5 Because of a deficiency in antidiuretic hormone, diabetes *insipidus* results in massive diuresis and dehydration. DDAVP is administered to promote fluid retention and achieve fluid balance. Oral fluids are encouraged, and hypotonic fluids are administered IV if necessary. Monitoring urine output evaluates the therapeutic effect of the DDAVP and determines the need for additional fluid replacement. Glucose levels are monitored for diabetes *mellitus*.
Cognitive Level: Analysis **Client Need:** Physiological Integrity: Physiological Adaptation **Integrated Process:** Nursing Process: Implementation **Content Area:** Adult Health: Endocrine and Metabolic **Strategy:** Distinguish between diabetes insipidus and diabetes mellitus. What is the pathophysiology in this client? **Reference:** Porth, C. M. (2005). *Pathophysiology: Concepts of altered health states* (7th ed.). Philadelphia, PA: Lippincott Williams & Wilkins, p 759.

9 Answer: 1 Hypertension with systolic blood pressures reaching up to 300 mmHg is possible with pheochromocytoma, making this disorder a life-threatening event. Monitoring blood pressure is a priority. Urine output and neurological status would follow blood pressure, and there is no indication to monitor glucose levels. The treatment of choice for this disorder is an adrenalectomy.
Cognitive Level: Application **Client Need:** Physiological Integrity: Physiological Adaptation **Integrated Process:** Nursing Process: Implementation **Content Area:** Adult Health: Endocrine and Metabolic **Strategy:** What is the life-threatening complication for this client? Monitor for that first. **Reference:** Lemone, P., & Burke, K. (2008). *Medical-surgical nursing: Critical thinking in client care* (4th ed.). Upper Saddle River, NJ: Pearson/Prentice Hall, p. 557.

10 Answer: 4 The client should inform the health care provider of illness, and then should follow "sick-day rules" as prescribed by health care provider, which include taking insulin as prescribed, or increasing insulin as prescribed, consuming extra fluids, resting, and self-monitoring glucose every two to four hours. Options 1, 2, and 3 are all correct responses by the client.
Cognitive Level: Analysis **Client Need:** Physiological Integrity: Physiological Adaptation **Integrated Process:** Teaching/Learning **Content Area:** Adult Health: Endocrine and Metabolic **Strategy:** The wording of the question indicates that the correct option is a negative or incorrect statement by the client. Choose the "wrong" statement, reading each option carefully. **Reference:** Lemone, P., & Burke, K. (2008). *Medical-surgical nursing: Critical thinking in client care* (4th ed.). Upper Saddle River, NJ: Pearson/Prentice Hall, p. 580.

References

Ignatavicius, D., & Workman, M. (2006). *Medical-surgical nursing: Critical thinking for collaborative care* (5th ed.). Philadelphia), PA: W. B. Saunders.

Kee, J. (2006). *Laboratory and diagnostic tests with nursing implications* (7th ed.). Upper Saddle River, NJ: Pearson/Prentice Hall.

Lemone, P., & Burke, K. (2008). *Medical surgical nursing: Critical thinking in client care* (4th ed.). Upper Saddle River, NJ: Prentice Hall.

McCance, K., & Huether, S. (2005). *Pathophysiology: The biologic basis for disease in adults and children* (5th ed.). St. Louis, MO: Mosby, pp. 450–501.

Porth, C.M. (2005). *Pathophysiology: Concepts of altered health states* (7th ed.). Philadelphia, PA: Lippincott Williams & Wilkins.

Ralph, S., & Taylor, C. (2005). *Sparks and Taylor's nursing diagnosis reference manual* (6th ed.). Philadelphia, PA: Lippincott William & Wilkins.

Venes, D., & Thomas, C. L. (Eds.). (2006). *Taber's cyclopedic medical dictionary* (21st ed.). Philadelphia, PA: F. A. Davis.

Wilson, B. A., Shannon, M. T., & Stang, C. L. (2006). *Nursing drug guide: 2006.* Upper Saddle River, NJ: Prentice Hall.

ANSWERS & RATIONALES

Renal and Urinary Health Problems

10

Chapter Outline

Risk Factors Associated with Renal and Urinary Health Problems

Urinary Tract Infection (UTI)

Urinary Calculi

Polycystic Kidney Disease

Pyelonephritis

Glomerulonephritis

Acute Renal Failure

Chronic Renal Failure

Bladder Cancer

Kidney Cancer

Objectives

➤ Define key terms associated with renal and urinary health problems.

➤ Identify risk factors associated with the development of renal and urinary health problems.

➤ Explain the common etiologies of renal and urinary health problems.

➤ Describe the pathophysiologic processes associated with specific renal and urinary health problems.

➤ Distinguish between normal and abnormal renal and urinary findings obtained from nursing assessment.

➤ Prioritize nursing interventions associated with specific renal and urinary health problems.

NCLEX-RN® Test Prep

Use the CD-ROM enclosed with this book to access additional practice opportunities.

Review at a Glance

acute renal failure (ARF) sudden decrease, over days to weeks, in renal function, resulting in retention of urea, nitrogen, and creatinine in blood

azotemia increased blood levels of nitrogenous waste products

calculi masses of crystals composed of minerals normally excreted in urine

chronic renal failure (CRF) progressive inability of kidneys, over months to years, to respond to changes in body fluid and electrolyte composition, GFR < 20% of normal, serum creatinine > 5 mg/dL

cystitis inflammation of urinary bladder

glomerulonephritis inflammation of capillary loops of glomeruli

hematuria blood in urine

nephrolithiasis stones in kidney

oliguria urine output less than 400 ml in 24 hours

polycystic kidney disease a hereditary disease characterized by cyst formation and massive kidney enlargement

prostatitis inflammation of prostate

pyelonephritis inflammatory disorder affecting renal pelvis and functional portion of kidney

pyuria presence of pus in urine

uremia syndrome of renal failure that includes increased blood urea and creatinine levels accompanied by fatigue, anorexia, nausea, vomiting, pruritis, and neurologic changes

urethritis inflammation of urethra

urinary tract infection (UTI) infection of urinary bladder, kidney, urethra, or prostate

urolithiasis stones in urinary bladder

PRETEST

1 A 25-year-old male college student is diagnosed with an upper urinary tract infection. The nurse anticipates that which of the following diagnoses is likely to be documented on the medical record?

1. Cystitis
2. Pyelonephritis
3. Urethritis
4. Prostatitis

2 The nurse would expect to see which pathogen on the urine culture and sensitivity (C & S) of a female client with an uncomplicated urinary tract infection?

1. *Streptococcus*
2. *Staphylococcus*
3. *E. coli*
4. *Klebsiella*

3 The nurse would consider that a urinary tract infection (UTI) is complicated when it is present in which of the following clients?

1. Teenage girl who has recently become sexually active
2. 2-year-old child
3. Elderly, bedridden client
4. Male client

4 The client with cystitis has a routine urinalysis (UA) and pyuria is noted on the report. The nurse concludes the client has:

1. Kidney damage.
2. A host response to the infection.
3. Infection with a gram negative organism.
4. Foul-smelling urine.

5 An adult client has passed a kidney stone and wants to prevent a recurrence. The nurse would include which of the following measures in a teaching plan to prevent recurrence of stones? Select all that apply.

1. Limit fluids, coffee, and milk to concentrate the urine
2. Limit foods high in dietary calcium oxalate like spinach, cocoa, and peanuts to prevent calcium oxalate stones
3. Lower pH of the urine to acidify the urine and reduce stone formation
4. Provide adequate fluids to reduce risk of crystals forming
5. Take vitamin D and calcium tablets to strengthen bones and kidneys

6 Which of the following laboratory findings should alert the nurse to the presence of glomerular injury and the increased risk of renal failure for a client?

1. Cystitis with a urine culture positive for *E. coli*
2. Presence of red blood cell casts in the urine
3. Blood urea nitrogen (BUN) level of 15 mg/dl
4. Hypotension and increased volume of very dilute urine

7 The nurse would conclude that which of the following is an iatrogenic cause of acute renal failure in an adult client?

1. Alcohol
2. Diet
3. Nephrotoxic medications
4. Exercise

8 A client has been told that the glomerular filtration rate (GFR) is less than 20% of normal. The nurse's discussion with this client will take into account that this level of filtration is seen in:

1. Urinary tract infection.
2. Kidney cancer.
3. Renal failure.
4. Polycystic kidney disease.

9 The nurse is reviewing laboratory results for an adult client. The nurse would look to the results of which laboratory test as the best measure of the client's renal function?

1. Complete blood count (CBC)
2. Blood urea nitrogen (BUN) and creatinine
3. Electrolytes and glucose levels
4. Alanine aminotransferase (ALT)

10 In intershift report the nurse hears that a client is in end-stage renal disease (ESRD). The nurse should anticipate that what treatment will be planned?

1. Postmortem care since death is near
2. Dialysis or kidney transplantation
3. No treatment is indicated until renal function deteriorates further
4. Loop diuretics and measures to lower the potassium

➤ *See pages 314–316 for Answers & Rationales.*

I. RISK FACTORS ASSOCIATED WITH RENAL AND URINARY HEALTH PROBLEMS

A. Urinary tract infection: female, geriatric clients; strictures; impaired bladder innervation; chronic disease such as diabetes, prostatic hypertrophy, and prostatitis; diaphragm use; instrumentation; and impaired immune response

B. Urinary calculi: male, Caucasian race, young and middle adulthood; prior personal or family history of calculi; diseases such as gout, hyperparathyroidism, urinary stasis, repeated infections; medications such as vitamins (A, C, and D), loop diuretics, calcium-containing antacids; frequent cola ingestion

C. Polycystic kidney disease: genetics; dialysis

D. Pyelonephritis: pregnancy; urinary tract obstruction; congenital malformation; urinary tract trauma; scarring; calculi; other kidney disorders; vesicoureteral reflux (urine moves from bladder back toward kidney); diabetes; and sickle cell disease

E. Glomerulonephritis: systemic diseases; poststreptococcal infections; staphylococcal or viral infections

F. Acute renal failure: major trauma or surgery; African Americans; predominantly males; infection; hemorrhage; diseases such as severe heart failure; severe liver disease; lower urinary tract obstruction; nephrotoxic medications; radiologic contrast dye; and shock

G. Chronic renal failure: African Americans, Native Americans, Asians, and European Americans; circulatory failure; urinary tract obstruction; analgesic abuse; diseases such as untreated hypertension (HTN) and diabetes; and cigarette smoking

H. **Bladder cancer:** geographic (heavily industrialized areas and northern regions); men; cigarette smoke; chemicals and dyes used in plastics, rubber, and cable industries; substances in work environment of textile workers, leather finishers, spray painters, hairdressers, petroleum workers; and chronic use of phenacetin-containing analgesics

I. **Kidney cancer:** males, over 50; smoking; obesity; chronic irritation caused by renal calculi; urban environment; industrial chemicals; phenacetin or analgesic abuse

II. URINARY TRACT INFECTION (UTI)

A. Overview

1. **Urinary tract infection** is defined as an infection of bladder, kidney, urethra, or prostate

2. Urinary tract is normally sterile above urethra, maintained by a free flow of urine from kidneys to meatus and by emptying bladder completely

3. UTIs are classified according to region and primary site affected

   a. Lower UTIs include **urethritis** (inflammation of urethra), **prostatitis** (inflammation of prostate) and **cystitis** (inflammation of urinary bladder); cystitis is most common form of UTI

   b. Upper UTIs include **pyelonephritis** (inflammation of kidney and renal pelvis)

4. Causes include bowel incontinence, procedures requiring instrumentation, sexual activity, urinary obstruction or calculi, and improper cleaning (especially in children)

B. Pathophysiology

1. Pathogens enter urinary tract by one of two routes

   a. Ascending from mucous membranes of perineal area to lower urinary tract (most common type); gram-negative bacteria, usually *E. coli,* is present in 90% of cases; it is most frequent in adult females because of colonization of bacteria found in the lower gastrointestinal tract gaining entry by ascending the short, straight female urethra

   b. Hematogenously from blood; this type is rare and usually associated with previous damage or scarring of urinary tract

2. A UTI can be categorized as:

   a. *Uncomplicated:* isolated incidence of UTI

   b. *Complicated:* more than two UTIs per year, related to functional, anatomic, metabolic, or neurological disorders, related to an antibiotic-resistant pathogen or pregnancy

3. Any UTI in a male client is considered complicated

4. Signs and symptoms include dysuria (painful or difficult urination), urinary frequency and urgency (sudden, compelling need to urinate) and nocturia (two or more awakenings at night to urinate); urine may have a foul odor and appear cloudy; presence of **pyuria** (excess mucus and white cells in urine) or **hematuria** (bloody urine) caused by bleeding of inflamed bladder wall; older clients may not experience classic symptoms, but instead present with nocturia, incontinence, confusion, behavior change, lethargy, anorexia, or "just not feeling right"

C. Nursing assessment

1. Assessment

   a. Subjective data: duration of symptoms, history of kidney stones, previous urinary, kidney or prostate problems, history of diabetes or hypertension;

inquire about last menstrual period (LMP), pregnancy, and birth control methods; question client regarding allergies, medications, and recent antibiotic use; review diet such as increased caffeine, carbonated drinks, and water intake; pain and tenderness (see Box 10-1)

b. Objective data: vital signs (VS), observe urine (color, consistency, odor), associated symptoms

c. Older adults may present with atypical signs, such as behavior changes, confusion, incontinence, or general deterioration

2. Diagnostic tests

a. Dipstick urinalysis is usually adequate for diagnosis and management of isolated acute UTI

b. A culture and sensitivity (C&S) of urine should be performed if UTI is thought to be complicated, caused by recent instrumentation, antibiotic sensitivities, or previous treatment failures

c. Urinalysis (UA) may show presence of blood cells or bacteria in urine; bacteria counts of 100 to 100,000 (normal is none) are indicative of infection; many red blood cells (RBCs) are often present as well as casts

D. Nursing management

1. Medications

a. Short term (3- to 5-day) antibiotic therapy for uncomplicated UTI; first-line therapy is trimethoprim-sulfamethoxazole (Bactrim), ciprofloxacin (Cipro) or ofloxacin (Floxin), and nitrofurantoin (Macrobid); alternate first-line therapy includes amoxicillin (Amoxil) and cephalexin (Keflex)

b. Second-line quinolones are more expensive, however, and can promote resistant strains of bacteria

c. Phenazopyridine hydrochloride (Pyridium) may be prescribed for comfort measures only (no antibacterial activity); clients should be warned that this drug can stain semen or urine orange

2. Instruct to take antibiotics at nighttime if possible as drug will remain in bladder longer

3. Instruct to increase fluid intake unless contraindicated

4. Assess pain levels and note any change, which may indicate additional disease processes

5. Teach client to avoid caffeinated drinks and alcoholic beverages that can increase bladder spasms and mucosal irritation

6. Teach preventive measures such as emptying bladder every 2 to 4 hours while awake and maintaining fluid intake of 8 to 10 glasses of fluid per day

7. Teach women to cleanse the perineal area front to back; void before and after intercourse; avoid bubble baths, feminine hygiene sprays, douching, and whirl pools and spas; and to wear cotton briefs

▶ **Practice to Pass**

A client tells the nurse that she has had frequency and burning on urination. What assessment should the nurse make? What instructions should the nurse give her?

Box 10-1		
Common Signs and Symptoms of Urinary Tract Infection	Dysuria	Urinary frequency
	Pyuria	Hematuria
	Nocturia	Suprapubic tenderness

8. Unless contraindicated, teach client measures to maintain acidic urine (pH = 5 or less) such as drinking cranberry juice or taking vitamin C daily; avoid excess intake of milk products, fruit juices, and sodium bicarbonate; acidity of urine inhibits bacterial growth by preventing adherance to bladder wall

9. Stress importance of taking all prescribed medication and keeping follow-up appointments

III. URINARY CALCULI

A. Overview

1. **Calculi** are defined as masses of crystals composed of minerals that are normally excreted in urine; majority are composed of calcium; other calculi may be made up of magnesium ammonium phosphate, uric acid, or cystine

2. Stones may develop and cause obstruction at any point in urinary system

3. Termed **urolithiasis** (stones in urinary tract) or **nephrolithiasis** (stones formed within kidney)

4. Causes include dehydration, immobility, excess dietary intake of calcium, oxalate, or protein

B. Pathophysiology

1. Urolithiasis involves precipitation of a poorly soluble salt around a mucoprotein to form a crystalline structure; when concentration of salt in urine is high, crystallization or precipitation is minimal

2. Ingesting an increased amount of involved mineral or decreasing fluid intake (such as during the night), allows an increased concentration where precipitation occurs and stones are formed; when fluid intake is adequate, no stone growth occurs

3. Stone formation is also affected by acidity or alkalinity of urine and presence or absence of calculus-inhibiting compounds such as pyrophosphate and nephrocalcin in urine

4. A majority of kidney stones are composed of calcium oxalate or calcium phosphate, which are associated with increased calcium levels in blood or urine

5. Signs and symptoms vary with their location and size

   a. Renal calculi may be associated with a dull, aching flank pain

   b. Bladder calculi may cause a dull, suprapubic pain

   c. Renal colic causes an acute, severe, intermittent pain of flank and upper outer abdomen on affected side; pain may radiate to suprapubic region, groin, and external genitalia; renal colic may be associated with nausea and vomiting, pallor, and cool, clammy skin

C. Nursing assessment

1. Assessment includes symptom analysis, pain (severity, quality, onset, duration, location, and intensity); urinalysis for presence of blood, protein, or leukocytes; previous history of stones and treatments and family history of calculi; review dietary intake, milk, calcium-rich foods, and antacids; question client about hematuria, recent injury or trauma; assess VS; inspect, palpate, and auscultate abdomen and inspect external genitalia; and assess for vaginal discharge and pelvic pain

2. Diagnostic tests

   a. Urinalysis is useful in diagnosis; gross or microscopic hematuria is generally present

    b. Other diagnostic tests may be necessary including urine calcium, uric acid studies, urine oxalate, culture and sensitivity, serum calcium, and phosphorus

    c. Radiographic studies include kidney, ureter, and bladder (KUB), intravenous pyelography (IVP), ultrasound, CT scan, and cystoscopy

D. Nursing management

    1. Medications include pain medications as ordered and needed; antiemetics to control nausea

    2. Increase fluid intake to increase urine output, which facilitates movement of stone

    3. Monitor urine output and strain urine for stones; document presence of hematuria

    4. Maintain patency and functioning of catheter system if in place

    5. Teach client about all diagnostic tests and interventions, such as lithotripsy, and to strain urine, saving all stones for analysis

    6. Maintain frequent telephone contact with client until stone passes if discharged

    7. Instruct client on preventive measures: fluid intake 2,500 to 3,000 mL/day, dietary modifications (low purine, limiting vitamin D and calcium [see Table 10-1]), promote activity level to prevent urinary stasis and to take all medications as prescribed

    8. Teach client that presence of a stone increases risk for developing UTIs; teach client signs and symptoms of infection and preventive measures

> **Practice to Pass**
>
> What self-management instructions should be given to the client with urolithiasis?

IV. POLYCYSTIC KIDNEY DISEASE

A. Overview

    1. **Polycystic kidney disease** is defined as a hereditary disease (genetic predisposition) characterized by cyst formation and massive kidney enlargement

    2. There are two forms: autosomal dominant (affects adults) and autosomal recessive (typically affects children)

    3. Genetics is the primary cause

B. Pathophysiology

    1. Adult polycystic kidney disease is a slow, progressive disease that is relatively common, accounting for 10% of clients with end-stage renal disease who require dialysis and/or kidney transplant; those individuals with polycystic kidney disease often develop cysts elsewhere in body, including liver, spleen, and pancreas

    2. Of those affected, 9% to 10% experience subarachnoid brain hemorrhage from a congenital aneurysm; there is also an increased incidence of incompetent cardiac valves in clients with polycystic kidney disease

Table 10-1	Food Group	Samples of Foods
Foods to Avoid with Urolithiasis	Acidic	Cheese, cranberries, eggs, grapes, plums, prunes
	Alkaline	Green vegetables, fruit except those listed above, legumes, milk products
	High calcium	Beans, chocolate, dried fruits, canned fish except tuna, milk products
	High purine	Organ meats, sardines, venison, chicken, crab, pork, salmon, veal
	High oxalate	Asparagus, beer, colas, celery, cabbage, green beans, nuts, tea, tomatoes

Adapted from: Lemone, P., & Burke, K. (2004). *Medical-surgical nursing: Critical thinking in client care* (3rd ed.). Upper Saddle River, NJ: Prentice Hall, p. 718.

3. Renal cysts are fluid-filled sacs affecting nephrons of kidneys, which may vary in size; as cysts fill and enlarge, kidneys will enlarge; renal blood vessels and nephrons become obstructed and functional tissue is destroyed

4. Signs and symptoms include flank pain, hematuria, proteinuria, polyuria, and nocturia; UTI and calculi are common as cysts interfere with urine drainage; most clients develop hypertension due to obstruction of blood vessels; kidneys become palpable, enlarged, and knobby as fluid-filled cysts replace functional tissue

C. Nursing assessment

1. Assessment includes presence, location, and duration of symptoms; fluid intake; VS; urination practices; polyuria and nocturia; family history and/or previous history of kidney disease and hypertension; review present and past medications and allergies; assess pain levels and intensity

2. Diagnostic tests: renal ultrasonography, IVP, CT scan of kidney, UA

D. Nursing management

1. Medications include angiotensin-converting enzyme (ACE) inhibitors to control hypertension

2. Instruct and teach client about diagnostic testing

3. Instruct client on signs and symptoms of UTIs and obstruction to avoid further damage to kidney

4. Fluid intake of 2,000 to 2,500 mL/day is encouraged as a preventive measure

5. Stress importance of monitoring BP to identify hypertension for pharmacological intervention

6. Instruct client to avoid medications that may be nephrotoxic and to check with a health care provider before taking any over-the-counter (OTC) medications

7. Discuss genetics and optional screening of family members especially if renal transplantation is contemplated

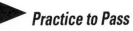

Practice to Pass

A client has just been diagnosed with polycystic kidney disease. How should the nurse explain this disorder to the client?

V. PYELONEPHRITIS

A. Overview

1. Pyelonephritis is defined as an inflammatory disorder affecting renal pelvis and functional portion of kidney tissue

2. Classification

   a. *Acute pyelonephritis,* a bacterial infection of kidney

   b. *Chronic pyelonephritis,* associated with nonbacterial infections and processes that may be metabolic, chemical, or immunological

3. Causes include an ascending bladder infection, blood-borne infections, frequent calculi, or other obstructions

B. Pathophysiology

1. The ascending route from lower urinary tract is most common pathway; infection develops in patchy areas spreading to cortex with WBC infiltration and inflammation

2. Kidney becomes grossly edematous and localized abscesses may form; tissue damage may occur primarily to tubules; scar tissue replaces infected/inflamed areas

3. *E. coli* is responsible in 85% of cases; other common pathogens are *proteus* and *klebsiella*

! **4.** Onset of pyelonephritis is typically rapid with chills and fever, malaise, and vomiting along with flank pain, costovertebral tenderness, urinary frequency, and dysuria

5. As with UTIs, older clients may present with behavior changes, confusion, incontinence, or general deterioration

! **6.** Chronic renal failure and end-stage renal disease may develop with chronic pyelonephritis; hypertension may develop as renal tissue is destroyed

C. Nursing assessment

1. Assessment includes onset and duration of symptoms and any associated symptoms including pain (description, severity, frequency); rule out pregnancy; review previous history of urinary tract problems, treatments and testing; review present medications and allergies; VS; inspect respiratory and cardiac status; hydration status; inspect external genitalia and abdomen for tenderness, masses, or pain; evaluate urinalysis (preferably by a midstream specimen); I&O, urinary frequency, urgency, and nocturia; assess urine for blood, odor, and appearance; question client about family history of kidney disease, infections, diabetes, and hypertension

2. Diagnostic tests: UA (midstream, clean-catch or catheterization), gram stain of urine, urine C&S, WBC, IVP, voiding cystourethrography (after contrast medium instilled into bladder), cystoscopy (direct visualization of urethra and bladder), pelvic/prostate exam

D. Nursing management

1. Medications

a. Analgesics

b. 7 to 10 days of oral antimicrobial therapy: sulfonamides, trimethoprim-sulfamethoxazole (TMP-SMZ, Bactrim, Septra), ciprofloxacin hydrochloride (Cipro), or ofloxacin (Floxin)

c. Urinary anti-infectives: methenamine (Hiprex), nalidixic acid (Neg Gram), nitrofurantoin (Macrodantin)

d. Urinary analgesics: phenazopyridine (Pyridium)

2. Alleviate pain using medication and nonpharmalogic measures such as heating pads or warm baths, rest, and balanced activity

! **3.** Unless contraindicated, increase fluid intake to 8 to 10 glasses/day to dilute urine, lessening irritation of mucosa

! **4.** Teach preventive measures of UTI such as emptying bladder every 2 to 4 hours and increased fluids; for women, proper perineal hygiene, voiding before and after intercourse, avoiding bubble baths, douching, spas, hot tubs, and whirlpools

5. Teach client on obtaining a midstream clean-catch specimen

6. Teach to maintain acidic urine (inhibits bacterial growth) by drinking cranberry juice, taking vitamin C, avoiding excess milk products, and avoiding sodium bicarbonate

7. Instruct to complete full course of prescribed medications even if symptoms have resolved

8. Instruct to keep follow-up appointments as scheduled

9. Referral to a urologist may be necessary

10. Teach about common side effects of antibiotics: nausea and superinfections (candidiasis); also teach about others specific to that medication, such as photosensitivity with sulfa medications

VI. GLOMERULONEPHRITIS

A. Overview

1. **Glomerulonephritis** is defined as an inflammation of capillary loops of glomeruli

2. It is classified as acute, rapidly progressive, or chronic glomerulonephritis

3. Acute poststreptococcal glomerulonephritis is most common form

4. Rapidly progressive glomerulonephritis may either be *idiopathic* or *secondary* to an acute infection or a multisystem disease with a greater incidence in males than females

5. Chronic glomerulonephritis is the end stage of glomerular disorders

6. Causes

    a. Acute: systemic diseases such as systemic lupus erythematosus (SLE) or primary glomerular disease, but a *beta hemolytic strep* infection of pharynx or skin is most common precipitating factor; *staphylococcal* or viral infections can also lead to postinfectious acute glomerulonephritis

    b. Rapidly progressive: unknown, vasculitis, SLE, or acute glomerulonephritis

    c. Chronic: unknown, lupus nephritis, diabetic nephropathy, rapid, progressive glomerulonephritis

B. Pathophysiology

1. In *acute* glomerulonephritis, circulating antigen-antibody immune complexes are formed and trapped in glomerular membrane; these cause an inflammatory response activating the complement system and releasing vasoactive substances and inflammatory mediators; edema and inflammation increase the porosity of glomerular capillaries allowing plasma proteins and blood cells to escape into urine; the renin-angiotensin-aldosterone (RAA) system is disrupted, which could lead to hypertension

    a. Symptoms usually subside in 10 to 14 days and 60% completely recover

    b. The remaining 40% may have persistent impaired renal function, continued proteinuria and/or hematuria leading to chronic glomerulonephritis or renal failure

2. In *rapidly progressive* glomerulonephritis, glomerular cells proliferate along with macrophages forming crescent-shaped lesions that obstruct Bowman's space

    a. More than 70% of glomeruli are affected with a rapid decrease in glomerular filtration rate (GFR)

    b. Up to 50% of clients will require maintenance dialysis and/or kidney transplant

3. *Chronic* glomerulonephritis involves a slow, progressive destruction of glomeruli with impaired renal function; kidneys decrease in size symmetrically and become granular or roughened; eventually, all nephrons are destroyed

4. Signs and symptoms (see Figure 10-1)

    a. Acute: hematuria-brown tinged, proteinuria, salt and water retention, red blood cell casts, hypertension, **azotemia,** fatigue, anorexia, nausea and vomiting, and headache

    b. Rapidly progressive: weakness, nausea and vomiting, flu-like symptoms, oliguria, abdominal or flank pain

    c. Chronic: develops insidiously and is often unrecognized until renal failure is evident

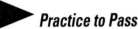

Practice to Pass

A client recovering from Hepatitis B begins to exhibit signs and symptoms of rapid, progressive glomerulonephritis. What is the significance of this disease on the GFR?

Figure 10-1

Critical pathway of glomerulonephritis.

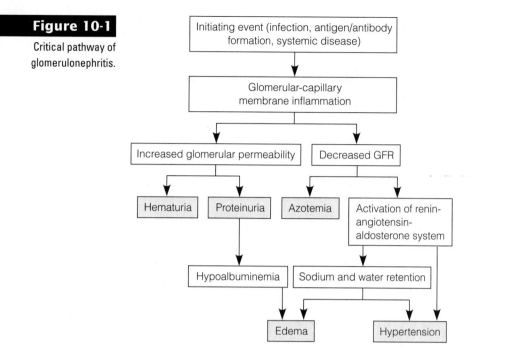

C. Nursing assessment

1. Assessment includes VS, remembering that increased fluid volume increases cardiac workload; weight and presence of edema; I&O; assess energy, activity and fatigue status; signs and symptoms of infections including the skin, throat, and lungs; client's knowledge of disease, coping abilities, support system, lifestyle changes, and need for additional interventions or support

2. Diagnostic tests: throat or skin cultures, antistreptolysin (ASO) titer, sedimentation rate, antinuclear antibody (ANA), blood urea nitrogen (BUN), creatinine, electrolytes, urinalysis, 24–hour urine for creatinine clearance; x-ray studies including abdominal x-rays, kidney scan, and biopsy

D. Nursing management

1. Medications (treat symptoms since no cure exists)

    a. Immunosuppressive therapy (to decrease risk of end-stage renal disease): cyclophosphamide (Cytoxan), azathioprine (Imuran), chlorambucil (Leukeran)

    b. Glucocorticoids (to enhance remission of nephrotic syndrome): prednisone—these may worsen certain types of glomerulonephritis, such as poststreptococcal

    c. ACE inhibitors and nonsteroidal anti-inflammatory drugs (NSAIDs) that decrease protein loss

    d. Antibiotics: penicillin

    e. Antihypertensives

2. Educate client and family regarding disease process

3. Instruct client on prescribed medications and side effects of immunosuppressive or steroid therapy

4. Instruct client and family regarding activity level and dietary restrictions; arrange for a dietary consultation if necessary

5. Teach about signs and symptoms of improving or declining renal function

6. Instruct on signs and symptoms of infectious processes

7. Instruct client to weigh self daily on same scale, at same time, and with same amount of clothing; and report weight gains to provider

8. Instruct on fluid restriction if ordered and importance of measuring I&O

9. Monitor IV fluids and monitor diuretic effect

10. Assess catheter system if indicated

11. Assist with problem solving and support services as needed

VII. ACUTE RENAL FAILURE

A. Overview

1. **Acute renal failure (ARF)** is defined as a rapid decrease in renal function

2. ARF is generally recognized by a fall in urine output and increase in BUN and/or creatinine; oliguria is common but high output failure is possible

3. Most common causes of ARF are ischemia and nephrotoxins; a fall in BP or volume can cause ischemia of kidney tissue; exposure of renal tissue is great when nephrotoxins (such as contrast media) are present in blood (see Figure 10-2)

4. ARF may have iatrogenic causes such as nephrotoxic medications, radiologic contrast dye, and surgical shock

5. Causes are categorized as prerenal, intrarenal, and postrenal (see Box 10-2)

B. Pathophysiology

1. Ischemia is primary cause of ARF; if allowed to continue longer than 2 hours, ischemia leads to severe and irreversible damage to tubules with patchy necrosis;

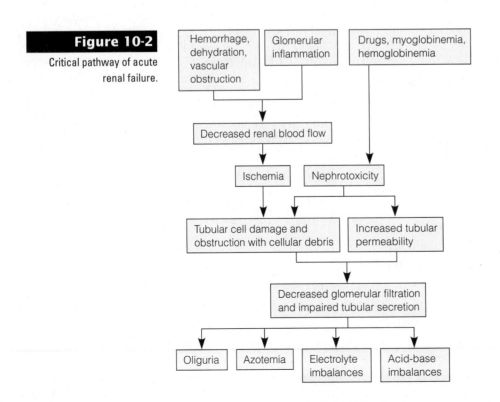

Figure 10-2

Critical pathway of acute renal failure.

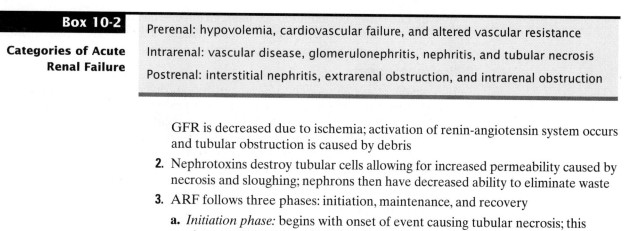

Box 10-2	Prerenal: hypovolemia, cardiovascular failure, and altered vascular resistance
Categories of Acute Renal Failure	Intrarenal: vascular disease, glomerulonephritis, nephritis, and tubular necrosis
	Postrenal: interstitial nephritis, extrarenal obstruction, and intrarenal obstruction

GFR is decreased due to ischemia; activation of renin-angiotensin system occurs and tubular obstruction is caused by debris

2. Nephrotoxins destroy tubular cells allowing for increased permeability caused by necrosis and sloughing; nephrons then have decreased ability to eliminate waste

3. ARF follows three phases: initiation, maintenance, and recovery

   a. *Initiation phase:* begins with onset of event causing tubular necrosis; this phase ends when tubular injury occurs

   b. *Maintenance phase:* begins within hours of initiation phase and typically lasts 1 to 2 weeks; it is characterized by persistent reduction in GFR and tubular necrosis

   c. *Recovery phase:* begins when GFR and tubular function have recovered and there is no further elevation of BUN and creatinine; renal function improves rapidly the first 5 to 25 days and continues up to 1 year

4. Signs and symptoms

   a. Initiation: has few manifestations and often is identified after later manifestations have occurred

   b. Maintenance:

      1) **Oliguria** (decreased urine output) is usually present during early maintenance phase; kidney cannot eliminate waste products during this phase, leading to azotemia, fluid retention, electrolyte imbalance, and metabolic acidosis; salt and water retention leads to edema and increased risk for congestive heart failure and pulmonary edema; impaired renal elimination leads to hyperkalemia, hyperphosphatemia, and hypocalcemia; infection is a leading cause of death but other complications include hypertension, neurologic symptoms, GI manifestations, and **uremia,** a syndrome of renal failure (see Table 10-2)

Table 10-2	System	Symptoms
The Multisystem Effects of Uremia	Respiratory	Pulmonary edema, pleuritis, respiratory distress
	Urinary	Hematuria, proteinuria, oliguria, nocturia
	Gastrointestinal	Anorexia, nausea, vomiting, abdominal pain, GI bleeding, uremic fetor
	Endocrine	Hyperparathyroidism, intolerance to glucose
	Musculoskeletal	Bone pain, fractures
	Neurologic	Apathy, lethargy, headache, impaired cognition, insomnia, paresthesias, decreased level of consciousness
	Cardiovascular	Elevated blood pressure, cardiac dysrhythmias, congestive heart failure
	Hematologic	Anemia, difficulty clotting
	Reproductive	Females experience amenorrhea, males experience impotence
	Integumentary	Pallor, uremic frost, dry skin, pruritis, ecchymosis

2) The end of the maintenance phase in oliguric clients is characterized by a progressive increase in urine volume; damaged tubules are repaired; diuresis indicates nephrons are sufficiently recovered

C. Nursing assessment

1. Assessment includes weight; VS (note orthostatic hypotension due to diuretics); hydration status; I&O; identify any underlying causes; assess client's knowledge of disease process, coping methods, and needs; pain status and effect of medications; question client about signs and symptoms of illness as well as past medical history, present and past medications, and family history of kidney disease; common signs and symptoms of renal failure include:

   a. Skin: yellow skin, edema, ecchymosis, uremic frost

   b. ENT: urinous breath

   c. Pulmonary: crackles, effusion, tachypnea

   d. Cardiovascular: hypertension, S_3 or S_4 heart sound, cardiac dysrhythmia

   e. Gastrointestinal: GI bleeding

   f. Neurologic: change in LOC

   g. Neuromuscular: tremors, hyperreflexia

2. Diagnostic tests: electrolytes (hyperkalemia, hyponatremia, hyperphosphatemia), BUN (elevated) and creatinine (elevated), ABGs (metabolic acidosis), CBC (anemia), UA (fixed specific gravity, protein, casts), bladder catheterization, renal ultrasonography, tomography, IVP, renal biopsy

3. Creatinine is more accurate than BUN because it is not affected by dietary protein or fluid status; BUN to creatinine ratio should be 10:1; creatinine does not increase unless 25% of nephrons are not functioning

D. Nursing management

1. Medications

   a. Renal blood flow enhancer: dopamine (Intropin)

   b. Diuretics: furosemide (Lasix) or mannitol (Osmitrol)

   c. Antihypertensives if necessary: ACE inhibitors

   d. Antacids and H_2-receptor blockers to prevent GI ulcer

   e. Potassium-binding exchange resin: polystyrene sulfonate (Kayexelate)

   f. Specific antacid: calcium carbonate (Tums) to control hyperphosphatemia

2. Weigh client at same time daily to document fluid volume status; restrict fluids as ordered

3. Treat infections as soon as possible

4. Record VS and monitor for development of congestive heart failure or pulmonary edema; use semi-Fowler's position to enhance cardiac and respiratory function

5. Monitor lab values

6. Monitor skin status since edema can decrease tissue perfusion and increase risk for skin breakdown

7. Administer medications cautiously as ordered and document effectiveness; avoid any medications that are nephrotoxic or contraindicated in ARF, such as metformin (Glucophage)

8. Document food intake and arrange for a dietary consultation to incorporate requirements (low protein, high carbohydrate [CHO]), restrictions, and client's preferences

9. Explain and answer questions regarding disease process and concerns

10. Teach client to monitor weight, BP, and pulse to assess fluid status

11. Teach client about medications that are nephrotoxic such as NSAIDs, some antibiotics, x-ray contrast, and heavy metals; instruct to avoid magnesium-containing antacids; explain that alcohol ingestion may increase nephrotoxic effects of medications

12. Stress importance of follow-up visits, urinalysis, and bloodwork

VIII. CHRONIC RENAL FAILURE

A. Overview

1. **Chronic renal failure (CRF)** is defined as a progressive inability, over months to years, of kidneys to respond to changes in body fluids and electrolyte composition and an inability to produce sufficient urine; GFR is less than 20% of normal and serum creatinine is greater than 5 mg/dL

2. There are four stages of chronic renal failure (see Box 10-3)

   a. *Early stage* (decreased renal reserve): unaffected nephrons compensate for lost nephrons

   b. *Second stage* (renal insufficiency): more than 25–50% of functional renal tissue is destroyed

   c. *Third stage* (renal failure): GFR is less than 20%

   d. *Fourth stage* (end-stage renal disease [ESRD]): GFR is less than 5%

3. Ideally, conservative treatment is used; educate client and family and explore options for long-term management; when conservative treatment is no longer effective, dialysis or renal transplantation is considered

4. Most common causes of CRF are diabetic nephropathy, hypertension, glomerulonephritis, cystic kidney disease, and urologic disease

B. Pathophysiology

1. Pathophysiologic process of CRF appears as a gradual loss of entire nephron units

2. As functional capacity of entire nephron is lost and renal mass is reduced, there is progressive deterioration of glomerular filtration, tubular secretion and reabsorption; eventually, kidneys are unable to excrete metabolic waste and regulate fluid and electrolyte balance

3. Signs and symptoms

   a. Early stage: clients remain free of symptoms and BUN and creatinine are normal

   b. Second stage: there is a slight rise in BUN and creatinine; few symptoms may be present including oliguria or polyuria, hypertension, and azotemia

Box 10-3	
Stages of Chronic Renal Failure	First: decreased renal reserve (BUN and creatinine are normal)
	Second: renal insufficiency (BUN 20–50 mg/dL)
	Third: renal failure (BUN > 100 mg/dL; Cr > 4 mg/dL)
	Fourth: end-stage renal disease (BUN > 200 mg/dL; Cr > 5 mg dL)

c. Third stage: there is a sharp increase in BUN and creatinine; symptoms of oliguria and uremia are present; there are usually multisystem effects of renal failure such as uremia, metabolic acidosis, and increasing azotemia

d. Fourth stage: there is extreme elevation in BUN and creatinine; client has overt uremia; survival depends on dialysis or transplant

C. Nursing assessment

1. Assessment includes VS, I&O, edema, daily weight, measurement of abdominal girth daily; fluid and dietary restrictions; client's knowledge of disease and support system; knowledge of treatment options; activity level and fatigibility; medication effect and any side effects; and question client regarding end-of-life care

2. Diagnostic tests: BUN (elevated), creatinine (elevated), electrolytes (hyponatremia [may be normal], hyperkalemia, hyperphosphatemia, hypocalcemia), CBC (severe anemia and thrombocytopenia), UA (fixed specific gravity, proteins, blood cells, casts), urine C&S, creatinine clearance (decreased), ABGs (metabolic acidosis), renal ultrasonography, and kidney biopsy

D. Nursing management

1. Medications
   a. Diuretics: usually loop diuretics
   b. Antihypertensives: ACE inhibitors: minoxidil (Loniten), clonidine (Catapress)
   c. Sodium bicarbonate, calcium carbonate (Tums), phosphate-binding agents, calcium supplements, vitamin D
   d. Iron and folic acid supplements; epoetin alfa (Epogen) for anemia
   e. Potassium-binding exchange resin: polystyrene sulfonate (Kayexelate)

2. Maintain fluid and dietary restrictions; refer for dietary consultation if necessary; limit Na^+ and protein, high CHO

3. Administer and document effects/side effects of medications; meds should be administered cautiously; phosphate-binding agents should be avoided

4. Monitor lab values

5. Use standard precautions and good handwashing at all times to decrease transfer of organisms to client

6. Provide oral hygiene at least every 4 hours

7. Monitor activity level and fatigibility

8. Arrange mealtime and activities around procedures and per client preferences

9. Encourage expression of feelings or concerns and assist client in developing realistic goals and coping strategies; refer to mental health counselor if necessary

10. Whether client has arteriovenous fistula or peritoneal dialysis, assess site for signs and symptoms of infection, patency, and check tubing for kinks

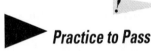

Practice to Pass

A client with CRF asks why he cannot have a drink with his meal tray and why proteins are limited. How should the nurse respond?

IX. BLADDER CANCER

A. Overview

1. Defined as a tumor of bladder; majority of tumors affecting urinary tract arise from epithelial tissue and most common site is urinary bladder

2. Bladder cancer is the fifth most common malignancy and the tenth leading cause of cancer deaths

3. Causes include cigarette smoke, exposure to chemicals and dyes, chronic use of phenacetin-containing analgesic agents

B. Pathophysiology

1. Two major factors are implicated in development of bladder cancer: presence of carcinogens in urine and chronic inflammation or infection of bladder mucosa

2. Urinary tract tumors begin as nonspecific cellular alterations that develop either as flat or papillary lesions that may be invasive or superficial; papillary lesions are characterized by a polyplike structure attached by a stalk to bladder mucosa; papillomas are superficial noninvasive tumors that frequently recur; carcinoma in situ is a poorly differentiated flat tumor that invades directly and has a poor prognosis

3. Signs and symptoms include painless hematuria (most common), which is gross or microscopic, constant or intermittent; symptoms of UTI, and colicky pain

C. Nursing assessment

1. Assessment includes urinary pattern, history of hematuria, pain

   a. Preoperative assessment: assess client's coping mechanisms and concerns; urine output and change in color; fluid intake to keep urine dilute; activity level; urinary catheters, tubing, and drainage system for patency and obstruction; signs and symptoms of infection

   b. Postoperative assessment: I&O; color and consistency of urine (bright red blood may indicate hemorrhage); stoma and surrounding skin (with cystectomy); and pain level

2. Diagnostic tests: UA, urine cytology, IVP, renal ultrasound, CT scan, cystoscopy, and ureteroscopy

D. Nursing management

1. Medications and treatment

   a. Chemotherapy agents may be used either as primary treatment or prophylactically to prevent recurrence; doxorubicin (Adriamycin), mitomycin C (Mutamycin), bacille calmette guerin (BCG Live)

   b. Radiation can reduce tumor size prior to surgery

   c. Surgical procedures range from simple resection to removal of bladder

2. Teach client about disease process, interventions, and postoperative care

3. Monitor I&O carefully, notify health care professional if urine output < 30 mL/hr; irrigate catheter as ordered

4. Monitor lab values, electrolyte, and renal function tests

5. Encourage fluid intake to 3,000 mL/day to dilute urine and decrease irritation

6. Teach family and client about stomal care and catheter care

7. Discuss family/client concerns about activity, sexual relations, and employment; initiate support group or counseling if necessary

8. Teach client/family about signs and symptoms of infection and preventive measures

9. Instruct client on toiletry care after receiving bacille Calmette Guerin (BCG live)

X. KIDNEY CANCER

A. Overview

1. Defined as a tumor of kidney; renal cell cancer is most common primary tumor; another primary tumor is a tumor of renal pelvis; these tumors arise in epithelium of proximal convoluted tubules

    2. Causes include metastasis from lung and breast cancer, melanoma, and malignant lymphoma

B. Pathophysiology

    1. Renal cell tumors metastasize most commonly to lungs, mediastinum, bone, lymph nodes, liver, and central nervous system

    2. Tumor may produce hormones or hormone-like substances, including parathyroid hormones, prostaglandins, prolactin, renin, gonadotropins, and glucocorticoids

    3. Classic triad of symptoms (gross hematuria, flank pain, and a palpable abdominal mass) are seen in only 10% of people with renal cell cancer

    4. Signs and symptoms include microscopic or gross hematuria, flank pain, palpable abdominal mass, fever, fatigue, weight loss, and anemia and/or polycythemia

C. Nursing assessment

    1. Assessment includes pain (level, location, intensity, and character); client's knowledge and understanding of disease and procedures to be performed; lab values; VS; urine output; fluid intake (oral and IV); activity level and fatigue

    2. Postoperative assessment includes incision site for signs/symptoms of inflammation or infection; drainage catheters and tubes for patency; respiratory status and GI function to prevent major complications; potential complications of surgery such as paralytic ileus, thrombosis, and embolus

    3. Diagnostic tests: renal ultrasound (first diagnostic evidence of a kidney tumor); CT scans (provide information about tumor density, extension of tumor and regional lymph node or vascular involvement); chest x-ray, bone scan, and liver function studies are done prior to intervention to evaluate potential metastasis of disease

D. Nursing management

    1. Medications and treatment

        a. Chemotherapy: immunotherapy such as interferon alpha (Roferon-A)

        b. Radiation therapy

        c. Radical nephrectomy (usual treatment); transabdominal approach

    2. Instruct on signs and symptoms of infection

    3. Teach client to maintain fluid intake 2,000 to 2,500 mL/day and increase during hot weather or exercise

    4. Instruct client to void when urge is experienced, and before and after intercourse

    5. Teach client to avoid trauma to remaining kidney

    6. Continue to encourage family and client to discuss feelings and concerns

    7. Instruct about home medications, wound care, diet, and activity

    8. Refer to support services if appropriate

    9. Stress importance of follow-up visits and scheduled bloodwork; instruct to report decreased urine output, fever, or abdominal pain

Case Study

L. J. is a 45-year-old construction worker who experienced a large myocardial infarction with cardiovascular complications. On day 3 of his hospital stay, the nurse notices his urine output is being maintained at 20 to 25 mL/hr. Another symptom is edema. His potassium (K^+) is 5.2 mg/L, sodium (Na^+) is 125 mEq/L, ABGs show pH 7.25, PCO_2 38, HCO_3^- 21). The BUN is 28, Cr is 2.5 mg/dL, and lung sounds reveal soft crackles. He is diagnosed with acute renal failure (ARF).

1. What do L. J.'s ABGs show and is this common with ARF? Why or why not?

2. What is significant about his electrolytes in relation to his cardiac condition?

3. What phase of ARF is L. J. in, and what can the nurse tell him is the expected time frame until the kidneys are hopefully working properly again?

4. Considering his initial diagnosis, presenting signs and symptoms, and the known complications of ARF, what is the greatest cardiovascular concern for L. J.?

5. Should L. J. be given a low-sodium or high-sodium diet? Why or why not?

For suggested responses, see page 536.

POSTTEST

1 A urinalysis is ordered for a client with urinary calculi. The nurse anticipates that which of the following is usually positive on the urinalysis report?

1. Leukocytes
2. Nitrite
3. Protein
4. Blood

2 The nurse considers that a 40-year-old male client is at high risk for which of the following disorders if his father also experienced this problem?

1. Glomerulonephritis
2. Renal failure
3. Polycystic kidney disease
4. Urinary tract infection

3 The client has a temperature of 102 degrees F and the urinalysis reveals a white blood count of 14,000/mm^3. Further diagnostic testing pinpoints the origin in the kidney. The nurse concludes the client most likely has which of the following disorders?

1. Acute pyelonephritis
2. Renal failure
3. Chronic pyelonephritis
4. Urinary calculi

4 A client is diagnosed with chronic pyelonephritis. The nurse explains to the client that it will be important to have ongoing monitoring for which of the following? Select all that apply.

1. Severely high blood pressure
2. Elevated body temperature
3. Hyperlipidemia
4. Renal failure
5. Sexually transmitted diseases

5 A client with pharyngitis has had a throat culture done. After the health care provider prescribes oral penicillin, the nurse explains that this medication will help to prevent development of acute glomerulonephritis from which of the following microorganisms?

1. *Group-A beta Hemolytic-streptococcus*
2. *Staphylococcus*
3. *E. coli*
4. *Proteus*

POSTTEST

6 The nurse interprets that which of the following clients is at highest risk for a urinary tract infection (UTI)?

1. 79-year-old female
2. 45-year-old male
3. 14-year-old female
4. 27-year-old male

7 During interdisciplinary rounds on a client with rapidly progressive glomerulonephritis, the health care provider describes that crescent-shaped lesions form and obliterate Bowman's space. During subsequent nursing care, what problem or problems should the nurse alert for?

1. Azotemia and hematuria
2. Renal colic and flank pain
3. Hypotension and tachycardia
4. Polyuria with urgency and frequency

8 A 19-year-old female client is diagnosed with an uncomplicated urinary tract infection. In addition to antibiotic therapy, the nurse will encourage which of the following?

1. Tub baths or saunas for relaxation and comfort
2. Increasing fluids to 2 to 2.5 liters per day
3. Avoiding sexual intercourse
4. Using acetaminophen (Tylenol) for pain

9 Because an older adult may not complain of dysuria with a urinary tract infection (UTI), the nurse should be alert for what other manifestations of infection? Select all that apply.

1. Incontinence
2. Cloudy urine
3. Diluted, clear urine
4. Foul-smelling urine
5. Ketonuria

10 The nurse would teach the client who has a urinary tract infection about which of the following helpful self-care measures?

1. Taking medication until feeling better
2. Restricting fluids
3. Decreasing caffeine drinks and alcohol
4. Douching daily

➤ *See pages 316–317 for Answers & Rationales.*

ANSWERS & RATIONALES

Pretest

1 **Answer: 2** Pyelonephritis is an upper urinary tract infection, involving the kidney tissue. Lower urinary tract infections include urethritis, prostatitis, and cystitis. The most common upper urinary tract infection is pyelonephritis.
Cognitive Level: Application **Client Need:** Physiological Integrity: Physiological Adaptation **Integrated Process:** Nursing Process: Analysis **Content Area:** Adult Health: Renal and Genitourinary **Strategy:** A critical word in the stem is *upper*. Review anatomy of the urinary tract and eliminate the options that apply to the lower urinary tract. **Reference:** Lemone, P., & Burke, K. (2008). *Medical-surgical nursing: Critical thinking in client care* (4th ed.). Upper Saddle River, NJ: Pearson/Prentice Hall, pp. 847–849.

2 **Answer: 3** *E. coli* from the lower GI tract is the infective organism in over 90% of first-time infections. The nurse should check that the organism is sensitive to the antibiotic or notify the health care provider.

Cognitive Level: Application **Client Need:** Physiological Integrity: Reduction of Risk Potential **Integrated Process:** Nursing Process: Assessment **Content Area:** Adult Health: Renal and Genitourinary **Strategy:** Consider the anatomy of a female and the proximity of the urinary meatus to the anus. **Reference:** Lemone, P., & Burke, K. (2008). *Medical-surgical nursing: Critical thinking in client care* (4th ed.). Upper Saddle River, NJ: Pearson/Prentice Hall, pp. 846–847.

3 **Answer: 4** Due to the anatomic structure of the male urethra and bacteriostatic effect of prostatic fluid, all urinary tract infections in the male client should be considered complicated. UTIs are more likely to be uncomplicated in females.
Cognitive Level: Application **Client Need:** Physiological Integrity: Physiological Adaptation **Integrated Process:** Nursing Process: Analysis **Content Area:** Adult Health: Renal and Genitourinary **Strategy:** Consider the normal anatomy of the GU system. Which client is least likely to be infected? That client's infection has contributing factors. **Reference:** Porth, C. M. (2005). *Pathophysiology:*

Concepts of altered health states (7th ed.). Philadelphia, PA: Lippincott Williams & Wilkins, pp. 818–821.

4 **Answer: 2** The presence of leukocytes (pyuria) means the host has an immune response to the infection instead of just an asymptomatic bacterial colonization. A gram stain is needed to determine the type of bacteria (gram + or −). Urine may have a foul odor and appear cloudy because of the presence of mucus and excess white cells, but the presence of pyuria does not mean the urine will have the characteristic in option 4. **Cognitive Level:** Analysis **Client Need:** Physiological Integrity: Physiological Adaptation **Integrated Process:** Nursing Process: Analysis **Content Area:** Adult Health: Renal and Genitourinary **Strategy:** First define pyuria (WBCs in the urine) and then determine what biological response is needed to get WBCs in the urine. Recognize that a clinical clue is in the diagnosis given in the question. **Reference:** Porth, C. M. (2005). *Pathophysiology: Concepts of altered health states* (7th ed.). Philadelphia, PA: Lippincott Williams & Wilkins, p. 820.

5 **Answers: 2, 3, 4** Prevention requires analysis of the stone to determine the formation. Depending on the type, dietary changes to limit calcium oxalates and measures to acidify pH will lower the risk of recurrence. Adequate fluid makes the dilute urine less likely to form crystals. Concentrated urine and high doses of vitamin D increase the risk of renal calculi. **Cognitive Level:** Application **Client Need:** Physiological Integrity: Physiological Adaptation **Integrated Process:** Teaching/Learning **Content Area:** Adult Health: Renal and Genitourinary **Strategy:** Recall that when there are opposite options, they both cannot be correct. Apply knowledge of saturated solutions and crystal formation to the question. **Reference:** Porth, C. M. (2005). *Pathophysiology: Concepts of altered health states* (7th ed.). Philadelphia, PA: Lippincott Williams & Wilkins, pp. 815, 817.

6 **Answer: 2** Red blood cell casts are not present in the normal urinalysis but are present in glomerular diseases, which are the leading causes of chronic renal failure. Cystitis does not indicate glomerular involvement. Glomerulonephritis presents with hypertension, cola-colored urine, azotemia, and water retention. A BUN of 15 is normal and not indicative of azotemia. **Cognitive Level:** Application **Client Need:** Physiological Integrity: Physiological Adaptation **Integrated Process:** Nursing Process: Assessment **Content Area:** Adult Health: Renal and Genitourinary **Strategy:** Recall that normal renal glomeruli do not allow proteins and blood cells to filter into the urine. Review normal lab values if needed. **Reference:** Lemone, P., & Burke, K. (2008). *Medical-surgical nursing: Critical thinking in client care*

(4th ed.). Upper Saddle River, NJ: Pearson/Prentice Hall, p. 886.

7 **Answer: 3** Iatrogenic causes result from treatment from a physician or other health care provider. Examples include nephrotoxic medications, radiologic contrast dye, and shock after surgery. Alcohol use, diet, and exercise and client-related factors that may or may not apply. **Cognitive Level:** Application **Client Need:** Physiological Integrity: Physiological Adaptation **Integrated Process:** Nursing Process: Assessment **Content Area:** Adult Health: Renal and Genitourinary **Strategy:** Knowing the definition of *iatrogenic* helps to eliminate the incorrect options. Review medical terminology if this is a weak area. **Reference:** Lemone, P., & Burke, K. (2008). *Medical-surgical nursing: Critical thinking in client care* (4th ed.). Upper Saddle River, NJ: Pearson/Prentice Hall, p. 762.

8 **Answer: 3** In renal failure, 90% or more of the nephrons are destroyed and glomerular filtration rate (GFR) is < 20% of normal with increased creatinine and BUN, edema, and hyperkalemia. In end stage renal disease (ESRD), the GFR is < 5% of normal. Until now, this client has had renal insufficiency but was probably adapting without symptoms. The other options are not related to a reduced GFR. **Cognitive Level:** Application **Client Need:** Physiological Integrity: Physiological Adaptation **Integrated Process:** Nursing Process: Assessment **Content Area:** Adult Health: Renal and Genitourinary **Strategy:** Apply knowledge of GFR to aid in deciding what the client's problem is. **Reference:** Porth, C. M. (2005). *Pathophysiology: Concepts of altered health states* (7th ed.). Philadelphia, PA: Lippincott Williams & Wilkins, pp. 838–839.

9 **Answer: 2** Although it can be influenced by hydration status and protein intake, the BUN is a good indicator of kidney function because most renal diseases interfere with urea excretion and cause blood levels to rise. Creatinine is produced in relatively constant amounts, according to the amount of muscle mass, and is excreted entirely by the kidneys, making it an excellent indicator of renal function. CBC, ALT, and glucose do not indicate renal function. Although electrolytes are affected by renal function, other etiologies are possible. Note that the "Chem 6" lab test includes electrolytes, BUN, and creatinine. **Cognitive Level:** Application **Client Need:** Physiological Integrity: Reduction of Risk Potential **Integrated Process:** Nursing Process: Analysis **Content Area:** Adult Health: Renal and Genitourinary **Strategy:** Review the normal reference ranges for common laboratory tests if this question was difficult. What compounds do healthy kidneys eliminate, keeping the blood levels down? **Reference:** Porth, C. M. (2005). *Pathophysiology: Concepts* *of altered health states* (7th ed.). Philadelphia, PA: Lippincott Williams & Wilkins, p. 839.

10 Answer: 2 In ESRD with signs and symptoms of uremia, dialysis or organ transplantation is needed for survival. Loop diuretics will not be effective at this stage. Since medical treatment is available, it is premature to anticipate the imminent need to provide postmortem care. **Cognitive Level:** Application **Client Need:** Physiological Integrity: Physiological Adaptation **Integrated Process:** Nursing Process: Planning **Content Area:** Adult Health: Renal and Genitourinary **Strategy:** Recall that ESRD is a step worse than renal failure, and very few nephrons are functioning. With this in mind, select the option that provides a replacement mechanism for renal filtration and excretion of fluid and metabolic wastes. **Reference:** Porth, C. M. (2005). *Pathophysiology: Concepts of altered health states* (7th ed.). Philadelphia, PA: Lippincott Williams & Wilkins, p. 839.

Posttest

1 Answer: 4 Hematuria, either gross or microscopic, is generally present in clients with urinary calculi. Leukocytes, nitrites, and protein may be common with other urinary disorders. **Cognitive Level:** Application **Client Need:** Physiological Integrity: Reduction of Risk Potential **Integrated Process:** Nursing Process: Assessment **Content Area:** Adult Health: Renal and Genitourinary **Strategy:** Recall that calculi are not infections but cause trauma to the ureter. This trauma can cause bleeding, resulting in hematuria. **Reference:** Porth, C. M. (2005). *Pathophysiology: Concepts of altered health states* (7th ed.). Philadelphia, PA: Lippincott Williams & Wilkins, p. 816.

2 Answer: 3 Adult polycystic kidney disease is an autosomal dominant disorder. In children, it is caused by an autosomal recessive trait. Glomerulonephritis, renal failure, and urinary tract infections are not inherited disorders. **Cognitive Level:** Application **Client Need:** Physiological Integrity: Physiological Adaptation **Integrated Process:** Nursing Process: Assessment **Content Area:** Adult Health: Renal and Genitourinary **Strategy:** The core issue of the question is an understanding of which disorder is inherited. Eliminate the ones that are not. **Reference:** Porth, C. M. (2005). *Pathophysiology: Concepts of altered health states* (7th ed.). Philadelphia, PA: Lippincott Williams & Wilkins, p. 811.

3 Answer: 1 Acute pyelonephritis is a bacterial infection of the kidney. Infection is characterized by an elevation in WBC count and fever. Chronic pyelonephritis is associated with nonbacterial infections and noninfectious processes that may be metabolic, chemical, or immunological.

Cognitive Level: Application **Integrated Process:** Nursing Process: Analysis **Client Need:** Physiological Integrity: Physiological Adaptation **Content Area:** Adult Health: Renal and Genitourinary **Strategy:** Recall that elevated WBCs are seen with infection and that the suffix *–itis* refers to inflammation and/or infection. Note the high temperature to determine that this is an acute process rather than a chronic one. **Reference:** Porth, C. M. (2005). *Pathophysiology: Concepts of altered health states* (7th ed.). Philadelphia, PA: Lippincott Williams & Wilkins, pp. 828–829.

4 Answers: 1, 4 Severe hypertension may develop as renal tissue is destroyed (secondary hypertension). Chronic pyelonephritis is a significant etiology of renal failure. It is a condition of inflammation and scarring, not bacterial infection, and will not have impact on body temperature. STDs and lipid abnormalities are not consequences. **Cognitive Level:** Application **Client Need:** Physiological Integrity: Physiological Adaptation **Integrated Process:** Teaching/Learning **Content Area:** Adult Health: Renal and Genitourinary **Strategy:** Note the critical word *chronic,* which differentiates the client's problem from an acute problem. Recall the difference in pathophysiology between these to make an accurate selection. **Reference:** Porth, C. M. (2005). *Pathophysiology: Concepts of altered health states* (7th ed.). Philadelphia, PA: Lippincott Williams & Wilkins, p. 829.

5 Answer: 1 Infection of the pharynx or skin with *group-A beta Hemolytic-streptococcus* is the common precipitating factor for acute glomerulonephritis. **Cognitive Level:** Application **Client Need:** Physiological Integrity: Physiological Adaptation **Integrated Process:** Teaching/Learning **Content Area:** Adult Health: Renal and Genitourinary **Strategy:** Apply knowledge of microbiology in identifying the pathogen. This is a critical point and one that should be committed to memory if this question was difficult. **Reference:** Lemone, P., & Burke, K. (2008). *Medical-surgical nursing: Critical thinking in client care* (4th ed.). Upper Saddle River, NJ: Pearson/Prentice Hall, p. 886.

6 Answer: 1 Risk factors for UTIs include female gender, older age, urinary obstruction or calculi, strictures, chronic disease, prostatic hyperplasia and prostatitis, diaphragm use, instrumentation, and impaired immune system. Although children and teenagers can contract a UTI, incontinence and disease conditions in the elderly make them a higher risk population. **Cognitive Level:** Analysis **Client Need:** Physiological Integrity: Physiological Adaptation **Integrated Process:** Nursing Process: Assessment **Content Area:** Adult Health: Renal and Genitourinary **Strategy:** The difference in the options are ages of the client and the genders. Determine which age or gender is at highest risk. **Reference:** Lemone, P., & Burke, K. (2008). *Medical-surgical nursing: Critical thinking in client care* (4th ed.). Upper Saddle River, NJ: Pearson/Prentice Hall, p. 846.

7 **Answer: 1** Glomerular cells proliferate along with macrophages to form crescent-shaped lesions obliterating Bowman's space, resulting in a rapid decline in glomerular filtration rate (GFR), which leads to azotemia and many of the complications of severe glomerular injury such as hypertension, oliguria, and hematuria. Renal colic and flank pain would occur with renal calculi. Hypertension, not hypotension, is more likely to affect a client with renal disease. Polyuria is the opposite of what occurs with glomerulonephritis, and urgency and frequency would accompany urinary tract infection. **Cognitive Level:** Analysis **Client Need:** Physiological Integrity: Physiological Adaptation **Integrated Process:** Nursing Process: Assessment **Content Area:** Adult Health: Renal and Genitourinary **Strategy:** Recall the physiology of Bowman's space and the pathophysiology of glomerulonephritis. With these concepts in mind, consider that the correct answer would reflect declining renal function as well as hematuria because of the suffix *–itis*. **Reference:** Porth, C. M. (2005). *Pathophysiology: Concepts of altered health states* (7th ed.). Philadelphia, PA: Lippincott Williams & Wilkins, pp. 823–824.

8 **Answer: 2** Increasing fluid intake may relieve signs and symptoms of UTI as an adjunct to the antibiotics. Tub baths may contribute to the infection. Although some data suggests sexual intercourse may contribute to UTIs, the risk can be lowered by emptying the bladder after intercourse. Antibiotic therapy, not acetaminophen, will be effective in relieving the pain associated with UTIs. **Cognitive Level:** Application **Client Need:** Physiological Integrity: Physiological Adaptation **Integrated Process:** Nursing Process: Planning **Content Area:** Adult Health: Renal and Genitourinary **Strategy:** Consider what action

helps to eliminate the bacteria from the bladder and what actions are contraindicated. **Reference:** Porth, C. M. (2005). *Pathophysiology: Concepts of altered health states* (7th ed.). Philadelphia, PA: Lippincott Williams & Wilkins, pp. 820–821.

9 **Answer: 1, 2, 4** Immune responses diminish with aging, reducing the irritative symptoms of a UTI. The nurse must be alert for cloudy, malodorous urine or incontinence. Ketones would be present when there is fat breakdown, usually as a result of diabetic ketoacidosis, dieting with severe calorie restriction, or starvation. **Cognitive Level:** Application **Client Need:** Physiological Integrity: Physiological Adaptation **Integrated Process:** Nursing Process: Assessment **Content Area:** Adult Health: Renal and Genitourinary **Strategy:** Eliminate one of the options that represents opposites and choose findings consistent with a UTI. **Reference:** Lemone, P., & Burke, K. (2008). *Medical-surgical nursing: Critical thinking in client care* (4th ed.). Upper Saddle River, NJ: Pearson/Prentice Hall, p. 873.

10 **Answer: 3** Caffeine and alcohol can increase bladder spasms and mucosal irritation, thus increase the signs and symptoms of a urinary tract infection (UTI). Fluids should be increased rather than restricted, and douches will not help a UTI. Antibiotics should be taken completely for the full course of therapy to prevent development of resistant strains of organisms. **Cognitive Level:** Application **Client Need:** Health Promotion and Maintenance **Integrated Process:** Teaching/Learning **Content Area:** Adult Health: Renal and Genitourinary **Strategy:** Recall the prime treatment for UTI includes antibiotic therapy and that classic adjunct measures are increasing fluid intake, acidifying the urine, and preventing further irritation. Evaluate each option in light of these and use the process of elimination to make a selection. **Reference:** Lemone, P., & Burke, K. (2008). *Medical-surgical nursing: Critical thinking in client care* (4th ed.). Upper Saddle River, NJ: Pearson/Prentice Hall, pp. 852–854.

References

Corbett, J. V. (2004). *Laboratory tests and diagnostic procedures* (6th ed.). Upper Saddle River, NJ: Prentice Hall.

Lemone, P., & Burke, K. (2008). *Medical-surgical nursing: Critical thinking in client care* (4th ed.). Upper Saddle River, NJ: Prentice Hall.

Porth, C. (2005). *Pathophysiology: Concepts of altered health states* (7th ed.). Philadelphia: Lippincott Williams & Wilkins, pp. 809–865.

Wilson, B. A., Shannon, M. T., & Stang, C. L. (2006). *Nursing drug guide: 2006.* Upper Saddle River, NJ: Prentice Hall.

ANSWERS & RATIONALES

11 Male and Female Reproductive Health Problems

Chapter Outline

Risk Factors Associated with Male and Female Reproductive Health Problems

Male Reproductive Health Problems

Female Reproductive Health Problems

Sexually Transmitted Infections (STIs)

Objectives

➤ Define key terms associated with male and female reproductive health problems.

➤ Identify risk factors associated with the development of male and female reproductive health problems.

➤ Explain the common etiologies of male and female reproductive health problems.

➤ Describe the pathophysiologic processes associated with specific male and female reproductive health problems.

➤ Distinguish between normal and abnormal male and female reproductive findings obtained from nursing assessment.

➤ Prioritize nursing interventions associated with specific male and female reproductive health problems.

NCLEX-RN® Test Prep

Use the CD-ROM enclosed with this book to access additional practice opportunities.

Review at a Glance

adenomyosis condition in which endometrium is present between myometrial cells

balanitis infection or inflammation of foreskin

benign prostatic hyperplasia (BPH) enlargement of prostate gland from noncancerous hyperplasia

cryptorchidism undescended testicle

dysfunctional uterine bleeding (DUB) condition causing irregular menstrual bleeding from lack of progesterone

dysmenorrhea painful menstruation

dyspareunia painful intercourse

endometriosis condition in which endometrium implants are present outside uterus

epispadias condition in which urethral meatus is located on upper (dorsal) aspect of penis instead of tip of shaft; may be located just above penile tip or anywhere along shaft

hypospadias condition in which urethral meatus is located on lower (ventral) aspect of penis instead of tip of shaft; may be located just below penile tip or anywhere along shaft

menorrhagia excessive or heavy menstrual flow

metrorrhagia irregular, frequent menstrual bleeding of abnormal amounts

myoma uterine muscle tumor

orchiectomy removal of a testicle

pelvic inflammatory disease (PID) inflammation of uterus, fallopian tubes, and ovaries

phimosis unretractable foreskin that may impede or prohibit urine flow

prostate specific antigen (PSA) blood test to measure antigen produced by prostate cancer

PRETEST

1 The nurse would question a client with balanitis about complaints of which of the following?

1. Vaginal discharge
2. Pain with urination
3. Spontaneous urethral discharge
4. Back pain

2 The nurse would assess the client experiencing prostatitis for which of the following symptoms?

1. Urinary retention or incontinence
2. Painful blisters and crater-like lesions, enlarged groin nodes, fever
3. Brownish rash on palms, painful crater-like lesions, malaise, and fever
4. Rectal pain, pain with erection, low abdominal pain, and low back pain

3 A male client in the ambulatory clinic reports that a female sexual partner from about five months ago has been diagnosed with syphilis. If the client became infected during this relationship, the nurse would expect him to have which of the following at this time?

1. Painless sore that healed and a rash on the palms of his hands
2. Negative VDRL, negative rapid plasma reagin (RPR), and positive fluorescent treponemal antibody absorption (FTA-ABS)
3. Night sweats, cough, low-grade fever, and elevated white count
4. Penile discharge, dysuria, and urinary frequency

4 The nurse concludes that teaching has been effective when the mother of an infant born with hypospadias says, "Our son will:

1. Need surgical correction so that he looks like the other boys."
2. Require circumcision now to prevent complications later."
3. Have surgical correction so he will be fertile as an adult."
4. Likely have other reproductive tract anomalies we can't see."

5 The nurse is preparing to teach a client who has dysfunctional uterine bleeding (DUB). Which medication would the nurse expect to include in the teaching plan?

1. Testosterone
2. Estrogen
3. Steroids
4. Progesterone

6 In preparing to discharge a client with gonococcal pelvic inflammatory disease (PID), the nurse determines that teaching was successful if the client makes which statement(s)? Select all that apply.

1. "I should douche after every episode of intercourse."
2. "Using condoms will decrease the risk of this happening again."
3. "My boyfriend and I should be monogamous."
4. "The sexual position I use won't prevent this infection."
5. "Voiding after intercourse will help prevent PID."

7 A 23-year-old male client has been diagnosed with testicular cancer. Which of the following should the nurse include in his teaching plan?

1. Future fertility is not affected by treatment
2. Impotence often results from needed treatments
3. Sperm banking should be done prior to treatment
4. Sexual interest is likely to increase as a result of successful treatment

8 The nurse working with a female client who has fibrocystic breast disease expects the client to report a diet high in which of the following?

1. Bacon, sausage, and ground meat
2. Fresh fruits and whole grain cereal
3. Cheese and milk
4. Coffee and cola

9 A male client has been diagnosed with *Chlamydia trachomatis* infection. The nurse should include which of the following when developing the plan of care?

1. Instructions to take all of the doxycycline (Vibra-tabs) that was ordered
2. Encouragement to use condoms with most episodes of intercourse
3. Obtaining the names of sexual contacts if client desires
4. Teaching testicular self-exam (TSE) for self-diagnosis

10 The client has a diagnosis of primary dysmenorrhea. Which of the following would the nurse expect to find when taking the client's history?

1. Heavy flow and clots for at least three months
2. Irregular menses with breakthrough bleeding
3. Painful periods since menarche
4. No periods for the last seven months

➤ *See pages 341–343 for Answers & Rationales.*

I. RISK FACTORS ASSOCIATED WITH MALE AND FEMALE REPRODUCTIVE HEALTH PROBLEMS

A. **Multiple sexual partners** increase risk of sexually transmitted infections and subsequent problems

B. **Smoking creates endothelial cell changes** that predispose cells to more radical changes from viruses such as human papilloma virus (HPV) or precancerous conditions and cancer

C. **Obesity increases amount of fat-soluble hormones** (such as estrogen), chemicals, and illicit drugs in tissues, which increases risk of cellular changes in reproductive tract

D. **Alcohol use** is associated with increased numbers of sexual partners and sexual assault

E. **Illicit drug use** is also associated with increased numbers of sexual partners and sexual assault, and some drugs (marijuana, cocaine, heroin) are fat-soluble, leading to long-term storage of drugs in fatty tissues of body for weeks to months after last ingestion of drug; this can lead to greater effects on reproductive tract such as decreased spermatogenesis

F. **Ionizing radiation** can disrupt normal cell division associated with oogenesis and spermatogenesis, leading to changes in genetic structure of gametes

G. **Chemical exposure** from occupational hazards or misuse of household chemicals can decrease sperm count, motility, and change morphology, as well as cause menstrual cycle changes

H. **Specific conditions**

1. Urethral disorders: congenital

2. Prostatitis: urinary catheterization or similar procedures, consumption of alcohol, caffeine, and spicy foods

3. Benign prostatic hyperplasia: age

4. Prostate cancer: age, ethnicity, chemical/environmental exposures

5. Testicular cancer: history of **cryptorchidism** (undescended testicle), trauma, estrogen administration to mother during pregnancy such as diethylstilbestrol (DES), decreased birth weight, prematurity, family history

6. Uterine bleeding: age, family history, stress, weight change, oral contraceptives, intrauterine device (IUD)

7. Dysmenorrhea: smoking, non-use of oral contraception, early menarche

8. Pelvic inflammatory disease (PID): use of IUD, oral contraceptives, and condoms, sexually transmitted infections (STI), multiple sex partners, previous PID

9. Endometriosis: nulliparity, family history

10. Benign breast disease: age

11. Breast cancer: age, family history (first-degree relative with breast cancer), ethnicity (Caucasian or African American), previous chest area radiation (i.e., treatment for Hodgkin's disease), menarche before age 12 or menopause after age 50, use of hormone replacement therapy over 5 years, nulliparous or first pregnancy after age 30, never breastfed, daily alcohol use, obesity

12. Sexually transmitted infections: unprotected sex, multiple sex partners, intravenous (IV) drug use, use of street drugs

II. MALE REPRODUCTIVE HEALTH PROBLEMS

A. **Urethral disorders**

1. Overview

   a. **Hypospadias:** urethral meatus is located on lower (ventral) aspect of penis instead of tip of shaft; may be located just below penile tip or anywhere along shaft

   b. **Epispadias:** urethral meatus is located on upper (dorsal) aspect of penis instead of tip of shaft; may be located just above penile tip or anywhere along shaft

   c. **Phimosis:** unretractable foreskin, which impedes or prohibits urine flow

   d. **Balanitis:** infection or inflammation of foreskin

   e. Urethritis: inflammation of urethra

   f. Causes

      1) Hypospadias and epispadias: congenital

      2) Phimosis: congenital or secondary to infection or injury

      3) Balanitis: improper hygiene

      4) Urethritis: insertion of an instrument/catheter, gonococcal infection

2. Pathophysiology

    a. Developmental anomalies

        1) Hypospadias and epispadias develop when urinary tract forms during embryological development

        2) Eight percent of men have a father or brother with same condition

        3) Occurs in about 1 in 250 males

        4) Phimosis is an acquired stenosis of intact foreskin resulting in an inability to retract foreskin

    b. Inflammatory processes

        1) Balanitis occurs as a result of overgrowth of normal flora under intact foreskin caused by lack of hygiene

        2) Urethritis is most common urinary tract infection (UTI)

    c. Signs and symptoms

        1) Hypospadias and epispadias: visual deformity noted

        2) Phimosis: secondary infections and scarring; edema and pain of glans penis (if constriction occurs); necrosis of glans

        3) Balanitis: redness, swelling, and pain of penis; foul odor and purulent drainage; dysuria

        4) Urethritis: painful urination; discharge from penis

3. Nursing assessment

    a. Assessment includes: physical examination of urethral meatus, color and retractability of foreskin; characteristics of urine; VS (especially temperature); amount of urine; report of discomfort during voiding; presence of discharge

    b. Diagnostic tests: urinalysis or UA (preferably clean catch); culture and sensitivity (C&S)

4. Nursing management

    a. Medications

        1) Urethritis: oral antibiotics, analgesics

        2) Balanitis: topical or oral antibiotic or antifungal

        3) Phimosis: topical steroid application

    b. Teach client about cause of problem

    c. Teach client hygiene measures to prevent recurrence

    d. Males with intact foreskin should be taught to retract foreskin prior to voiding, wipe glans dry after voiding, and then replace foreskin; additionally, glans of penis should be retracted, cleansed, dried, and replaced after intercourse and during daily bathing

    e. Instruct client in proper use of medications, including route, amount, and frequency of use

    f. Surgical correction may be undertaken in early childhood if urethral opening is along shaft of penis, primarily to promote fertility in adulthood

    g. Treatment of phimosis may consist of stretching under local anesthetic; circumcision may be required

B. Prostatitis

    1. Overview

        a. Most common form is acute prostatitis, a bacterial infection

> **▶ Practice to Pass**
>
> The client with hypospadias asks if his sons will have the condition. How should the nurse respond?

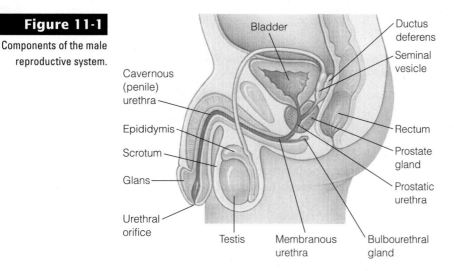

Figure 11-1

Components of the male reproductive system.

Labels: Bladder, Ductus deferens, Seminal vesicle, Cavernous (penile) urethra, Epididymis, Scrotum, Glans, Urethral orifice, Testis, Membranous urethra, Rectum, Prostate gland, Prostatic urethra, Bulbourethral gland

    b. Chronic prostatitis can be bacterial or noninfectious

    c. Can be acute or chronic bacterial or nonbacterial that is chronic in nature

    d. Causes include trauma, autoimmune response, gonorrhea, bacterial infection

2. Pathophysiology

    a. Prostate gland (see Figure 11-1) secretes a thin, alkaline fluid that is part of seminal secretion

    b. Is not well-understood; bacteria from rectum or infected urine invade prostate

    c. Not considered sexually transmitted

    d. Signs and symptoms

        1) Acute: chills, fever, urinary (dysuria, frequency, urgency, hematuria); pain (suprapubic, perineal, scrotal, lower back, rectal); discharge; enlarged prostate that is tender and warm; palpable seminal vesicles; blood and pus in urine; pain during ejaculation

        2) Chronic and nonbacterial: may be asymptomatic; low-grade fever; pain; nocturia; dysuria

3. Nursing assessment

    a. Assessment includes obtaining a history on onset, severity, and precipitating factors of symptoms; inspection of urine; VS; symptom analysis of pain

    b. Diagnostic tests: urinalysis, physical examination, urine C&S

4. Nursing management

    a. Medications include antibiotics

    b. Educate client about cause and treatment plan

    c. Instruct client to avoid caffeine and alcohol (irritants)

C. Benign prostatic hyperplasia (BPH)

    1. Overview

        a. **Benign prostatic hyperplasia (BPH)** is defined as a noncancerous enlargement of prostate gland because of hyperplasia or hypertrophy (see Figure 11-2)

        b. Begins around age 40 but usually not symptomatic until 60 years and older

        c. Causes include aging process

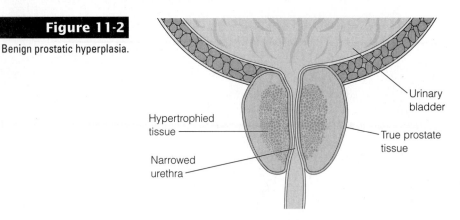

2. Pathophysiology
   a. Results from decreased testosterone and increased estrogen levels
   b. Prostate cells increase in size and in number
   c. Causes pressure on and decreases diameter of urethra
   d. Although androgen levels decrease as male ages, the prostate gland is still sensitive to presence of dihydrotestosterone (DHT), which causes growth of prostate gland
   e. May be asymptomatic until acute onset inhibits opening of bladder sphincter; excess alcohol intake can be a trigger
   f. Signs and symptoms include incomplete bladder emptying, difficulty starting the stream and weak stream; nocturia; feeling of fullness in bladder; increased urinary time; dribbling of urine

3. Nursing assessment
   a. Assessment includes client history related to urinating; symptom analysis of urinary problems; characteristics of urine
   b. Diagnostic tests: biopsy of prostate; physical examination; ultrasonography; urinalysis; serum creatinine (Cr) and blood urea nitrogen (BUN)

4. Nursing management
   a. Medications include finasteride (Proscar), which inhibits testosterone conversion to dihydrotestosterone; alpha-adrenergic antagonist; phytotherapy (newer treatment) with saw palmetto berry, echinacea, and hypoxis rooperi
   b. Instruct client to avoid alcohol use, and report increased urinary symptoms
   c. If transurethral resection of prostate (TURP) is indicated, educate client as to
      1) Nature of surgical procedure and regional anesthesia
      2) Recovery, including continuous bladder irrigation (to prevent clotting) and going home with an indwelling urinary catheter
      3) Potential for bladder spasms
      4) Avoidance of nonsteroidal antiinflammatory drugs (NSAIDs) for 10 days preoperative
      5) Newer treatments that are less invasive: balloon urethroplasty, laser energy microwave hyperthermia, intraurethral stents

D. **Prostate cancer**
   1. Overview
      a. Average age at diagnosis is 65

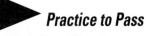

Practice to Pass

The client with benign prostatic hyperplasia with transurethral resection of the prostate (TURP) scheduled in 1 week calls to ask if there are any over-the-counter (OTC) medications that he shouldn't take. How should the nurse reply?

      b. Usually slow growing, often asymptomatic in early stages

      c. African-American men are 50% more likely to develop prostate cancer than Caucasian men; incidence is increased if first-degree relative has prostate cancer

      d. Causes include genetic disposition, history of STIs, high-fat diet; hormones; often unknown

2. Pathophysiology

      a. Single or multiple areas within prostate gland develop proliferative cancer and enlarge gland both outward toward capsule and then inward toward urethra (see Table 11-1)

      b. Causes are similar to benign prostatic hyperplasia

      c. Extension of cancer outside of prostate gland capsule may also occur, first into seminal vesicles

      d. Compression of urethra by tumor may cause urinary symptoms

      e. Common sites of metastases: lymph nodes, bones, lungs, liver

      f. Cancer of prostate is testosterone-dependent early in course of disease

      g. Signs and symptoms include urinary problems (increased frequency, urgency, reduction in stream, nocturia, hematuria); blood during ejaculation; back pain; pain of joints and bone if metastasis occurs; weight loss; fatigue; client may be asymptomatic

3. Nursing assessment

      a. Assessment includes

         1) History of urinary symptoms as in BPH; question client for known risk factors

         2) Symptom analysis of pain (hips, low back, abdomen, pelvis)

         3) Assess weight, energy level, sexual function/problems

         4) Symptom analysis on urinary status

      b. Diagnostic tests

         1) Screening utilizes **prostate specific antigen (PSA)** blood tests (PSA should be less than or equal to 4.0)

Table 11-1	Stages of Prostate Cancer		
Stage	**Location of Cancer**	**Symptoms**	**Diagnosis**
1	Prostate only	Asymptomatic	Accidental discovery (i.e., during transuretheral resection of prostate for benign prostatic hyperplasia)
2	Prostate only	Mild urinary symptoms of enlarged prostate or asymptomatic	Prostate specific antigen (PSA) elevated or gland palpated during rectal exam
3	Outside capsule of prostate; may also be in seminal vesicles	Urinary symptoms, rectal or pelvic pain	PSA elevated or gland palpated during rectal exam
4	Lymph nodes involvement and metastasis	Urinary symptoms, rectal or pelvic pain; plus pain in affected tissue	PSA elevated or gland palpated during rectal exam
Recurrent	Anywhere in body after previous treatment	Determined by tissue involved	PSA elevated after treatment

      2) Digital rectal exams recommended yearly for men over 45

      3) Urinalysis

      4) Transrectal ultrasonography (TRUS) if PSA is elevated

      5) Tissue biopsy: diagnosis is through rectal or perineal fine-needle aspiration after increased PSA or rectal exam detects hard nodules on prostate

      6) Magnetic resonance imagery (MRI), bone scan, or computerized tomography (CT) for possible metastasis

4. Nursing management

  a. Medications/treatment

      1) Hormone therapy (via bilateral orchiectomy or monthly injections)

      2) Surgery (transurethral resection of prostate [TURP] or radical abdominal prostatectomy)

      3) Chemotherapy

      4) Internal or external radiation

  b. Education needed that most men will be impotent after abdominal prostatectomy, and 40% will experience urinary incontinence, which can be treated in some men with an artificial urinary sphincter

  c. Age of client at diagnosis, concurrent medical conditions, and stage of cancer determine recommended treatment regimen

  d. If receiving chemotherapy or radiation therapy, assess mouth for stomatitis, skin condition at radiation site, and signs of dehydration

  e. Educate client as to what his cancer stage means and assess for suicidal tendencies

  f. Provide support for body image disturbance and sexual dysfunction issues, including referral to support groups for client and family

E. Testicular cancer

1. Overview

  a. Most common cancer in males age 15 to 35

  b. Many forms exist

  c. Types

      1) Germinal cell tumor

      2) Seminomas (most common)

  d. Cause is unknown

2. Pathophysiology

  a. Types:

      1) Germ cell (95%): originating in sperm-producing cells of testes

      2) Seminomas (40%): slow-growing and remain localized within a testis

      3) Nonseminoma (60%) are more aggressive

      4) Other forms may be leydig, sertoli, leiomyosarcoma, rhabdomyosarcoma, mesothelioma, or stromal cell

  b. Cancer cells grow within testicle, replacing parenchymal tissue

  c. Spread of disease is usually by lymphatic (lymph nodes) and vascular channels (to lungs, bone, or liver), even before any large mass appears in scrotum

Table 11-2	Stage	Location
Stages of Testicular Cancer	I	Confined to testicle
	II	Retroperitoneal lymph nodes and testicle
	III	Beyond lymph nodes; metastasis

> **d.** Signs and symptoms
>
> **1)** Painless, hard nodule or swelling (usually on only one side of testis), dull ache in testes
>
> **2)** Metastatic symptoms include respiratory problems (coughing, dyspnea), back or bone pain, or gastrointestinal problems
>
> **e.** There are three stages of testicular cancer (see Table 11-2)

3. Nursing assessment

   a. Assessment

      1) Obtain client history of testicular or groin pain, change in size, shape, or consistency of testis, and size and consistency of palpable lumps, presence of cryptorchidism with or without surgical correction

      2) Other: symptom analysis of any pain, respiratory or GI problems

   b. Diagnostic tests

      1) Radioimmunoassay studies for tumor markers (human chorionic gonadotropin [hCG] and alpha-fetoprotein [AFP])

      2) Serum lactic acid dehydrogenase (LDH)

      3) Metastasis: liver function tests, x-ray, and CT scan

      4) Diagnosis made via pathology examination following inguinal **orchiectomy** (removal of a testis) on affected side

4. Nursing management

   a. Medications include chemotherapy

      1) Cisplatin (Platinol), bleomycin (Blenoxane), and etoposide (VePesid)

      2) Etoposide (VePesid) plus cisplatin (Platinol)

   b. Treatment after orchiectomy involves radiation and/or chemotherapy

   c. Monitor VS during chemotherapy or radiation therapy and fluid balance assessment because of nausea, vomiting, and diarrhea from treatment modalities

   d. Provide client education on expected client experience with treatment

   e. If client desires fertility, inform him of sperm banking prior to chemotherapy

   f. Teach client monthly testicular self-examination (TSE) of remaining testis and to have annual visits to physician; education about TSE should begin at age 15

Practice to Pass

The client with a testicular lump is scheduled for an inguinal orchiectomy and asks why the doctor doesn't just remove the lump "like they do with breast lumps." How should the nurse respond?

III. FEMALE REPRODUCTIVE HEALTH PROBLEMS

A. Uterine bleeding disorders

1. Overview

   a. **Dysfunctional uterine bleeding (DUB)** is a nonspecific condition from lack of progesterone, where menstruation is

      1) Irregular, frequent (**metrorrhagia**)

        2) Excessive (**menorrhagia**)

        3) Both (metromenorrhagia)

    b. Occurs mostly in adolescents and in premenopausal women

    c. 25 to 50% of women will develop fibroid tumors (**myomas,** leiomyomas), usually in their 30s and 40s, which can also create bleeding disorders

    d. Causes

        1) Adenomyosis (a condition in which endometrium is present between myometrial cells) can also cause irregular or heavy menstrual bleeding

        2) Over 90% caused by anovulatory cycles

        3) Other: blood dyscrasias, endocrine problems, pelvic inflammatory disease, endometrial cancer or polyps, exogenous estrogen, pregnancy, menopause, athletic training or excessive athletic activity, or no known cause

2. Pathophysiology

    a. Dysfunctional uterine bleeding results from a lack of progesterone

        1) This causes proliferation of fragile endometrium that does not mature into secretory endometrium

        2) Endometrium sheds at irregular times

    b. If proliferative phase of menstrual cycle is shortened because of a defect in follicular phase, spotting and breakthrough bleeding may occur

    c. Excessive flow may be a result of defects during luteal phase

    d. Disorders of DUB

        1) Amenorrhea (absence of menstruation)

            a) Primary (by age 17)

            b) Secondary (absence in a previously menstruating woman)

        2) Oligomenorrhea (scant menses)

        3) Menorrhagia

        4) Metrorrhagia

        5) Postmenopausal bleeding

    e. Uterine myomas form in several areas (see Figure 11-3)

        1) In myometrial wall (intramural)

        2) Pedunculated and into uterine cavity (submucosal)

        3) Pedunculated (having a stalk) and outwards into pelvis (subserosal)

Figure 11-3

Myomas of the uterus.
A. Intramural; *B.* Submucosal;
C. Subserosal.

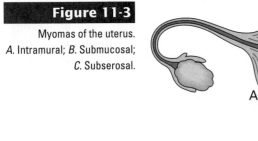

    f. Adenomyosis is endometrium in the myometrium, which enlarges each month under hormonal influence but is unable to be shed because it is trapped between myometrial cells

    g. Signs and symptoms include change in menstrual cycle (repetitive or long history), fatigue, anemia, hemorrhage, sexual dysfunction, cramping, water retention, anxiety, problems with reproduction; large tumors or presence of more than one tumor tend to cause more symptoms (enlarged uterus, metrorrhagia, **dysmenorrhea,** pelvic pressure or fullness, and increased urinary frequency)

3. Nursing assessment

    a. Obtain history of bleeding pattern

    b. BP and pulse sitting and standing

    c. Symptom analysis of pain or discomforts associated with problem

    d. Activity level

    e. Sexual and reproductive history

4. Nursing management

    a. Medications

        1) Analgesics for discomfort

        2) Nonsteroidal antiinflammatory drugs to inhibit prostaglandins

        3) Leuprolide acetate (Lupron) to decrease tumor size; gonadotropin-releasing hormone (GnRH) agonists

        4) Antibiotics for secondary form

    b. Educate clients about cause of their dysmenorrhea

    c. Teach how to take prescribed or OTC medications correctly

    d. Instruct clients to drink plenty of fluids and have an adequate calcium intake

    e. Application of heat to lower abdomen may help when discomfort occurs

B. Pelvic inflammatory disease (PID)

1. Overview

    a. Pelvic inflammatory disease (PID) is defined as an inflammation of uterus and fallopian tubes (salpingitis), endometrium (endometritis), pelvic peritoneum, and ovaries (oophoritis) usually resulting from infection

    b. Highest incidence occurs among women who have had more than one sexual partner in their lifetime, increasing with greater numbers of partners

    c. 20% of women will be infertile after infectious PID; 20% will have chronic pelvic pain; ectopic pregnancy occurs 10 times as often after PID

    d. Most prominent in women ages 15 to 24 who are nulliparous

    e. May be acute or chronic

    f. Causes: use of IUDs, oral contraceptives, or condoms; secondary infections are caused by appendicitis, peritonitis, STIs, douching

2. Pathophysiology

    a. Bacteria invade uterine and tubal tissues after migrating through cervix

    b. Migration occurs during ovulation, menstruation, forced through cervix with douching, childbirth, abortion, or surgery of reproductive tract

    c. Scar tissue is formed from infection, which obstructs uterine tubes

    d. Tubo-ovarian abscesses can form because of obstruction

    e. Bacterial infection causes inflammation, which in turn causes symptoms

　　f. Common infecting organisms include *Neisseria gonorrhea, Chlamydia trachomatis, E. coli, Gardnerella vaginalis,* or *Mycoplasma hominis*

　　g. Signs and symptoms include low abdominal pain, dysmenorrhea, **dyspareunia,** dysuria, and fever; vaginal discharge may be noted (green-yellow, green-gray, or yellow); nausea, malaise

　　h. Complications of PID include infertility, ectopic pregnancy, pelvic abscess, and dysmenorrhea

3. Nursing assessment

　a. Assessment

　　1) History for onset of symptoms, precipitating factors, known exposure to STIs, number of sexual partners, and amount of douching

　　2) Assess for VS (fever), activity level, any discharges

　　3) Symptom analysis of pain and GI symptoms

　　4) History of menstrual cycle and pregnancies

　b. Diagnostic tests

　　1) Cervical cultures

　　2) Ultrasound

　　3) Laparoscopy

　　4) CBC for elevated white blood count (WBC)

　　5) Review of client's symptoms

　　6) Pap smear, visualization of cervix will detect any discharge

4. Nursing management

　a. Medications include analgesics for fever and at least 2 broad spectrum antibiotics (may require inpatient intravenous [IV] form)

　　1) Tetracycline: doxycycline (Vibramycin)

　　2) Cephalosporin: cefoxitin (Mefoxin) or ceftriaxone (Rocephin)

　　3) Aminoglycoside: gentamicin (Garamycin)

　　4) Fluoroquinolone: ofloxacin (Floxin)

　　5) Antiprotozoal: metronidazole (Flagyl)

　　6) Antiinfective: clindamycin (Cleocin)

　b. Client education

　　1) Proper timing and use of oral antibiotics

　　2) Avoiding douching

　　3) Cause of PID

　c. Instruct client to take her temperature 3 times a day and call if elevated

　d. Instruct client to report PID to provider if she becomes pregnant so that ectopic pregnancy can be detected early

C. Endometriosis

1. Overview

　a. Endometriosis is defined as a growth of endometrium outside of uterus

　b. Most likely sites of growth include bladder, ovaries, fallopian tubes, bowel, and broad ligament

　c. Most often occurs in European American women of childbearing age

　d. Major complication is infertility

    e. Causes include unknown, theorized to be caused from embryonic epithelial cells; backflow of menstrual fluid through uterine tubes during menstruation; and spread of endometrial implants by way of lymphatic or vascular system

2. Pathophysiology

    a. Endometrial tissue is present outside of uterus, and responds to hormonal influence of menstrual cycle

    b. However, blood (that normally is shed from intrauterine endometrium) cannot escape and builds up causing scarring and further growth of endometriosis

    c. Bleeding results in inflammation and pain in tissues

    d. Infertility associated with endometriosis may be unexplained or occurs from mechanical blockage of tubes from endometrial implants

    e. Signs and symptoms include dysmenorrhea, dyspareunia, dysuria, constipation, and painful bowel movements during menses, tender masses that are palpable

3. Nursing assessment

    a. Assessment

        1) Obtain thorough history of symptoms including onset and when in menstrual cycle symptoms worsen or improve

        2) Symptom analysis of pain and related symptoms

        3) Assess bowel characteristics

    b. Diagnostic tests

        1) Diagnosis is made by laparoscopy

        2) CBC to identify low hemoglobin and hematocrit (H&H) and rule out infection (WBC)

        3) Pelvic ultrasonography

4. Nursing management

    a. Medications include analgesics for pain, NSAIDs for inhibiting prostaglandin synthesis; hormone therapy such as leuprolide (Lupron); gonadotropin-releasing hormone (GnRH) to raise estrogen and progesterone levels to control bleeding; danazol (Danocrine) to induce amenorrhea

    b. Educate client about endometriosis

    c. Provide education on treatment being utilized, including side effects of medications such as hot flashes

    d. Provide support and refer to support groups for infertility issues

D. Benign breast disorders

1. Overview

    a. Fibrocystic disease is defined as benign breast lesions

    b. Common in women 30 to 50 years of age

    c. Causes include hormonal changes, aging, and diet high in caffeine

2. Pathophysiology

    a. Mammary tissue retains fluid and forms a cyst during latter half of menstrual cycle, which resolves spontaneously with menstruation

    b. Inflammation from repetition of filling causes wall of cyst to fibrose and become hard, blocking drainage of fluid

    c. Cyst remains even after menses

      d. Classification

         1) Nonproliferative lesion: may be cystic or fibrous and may result in a mass in upper outer breast quadrant after an inflammatory response to irritation of ducts

         2) Proliferative lesion: lesions without atypical cells

         3) Atypical hyperplasia: lesions that are "borderline," possible morphologic characteristics of cancer cells

      e. Signs and symptoms: painful, mobile, round or oval, smooth lump in the breast tissue that enlarges or becomes more painful premenstrually; nipple discharge (clear, milky, straw-colored, green)

   3. Nursing assessment

      a. Assessment

         1) Obtain history on when the lump was first detected, with size, shape, location, mobility, tenderness, and cyclical changes

         2) Determine if ultrasound or mammogram has been previously performed

         3) Perform self breast exam (SBE) monthly

         4) Identify details of menstrual cycle and previous problems

      b. Diagnostic tests

         1) Mammogram

         2) Ultrasound examination

         3) Needle aspiration may be performed

         4) Excisional biopsy may be done to rule out cancer

         5) Breast examination

   4. Nursing management

      a. Medications include mild analgesics and Vitamin E

      b. There is no cure, but limiting caffeine, smoking, and chocolate usually improves or eliminates the condition

      c. Provide education on what is known about fibrocystic breast disease and explain the vagueness of prevention and treatment

      d. Reassure client that fibrocystic breast lumps are not precancerous

      e. Educate on monthly SBE and yearly exam by physician; mammograms for women over 40

E. Breast cancer

   1. Overview

      a. Defined as growth of abnormal cells in breast tissue that is irregular

      b. Affects 1 out of 9 women over course of a lifetime; 10% of cases linked to mutations in the BRCA1 or BRCA2 gene

      c. Involves mammary ducts, lobules, or both

      d. Cause: unknown, see risk factors

   2. Pathophysiology

      a. Two main locations: lobular (20%) and ductal (80%)

      b. Breast cancer is hormone-dependent; must have functioning ovaries

      c. Termed

         1) Noninvasive (in situ): proliferation of cancer cells are either ductal or lobular but do not invade surrounding tissue

> 2) Invasive (penetration of tumor into surrounding tissue); arise in terminal section of ductal tissue; five types
>
>> a) Infiltrating ductal carcinoma: stony hardness when palpated; metastasizes to axillary lymph nodes; most common; poor prognosis
>>
>> b) Tubular carcinoma or "well-differentiated"; less common
>>
>> c) Medullary carcinoma: bulky, large tumor that is well-circumscribed
>>
>> d) Mucinous carcinoma: bulky, slow-growing tumor with sharp edges
>>
>> e) Infiltrating lobular carcinoma: uncommon; thick, ill-defined area in breast
>
> d. May metastasize to bone, brain, lung, liver, skin, and lymph nodes
>
> e. Tumors are staged according to size of tumor, involvement of lymph node, and metastasis to other sites (see Table 11-3)
>
> f. Metastasis occurs as small masses of cells break away from tumor, enter lymphatic system where they remain, causing swelling of node or traveling to another node; lymphatic drainage has three pathways
>
>> 1) Axillary (most common route of spread)
>>
>> 2) Internal mammary
>>
>> 3) Transpectoral
>
> g. Signs and symptoms include hard, irregular, painless, fixed lump or thickening of a breast area; red, scaly patch of skin on breast; development of nipple inversion or calcifications detected on mammogram; possibly no palpable or visible symptoms initially

Table 11-3	Stage	Tumor	Node	Metastasis
Staging of Breast Cancer	0	Tis-Carcinoma in situ or Paget's disease of the nipple	N0-No regional lymph node metastasis	M0-No evidence of distant metastasis
	I	T1-Tumor no larger than 2 cm	N0	M0
	IIA	T0-No evidence of primary tumor	N1-Metastasis to movable ipsilateral axillary nodes	M0
		T1		
		T2-Tumor no larger than 5 cm	N0	M0
	IIB	T2	N1	M0
		T3-Tumor larger than 5 cm	N0	M0
	IIIA	T0	N2-Metastasis to ipsilateral fixed axillary nodes	M0
		T1		
		T2		
		T3	N1	M0
			N2	M0
	IIIB	T4-Tumor of any size with direct extension to chest wall or skin	Any N	M0
		Any T	N3-Metastasis to ipsilateral internal mammary lymph nodes	M0
	IVA	Any T	N0 and N1	M1-Distant metastasis

Source: LeMone, P., & Burke, K. (2008). *Medical-surgical nursing: Critical thinking for client care* (4th ed.). Upper Saddle River, NJ. Pearson Education, p. 1583.

!▷   **h.** *Inflammatory carcinoma* is a systemic disease of breast and most malignant form of breast cancer

          1) Signs and symptoms include skin erythema, redness, warmth, and induration of breast; *peau d'orange* sign (edema of skin with orange peel look) is present

          2) Prognosis is poor

!▷   **i.** *Paget's disease* is a rare type of breast cancer that involves epithelium of nipple

          1) Signs and symptoms include itching, burning of nipple; crusting or ulceration of nipple

          2) Excellent prognosis if confined to nipple

3. Nursing assessment

    a. Assessment includes history on lump: size, shape, location, fixed or mobile, presence of pain, when discovered; family history of breast cancer; date and location of last mammogram (if any); client's fear and knowledge of cancer

    b. Diagnostic tests

       1) Screening mammography

       2) Clinical breast examination

       3) Ultrasonography

       4) MRI

       5) Biopsy (fine needle, excisional, or stereotactic needle); with cytologic examination of fluid

       6) Ductal lavage and nipple aspiration

4. Nursing management

!▷   **a.** Medications include estrogen-antagonist medication (Tamoxifen)— may be ordered if tumor has estrogen receptors; chemotherapy used with large tumors, age less than 50, if nodes are positive, or metastasis present

!▷   **b.** Treatment: lumpectomy or mastectomy with axillary node dissection followed by radiation

    c. Breast reconstruction surgery, if desired by client, can be performed at time of mastectomy or later

!▷   **d.** Provide education as to

       1) Results of screening and diagnostic tests (mammogram, ultrasound, biopsy, pathology report following lumpectomy or mastectomy)

       2) Expected client experience with procedures ordered and anesthesia required for them

       3) Appropriate use of home medications

       4) Side effects of radiation or chemotherapy if utilized

       5) Placement of drains after surgery and their care post-discharge

    e. Provide support to client and family, and encourage client to attend support groups such as Reach for Recovery

▶ **Practice to Pass**

A 40-year-old client wants to know when she should start having mammograms. How should the nurse respond?

IV. SEXUALLY TRANSMITTED INFECTIONS (STIs)

A. Gonococcal infection

1. Overview

!▷   **a.** Defined as infection of cervix and male urethra with *Neisseria gonorrhea,* a gram-negative anaerobic diplococci; can also affect mouth, throat, and anus

      b. Second most common STI; incidence is decreasing, highest incidence in urban areas among men and women 15 to 24 years old

      c. Also known as GC or "clap"

      d. Cause: direct sexual contact with infected person or by an infected mother to a fetus during delivery

2. Pathophysiology

      a. Bacteria present in semen, vaginal, and cervical secretions are distributed during unprotected intercourse to mucous membranes, causing damage to cells

      b. Damage to cells triggers inflammatory response, accounting for symptoms

      c. Infection occurs at site of contact (i.e., vagina, rectum, urethra, oropharynx)

      d. Incubation period is 2 to 8 days with symptoms appearing about day 10 after exposure

      e. Signs and symptoms

          1) Female: often asymptomatic; if symptomatic, presents with thick yellow or greenish-yellow vaginal discharge, new onset of dysmenorrhea and/or dyspareunia, pelvic pain, enlarged groin nodes, possible rectal pain or urethral discharge; pharyngitis; purulent exudate from urethra or Bartholin's duct

          2) Males: dysuria, thick yellow or greenish-yellow spontaneous penile discharge, pain with ejaculation, rectal pain if engage in rectal intercourse; (oropharynx)—extremely sore throat, reddened oropharynx with copious adherent yellow discharge, fever, enlarged neck nodes

      f. Complications: female—spontaneous abortion if pregnant, premature delivery, salpingitis, PID, infertility secondary to scarring and blockage of fallopian tubes or vas deferens, ectopic pregnancy or chorioamnionitis, abscess of Bartholin's gland

3. Nursing assessment

      a. Assessment

          1) Obtain sexual history including unprotected intercourse, onset and severity of symptoms, any known exposure to gonorrhea; menstrual history

          2) Assess VS, palpate lymph nodes, visually inspect any discharge, perform oral exam

          3) Symptom analysis of any pain

      b. Diagnostic tests

          1) Culture of cervix or urethra

          2) Urine specimen for polymerase chain reaction (PCR) testing

4. Nursing management

      a. Medications include antibiotic therapy

          1) Oral: ciprofloxacin hydrochloride (Cipro), a single or 7-day course of azithromycin (Zithromax), doxycycline (Vibra-tabs), or ceftriaxone sodium (Rocephin)

          2) Intramuscular (IM): ceftriaxone sodium (Rocephin)

      b. Client education

          1) Bacterial cause of gonorrhea and transmission through unprotected intercourse

          2) Use of condoms correctly for each episode of intercourse

3) Limit number of sexual partners or become abstinent

4) Use of oral antibiotics including need to finish all medication

c. Obtain names of sexual contacts for follow-up testing and treatment

B. Nongonococcal infection

1. Overview

a. Defined as a sexually transmitted infection known as chlamydial infection, which causes an acute infection of reproductive tract

b. *Chlamydia trachomatis,* a very small anaerobic, obligate intracellular bacteria; the most common STI among men and women 15 to 24 years of age

c. Incidence is increasing across United States

d. Causes: direct sexual contact, perinatally, mother-to-child transmission in delivery

2. Pathophysiology

a. Bacteria found in semen, vaginal, and cervical secretions are transported during sexual contact; bacteria replicate rapidly and can be spread within 24 hours of becoming infected

b. Organism usually invades urethra in men and cervix in women

c. Can cause conjunctivitis and blindness in newborn

d. Incubation period is about 2 weeks after exposure

e. Permanent tissue scarring can result from infection

f. Symptoms: often asymptomatic, and may remain so for years

1) Females: greenish or yellowish vaginal discharge that will be visualized in cervical os, sudden onset of dysmenorrhea or dyspareunia, dysuria, or midcycle postcoital bleeding, pelvic pain, pain with orgasm

2) Males: more likely to be symptomatic than females; dysuria, expressed yellowish penile discharge, pain with ejaculation

g. Complications include pneumonitis if client is immunocompromised, endocarditis, and meningoencephalitis

1) Females: PID, endometritis, salpingitis, infertility, ectopic pregnancy

2) Males: epididymitis, prostatitis, sterility

3. Nursing assessment

a. Assessment

1) Obtain sexual history including unprotected intercourse, onset and severity of symptoms, known exposure to chlamydia, menstrual history

2) Assess VS, discharge

3) Symptom analysis of pain

b. Diagnostic tests

1) Cultures of tissue

2) Antibody tests: direct fluorescent antibody test (DEA), enzyme-linked immunosorbent assay (ELISA)

3) Urine specimen for polymerase chain reaction (PCR) testing

Practice to Pass

When instructing the female client on taking doxycycline (Vibra-tabs) for her *Chlamydia trachomatis* cervicitis, the client states that she thinks she may be pregnant. What should the nurse do?

4. Nursing management

    a. Medications include oral antibiotics such as azithromycin (Zithromax), or doxycycline (Vibra-tabs)

    b. Client education

        1) Bacterial cause of chlamydia and transmission through unprotected intercourse

        2) Use of condoms correctly with each episode of intercourse

        3) Limiting number of sexual partners or becoming abstinent

        4) Use of oral antibiotics including need to finish all medication

    c. Obtain names of sexual contacts for follow-up testing and treatment

C. Syphilis

1. Overview

    a. Defined as a chronic form of STI caused by a spirochete bacteria, *Treponema pallidum*

    b. Four stages: primary, secondary, latent, and tertiary

    c. Often occurs with other STIs such as chlamydial infection or gonorrhea

    d. Highest incidence in African American men in southeast United States

    e. Cause: transmission during sexual contact; through blood; mother-to-child transfer during childbirth

2. Pathophysiology

    a. Distinct stages, onset/timing, symptoms, and transfer are described in Table 11-4

        1) Primary stage: initial chancre (typical lesion) appears

        2) Secondary stage: development of a systemic illness

        3) Latent stage: period until manifestations of tertiary stage begin; no clinical manifestations occur

Table 11-4	**Syphilis**		
Stage	**Onset/timing**	**Symptoms**	**Transfer**
Primary	10 to 90 days after exposure; average 21 days, lasts 3 to 6 weeks	Firm, round, small, crater-like chancre at site of bacterial entry that heals spontaneously, lymphadenopathy	Contact with lesion, sexual contact, or blood
Secondary	2 weeks to 6 months after chancre appears; may come and go up to 2 years	Brownish rash especially on palms of hands and soles of feet that does not itch; malaise; may have patchy hair loss; mild swollen glands, glomerulonephritis, nephrotic syndrome, oral mucous patches, arthralgia, alopecia	Contact with rash, sexual contact, blood
Latent	Disappearance of symptoms of secondary stage; lasts for years	None	No
Tertiary	Onset may be several years from initial infection; can be fatal	Depends on site of bacterial invasion: heart valve or aortic stenosis Neurosyphilis leads to CNS involvement, leading to dementia, blindness, paralysis	No

        4) Tertiary stage: systemic manifestations occur and complications in this stage may result in death

    b. Infestation can occur in any body tissue or organ

    c. Incubation period ranges from 10 to 90 days

    d. Upon entering body, spirochete is spread by way of blood and lymphatic system

    e. See Table 11-4 for signs and symptoms

    f. Complications include blindness, paralysis, mental illness, cardiovascular damage, encephalitis, and death; pregnant women with syphilis can transmit infection to their fetus, resulting in congenital syphilis, causing intrauterine fetal death or numerous central nervous system (CNS) defects

  3. Nursing assessment

    a. Assessment

      1) Obtain sexual history including unprotected intercourse, onset and severity of symptoms, and known exposure to syphilis

      2) Assess for IV drug use

      3) Assess VS, mental clarity, lung and heart sounds, activity level

      4) Visual inspection for lesions

    b. Diagnostic tests

      1) Dark field microscopy of scraping from lesion

      2) Blood work: if venereal disease research laboratory (VDRL) or rapid plasma reagin (RPR) are positive, more specific fluorescent treponemal antibody absorption (FTA-ABS) is performed; VDRL will remain positive for life after infection

      3) Immunofluorescent staining

  4. Nursing management

    a. Medications include long-term IV and/or IM penicillin; weekly then monthly; dose depending on stage; doxycycline may also be used

    b. Educate client about cause of syphilis and potentially long duration of infection

    c. Encourage client to use condoms during every episode of intercourse and to avoid sharing needles

    d. Obtain names of sexual contacts for follow-up testing and treatment

    e. Instruct about need for compliance with follow-up testing and antibiotic treatment

    f. Assess if allergic to penicillin; educate on expected client experience with desensitization to penicillin in an intensive care unit if penicillin-allergic

D. Herpes

  1. Overview

    a. Defined as a common STI involving transmission of herpes virus

    b. Second most common viral STI (*human papilloma* virus or HPV is most common)

    c. Two types

      1) HSV1 is more likely to be present orally

      2) HSV2 more likely to cause genital infection

    d. Cause: sexual transmission, blood borne; and mother-to-fetus during delivery

2. Pathophysiology

   a. Retrovirus infection develops at site of viral entry into body; virus will travel along dermatome to nerve root and remain dormant there until next outbreak, which will occur at same site as primary lesion

   b. Transmission can occur during genital contact, oral-genital contact, or digital contact after contact with lesions

   c. Asymptomatic viral shedding also occurs

   d. Incubation period ranges from 1 to 26 days

   e. Reactivation occurs at any time; vesicles will reappear

   f. Reactivation is often caused by physical or emotional stress; hormone changes

   g. Signs and symptoms

      1) Primary infection symptoms: extremely painful blisters that progress to crater-like lesions lasting up to 3 weeks, malaise, enlarged groin nodes, low-grade temperature

      2) Recurrent infection: extremely painful blisters progressing to crater-like lesions that heal within 10 days

   h. Complications include meningitis, encephalitis, arthritis, hepatitis, prostatitis, neonatal transmission can occur transplacentally if primary infection occurs during pregnancy or birth while in primary stage or during recurrent infection, causing systemic neonatal herpes, which has high morbidity (from CNS involvement) and mortality

3. Nursing assessment

   a. Assessment

      1) Obtain sexual history including unprotected intercourse or oral-genital intercourse with partner having oral herpes lesions ("cold sores"), onset and severity of symptoms, and known exposure to herpes

      2) Assess VS

      3) Symptom analysis of pain

   b. Diagnostic tests

      1) Cultures

      2) Diagnosed primarily by symptoms and physical examination

4. Nursing management

   a. Medications include oral antiviral medications: acyclovir (Zovirax) or valacyclovir Hcl (Valtrex) started with diagnosis for primary infection, or with onset of symptoms with recurrence; valacyclovir Hcl may be used for suppressive therapy; penciclovir (Danavir) and famcyclovir (Famvir) may be used

   b. Client education

      1) Transmission of herpes simplex virus infections

      2) Appropriate use of medications prescribed

   c. Encourage client with primary infection to report headache or stiff neck immediately

   d. Instruct client with urinary hesitancy to run water while trying to void or pour warm water over perineum or glans of penis

Case Study

T. J. is a 45-year-old client who has been diagnosed with prostate cancer. He will be having abdominal prostatectomy surgery next week for the condition.

1. How should the nurse describe the expected client experience with this surgery?

2. T. J. asks the nurse how the doctor determines if the cancer has spread beyond the prostate gland. How should the nurse reply?

3. T. J. asks why his surgery will be abdominal when his 82-year-old uncle had transurethral surgery. What is a correct answer?

4. Describe the treatments T. J. will most likely undergo after recovering from his surgery.

5. The pathology report indicates that T. J.'s cancer is stage 3. Describe what this means.

For suggested responses, see page 536–537.

POSTTEST

1 The nurse who is triaging clients in the ambulatory clinic determines that which client should be seen first? The client with:

1. Genital herpes infection diagnosed yesterday, with a severe headache.
2. Recurrent herpes infections for three years, with burning during urination.
3. Chlamydia diagnosed yesterday, now with worsening pelvic pain.
4. Secondary syphilis diagnosed last month, due for penicillin injection.

2 Which of the following statements should be presented by the nurse teaching in a breast cancer detection program for the community?

1. Mammograms should be started when women become age 50.
2. Self-breast exams should be performed weekly.
3. Birth control pills may prevent breast cancer.
4. Estrogen replacement may increase breast cancer risk.

3 The client with benign prostatic hyperplasia has undergone transurethral resection of the prostate (TURP) and is asking why he needs continuous bladder irrigation (CBI). The nurse's best response would be:

1. "The irrigation prevents blood from clotting and blocking the catheter."
2. "Your bladder needs to be kept full to promote healing after this surgery."
3. "The urine would be very concentrated without the irrigation."
4. "The saline running through the bladder helps keep you hydrated."

4 The nurse is caring for a female client who has endometriosis and wants to start a family. If she has the classic triad of symptoms, the nurse anticipates that which of the following will be the goals of her treatment? Select all that apply.

1. Relief from dysmenorrhea
2. Less painful sexual intercourse
3. Menstrual periods regularly every 28 days
4. Restoration of fertility
5. Relief of headache and constipation

5 The nurse interprets that which male client is at the highest risk for developing balanitis?

1. 1-year-old with intact foreskin
2. Circumcised 40-year-old
3. 22-year-old with intact foreskin
4. Circumcised 6-year-old

6 Which client is at lowest risk for developing breast cancer?

1. Client with BRCA1 gene mutation
2. Client who had Hodgkin's disease
3. First child at age 18, breastfed for two years
4. Smoker, age 74

7 The clinic nurse anticipates that female clients with *Chlamydia trachomatis* infections will most likely present with which signs and symptoms?

1. Painful perineal blisters and high fever of sudden onset
2. Painless crater-like lesion on the labia that lasts six weeks
3. Rapidly progressing pruritic rash on labia and buttocks
4. Yellow-green vaginal discharge, dyspareunia, pelvic pain

8 The client with a new diagnosis of genital herpes simplex virus 1 (HSV1) wants to know how she contracted the infection. The nurse's best answer is based on which of the following?

1. Inanimate objects can harbor HSV1 for several hours
2. HSV1 is found only in the genital tract and not orally
3. Sexual contact is the most common mode of transmission
4. Immune system suppression is needed to contract the infection

9 The nurse is assessing a client diagnosed with benign prostatic hyperplasia (BPH). What findings would the nurse expect to note? Select all that apply.

1. Forceful urinary stream
2. Frequency and urgency
3. Increased time to void
4. Incomplete bladder emptying
5. Nocturia

10 The nurse would assess the client with multiple subserosal uterine myomas for which of the following?

1. Uterine enlargement, urinary frequency, and pelvic pressure
2. Uterine enlargement, pain with urination, and vaginal discharge
3. Uterine atrophy, heavy and painful menses, and decreased libido
4. Uterine atrophy, pain with intercourse, and vaginal dryness

➤ *See pages 343–344 for Answers & Rationales.*

POSTTEST

ANSWERS & RATIONALES

Pretest

1 **Answer: 2** Balanitis, or inflammation of the foreskin and prepuce, would cause edema and pain of the penile glans, leading to dysuria. Option 1 is inappropriate for balanitis because this affects males not females; a urethral discharge (option 3) may occur in gonorrhea; and back pain (option 4) could indicate many disorders, but not balanitis.
Cognitive Level: Application **Client Need:** Physiological Integrity: Physiological Adaptation **Integrated Process:**

Nursing Process: Assessment **Content Area:** Adult Health: Renal and Genitourinary **Strategy:** Use nursing knowledge and the process of elimination to make a selection. If you need to make an educated guess, go with an option that fits an inflammatory problem—bala*nitis.*
Reference: LeMone, P., & Burke, K. (2008). *Medical-surgical nursing: Critical thinking in client care* (4th ed.). Upper Saddle River, NJ: Pearson/Prentice Hall, p. 1749.

2 **Answer: 4** Prostatitis creates pain in the tissues surrounding the prostate gland, and may manifest as rectal pain or pain with erection, as well as low back or rectal

ANSWERS & RATIONALES

pain. Option 1 is not related to prostatitis; rather urinary retention or incontinence would indicate problems with control of the urinary bladder. Option 2 is characteristic of infection with herpes virus; and option 3 represents syphilis (secondary stage).
Cognitive Level: Application **Client Need:** Physiological Integrity: Physiological Adaptation **Integrated Process:** Nursing Process: Assessment **Content Area:** Adult Health: Renal and Genitourinary **Strategy:** Differentiate prostatitis from sexually transmitted infections or other problems. Use nursing knowledge and the process of elimination to make a selection. **Reference:** LeMone, P., & Burke, K. (2008). *Medical-surgical nursing: Critical thinking in client care* (4th ed.). Upper Saddle River, NJ: Pearson/Prentice Hall, p. 1776.

3 **Answer: 1** Secondary syphilis begins with the healing of the chancre, and ends when the rash disappears, which can take up to six months from time of infection. The latent stage of syphilis then starts, which can last for years. VDRL and RPR would need to be positive for syphilis (option 2); option 3 could indicate TB or HIV; option 4 lists signs and symptoms of a bacterial infection such as chlamydia.
Cognitive Level: Application **Client Need:** Physiological Integrity: Physiological Adaptation **Integrated Process:** Nursing Process: Assessment **Content Area:** Adult Health: Renal and Genitourinary **Strategy:** Review the manifestations of sexually transmitted infections. Which relate to syphilis? Note that the timeframe given in the question is a big clue! **Reference:** LeMone, P., & Burke, K. (2008). *Medical-surgical nursing: Critical thinking in client care* (4th ed.). Upper Saddle River, NJ: Pearson/Prentice Hall, pp. 1609, 1846–1850.

4 **Answer: 3** Hypospadias repair is undertaken using the foreskin to create a channel through the penis to the tip of the glans so that he will deposit his sperm near his partner's cervix. Although option 1 may also be an appropriate answer, it is not the best answer to demonstrate effective teaching. Options 2 and 4 are incorrect statements.
Cognitive Level: Application **Client Need:** Health Promotion and Maintenance **Integrated Process:** Teaching/Learning **Content Area:** Child Health **Strategy:** If the problem is unfamiliar, use clues to help choose the correct option. Note the age of the child, the gender, and the prefix *hypo-* in the question. **Reference:** Porth, C. M. (2005). *Pathophysiology: Concepts of altered health states* (7th ed.). Philadelphia, PA: Lippincott Williams & Wilkins, pp. 1031–1032.

5 **Answer: 4** DUB most commonly results from a progesterone deficiency that causes a fragile endometrium that fails to mature from proliferative stage to secretory. This causes irregular menstrual bleeding. Treatment is aimed at correcting the cause, thus progesterone supplementation is prescribed.
Cognitive Level: Application **Client Need:** Physiological Integrity: Pharmacological and Parenteral Therapies **Integrated Process:** Nursing Process: Planning **Content Area:** Adult Health: Renal and Genitourinary **Strategy:** Recall which hormone regulates uterine bleeding. If guessing, eliminate the hormones that are not predominantly female ones. **Reference:** LeMone, P., & Burke, K. (2008). *Medical-surgical nursing: Critical thinking in client care* (4th ed.). Upper Saddle River, NJ: Pearson/Prentice Hall, pp. 1802–1805.

6 **Answers: 2, 3, 5** Douching should be avoided in order to prevent bacteria present in the lower reproductive tract from being forced upwards into the uterus, potentially causing PID. Condoms and monogamy help prevent reinfection. Position does not affect the spread of STIs. Voiding after intercourse will help prevent urinary tract infection.
Cognitive Level: Application **Client Need:** Physiological Integrity: Physiological Adaptation **Integrated Process:** Teaching/Learning **Content Area:** Adult Health: Renal and Genitourinary **Strategy:** The critical words in the question are *teaching* and *successful*. With this in mind, choose the options that prevent STIs. **Reference:** LeMone, P., & Burke, K. (2008). *Medical-surgical nursing: Critical thinking in client care* (4th ed.). Upper Saddle River, NJ: Pearson/Prentice Hall, pp. 1850–1852.

7 **Answer: 3** Chemotherapy and radiation used in the treatment of testicular cancer often cause a radically decreased sperm count. If the client desires children, he should consider sperm banking prior to beginning treatment. Impotence is not a key concern, and the client's increase in sexual activity may return to normal, but not directly because of successful treatment.
Cognitive Level: Application **Client Need:** Health Promotion and Maintenance **Integrated Process:** Nursing Process: Planning **Content Area:** Adult Health: Renal and Genitourinary **Strategy:** Consider the client's age, type of cancer, and the side effects of cancer treatments. **Reference:** LeMone, P., & Burke, K. (2008). *Medical-surgical nursing: Critical thinking in client care* (4th ed.). Upper Saddle River, NJ: Pearson/Prentice Hall, p. 1775.

8 **Answer: 4** Xanthines (caffeine) can precipitate or worsen fibrocystic breast disease, and elimination of coffee, tea, cola, and chocolate in the diet can decrease the symptoms. No other dietary factors have been identified.
Cognitive Level: Application **Client Need:** Health Promotion and Maintenance **Integrated Process:** Nursing Process: As-

sessment **Content Area:** Adult Health: Renal and Genitourinary **Strategy:** If you were thinking high fat diet was the answer, note that two options contain high fat foods. Look for another food culprit since there is only one answer to this question. **Reference:** LeMone, P., & Burke, K. (2008). *Medical-surgical nursing: Critical thinking in client care* (4th ed.). Upper Saddle River, NJ: Pearson/Prentice Hall, p. 1822.

9 **Answer: 1** Doxycycline (Vibra-tabs) is a commonly utilized treatment for chlamydia infections and, like all antibiotics, must be taken until the medication is gone. Use of condoms with every sexual encounter decreases the transmission of sexually transmitted infections. Sexual contacts should be notified of the infection so that appropriate testing can be obtained. This is especially important with chlamydia because it is often asymptomatic in women, and early detection can prevent complications such as pelvic inflammatory disease. Testicular self-exam is a screening measure for testicular cancer.

Cognitive Level: Application **Client Need:** Physiological Integrity: Physiological Adaptation **Integrated Process:** Nursing Process: Planning **Content Area:** Adult Health: Renal and Genitourinary **Strategy:** Consider which action cures the infection or prevents reinfection. **Reference:** LeMone, P., & Burke, K. (2008). *Medical-surgical nursing: Critical thinking in client care* (4th ed.). Upper Saddle River, NJ: Pearson/Prentice Hall, p. 1845.

10 **Answer: 3** Primary dysmenorrhea begins at menarche and is usually a lifelong condition. Options 1, 2, and 4 can occur with secondary dysmenorrhea or endometriosis.

Cognitive Level: Application **Client Need:** Physiological Integrity: Physiological Adaptation **Integrated Process:** Nursing Process: Assessment **Content Area:** Adult Health: Renal and Genitourinary **Strategy:** Note the critical words *primary* in the question and *since menarche* in the correct option and make an association. Alternatively, eliminate at least two options after noting three months and seven months as timeframes. **Reference:** LeMone, P., & Burke, K. (2008). *Medical-surgical nursing: Critical thinking in client care* (4th ed.). Upper Saddle River, NJ: Pearson/Prentice Hall, p. 1800.

Posttest

1 **Answer: 1** The primary genital herpes infection involves systemic viremia, and encephalitis is a possible complication. Headache and stiff neck may indicate encephalitis and requires further investigation. Herpes encephalitis is a life-threatening disorder needing prompt treatment with an antiviral agent. Option 2 rep-

resents a chronic herpes infection, while options 3 and 4 indicate other sexually transmitted infections.

Cognitive Level: Analysis **Client Need:** Safe Effective Care Environment: Management of Care **Integrated Process:** Nursing Process: Planning **Content Area:** Adult Health: Renal and Genitourinary **Strategy:** Consider which problem may be life threatening if prompt treatment is not given. Note the critical word *headache* in the correct option, which is an atypical or nonlocal symptom of a new genital herpes infection. **Reference:** LeMone, P., & Burke, K. (2008). *Medical-surgical nursing: Critical thinking in client care* (4th ed.). Upper Saddle River, NJ: Pearson/Prentice Hall, p. 1839.

2 **Answer: 4** Breast cancer detection begins with monthly self-breast exams. Mammograms should be performed yearly after age 40. Birth control pills do not increase nor decrease breast cancer risk, but the longer a woman is on estrogen replacement therapy, the greater her risk for developing the disease.

Cognitive Level: Application **Client Need:** Health Promotion and Maintenance **Integrated Process:** Nursing Process: Implementation **Content Area:** Adult Health: Oncology **Strategy:** Read the question and the options carefully. Some options are incorrect because one word or number changes the meaning. **Reference:** LeMone, P., & Burke, K. (2008). *Medical-surgical nursing: Critical thinking in client care* (4th ed.). Upper Saddle River, NJ: Pearson/Prentice Hall, pp. 1822–1823.

3 **Answer: 1** Continuous bladder irrigation serves to flush out the blood that will be oozing from the raw edges of the TURP site before the blood can clot. Clots in the bladder would obstruct the urine flow through the catheter. The resulting bladder distention increases the risk of bleeding.

Cognitive Level: Application **Client Need:** Physiological Integrity: Physiological Adaptation **Integrated Process:** Communication and Documentation **Content Area:** Adult Health: Renal and Genitourinary **Strategy:** Rationales for actions are often tested on NCLEX. Review "why" as well as "how" procedures are done. **Reference:** LeMone, P., & Burke, K. (2008). *Medical-surgical nursing: Critical thinking in client care* (4th ed.). Upper Saddle River, NJ: Pearson/Prentice Hall, pp. 1779–1780.

4 **Answers: 1, 2, 4** The classic triad is dysmenorrhea (painful menses), dyspareunia (painful intercourse), and infertility. The treatment goals are pain management and restoration of fertility. Headache and constipation are not symptoms of endometriosis. The length of the menstrual cycle is not relevant.

Cognitive Level: Analysis **Client Need:** Physiological Integrity: Physiological Adaptation **Integrated Process:**

Nursing Process: Planning **Content Area:** Adult Health: Renal and Genitourinary **Strategy:** A clue in the question is the client's goal of pregnancy. The other correct options relate to relieving symptoms of the disease. **Reference:** Porth, C. M. (2005). *Pathophysiology: Concepts of altered health states* (7th ed.). Philadelphia, PA: Lippincott Williams & Wilkins, p. 1075.

5 Answer: 3 Balanitis, inflammation of the foreskin, occurs in uncircumcised males with phimosis or poor hygiene, which predisposes them to bacterial growth in the secretions. It occurs after the foreskin becomes retractable (at about age 3). Options 2 and 4 are incorrect because of the circumcision. **Cognitive Level:** Analysis **Client Need:** Physiological Integrity: Physiological Adaptation **Integrated Process:** Nursing Process: Assessment **Content Area:** Adult Health: Renal and Genitourinary **Strategy:** If the name of the problem is unfamiliar, look for a clue in the root or suffix (-*itis* means inflammation). Rule out options that are not clients with higher risk of inflammatory process. **Reference:** Porth, C. M. (2005). *Pathophysiology: Concepts of altered health states* (7th ed.). Philadelphia, PA: Lippincott Williams & Wilkins, p. 1032.

6 Answer: 3 Early childbearing with breastfeeding for a total of two years or more decreases a woman's lifetime risk of developing breast cancer. BRCA1 or BRCA2 gene mutations increase risk. Hodgkin's disease treatment usually involves chest radiation, which increases breast cancer risk and breast cancer mortality. Aging is another factor. The older a woman becomes, the more likely she is to develop breast cancer. **Cognitive Level:** Analysis **Client Need:** Physiological Integrity: Physiological Adaptation **Integrated Process:** Nursing Process: Analysis **Content Area:** Adult Health: Oncology **Strategy:** Consider the risk factors for breast cancer and select the option that has the fewest risks. **Reference:** Porth, C. M. (2005). *Pathophysiology: Concepts of altered health states* (7th ed.). Philadelphia, PA: Lippincott Williams & Wilkins, p. 1090–1091.

7 Answer: 4 Chlamydia, although often silent and asymptomatic, will eventually present symptoms including new occurrence of dyspareunia, dysmenorrhea, low abdominal and pelvic pain, with yellow or yellow-green vaginal discharge. Options 1, 2, and 3 describe symptoms of different sexually transmitted infections. **Cognitive Level:** Application **Client Need:** Physiological Integrity: Physiological Adaptation **Integrated Process:** Nursing Process: Analysis **Content Area:** Adult Health: Renal and Genitourinary **Strategy:** Eliminate options that describe other diseases. **Reference:** LeMone, P., & Burke, K. (2008). *Medical-surgical nursing: Critical*

thinking in client care (4th ed.). Upper Saddle River, NJ: Pearson/Prentice Hall, p. 1844.

8 Answer: 3 HSV1 is transmitted by oral secretions and may be spread to the genital area by autoinoculation after poor handwashing or by oral intercourse. HSV2 is spread by sexual contact or to the newborn passing through an infected birth canal. Sexual partners may not know they are infected and shedding virus. The virus is inactivated by room temperature and drying so inanimate objects are seldom the means of transmission. Persons with intact immune systems can contract the infection. **Cognitive Level:** Application **Client Need:** Safe, Effective Care Environment: Safety and Infection Control **Integrated Process:** Nursing Process: Analysis **Content Area:** Adult Health: Renal and Genitourinary **Strategy:** Watch for extreme words (e.g. *only*) since they allow no exceptions. **Reference:** Porth, C. M. (2005). *Pathophysiology: Concepts of altered health states* (7th ed.). Philadelphia, PA: Lippincott Williams & Wilkins, pp. 1101–1102.

9 Answers: 2, 3, 4, 5 Manifestations are seen from obstruction such as weak urinary stream, incomplete bladder emptying, and increased time to void. Manifestations from the resulting irritation include frequency, urgency, dysuria, and nocturia. Chronic retention can lead to overflow incontinence. **Cognitive Level:** Application **Client Need:** Physiological Integrity: Physiological Adaptation **Integrated Process:** Nursing Process: Assessment **Content Area:** Adult Health: Renal and Genitourinary **Strategy:** Choose symptoms of obstruction and irritation. **Reference:** LeMone, P., & Burke, K. (2008). *Medical-surgical nursing: Critical thinking in client care* (4th ed.). Upper Saddle River, NJ: Pearson/Prentice Hall, p. 1778.

10 Answer: 1 Subserosal uterine myomas are located on the outer surface of the uterus and tend to cause fewer menstrual disorders than submucosal or intramural myomas. However, they do cause mechanical pressure on the pelvic contents from their size and weight, including bladder pressure that results in urinary frequency and urgency. **Cognitive Level:** Analysis **Client Need:** Physiological Integrity: Physiological Adaptation **Integrated Process:** Nursing Process: Assessment **Content Area:** Adult Health: Renal and Genitourinary **Strategy:** If unfamiliar with the disorder in the question, try "decoding" the terms. *Subserosal* (just below the outer serous layer) tells where the -*oma* (tumor) is located on the uterus. Now determine what manifestations a growth in that location may cause. **Reference:** Porth, C. M. (2005). *Pathophysiology: Concepts of altered health states* (7th ed.). Philadelphia, PA: Lippincott Williams & Wilkins, p. 1077.

References

Endo-online, the Voice of the Endometriosis Association (2005). Retrieved October 31, 2005 from http://www.endometriosisassn.org/endo.html

Gonorrhea Fact Sheet. Centers for Disease Control and Prevention, National Center for Infectious Diseases, Bacterial STD Branch of the Division of AIDS, STD, and TB Laboratory Research. Retrieved October 31, 2005 from http://www.cdc.gov/std/healthcomm/fact-sheets.htm.

LeMone, P., & Burke, K. (2008). *Medical-surgical nursing: Critical thinking in client care* (3rd ed.). Upper Saddle River, NJ: Pearson/Prentice Hall.

Lowdermilk, D., Perry, S., & Boback, I. (2004) *Maternity and women's health care* (8th ed.). St. Louis, MO: Mosby.

Office on Women's Health in the Department of Health and Human Services. *Uterine fibroids.* Retrieved October 31, 2005 http://womenshealth.about.com/od/fibroidtumors/f-lufibroidtumors.htm.

O'Hara Smith, N. (2003). *Testicular cancer: The pathology report.* Retrieved on Oct. 31, 2005 from Testicular Cancer Resource Center website: http://www.acor.org/pathology_report.html

Pilliteri, A. (2005). *Maternal and child health nursing* (5th ed.). Philadelphia, PA: Lippincott.

Prostate Enlargement: Benign Prostatic Hyperplasia. (2004). Retrieved Oct. 31, 2005 from National Kidney and Urologic Diseases Information Clearinghouse of the National Institute for Health: http://kidney.niddk.nih.gov/kudiseases/pubs/prostateenlargement/index.htm

Prostate.org. (2005). Retrieved Oct. 31, 2005 from Prostatitis Foundation website: http://www.prostatitis.org.

Porth, C. (2005). *Pathophysiology: Concepts of altered health states* (7th ed.). Philadelphia, PA: Lippincott Williams & Wilkins.

U.S. Department of Health and Human Services, Public Health Service, Centers for Disease Control and Prevention Division of STD Prevention. *Sexually transmitted disease surveillance, 2003.* Atlanta, GA. Retrieved Oct. 31, 2005 from http://www.cdc.gov/nchstpidstd/dsta/stats-trends/stats_and_trends.htm

U.S. Preventive Services Task Force, U.S. Department of Health and Human Services, Office of Disease Prevention and Health Promotion. *Guide to Clinical Preventive Services,* (2nd ed.). Genital Herpes Simplex. (1996). Retrieved Oct. 31, 2005 from http://cpmcnet.columbia.edu/texts/gcps/gcps0040.html

Wilson, B., Shannon, M., & Stang, C. (2006). *Nurses drug guide 2006.* Upper Saddle River, NJ: Prentice Hall.

12 Immunological Health Problems

Chapter Outline

Risk Factors for Immunological Health Problems

Allergies

Latex Allergy

Anaphylaxis

Acquired Immunodeficiency Syndrome (AIDS)

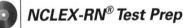

NCLEX-RN® Test Prep

Use the CD-ROM enclosed with this book to access additional practice opportunities.

Objectives

➤ Define key terms associated with immunological health problems.

➤ Identify risk factors associated with the development of immunological health problems.

➤ Explain the common etiologies of immunological health problems.

➤ Describe the pathophysiologic processes associated with specific immunological health problems.

➤ Distinguish between normal and abnormal immunological findings obtained from nursing assessment.

➤ Prioritize nursing interventions associated with specific immunological health problems.

Review at a Glance

acquired immunodeficiency syndrome (AIDS) disease syndrome characterized by infection with human immunodeficiency virus (HIV) and opportunistic infections or neoplasms

allergen substance, foreign protein, or cell capable of causing alterations in sensitivity

antibody immune or protective protein, evoked by an antigen; capable of reacting with a certain antigen

antigen substance that as a result of coming in contact with certain tissues induces a state of sensitivity or resistance

autoimmune disorders disorders resulting when one's own tissues are subject to destructive effects of immune system

cell-mediated immune response an immune system response to antigens, which do not evoke antibody-mediated response because they live in-side body's cells (viruses and mycobacteria are examples of such antigens)

cytokines agents of lymphoid system (interferons and interleukins) that act to modify body's response to cancerous cells; they may also be cytotoxic

graft-versus-host disease (GvHD) frequent and potentially fatal complication of bone marrow transplant; grafted tissue recognizes host tissue as foreign and mounts a cell-mediated immune response

humoral immune response antibody-mediated immune response produced by B-lymphocytes

hypersensitivity altered immune response in a client that results in harm to client

immunodeficiency a state in which client's immune system is incompetent or unable to respond effectively

immunotherapy natural and/or synthetic substances used to stimulate or suppress response of immune system

latex allergy allergic response to latex; common in health care workers and others who routinely use latex gloves as barrier protection

lymphocytes small, nondescript cells that account for 20 to 40% of circulating leukocytes; are principal effector and regulator cells of specific immune response

macrophage mature monocytes that actively phagocytize large foreign particles and cell debris

opportunistic disease any infection resulting from a deficient immune system

viral load number of circulating human immunodeficiency virus (HIV) particles per milliliter

PRETEST

1 An adult male client is admitted to the hospital with symptoms of pneumonia. He has not improved clinically and has not responded well to antibiotics. When the sputum culture and sensitivity (C&S) and his chest x-ray (CXR) results are available, a diagnosis of *pneumocystis carinii* pneumonia is made. The nurse should conclude that this client has:

1. Become infected recently with the human immunodeficiency virus (HIV).
2. Acquired immunodeficiency syndrome (AIDS).
3. Tuberculosis (TB).
4. An infection of unknown origin.

2 A child contracts and recovers from chickenpox at age 5. The nurse explains to the mother that the child will not need the varicella vaccine since the child has developed which type of immunity?

1. Active acquired, natural
2. Passive acquired, natural
3. Passive acquired, artificial
4. Active acquired, artificial

3 A person who is HIV-positive starts to exhibit signs of AIDS. The nurse would accurately interpret that the client now has AIDS, defining illness after noting which of the following?

1. Low viral load and a high white blood cell count (WBC)
2. High CD4 count and symptoms of immunodeficiency
3. High white blood count (WBC) and anemia
4. High viral load and CD4 count below 200 cells/mm^3

4 The health care provider tells a sexually active 16-year-old female with flulike symptoms that a negative enzyme linked immunosorbent assay (ELISA) will need to be repeated in several weeks. When the client asks the nurse why the second test is necessary, what is the best explanation by the nurse?

1. First test may be inaccurate
2. Antibodies do not always show up initially
3. Test is sensitive and can give false positives
4. It is standard practice

5 A client experiences an anaphylactic reaction after taking the first dose of a newly prescribed antibiotic. The client history reveals that the client had taken the antibiotic once before without a problem. The nurse's explanation to the client will be based on what knowledge of hypersensitivity response?

1. Histamine precursor causes anaphylaxis and a life-threatening situation.
2. IgE antibodies destroy mast cells, releasing substances that cause hypotension and vascular collapse.
3. Cell-mediated response, or delayed hypersensitivity, is caused by sensitized T lymphocytes and can lead to tissue injury.
4. Massive numbers of red blood cells are lysed because of an incompatibility with the medication that requires discontinuing the medication.

6 A female client who has recently been diagnosed with type 1 diabetes mellitus (DM) asks the nurse how she developed this because no one in her family is a diabetic. The nurse's best response is, "DM is an autoimmune disease characterized by:

1. Failure of the immune system to recognize self."
2. Exacerbations and remissions."
3. Accelerated production of killer T-cells."
4. Immunosuppression and altered cortisol levels."

7 A mother of twins calls the office and speaks to the nurse about a rash that has developed on both children since taking an antibiotic prescribed seven days ago. The twins also have edema of the face and neck, joint pain, and fever. What conclusion does the nurse draw about the problem and the appropriate nursing action?

1. Type I hypersensitivity reaction—get an order for diphenhydramine (Benadryl) and stop the medication
2. Type II hypersensitivity reaction—monitor renal function after stopping the drug
3. Type III hypersensitivity reaction (serum sickness)—stop the drug and notify the physician
4. Type IV hypersensitivity reaction—get order to change to another drug and recommend calamine lotion for the rash

8 The nurse is working with a client who has been asymptomatic with human immunodeficiency virus (HIV) until recently when he developed *pneumocystis carinii* pneumonia (PCP). The CD4 T-cell counts have dropped to below 200/mm^3 (Diagnostic Category 3). The nurse then assesses the client for the presence of what clinical problems that would also place this client in Clinical Category C? Select all that apply.

1. HIV encephalopathy
2. Kaposi's sarcoma
3. Persistent generalized lymphadenopathy
4. HIV wasting syndrome
5. Flulike symptoms of fever, sore throat, myalgia, and headache

9 The ambulatory care nurse concludes that which of the following clients is at highest risk of contact with the HIV virus? A client who:

1. Counsels HIV victims and their families.
2. Works with athletes who perspire a lot.
3. Collects blood donations via a mobile blood unit.
4. Gives flu shots in a doctor's office.

10 A client is brought to the Emergency Department with anaphylaxis after taking a dose of penicillin. The nurse delivers care based on which of the following nursing diagnoses that has highest priority?

1. Ineffective breathing pattern
2. Decreased cardiac output
3. Risk for injury
4. Anxiety

➤ *See page 367–369 for Answers & Rationales.*

I. RISK FACTORS FOR IMMUNOLOGICAL HEALTH PROBLEMS

A. Overview

1. Immunity is a specific bodily response to invasion by microorganisms and foreign protein and, with other defenses of body, constitutes an essential protective mechanism

2. Immune system is a complex network of specialized cells and organs that defend body against attack from foreign pathogens

3. The major **lymphocytes** (a white blood cell [WBC] accounting for 20 to 30% of total count) involved in protecting body against potential infections are B and T cells, which also play an important role in combating tumor growth

4. Cells of immune system patrol tissues and organs through both blood and lymphatic vessels

5. Immune system functions

   a. Defend and protect body from infection by bacteria, viruses, fungi, and parasites

   b. Remove and destroy damaged or dead cells

   c. Identify and destroy malignant cells, thereby preventing their development into tumors

6. Immune system components

   a. Human blood is made up of red blood cells (RBCs or erythrocytes) that transport oxygen, platelets (thrombocytes) that trigger clotting, and white blood cells (WBCs or leukocytes); WBCs are an important element of immune system that defends human body against attack from foreign pathogens

   b. WBCs originate in bone marrow from hemocytoblasts (stem cells) that give rise to lymphoid and myeloid stem cells (see Figure 12-1)

   1) *Leukocytes* or WBCs are the principal cells involved in immune response; normal number of leukocytes is 4,000 to 10,000 cells per cubic millimeter of blood

   2) *Granulocytes* compose 60 to 80% of total number of normal leukocytes; have a relatively short life span (hours to days) and are key defenders in protecting body from harmful microorganisms during acute inflammation and infection; there are three types

   a) Neutrophils or polymorphonuclear leukocytes (or polys) comprise largest percentage (55 to 70%); are phagocytic (responsible for engulfing and destroying pathogens) and arrive first at site of invasion (because of release of chemical triggers from damaged tissues and invading pathogens)

   b) Eosinophils account for 1 to 4% of total number of circulating leukocytes; mature in bone marrow shortly before being released into circulation where they are very short-lived; are less efficient phagocytic cells than neutrophils; are commonly found in higher numbers in respiratory and gastrointestinal tracts

   c) Basophils constitute about 0.5 to 1.0% of circulating leukocytes; not phagocytic; granules within basophils contain proteins and chemicals such as heparin, histamine, bradykinin, serotonin, and a slow-reacting substance of anaphylaxis (leukotrienes); these substances are released

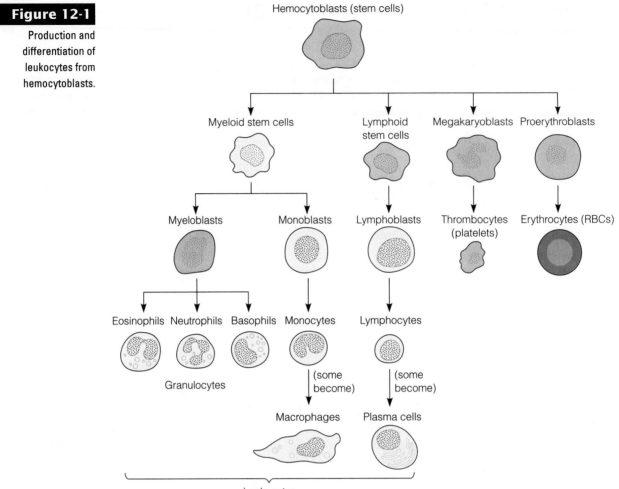

into bloodstream during an acute **hypersensitivity** (abnormally sensitive to a stimulus) reaction or stress response

3) *Monocytes and macrophages*

    a) Monocytes are largest of leukocytes and comprise 2 to 3% of total circulating leukocytes; released from bone marrow and circulate for 1 to 2 days before they attach to various tissues, where they remain for months to years before they are activated

    b) Monocytes mature into **macrophages** (mature monocytes that actively phagocytize large foreign particles and cell debris) after settling into tissues

    c) Both types are actively phagocytic with capacity to engulf large foreign particles and cell debris

    d) Monocytes and macrophages are particularly important in fight against chronic infections such as viral infections, tuberculosis, and certain intracellular parasitic infections

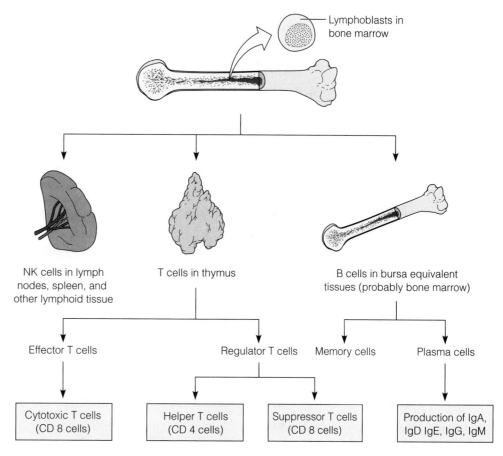

Figure 12-2

Development and differentiation of lymphocytes from lymphoblast in bone marrow.

4) Lymphocytes are small cells that account for 20 to 40% of circulating lymphocytes; are principal effectors and regulators of specific immune response (see Figure 12-2)

   a) Monitor body for cancerous cells in a process known as immune surveillance

   b) Lymphocytes constantly circulate, but in a homing pattern return to lymphoid tissues

   c) On contact with an **antigen** (substance capable of producing a specific immune response), lymphocytes are activated and mature into either effector cells (plasma cells or cytotoxic cells), which are instrumental in destruction of antigens, or memory cells

   d) Memory cells activate immediately upon subsequent exposure to same antigen; are responsible for providing acquired immunity

   e) There are three types of lymphocytes: T lymphocytes (T cells), B lymphocytes (B cells), and natural killer cells (NK cells)

   f) T and B cells are integral to specific immune response

   g) NK cells are large, granular cells found in spleen, lymph nodes, bone marrow, and blood that provide immune surveillance and resistance to infection and play an important role in destruction of early malignant cells

7. Lymphoid system

   a. Lymphocytes concentrate in lymphoid tissues, which include lymph nodes, spleen, thymus, tonsils, lymphoid tissue scattered in connective tissues and mucosa, and bone marrow

   b. Thymus and bone marrow, in which T and B cells mature, are considered primary lymphoid organs

   c. Spleen, lymph nodes, tonsils, and other peripheral lymphoid tissues are considered secondary lymphoid organs

   1) Lymph nodes are most numerous of lymphoid tissues and are distributed throughout body as small round or bean-shaped nodules that vary in size from 1 mm to 2 cm, which filter foreign products or antigens from lymph, storing and supporting proliferation of lymphocytes and macrophages

   a) Lymph, a clear, protein-filled fluid, is transported by lymph vessels

   b) The presence of a foreign protein stimulates lymphocytes and macrophages to proliferate in lymph nodes

   2) The spleen, the largest lymphoid organ, is only part of system able to filter blood

   a) Located in upper left quadrant of abdomen

   b) Composed of white pulp, which serves as a site for lymphocyte proliferation and immune surveillance

   c) B cells predominate in white pulp; blood filtration occurs in red pulp

   d) Spleen also stores blood and breakdown products of RBCs for future use

   e) Spleen is not essential for life; when removed or damaged, liver and bone marrow assume its functions

   3) Thymus gland is located in superior anterior mediastinal cavity beneath sternum

   a) It reaches maximum size at puberty and begins to atrophy slowly; in adult, it is difficult to differentiate from other tissue

   b) Main function of thymus is to serve as a site for maturation and differentiation of T cells

   c) Thymosin, an immunoregulatory hormone, stimulates lymphopoiesis, the formation of lymphocytes or lymphoid tissue

   4) Bone marrow is soft tissue found in hollow cavity of long bones, as well as flat bones of skull, sternum, ribs, and vertebrae; produces and stores stem cells (from which all cellular components of blood are derived)

   5) Lymphoid tissues are also located at key sites of potential invasion by microorganisms: the genitourinary, respiratory, and gastrointestinal tracts

8. Bodily response

   a. Nonspecific inflammatory response: when first-line defenses are breached, the resulting damage or invasion produces a nonspecific immune response known as inflammation

   b. Specific immune response: occurs with introduction of foreign substances, or antigens, into body; specific immune response has the following properties:

   1) Typically directed against materials recognized as foreign and is not usually directed against self (because of self-recognition)

   2) Response is specific; it is initiated by and directed against particular antigens

3) Response is systemic, not localized

4) Immune response has memory; repeated exposures to an antigen produce a more rapid response

5) Recognition of self: effectiveness of immune system depends on its ability to differentiate normal host tissue from abnormal or foreign tissue

    a) Body's components have antigenic properties that are unique and are recognized by immune system as self

    b) External agents have antigenic properties which are identified by immune system as non-self

9. Antigens

    a. Antigens are substances recognized as foreign or non-self and provoke a specific immune response when introduced into body

    b. Typically, antigens are large protein molecules although other substances (polysaccharides, polypeptides, and nucleic acids) may be antigenic

    c. Other antigens include transplanted tissue or organs; incompatible blood cells, vaccines, pollen, egg white, and toxins such as snake or bee venom

    d. When an antigen is introduced into body, it is recognized by a specific receptor on a lymphocyte and an immune response is initiated

B. Humoral immune response

1. Humoral immune response is defined as an antibody-mediated immune response produced by B lymphocytes

2. Antigens such as bacteria, bacterial toxins, and free viruses usually activate B cells to produce **antibodies** (immune or protective protein evoked by an antigen)

3. An antibody-mediated response is characterized by:

    a. Phagocytosis of antigen by neutrophils

    b. Precipitation: combining of soluble antigens to form insoluble forms (precipitates)

    c. Neutralization: combining with a toxin to neutralize its effects; followed by destruction by phagocytosis

    d. Lysis of antigen cell membrane

    e. Agglutination or clumping of antigens to form a noninvasive aggregate

    f. Opsonization: coating of antigen with antibodies and complement, making it more susceptible to phagocytosis

C. Cell-mediated immune response

1. Cell-mediated immune response is defined as an immune system response to antigens that do not evoke antibody-mediated response because they live inside body cells (viruses and mycobacterium are examples of such antigens)

2. Antigens, such as viral infected cells, cancer cells, and foreign tissue, activate T cells, which are primary agents of cell-mediated [cellular] response

3. T cells are antigen specific and are much more complex than B cells

    a. Killer T cells bind with cell surface antigens on infected or foreign cells and then either destroy cell membrane or release cytotoxic substances into cell

    b. Regulator T cells, (majority of which are T helper cells [CD4 cells]), play a key role in controlling immune response by:

        1) Stimulating proliferation of other T cells

        2) Amplifying cytotoxic activity of killer T cells

        3) Activating B cells to proliferate and differentiate

        4) Interacting directly with B cells to promote their conversion into plasma cells capable of producing antibodies

    c. Other regulatory T cells (suppressor T cells) provide negative feedback, making immune response a self-limiting process; they are also important in preventing autoimmune disorders

    d. T cells synthesize and release lymphokines, which stimulate:

        1) B cells to become plasma cells and produce antibodies

        2) Macrophages to become activated macrophages (most aggressive phagocyte)

        3) Proliferation of killer T cells

D. The processes of antibody-mediated and cell-mediated immunity result in development of acquired immunity or active immunity

    1. *Active immunity* occurs when body produces antibodies or develops immune lymphocytes against specific antigens

        a. Memory cells, which can produce an immediate immune response on re-exposure to an antigen, provide long-term immunity

        b. Active immunity can be *naturally acquired* resulting from contact with a disease-producing antigen and subsequent development of disease; this is common for diseases such as chickenpox and hepatitis A

        c. Active immunity can be *artificially acquired* through immunization or vaccinations

    2. *Passive immunity* provides temporary protection against disease-producing antigens

        a. *Naturally acquired* passive immunity is provided by transfer of maternal antibodies via placenta and breast milk to infant

        b. *Artificially acquired* passive immunity is provided by immune globulins and serums

E. Risk factors

    1. Allergies: inherited or acquired sensitivity with repeated exposures; diseases (asthma, AIDS, immunodeficient states); individuals in contact with venomous animals; environment

    2. Latex allergy: acquired sensitivity with repeated exposures, employees required to use gloves often (health care professionals, rescue workers, firefighters, police officers, food service workers, housekeeping staff, etc.); clients identifying atopic conditions; spina bifida clients; clients with a history of multiple surgeries when young

    3. Anaphylaxis: history of known allergens; injection of antigenic material (allergy shots, serum from a sensitized animal); children receiving immunizations; blood transfusion; food; contrast media

    4. Acquired immunodeficiency syndrome (AIDS): health care professionals (contact, blood products, needle sticks); homosexual practice; homeless state; blood transfusion; IV drug abusers; link to sexually transmitted diseases

II. ALLERGIES

A. Overview

    1. An allergy is defined as an abnormal response of immune system to an **allergen** (substance, foreign protein or cell, capable of causing alterations in sensitivity)

2. When antigen is environmental or external it is called an allergy, and antigen is referred to as an allergen

3. Hypersensitivity reactions are classified by type of immune response that occurs on contact and may also be classified by timing of response

   a. Anaphylaxis and transfusion reactions are examples of immediate hypersensitivity reactions

   b. Contact dermatitis is a typical delayed reaction

4. Allergens are introduced by contact, inhalation, or ingestion

5. Causes are numerous and include plants, animals, chemicals, molds, grasses, trees, pests, dust, food, drugs, latex, cosmetics, and perfumes

B. Pathophysiology

1. An initial contact or exposure to an allergen is required to produce sensitization

2. Following sensitization, subsequent contact with allergen produces symptoms; this may occur with next contact or years later

3. Classified as four types of hypersensitivity responses

   a. *Type I* or *IgE-mediated hypersensitivity reaction*

      1) Produces an immediate reaction; local or systemic

      2) Examples are: immediate—allergic asthma, allergic rhinitis (hayfever), allergic conjunctivitis, and hives; rapid—anaphylactic

      3) Occurs when an allergen interacts with IgE bound to mast cells and basophils; this complex prompts release of histamine and other chemicals such as complement, acetylcholine, kinins, and chemotactic factors

      4) Histamine is responsible for most inflammatory symptoms: peripheral vasodilation, increased vascular permeability, vascular congestion, and edema

      5) Leukotrienes and **cytokines** (agents of lymphoid system that act to modify body's response to cancerous cells) involve T lymphocytes, monocytes, eosinophils, and neutrophils, producing symptoms of contraction of smooth muscle causing bronchiolar constriction and edema

   b. *Type II* or *cytotoxic hypersensitivity* reaction

      1) Characterized by IgG or IgM type antibodies that react to foreign tissues or cells; are usually immediate responses

      2) Examples include hemolytic transfusion reaction of an incompatible blood type or a drug reaction (where drug forms an antigenic complex on surface of a blood cell)

      3) In this reaction, lysis of blood cells (platelets, erythrocytes, and leukocytes) occurs because of activation of complement

      4) Transfusion reactions: antibodies in recipient's serum react against antigens in donor's RBCs

         a) Results in hemolysis of donor RBCs, unconjugated bilirubin from broken-down hemoglobin, and precipitation of large amounts of hemoglobin

         b) Symptoms include fever, chills, low back pain, hypotension, tachycardia, nausea, vomiting, urticaria, red-colored urine, shock, and renal failure

      5) Other conditions caused by a Type II reaction include erythroblastosis fetalis (Rh incompatibility in mother and child); autoimmune hemolytic anemia and drug induced hemolysis

c. *Type III immune complex-mediated hypersensitivity* reaction

        1) Results from formation of IgG or IgM antibody-antigen complexes that circulate in blood; are usually immediate responses

        2) Complexes adhere to walls of vessels and cause inflammation and leads to intravascular, synovial, endocardial, or other organ complications

        3) Examples include serum sickness, arthus (joint) reactions, and autoimmune conditions

        4) Symptoms are specific to reaction: serum sickness—fever, joint and muscle pain, urticaria, rash; arthus (joint) reaction—acute, localized edema, tissue inflammation

    d. *Type IV delayed hypersensitivity reaction*

        1) These reactions are cell-mediated, rather than antibody-mediated, involving T cells of immune system

        2) Are delayed rather than immediate; with an onset 24 to 48 hours after exposure to antigen

        3) Result from an exaggerated interaction between an antigen and normal cell-mediated mechanisms

        4) Examples include contact dermatitis, infections, granulomatous inflammation, autoimmune diseases, transplant or graft rejection

        5) Symptoms are specific to type of response

            a) Contact dermatitis such as poison ivy: redness, induration, lesions, urticaria, weeping

            b) Positive TB skin testing: reddening and induration of > 5 mm at 72 hours for people who are immunosuppressed or have close contact with a client positive for TB

            c) Granulomatous inflammation: leprosy, syphilis, cat-scratch disease

4. Autoimmune disorders

    a. Occur when immune system's ability to recognize self is impaired and immune defenses are directed against normal host tissue

    b. Can affect any tissue in body; some disorders are tissue- or organ-specific and some are systemic, with neither antibodies nor inflammatory lesions confined to any one organ

    c. Mechanism that causes immune system to recognize host tissue as a foreign antigen is not clear

    d. Known characteristics

        1) Genetics plays a role

        2) More prevalent in females than males

        3) Onset of an immune disorder is frequently associated with an abnormal stressor, either physical or psychological

        4) Are frequently progressive relapsing-remitting disorders characterized by periods of exacerbation and remission

5. Tissue transplants

    a. Transplant success is closely tied to obtaining the best match of tissue antigens to recipient; an autograft (a transplant of client's own tissue) is most successful type of transplantation

    b. *Hyperacute tissue rejections* occur immediately or 2 to 3 days after transplant of new tissue and are due to preformed antibodies and T cells sensitized to

---

► **Practice to Pass**

The physician suggests weekly allergy shots for a child with asthma caused by seasonal allergies. How should the nurse explain how the shots will work to the mother?

antigens in donor organ; this type of rejection is most likely to occur in individuals who have had previous organ or tissue transplants

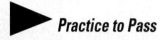

   c. *Acute tissue rejection* is most common and treatable type of rejection episode; it occurs between 4 days and 3 months following transplant

      1) It is mediated primarily by cellular immune response and results in transplant cell destruction

      2) Client demonstrates manifestations of inflammatory process, with fever, redness, swelling, and tenderness over graft site

      3) Signs of impaired function of transplanted organ may be noted

   d. *Chronic tissue rejection* occurs from 4 months to years after transplantation of new tissues or organs

      1) It is likely the result of an antibody-mediated immune response

      2) Antibodies and complement deposit in transplanted tissue vessel walls resulting in decreased blood flow and ischemia

   e. **Graft-versus-host disease** (GvHD) is a frequent and potentially fatal complication of bone marrow transplantation

      1) Defined as a disorder occurring when immunocompetent graft cells recognize host tissue as foreign and mount a cell-mediated immune response

      2) Host is usually immunocompromised and unable to fight graft cells, and host's cells are destroyed

      3) Other areas affected are skin, liver, and gastrointestinal tract

C. Nursing assessment

  1. Assessment includes skin, vital signs (VS), lung sounds, respiratory status, level of consciousness (LOC), fluid status, peripheral perfusion (pulses, capillary refill, temperature of extremities); any reports of discomfort; mental status (anxiety); history of events leading to allergic reaction

  2. Diagnostic tests

   a. WBC, high eosinophil level

   b. Radioallergosorbent test (RAST), to determine presence of IgE

   c. Type and crossmatch

   d. Indirect Coombs' test; agglutination occurs if antibodies to an RBC antigen are present

   e. Direct Coombs' test; antibodies are present on client's RBCs

   f. Immune complex assays, circulating immune complexes present

   g. Complement assay; complement levels are decreased

   h. Skin testing

      1) Skin prick test, positive test produces a wheal and erythema

      2) Intradermal, wheal of 5 mm or greater and erythema

      3) Patch, mild to severe erythema with papules or vesicles

      4) Food allergy testing, presence of symptoms within hours of eating particular food thought to cause reaction

D. Nursing management

  1. Medications include **immunotherapy** (natural and/or synthetic substances used to stimulate or suppress response of immune system such as allergy shots), antihistamines, epinephrine for severe symptoms, budesonide (Rhinocort) or cromolyn sodium (Nasalcrom) for allergic rhinitis and asthma, glucocorticoids, over-the-counter (OTC) nasal decongestants such as pseudoephedrine tablets

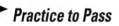

Practice to Pass

Explain in simple terminology how the body develops an autoimmune disease or rejects organ tissue.

Practice to Pass

Why should the nurse explain to the client who is scheduled for a skin prick test for allergies to avoid antihistamines for 3 days prior to the test?

2. Goal is to minimize exposure, prevent a hypersensitivity response, and provide quick interventions if a response occurs

3. Instruct clients to wear a Medic-alert bracelet

4. Airway management is highest priority if laryngeal edema occurs; administer oxygen (O_2); intubate or use nasopharyngeal/oropharyngeal airway if necessary

5. Other therapies consist of plasmapheresis (removal of components in plasma)

6. Monitor VS

7. Access an intravenous (IV) line and administer fluids as necessary; use a Foley catheter and monitor intake and output (I&O) as ordered and indicated

8. Administer blood products following hospital protocol

   a. Have a signed informed consent

   b. Check the blood for type, Rh factor (Rh− must have Rh− and Rh+ must have Rh+), expiration date, crossmatch with another licensed health care professional

   c. Monitor VS every 5 minutes for the first 15 minutes and every 30 minutes or 1 hour thereafter until blood has been infused according to policy

   d. Administer blood with normal saline (NS) only

   e. Stop the transfusion if any reaction occurs, send blood bag and tubing to lab for analysis; obtain urine speciment for urinalysis per protocol

9. Educate client on having a bee sting kit or an Epi-pen available at all times

III. LATEX ALLERGY

A. Overview

1. A **latex allergy** is defined as a reaction to contact with latex, producing an allergic contact dermatitis, immediate hypersensitivity, or anaphylaxis

2. Latex is extracted from tissue beneath bark of rubber tree; it is a cloudy white liquid composed of rubber particles, protein, water, and other substances

3. The method used to process latex affects amount of protein left in finished product

4. Produces a type I or type IV reaction

5. Prevention of latex allergy reactions should focus on both client and staff

6. Causes of latex allergy include exposure through cutaneous route (gloves, tapes, masks); mucous membranes (anesthesia, rectal examinations, eye and ear droppers); intrauterine devices; intravascular (IV fluids, injectables, IV devices); internal contact through surgery

B. Pathophysiology

1. An allergic reaction is triggered upon contact with latex (see Section II, Allergies)

2. Reactions usually manifest in three ways

   a. Allergic contact dermatitis (type IV delayed hypersensitivity): most common

      1) An allergic reaction to residues of chemical agents used in latex and in manufacturing plastics

      2) Symptoms include: dry, itchy red rash on hands and fingers; blistering and weeping of skin; swelling

   b. Immediate hypersensitivity (type I)

      1) Natural latex protein produces an IgE response

      2) Can cause severe, even fatal reactions

3) Symptoms develop within 5 to 30 minutes from exposure and diminish quickly when exposure is removed

4) Symptoms include immediate itching; intense swelling of fingers and hand; may proceed to anaphylaxis

c. Anaphylaxis

1) Occurs when there has been contact with latex through mucous membranes or body cavities such as in surgery

2) Symptoms include local or generalized itching; urticaria; angioedema; rhinitis; conjunctivitis; asthma; extreme anxiety; gastrointestinal (GI) complaints (nausea, vomiting, abdominal pain); tachycardia; hypotension; faintness; coma; cardiac arrest

C. Nursing assessment

1. Assessment includes color and moisture of skin; reports of itching; presence of wheals or urticaria; visual inspection of swelling; history concerning any prior problems (especially if client is going to surgery); history of reaction to fruits (especially banana and kiwi fruit); if anaphylaxis suspected, assess respiratory and cardiac status; LOC; VS; mentation

2. Diagnostic tests

a. Patch tests or skin prick test: positive for one or more latex accelerators

b. Blood sample for specific IgE test

D. Nursing management

1. Medications include topical steroids, same as for anaphylaxis (see Section IV)

2. Primary treatment is removal of irritant

3. Educate client on what caused reaction and to avoid future contact

4. Instruct client to wear a Medic-alert bracelet

5. Instruct client to use a non-irritating soap substitute and emollient creams while affected area is red and irritated

6. Supervise housekeeping practices to reduce latex-containing dust from environment

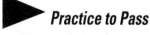

Practice to Pass

What symptoms would be present in an environmental service worker who is allergic to latex and why? Why should the gloves not be snapped upon removal?

IV. ANAPHYLAXIS

A. Overview

1. Anaphylaxis is defined as an allergic response when an antigen is introduced to a highly sensitive individual

2. Response is a type I allergic reaction and is a medical emergency

3. Categorized as local or systemic

4. May lead to anaphylactic shock (see Chapter 17)

5. Multiple causes exist and are individualized: pollens, foods, drugs (antibiotics are common), venom, insect bites, diagnostic agents (contrast medium), antiserum, enzymes, hormones, vitamins, occupational agents, iodine

B. Pathophysiology

1. An antigen is introduced and interacts with immunoglobulin E (IgE), which is bound to mast cells and basophils

2. This reaction causes mast cells to suddenly release histamines and other mediators throughout body or locally

3. Mast cells also release packets containing chemical mediators, which attract neutrophils and eosinophils

4. Local reactions include urticaria, vasodilation (warmth), edema, erythema

5. Systemic reactions include respiratory (bronchoconstriction, air hunger, stridor, wheezing, barking cough); cardiovascular (hypotension, tachycardia, impaired tissue perfusion); skin (same as local reaction); gastrointestinal system (nausea, vomiting); angioedema; anxiety

6. Systemic reactions can lead to anaphylactic shock when widespread vasodilation occurs

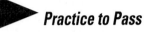

Practice to Pass

Why is an anaphylactic reaction considered an emergency?

C. Nursing assessment

1. Assessment includes VS, lung sounds, heart sounds, skin assessment, analysis of symptoms, respiratory status, presence of edema, LOC, history of past allergies

2. Diagnostic tests

    a. Initial laboratory tests focus on acute symptoms: complete blood count (CBC), arterial blood gases (ABGs), type and crossmatch (if blood transfusion involved), RAST, direct and indirect Coombs' Test, immune complex assay, complement assay

    b. Tests to determine cause of anaphylaxis would follow, after client is stabilized

D. Nursing management

1. Medications include antihistamines and epinephrine, vasopressors such as dopamine, and corticosteroids

2. Initial management and airway management are of highest priority

3. Client teaching

    a. Wear a Medic-alert bracelet

    b. Identify triggers and how to avoid these

    c. Know emergency management until client can be brought to an emergency room (bee sting kit, Epi-pen)

4. Initiate and maintain an IV line in order to access emergency drugs

5. Administer O_2 as needed

6. Monitor VS frequently, as often as every 15 minutes if needed

V. ACQUIRED IMMUNODEFICIENCY SYNDROME (AIDS)

A. Overview

1. **Acquired immunodeficiency syndrome (AIDS)** is defined as last stage of infection with human immunodeficiency virus (HIV) (a retrovirus of lentivirus family)

2. **Immunodeficiency** is a state in which client's immune system is incompetent or unable to respond effectively

3. Adult classification of HIV disease is based on clinical manifestations and T4 cell counts

    a. Category A: asymptomatic, primary HIV or persistent generalized lymphadenopathy (PGL)

    b. Category B: symptomatic, not category A or C conditions

    c. Category C: AIDS-defining characteristics

4. Diagnosis is made on presence of all of the following
   a. CD4 count of less than 200 cells/mm^3
   b. Two opportunistic pathogens
   c. Presence of an AIDS-defining malignancy
5. Two primary human immunodeficiency viruses
   a. HIV-1, prototype virus, mostly in United States
   b. HIV-2: primarily limited to West Africa
6. Transmission
   a. Adult to adult: unprotected sexual activity and blood-to-blood contact
   b. Adult to child: perinatal transmission and blood-to-blood contact
7. Causes
   a. Unprotected sexual activity: vaginal, anal, and oral intercourse
   b. Blood to blood: needles, blood transfusions, exposure of health care workers
   c. Perinatal transmission: placental or intrapartum transmission and via breast milk

B. **Pathophysiology**
   1. HIV is a retrovirus, which carries its genetic information in RNA; on entry into body virus infects cells that have CD4 antigen [primarily T helper cells] (see Figure 12-3)
   2. As with any virus, HIV is a parasite and must infect other cells in order to replicate
   3. Many target cells used by HIV to replicate are antigen-presenting cells needed for a normal immune response in body (CD4 lymphocytes, bone marrow CD4 precursor cells, monocytic T cell lines, etc.)
   4. Once inside cell, virus is transported to lymph nodes and attached by viral gp120 to host cell
   5. Once attached, virus enters host cell, reveals its RNA genome and uses an enzyme, reverse transcriptase, to convert viral RNA to viral DNA by using normal DNA
   6. This viral DNA insinuates itself into host cell DNA and is replicated during normal cell processes
   7. This process results in two major effects
      a. Viral number increases (viral load)
         1) **Viral load** is the number of circulating HIV particles per milliliter (should be zero)
         2) Viral loads of less than 10,000 = low risk; 10,000 to 100,000 = moderate risk; greater than 100,000 = high risk
      b. Infected CD4 cells die
         1) Competent immune system = T4 count of 650 to 1,200 cells/mm^3
         2) Suppressed immune system = T4 count of 500 to 200 cells/mm^3
         3) AIDS: indicator values = T4 count of less than 200 cells/mm^3
   8. Virus may lie dormant or become activated, producing new RNA and virions leading to destruction of host cells
   9. Although virus may remain inactive, antibodies are produced and detectable between 6 weeks and 6 months of infection; however, these antibodies are not able to fight HIV infection

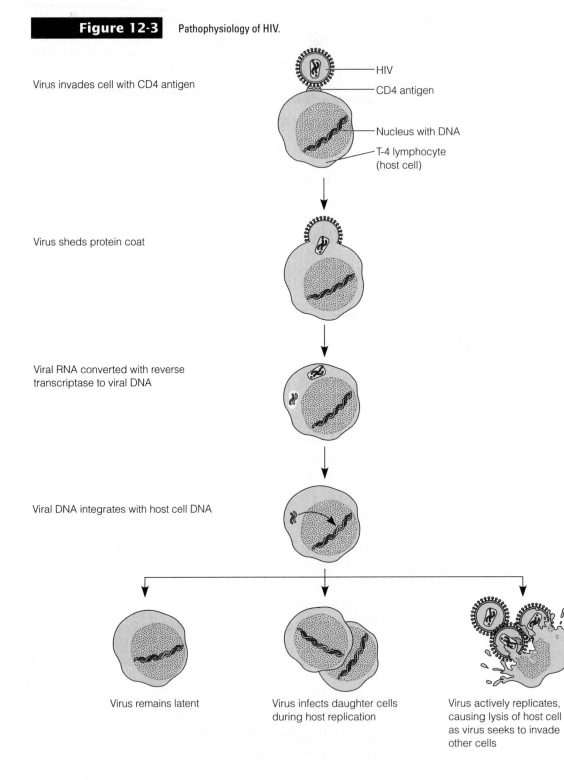

Figure 12-3 Pathophysiology of HIV.

Virus invades cell with CD4 antigen

- HIV
- CD4 antigen
- Nucleus with DNA
- T-4 lymphocyte (host cell)

Virus sheds protein coat

Viral RNA converted with reverse transcriptase to viral DNA

Viral DNA integrates with host cell DNA

Virus remains latent

Virus infects daughter cells during host replication

Virus actively replicates, causing lysis of host cell as virus seeks to invade other cells

10. A client may show negative on antibody test for HIV but still have virus; a seroconversion time exists (6 to 12 weeks) that allows an HIV positive client who has no symptoms to start producing antibodies; after seroconversion, antibodies will continue to be produced

11. Although T helper cells are primarily infected with HIV, other cells (including macrophages and cells of central nervous system [CNS]) are also infected

12. Classification of HIV infection and AIDS

   a. *Category A*

      1) Primary HIV infection: negative HIV antibody tests; influenza-like symptoms; rash; symptoms cease after a few days

      2) Asymptomatic: positive antibody tests, no disease processes

      3) Persistent generalized lymphadenopathy (PGL): positive antibody tests, lymphadenopathy present for more than 3 months

      4) CD4 T cell counts

         a) A1 = greater than or equal to 500/mm^3

         b) A2 = 200 to 499/mm^3

         c) A3 = less than 200/mm^3

   b. *Category B*

      1) Positive antibody tests

      2) Symptomatic: oral thrush, candidiasis, cervical dysplasia, leukoplakia, herpes zoster, pelvic inflammatory disease (PID), fever, or diarrhea for more than 1 month

      3) CD4 T cell counts

         a) B1 = greater than or equal to 500/mm^3

         b) B2 = 200 to 499/mm^3

         c) B3 = less than 200/mm^3

   c. AIDS-indicator conditions

      1) Positive antibody tests

      2) AIDS-defining conditions

         a) *Pneumocystis carinii* pneumonia

         b) Candidiasis

         c) Cytomegalovirus

         d) *Mycobacterium tuberculosis*

         e) Toxoplasmosis of brain

         f) Histoplasmosis

         g) Kaposi sarcoma

         h) Lymphomas

         i) AIDS dementia complex

         j) HIV wasting syndrome, weight loss of 10% or more of body weight within a 6-month period without intention

      3) CD4 T cell counts

         a) C1 = greater than or equal to 500/mm^3

         b) C2 = 200 to 499/mm^3

         c) C3 = less than 200/mm^3

13. Signs and symptoms range from no symptoms to severe immunodeficiency with multiple severe **opportunistic disease** (any infection resulting from a deficient immune system) and neoplasm, including:

    a. Flulike or mononucleosis-like illness lasting days to weeks after contracting HIV

    b. Fever, sore throat, joint and muscle pain, headache, rash, and swollen lymph nodes (often first symptom); this presentation is commonly mistaken for influenza, upper respiratory infection, or gastroenteritis

    c. Progression from asymptomatic infection to AIDS is not clearly defined; the client may report general malaise, fever, fatigue, night sweats, and unintentional weight loss; diarrhea is common, as are oral lesions of hairy leukoplakia, candidiasis/thrush, and gingival inflammation and ulceration

    d. Other symptoms include stiff neck; burning, numbness, and tingling of extremities; headache, lightheadedness, memory loss, mood swings; nausea and vomiting; pain; dyspnea

    e. AIDS dementia complex (ADC) is a dementia with cognitive, behavioral, and motor deficits that is common in untreated HIV disease and affects CNS; it is thought to be caused by infection of HIV in brain cells and symptoms include impaired concentration, mental slowing, forgetfulness, apathy, confusion, hallucinations, personality changes, unsteady gait, leg tremors, and motor difficulties

14. There is a long asymptomatic period following initial infection; host is capable of infecting others during this latent period

15. Seroconversion occurs when an HIV-infected individual starts producing detectable HIV antibodies; seroconversion window is that time when infection has occurred but HIV antibodies are not detectable; individuals are able to pass virus to others unknowingly during this period

16. Mean length of time from infection to symptomatology is currently estimated to be 8 to 10 years

C. Nursing assessment

1. Assessment includes common symptoms, weight analysis, GI disturbances, neurological manifestations; gait; LOC; reports of pain; history of recurring infections; skin assessment; palpation of lymph nodes; VS; lung sounds; oral cavity; vaginal and rectal exam

2. Diagnostic tests

    a. Enzyme-linked immunosorbent assays (ELISA) to screen for HIV antibodies; usually will run two different tests

    b. Western-blot test, to confirm a positive ELISA finding

    c. HIV viral load, high

    d. CBC, anemia, leukopenia, thrombocytopenia

    e. CD4 cell count, low

    f. Immune complex dissociated p24 assay, shows active reproduction of HIV, used for progression of disease

    g. Diagnostic tests for opportunistic infections include:

        1) TB skin tests

        2) Magnetic resonance imagery (MRI) of brain, lymphomas

        3) Cultures

Practice to Pass

Explain why an initial ELISA test could be negative in an HIV-positive client and why two ELISA tests are usually conducted, followed by a Western blot?

      4) Pap smears

      5) Chest x-ray for *Pneumocystis carinii* pneumonia

D. Nursing management

  1. Medications include

    a. Antiretroviral agents

      1) Nucleoside reverse transcriptase inhibitors (NRTIs): inhibit action of viral reverse transcriptase, which is necessary for introduction of viral RNA into cells' DNA and replication, resulting in an incomplete viral DNA; example: zidovudine (AZT)

      2) Protease inhibitors: inhibit protease, a viral enzyme necessary for production of mature viral particles; example: saquinavir (Invirase)

      3) Nonnucleoside reverse transcriptase inhibitors (NNRTIs): block making of DNA by getting on a part of virus called the reverse transcriptase enzyme; example: nevirapine (Viramune)

      4) Fusion inhibitor: interferes with entry of HIV-I into host cells by blocking fusion of virus and cell membranes: enfuvirtide (Fuzeon)

    b. Drug cocktails are a combination of above types in order to attack disease more aggressively; close monitoring is necessary

    c. Other agents include chemotherapy, antibiotics for infections, analgesics for pain and discomforts, antiemetics, antidiarrheals

    d. Consult Centers for Disease Control (CDC) for most accurate information on new drug development (http://www.cdc.gov/hiv/dhap.htm)

  2. At present, there is a reasonable life expectancy that requires attention to prevention of transmission and avoidance of secondary infections

  3. All persons should practice safe sex techniques and avoid contamination by body fluids or shared needles

  4. For clients with advanced disease, information about community resources, nonjudgmental care, and health promotion activities are essential

  5. Surgical treatments for abscesses and Kaposi's sarcoma may be indicated

  6. Counseling for psychological and social effects should be initiated

  7. Maintain clean perianal area if diarrhea is persistent

  8. Instruct client on foods to avoid that are GI irritants; avoid spicy, acidic foods and those hard to chew

  9. Educate client on common side effects of medications

  10. Offer and instruct on proper oral care; avoid toothbrushes; use mouthwash without alcohol

  11. Educate client about symptoms of candida and herpes and when to seek help

  12. If blood or body fluid spills occur, instruct client to use a 1:10 solution of bleach

  13. Allow client and family to talk about illness and discuss concerns; offer touch

  14. Monitor weight and nutritional status; assess caloric intake

  15. Encourage ambulation and exercise as tolerated with planned rest periods

  16. Offer O_2 as needed for dyspnea

Case Study

A 43-year-old man is brought to the emergency department after being stung multiple times by hornets while cutting grass. He has welts over most of his body, is itching all over, exhibits extreme anxiety, shows tachycardia of 150 on the cardiac monitor and BP 108/65. His frantic wife states that he is allergic to penicillin and has reacted to bee stings in the past.

1. What immediate assessment should the nurse make?

2. What additional information is needed from the client or his wife?

3. What drug therapy would the nurse expect the emergency room physician to institute?

4. The client's wife asks the nurse to explain to her what is going on. How should the nurse respond?

5. What discharge instructions should be given to this client, once he is stabilized and able to return home?

For suggested responses, see page 537

POSTTEST

1. The nurse concludes that medications taken by a client with acquired immunodeficiency syndrome (AIDS) are effective if, in addition to a viral load of 25,000, the client exhibits which of the following?

1. Rare occurrence of symptoms
2. Negative enzyme linked immunosorbent assay (ELISA)
3. CD4 T lymphocyte count of 490
4. White blood cell (WBC) count of 1,700 mm^3

2. The nurse anticipates that a child with asthma caused by allergies will have which of the following findings on a complete blood count (CBC) with differential report?

1. Eosinophils 21.9
2. White blood cells 10.9
3. Monocytes 4.0
4. Neutrophils 85.7

3. The mother of a child with swollen lymph nodes is extremely panic-stricken that the swelling means cancer. What is the best statement that the nurse could make to calm the mother?

1. "The finding is very alarming and could be serious, but you must remember it may be insignificant also."
2. "The lymph nodes filter foreign products and may only be swollen because of an infection."
3. "The lymph nodes will swell quite often and we may not ever know it."
4. "The lymph nodes are the major organ indicating a problem with the immune system."

4. A client in an allergy clinic asks the nurse why some allergic reactions affect only a small area while one in the past involved "my whole body and my breathing." The nurse offers which of the following as examples of reactions that could cause systemic immune responses? Select all that apply.

1. Extreme redness and swelling after being bitten by ants
2. Anaphylaxis after ingesting a certain food such as shellfish
3. Developing symptoms of systemic latex allergy
4. Severe bronchoconstriction and wheezing after playing football in the grass
5. Sprained ankle becoming swollen, bruised, and painful

5 A client reports to the clinic with reports of itching and weeping along the back of her legs. Upon inspection, wheals are evident that appear to be poison ivy. The client states that the symptoms developed a day after sitting in the car wearing shorts. She sat on the same seat as her husband, who had been working in a field of grass all day. The nurse concludes that the client is having which type of reaction?

1. Type I hypersensitivity
2. Type II hypersensitivity
3. Type III hypersensitivity
4. Type IV hypersensitivity

6 A family member of a client with type O− blood is concerned about the risk of allergic reaction when the client receives a needed transfusion. The nurse explains that which type of blood will be transfused to avoid an allergic reaction?

1. O+
2. O−
3. AB+
4. AB−

7 In assessing a client with a suspected latex allergy, the nurse should ask which of the following questions?

1. "Are your hands usually moist or dry?"
2. "What drug allergies do you have?"
3. "Do the elastic bands in your underwear cause rash and itching?"
4. "What types of surgeries have you had?"

8 The nurse would immediately assess for which of the following symptoms in the client suspected of having an anaphylactic reaction?

1. Elevated blood pressure of 180/94
2. Decreased apical pulse rate of 56
3. Onset of lung crackles
4. Onset of stridor or wheezing

9 A 31-year-old female who has progressed into advanced acquired immunodeficiency syndrome (AIDS) is concerned about developing a secondary cancer. What diagnostic test should the nurse explain will probably be ordered every six months?

1. Papanicolaou smear
2. Viral load
3. CD4 cell counts
4. CA 125 antigen level

10 The public health nurse considers that which of the following individuals is at increased risk of acquiring human immunodeficiency virus (HIV)?

1. Police officer who works the streets and responds to emergencies
2. Sexually active teenager
3. School nurse who examines children
4. Nurse working on a telemetry unit

➤ *See pages 369–371 for Answers Rationales.*

POSTTEST

ANSWERS & RATIONALES

Pretest

1 **Answer: 2** *Pneumocystis carinii* pneumonia is the most common opportunistic infection associated with acquired immunodeficiency syndrome (AIDS). The fungus responsible is not pathogenic in individuals with a normal immune system. Opportunistic infections are likely to be seen when the CD4 cell count falls below 200/mm³ in the more advanced stages of AIDS. **Cognitive Level:** Analysis **Client Need:** Physiological Integrity: Physiological Adaptation **Integrated Process:**

Nursing Process: Analysis **Content Area:** Adult Health: Immunological **Strategy:** Analyze the signs and symptoms and decide what disease is being described. Note this infection is associated with immunocompromised individuals. Next determine whether this finding would occur in late or early stages. **Reference:** LeMone, P., & Burke, K. (2008). *Medical-surgical nursing: Critical thinking in client care* (4th ed.). Upper Saddle River, NJ: Pearson/Prentice Hall, p. 353.

2 **Answer: 1** Active acquired immunity occurs when the body produces antibodies or develops immune lympho-

ANSWERS & RATIONALES

cytes against specific antigens, in this case chickenpox (varicella). Breastfeeding a child would offer passively acquired immunity; immune globulins offer passively acquired artificial immunity; immunizations offer actively acquired artificial immunity. This child should be immune to future infections of chickenpox.

Cognitive Level: Application **Client Need:** Health Promotion and Maintenance **Integrated Process:** Nursing Process: Planning **Content Area:** Child Health **Strategy:** Consider what immunologic mechanism occurs when a person recovers from a viral infection. **Reference:** LeMone, P., & Burke, K. (2008). *Medical-surgical nursing: Critical thinking in client care* (4th ed.). Upper Saddle River, NJ: Pearson/Prentice Hall, pp. 298–299.

3 **Answer: 4** A client with Category 3 (AIDS) will have a low CD4 count (< 200 cells/mm^3) and a high viral load. What is desired is to have a high CD4 count and a low viral load (which should normally be zero). The white blood count is not used in classifying HIV.

Cognitive Level: Analysis **Client Need:** Physiological Integrity: Reduction of Risk Potential **Integrated Process:** Nursing Process: Assessment **Content Area:** Adult Health: Immunological **Strategy:** Recall that for an option to be correct, everything in the option must be correct. Analyze each option completely, eliminating first the options that contain WBC counts. **Reference:** Porth, C. M. (2005). *Pathophysiology: Concepts of altered health states* (7th ed.). Philadelphia, PA: Lippincott Williams & Wilkins, pp. 431–432.

4 **Answer: 2** The symptoms in the question are consistent with early human immunodeficiency virus (HIV) infection. The ELISA test may be negative upon initial testing and positive at the time of seroconversion, which takes 6 to 12 weeks after infection. This time period when the antibodies are negative is called the seroconversion window and virally infected individuals may have negative antibody tests.

Cognitive Level: Analysis **Client Need:** Physiological Integrity: Reduction of Risk Potential **Integrated Process:** Communication and Documentation **Content Area:** Adult Health: Immunological **Strategy:** To answer this question accurately, it is necessary to know commonly performed diagnostic tests for the immune system. It is also helpful to know factors that will interfere with accurate diagnostic results—in this case time after exposure to develop antibodies. **Reference:** LeMone, P., & Burke, K. (2008). *Medical-surgical nursing: Critical thinking in client care* (4th ed.). Upper Saddle River, NJ: Pearson/Prentice Hall, pp. 354–356.

5 **Answer: 2** Type I hypersensitivity reactions are caused by widespread antigen-antibody reactions such as anaphylaxis. This person has been sensitized by a prior ex-

posure to the antigen and formed IgE antibodies, which reacted during a subsequent exposure. The anaphylactic response is usually immediate and leads to an antigen-antibody complex that causes the release of histamine and other substances. Option 4 is an explanation of what occurs with a blood transfusion reaction and may also happen with some medications. Option 3 is an explanation of a Type IV delayed hypersensitivity. The first part of option 1 is false.

Cognitive Level: Application **Client Need:** Physiological Integrity: Physiological Adaptation **Integrated Process:** Nursing Process: Analysis **Content Area:** Adult Health: Immunological **Strategy:** Review hypersensitivity reactions. This client situation clearly gives a history of past exposure to the antigen and an anaphylactic response this time. **Reference:** Porth, C. M. (2005). *Pathophysiology: Concepts of altered health states* (7th ed.). Philadelphia, PA: Lippincott Williams & Wilkins, pp. 412–416.

6 **Answer: 1** Type 1 diabetes is caused by the autoimmune destruction of pancreatic beta cells. Recognition of self as foreign is the definition of any autoimmune disease. Further explanation may be needed to explain that the immune system usually recognizes self and identifies what is foreign, targets foreign cells, and destroys them.

Cognitive Level: Application **Client Need:** Physiological Integrity: Physiological Adaptation **Integrated Process:** Nursing Process: Implementation **Content Area:** Adult Health: Immunological **Strategy:** Eliminate the options that do not relate to an autoimmune process. The key word is *autoimmune,* not diabetes mellitus. **Reference:** Porth, C. M. (2005). *Pathophysiology: Concepts of altered health states* (7th ed.). Philadelphia, PA: Lippincott Williams & Wilkins, p. 994.

7 **Answer: 3** Serum sickness, a reaction a week after ingestion of a drug, is a type III hypersensitivity reaction where formation of IgG or IgM antibody-antigen complexes occurs in the blood. The deposited immune complexes activate the inflammatory process causing focal tissue damage and edema. Urticaria, rash, extensive edema, and fever are usually temporary, resolving within a few days after the drug is stopped.

Cognitive Level: Analysis **Client Need:** Physiological Integrity: Physiological Adaptation **Integrated Process:** Nursing Process: Planning **Content Area:** Child Health **Strategy:** The core issue of the question is that the clients have developed an adverse drug reaction. Recall that antibiotics can cause hypersensitivity reactions to determine the correct option. **Reference:** Porth, C. M. (2005). *Pathophysiology: Concepts of altered health states* (7th ed.). Philadelphia, PA: Lippincott Williams & Wilkins, pp. 412–416.

ANSWERS & RATIONALES

8 **Answers: 1, 2, 4** The classification system (1993 CDC recommendations) for HIV and acquired immunodeficiency syndrome (AIDS) lists several clinical problems that place an HIV infected client into Clinical Category C. This is the most advanced category when the client develops significant disease with neurological manifestations (HIV encephalopathy), opportunistic infections, cancers (Kaposi's sarcoma), and possibly HIV wasting syndrome. Options 3 and 5 are seen in Clinical Category A.
Cognitive Level: Application **Client Need:** Physiological Integrity: Physiological Adaptation **Integrated Process:** Nursing Process: Assessment **Content Area:** Adult Health: Immunological **Strategy:** Select the problems seen in advanced AIDS. **Reference:** LeMone, P., & Burke, K. (2008). *Medical-surgical nursing: Critical thinking in client care* (4th ed.). Upper Saddle River, NJ: Pearson/Prentice Hall, p. 352.

9 **Answer: 3** Fluids containing blood or blood cells have been identified as a mode of transmission for HIV. Collecting blood, especially in a mobile unit (where the population is more diverse) is a risk for any health care worker. Appropriate gloving is essential. Counseling may require touch, which isn't a form of transmission; perspiration has not been identified as a form of contact. Using retractable syringes and disposing of used needles appropriately reduces the risk for nurses giving IM injections.
Cognitive Level: Analysis **Client Need:** Safe, Effective Care Environment: Safety and Infection Control **Integrated Process:** Nursing Process: Assessment **Content Area:** Adult Health: Immunological **Strategy:** Consider how the HIV virus is spread and which body fluid is known to contain the virus. **Reference:** LeMone, P., & Burke, K. (2008). *Medical-surgical nursing: Critical thinking in client care* (4th ed.). Upper Saddle River, NJ: Pearson/Prentice Hall, p. 349.

10 **Answer: 1** Because laryngeal spasms and bronchial constriction can occur with anaphylaxis, assessing the client's airway is top priority. The nurse should maintain and establish a patent airway first. Remember the ABCs (airway, breathing, and circulation), cardiac output would come next, followed by risk for injury and finally anxiety.
Cognitive Level: Analysis **Client Need:** Physiological Integrity: Physiological Adaptation **Integrated Process:** Nursing Process: Analysis **Content Area:** Adult Health: Immunological **Strategy:** Use the ABCs and Maslow's hierarchy to prioritize. Recall that airway takes priority in life-threatening situations. **Reference:** Porth, C. M. (2005). *Pathophysiology: Concepts of altered health states* (7th ed.). Philadelphia, PA: Lippincott Williams & Wilkins, p. 412.

Posttest

1 **Answer: 3** A client with AIDS will have exacerbations and remissions with opportunistic infections, therefore symptoms may vary. With a diagnosis of AIDS, an ELISA test would remain positive for antibodies. WBC of 1,700 shows neutropenia, which does not indicate improvement. A CD4 cell count between 200 and 500 is in the "suppressed immune state" but certainly above the 200 mark that is indicative of severe depression of the immune system.
Cognitive Level: Analysis **Client Need:** Physiological Integrity: Physiological Adaptation **Integrated Process:** Nursing Process: Evaluation **Content Area:** Adult Health: Immunological **Strategy:** Compare the desired response to the options. Determine what factors will not change even with the treatment. **Reference:** Porth, C. M. (2005). *Pathophysiology: Concepts of altered health states* (7th ed.). Philadelphia, PA: Lippincott Williams & Wilkins, pp. 438–440.

2 **Answer: 1** Eosinophils are usually elevated in an allergic response. The WBC in option 2 is barely above normal. The monocytes are normal in option 3 and the elevated neutrophils indicate an acute infection (option 4).
Cognitive Level: Analysis **Client Need:** Physiological Integrity: Reduction of Risk Potential **Integrated Process:** Nursing Process: Assessment **Content Area:** Adult Health: Immunological **Strategy:** Specific knowledge of laboratory values is needed to answer the question. Review common lab values such as CBC and differential if this question was difficult. **Reference:** Kee, J. (2006). *Laboratory and diagnostic tests with nursing implications* (7th ed.). Upper Saddle River, NJ: Pearson/Prentice Hall, pp. 457–459.

3 **Answer: 2** The mother is already alarmed enough, and the nurse should be careful with wording of the response. Option 2 is correct and is not alarming so that the mother may be able to focus on a different perspective besides cancer. The wording of options 1 and 4 may cause added concern for the mother. Option 3 does not provide definitive information or assurance in addressing the mother's concern.
Cognitive Level: Application **Client Need:** Physiological Integrity: Physiological Adaptation **Integrated Process:** Communication and Documentation **Content Area:** Adult Health: Immunological **Strategy:** The focus in this question is meeting the needs of the mother who is alarmed. Choose the response that best meets her needs for reassurance and yet gives correct information. **Reference:** Porth, C. M. (2005). *Pathophysiology: Concepts of altered health states* (7th ed.). Philadelphia, PA: Lippincott Williams & Wilkins, p. 377.

ANSWERS & RATIONALES

4 **Answers: 2, 3, 4** A nonspecific inflammatory response is evoked by any injury and is of short duration, occurring before the immune response is established. It is usually local and produces inflammation. In some cases, local injuries result in systemic manifestations that usually begin in hours or days generated by the release of cytokines causing fever, lethargy, and metabolic changes. Options 2, 3, and 4 are all systemic, leading to generalized symptoms. Options 1 and 5 are examples of local reactions.

Cognitive Level: Analysis **Client Need:** Physiological Integrity: Physiological Adaptation **Integrated Process:** Nursing Process: Implementation **Content Area:** Adult Health: Immunological **Strategy:** The critical word in the question is *systemic.* Separate local from systemic reactions and choose the options that are systemtic. **Reference:** Porth, C. M. (2005). *Pathophysiology: Concepts of altered health states* (7th ed.). Philadelphia, PA: Lippincott Williams & Wilkins, pp. 338, 393–394.

5 **Answer: 4** This type of contact dermatitis is commonly a delayed reaction and type IV hypersensitivity. This reaction is cell-mediated rather than antibody-mediated and delayed 24 to 48 hours.

Cognitive Level: Application **Client Need:** Physiological Integrity: Physiological Adaptation **Integrated Process:** Nursing Process: Analysis **Content Area:** Adult Health: Immunological **Strategy:** The clue in the question is the timing of the reaction. Only one hypersensitivity type happens in a delayed time frame. **Reference:** Porth, C. M. (2005). *Pathophysiology: Concepts of altered health states* (7th ed.). Philadelphia, PA: Lippincott Williams & Wilkins, pp. 312–314.

6 **Answer: 2** Remember the Rh (+ or −) must also match besides the type of blood (O in this case). If antigens are present in the donor blood, which can interact with antibodies in the recipient's blood, a type II hypersensitivity, hemolytic reaction follows. Type O negative blood can be given to any recipient (the "universal donor"). For all other types (options 1, 3, and 4) the blood given must match the client's blood type.

Cognitive Level: Application **Client Need:** Physiological Integrity: Pharmacological and Parenteral Therapies **Integrated Process:** Nursing Process: Implementation **Content Area:** Adult Health: Immunological **Strategy:** Recall principles of safely administering a blood transfusion including the type and crossmatch needed before transfusing. **Reference:** Porth, C. M. (2005). *Pathophysiology: Concepts of altered health states* (7th ed.). Philadelphia, PA: Lippincott Williams & Wilkins, pp. 312–313.

7 **Answer: 3** Exposure to latex can be via skin, mucous membrane, inhalation, or internal tissue. The allergy can be a type I or type IV hypersensitivity reaction. Diagnosis is based on evidence of skin reaction after exposure. The elastic band in most underwear contains latex. The degree of moistness of the skin might need to be assessed but will not determine a latex allergy. Although drug allergies should be asked, this information does not help in determining a latex allergy. Option 4 is also important information for an assessment, but the focus of the question for a latex allergy would be if there were any problems after the surgery similar to the one being exhibited now.

Cognitive Level: Application **Client Need:** Physiological Integrity: Physiological Adaptation **Integrated Process:** Nursing Process: Assessment **Content Area:** Adult Health: Immunological **Strategy:** Consider which option gives the best information in assessing for *latex* allergy. Do not be misled by options that sound good but assess for other problems. **Reference:** Porth, C. M. (2005). *Pathophysiology: Concepts of altered health states* (7th ed.). Philadelphia, PA: Lippincott Williams & Wilkins, p. 418.

8 **Answer: 4** A barking cough, wheezing, and stridor are clinical manifestations of the bronchoconstriction and airway edema that accompanies anaphylaxis. Lung crackles are not part of the clinical picture (option 4). The blood pressure is usually low (hypotension) because of vasodilation rather than high as in option 1. The pulse would be rapid (tachycardia) rather than slow (option 2).

Cognitive Level: Application **Client Need:** Physiological Integrity: Physiological Adaptation **Integrated Process:** Nursing Process: Assessment **Content Area:** Adult Health: Immunological **Strategy:** Remember that anaphylaxis results in a type of shock, so choose the option that fits assessment findings of a client in shock. **Reference:** Porth, C. M. (2005). *Pathophysiology: Concepts of altered health states* (7th ed.). Philadelphia, PA: Lippincott Williams & Wilkins, p. 412–413.

9 **Answer: 1** Cervical dysplasia is present in 40% of women with human immunodeficiency virus (HIV). Cervical cancer often develops and is aggressive. Younger women die from the cervical cancer rather than from AIDS. Papanicolaou (PAP) smears every six months are recommended with aggressive treatment of any cervical dysplasia. CD4 cell counts and viral loads monitor the progression of AIDS but do not check for cancer. The CA 125 antigen is useful for detecting ovarian cancer.

Cognitive Level: Analysis **Client Need:** Health Promotion and Maintenance **Integrated Process:** Nursing Process: Planning **Content Area:** Adult Health: Immunological **Strategy:** The question asks specifically for a diagnostic test for cancer, narrowing the options to two. Recall which cancer is seen in women with AIDS. **Reference:** LeMone, P., & Burke, K. (2008). *Medical-surgical nursing: Critical thinking in client care* (4th ed.). Upper Saddle River, NJ: Pearson/Prentice Hall, pp. 354–355.

10 **Answer: 2** The police officer and nurse on the telemetry unit should be using standard precautions, which include gloves any time body secretions are encountered. Although either of these may encounter blood accidentally, the percentage is low. A school nurse should not be coming into contact with body secretions that would

increase the risk factor. A sexually active teenager, especially if the act is unprotected, is at highest risk. **Cognitive Level:** Analysis **Client Need:** Health Promotion and Maintenance **Integrated Process:** Nursing Process: Assessment **Content Area:** Adult Health: Immunological **Strategy:** Consider the bloodborne transmission of the virus to analyze which person in the options is most likely to be exposed and unprotected. **Reference:** LeMone, P., & Burke, K. (2008). *Medical-surgical nursing: Critical thinking in client care* (4th ed.). Upper Saddle River, NJ: Pearson/Prentice Hall, p. 349.

References

Centers for Disease Control. Online at http://www.cdc.gov/hiv/dhap.htm

Kee, J. L. (2005). *Laboratory and diagnostic tests with nursing implications* (7th ed.). Upper Saddle River, NJ: Prentice Hall.

Latex Allergy Policy (retrieved Oct. 15, 2005). http://www.smtl.co.uk/MDRC/Latex/Latex-Allergy-Policy/latex-allergy-policy.html, pp. 1–7.

LeMone, P., & Burke, K. M. (2008). *Medical-surgical nursing: Critical thinking in client care* (4th ed.). Upper Saddle River, NJ: Prentice Hall.

Lilley, L., Harrington, S., & Snyder, S. (2005). *Pharmacology and the nursing process* (4th ed.). St. Louis, MO: Mosby, pp. 664–677.

McKenry, L., Tessier, E., & Hogan, M. (2006). *Mosby's pharmacology in nursing* (22nd ed.). St. Louis, MO: Mosby, pp. 1133–1160.

Porth, C. M. (2005). *Pathophysiology: Concepts of altered health states* (7th ed.). Philadelphia, PA: Lippincott Williams & Wilkins, pp. 365–445.

Venes, D. & Thomas, C. (Eds.). (2006). *Taber's cyclopedic medical dictionary* (20th ed.). Philadelphia, PA: F. A. Davis.

Wagner, K., Johnson, K., & Kidd, P. (Eds.). (2006). *High-acuity nursing* (4th ed.). Upper Saddle River, NJ: Prentice Hall.

Wilson, B. A., Shannon, M. T., & Stang, C. L. (2006). *Nurse's drug guide* 2006. Upper Saddle River, NJ: Prentice Hall.

13 Infectious Health Problems

Chapter Outline

Overview of Infectious Health
  Problems

Viral Infections

Bacterial Infections

Fungal Infections

Chlamydial Infections

Spirochetal Infections

Rickettsial Infections

Protozoal Infections

Helminthic Infections

Mycoplasmal Infections

Mycobacterial Infections

Prion Infections

NCLEX-RN® Test Prep

Use the CD-ROM enclosed with this book
to access additional practice opportunities.

Objectives

➤ Define key terms associated with infectious health problems.

➤ Identify risk factors associated with the development of infectious
  health problems.

➤ Explain common etiologies of infectious health problems.

➤ Describe the pathophysiologic processes associated with specific
  infectious health problems.

➤ Distinguish between normal and abnormal infectious findings
  obtained from nursing assessment.

➤ Prioritize nursing interventions associated with specific infectious
  health problems.

Review at a Glance

chain of infection the series of events or conditions that lead to development of a particular communicable disease

colonization establishment of an infectious agent in a host

epidemiology the study of the distribution of health and illness within the population

host organism capable of supporting growth and reproduction of another organism

iatrogenic infection disease acquired in a hospital or health care setting; formerly called nosocomial infection

opportunistic infection disease that occurs only when host defenses are impaired

pathogen microorganism capable of causing disease

pathogenicity the ability of a microorganism to cause pathologic changes and the process of developing disease

reservoir habitat in which a living organism lives and multiplies

resident (normal) flora relationship where parasites depend on the host's environment to grow and reproduce but prevent colonization of other microbes and may contribute to synthesis of beneficial substances

virulence the ease with which a pathogenic organism can overcome host defenses

PRETEST

PRETEST

1 A client has an opportunistic respiratory infection. The nurse considers that which of the following most likely represents the etiology of the client's infection?

1. Client consumed contaminated food or water
2. Client encountered an extremely virulent microorganism
3. Client's immune system is compromised
4. Client has likely become infected in a health care facility

2 A client presents to the Emergency Department with a fever of 102° F, malaise, and a productive cough. Which of the following should the nurse do first?

1. Administer prescribed antibiotic
2. Obtain ordered sputum culture
3. Administer dose of PRN acetaminophen to lower fever
4. Teach client importance of handwashing

3 The nurse is explaining why an antibiotic must be taken as directed to prevent the development of resistant bacterial strains. The nurse should utilize which of the following information in explaining to the client the concept of bacterial resistance? Select all that apply.

1. Production of enzymes, such as beta-lactamase, to inactivate antibiotics
2. Stimulation of host's immune system, producing leukocytosis
3. Genetic mutations altering bacterial binding sites
4. Alternate metabolic pathways bypassing antibiotic activity
5. Changes in bacterial cell wall preventing antibiotic from reaching intracellular target site

4 The nurse is explaining infectious disease terminology to unlicensed assistive personnel (UAPs) who are orienting to an infectious disease unit. One UAP asks what makes bacteria able to cause disease in a person. The nurse includes an explanation of what concept in a response?

1. Communicability
2. Pathogenicity
3. Toxogenicity
4. Latency

5 The nurse considers that a client with a fever and enlarged regional lymph nodes most likely has infection of which of the following etiologies?

1. Bacterial
2. Fungal
3. Protozoal
4. Rickettsial

6 The public health nurse explains to a community group that which of the following viruses is most likely to be acquired through casual contact with an infected individual?

1. Influenza virus
2. Herpes virus
3. Cytomegalovirus (CMV)
4. Human immunodeficiency virus (HIV)

7 A female prostitute enters the clinic for treatment of a sexually transmitted infection. The nurse anticipates preparing her and setting up the equipment to send culture and sensitivity testing for which of the following? Select all that apply.

1. Herpes virus
2. Chlamydia
3. Gonorrhea
4. Syphilis
5. Human papilloma virus (genital warts)

8 A female client is admitted to the hospital with hemorrhagic colitis. The etiology was found to be an exotoxin, the shiga toxin produced by *Escherichia coli*. The client asks the nurse what caused the problem. The nurse's best reply is:

1. Eating food from a can that was damaged or bulging.
2. Kissing someone who was infected with the organism.
3. Eating undercooked hamburger meat or drinking unpasteurized fruit juices.
4. The toxic shock-like symptoms came from a tampon used incorrectly.

9 After taking a client history, the nurse explains to a client exhibiting symptoms of a rickettsia infection that it was probably acquired through:

1. Respiratory droplets.
2. Mosquito bites.
3. Bites or feces of ticks, lice, or fleas.
4. Direct skin contact with infected animals.

10 The nurse is analyzing the development of an infectious disease in the community. The nurse incorporates each element of the chain of infection in the study because each gives information regarding:

1. The linkages between various forms of microorganisms.
2. The sequence required for transmission of disease.
3. The clustering of bacteria in a specific pattern.
4. Increasing virulence patterns among species of microorganisms.

➤ *See pages 400–401 for Answers & Rationales.*

I. OVERVIEW OF INFECTIOUS HEALTH PROBLEMS

A. Introduction

1. **Epidemiology** refers to the study of distribution and patterns of disease in populations

2. Infectious diseases are caused by invasion of **pathogens** (microorganisms capable of causing disease), including bacteria, viruses, fungi, protozoa, rickettsiae, and helminths

3. Types of pathogens
   a. Communicable (such as influenza, hepatitis, tuberculosis)
   b. Noncommunicable (such as cellulitis and endocarditis)

4. Injury of body cells can occur directly by microorganisms, by toxins released from microorganisms, or indirectly from the inflammatory response to microorganisms

B. Risk factors

1. Age (very young or very old)
2. Poor nutrition
3. Immune deficiency (congenital or acquired)
4. Impaired integrity of skin or mucous membranes

5. Circulatory disturbances
6. Alteration of normal flora by antibiotic therapy
7. Diabetes mellitus
8. Corticosteroid therapy
9. Chemotherapy
10. Smoking
11. Alcohol consumption

C. **Transmission of infection**

1. Occurs through the **chain of infection** (the series of events or conditions that lead to development of a particular communicable disease) (see Figure 13-1)
2. Causative agents include pathogens previously listed
3. **Reservoir** (or source) is the environment where the infectious agent can survive
   a. Human: individuals or groups of people
   b. Environment/fomites: contaminated food, water, air, or soil
   c. Animals: such as ticks, fleas, mosquitoes, or bats
4. Portal of exit is the route by which an agent leaves a reservoir
   a. Gastrointestinal (such as ingestion)
   b. Respiratory (such as coughing or sneezing)
   c. Genitourinary (such as sexual contact)
   d. Blood (such as insect bites, needles)

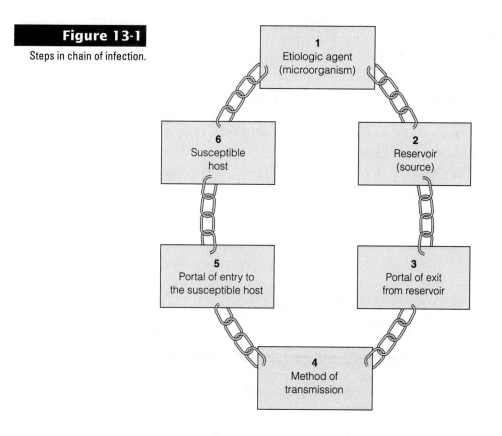

Figure 13-1

Steps in chain of infection.

5. Mode of transmission is the route of transmission of the agent

    a. Contact transmission may be direct or indirect

        1) Direct contact is person-to-person transmission accomplished through body fluids or through contaminated food or water

        2) Indirect contact is transmission accomplished through inanimate objects

    b. Airborne or droplet transmission involves transfer through droplets (from coughing, sneezing, or talking) or through droplet nuclei carried on air currents

    c. Vector transmission involves intermediaries such as flies, mosquitos, or other insects or rodents

6. Portal of entry is the location by which an agent enters the body

7. Susceptible **host** (organism capable of supporting growth and reproduction of another organism): individual who lacks resistance to this infectious agent

D. Relationship of host to parasite (host-parasite interaction)

1. **Resident (normal) flora** represent a symbiotic (balanced) relationship where parasites depend on the host's environment to grow and reproduce but prevent **colonization** (establishment of an infectious agent in a host) of other microbes

    a. May contribute to synthesis of beneficial substances

    b. Depends on maintenance of balance

2. **Opportunistic infection** occurs when immunity is compromised and normal flora become pathogenic

3. **Iatrogenic infections** (formerly nosocomial infections) are hospital-acquired and typically are caused by virulent or drug-resistant organisms and are often spread through poor handwashing

E. Factors affecting infection by pathogen

1. Mechanism of action: pathogen can damage normal cells or interfere with cellular metabolism by producing toxins

2. Infectivity: ability of the pathogen to invade and multiply in the host

3. **Pathogenicity** is the origin and process of developing disease

4. **Virulence:** the ease with which a pathogen can overcome host defenses; important components of virulence include invasiveness, adherence, and toxigenicity

5. Toxigenicity refers to the agent's ability to produce endotoxins or exotoxins

6. Defense mechanisms of the body

    a. Physical factors such as skin and mucous membranes

    b. Chemical factors such as the pH of skin, urine, stomach, etc.

    c. Normal flora, which helps to prevent colonization by transient organisms by competing for nutrients and contributing to a low pH

    d. Immunity/inflammatory response

    e. Individual factors such as nutrition, genetic makeup, and presence of other illnesses

F. Stages of infectious process

1. Incubation stage: pathogen is present and reproduces but host remains asymptomatic; could last from hours to years

2. Prodromal stage: initial (mild) symptoms appear, which may be nonspecific

3. Acute: pronounced symptoms are present; results from toxic by-products of the microorganism's metabolic processes and from tissue damage caused by the inflammatory response

Practice to Pass

Identify conditions that could lead to opportunistic infections.

   4. Convalescent: diminished symptoms with infection contained

   5. Resolution: elimination of pathogen

G. Clinical manifestations

   1. General symptoms of systemic infection include malaise, weakness, headache, anorexia, and weight loss

   2. Infection may also produce acute inflammatory reactions; the extent of tissue damage is determined by the number and the virulence of the organisms, the site of invasion, and host defenses

   3. General manifestations of specific types of infection

   a. Bacterial, viral, and mycoplasma infections

   1) Fever (may be low grade, especially with viral infection)

   2) Body aches

   3) Regional lymph node enlargement

   4) Site-specific manifestations (i.e., cough, earache, sore throat, etc.)

   b. Fungal infections

   1) Itching/redness of skin

   2) Nail thickening

   3) Thrush in mouth

   4) Vaginal discharge (thick, white)

   c. Protozoa and helminths

   1) Itcing and rash (skin infections)

   2) Diarrhea

   3) Fever (with malaria)

   d. Rickettsiae

   1) Skin rash

   2) Muscles aches

   3) Fever and chills

   4) Headache

II. VIRAL INFECTIONS

A. Overview

   1. Viruses are tiny intracellular organisms (20 to 100 times smaller than bacteria) that totally depend upon the living host for survival and the necessary materials to replicate

   2. Intracellular development allows viruses to bypass many body defense mechanisms

B. Pathophysiology

   1. Viral particles are called virions and consist of a single strand of DNA or RNA contained within a protein shell called a capsid

   2. Viruses are classified as either DNA or RNA viruses according to their genetic material; they are also categorized according to mechanism of replication, mode of transmission, or the type of disease produced

   3. Viruses produce specific diseases in specific tissues

   a. The protein covering of the virus is type-specific and attaches as a "lock and key" to the host cell membrane

      b. The virus must be able to use the host cell in production of nucleic acid in order to survive since they have no independent metabolism

      c. Mature virions are created within the host cell and released through cell lysis, direct passage to adjacent cells, or through reverse endocytosis

  4. Viruses may damage or kill cells they infect, causing disease

  5. The viral replication cycle can be relatively brief (minutes or hours) or as long as several days; includes 6 phases of adsorption, penetration, uncoating, replication, assembly, and release

      a. Some viruses enter the host cell and insert their genome into the host chromosome, remaining in a latent, nonreplicating state for long periods of time; examples include the herpes viruses (varicella zoster, chickenpox, genital herpes) and cytomegalovirus

      b. Influenza virus is transmitted by respiratory droplets

  6. Viruses bind to cell membrane receptors, leading to endocytosis of the virus; the virus then uses the cell's resources to synthesize new viral nucleic acids that are released from the host cell to infect other cells

  7. Retroviruses replicate in a unique process

      a. The viral RNA is translated into DNA by an enzyme, reverse transcriptase, and is then integrated into the host chromosome

      b. It then exists in a latent state until reactivated

      c. Replication requires reversal of the process

      d. HIV is an example of a retrovirus

  8. Bacteriophages are viruses that use bacteria as their hosts; these viruses attach to the bacteria and inject their DNA into the cell for replication

  9. Viral infections can be local or systemic and can be either acute or chronic; some viruses are thought to be agents of cancer (such as human papilloma virus [HPV] and cervical cancer), although the role of viruses in human cancers is still not well understood

  10. Viral infection stimulates antibody production primarily through cell-mediated immunity and production of interferon

      a. Antibodies coat particles to make them better targets of macrophages

      b. This coating prevents viruses from entering target cells

      c. Macrophages also secrete cytokines that initiate the inflammatory response

  11. Antiviral therapy is difficult to develop because of the large number of variant viruses that cause the same disease and inability of medications to destroy the virus without destroying normal cells

  12. Common viral infections and antiviral agents are listed in Table 13-1

C. Nursing assessment

  1. Assessment includes identifying factors that increase risk for infection, vital signs (VS), complaints of pain, palpation of lymph nodes, signs and symptoms specific to type of virus

  2. Diagnostic tests

      a. Complete blood count (CBC)

         1) Lymphocytes increase in many viral infections; normal lymphocyte count is 25 to 35% of the total white blood count (WBC)

Table 13-1	Common Viral Infections		
Virus	**Transmission**	**Pathological Considerations**	**Therapeutic Management**
Hepatitis Hepatitis A (HAV)	Transmitted through fecal-oral route and through contaminated food and water. Occurs in overcrowded and unsanitary conditions.	Acute onset with incubation of 2 to 6 weeks. Inflammatory process can result in destruction of hepatocytes. Signs and symptoms include anorexia, malaise, jaundice. Liver enzymes likely elevated. ALT liver enzyme usually rises sharply at the time of fever onset. Serologic markers include anti-HAV (which may persist for years) and IgM (which is short-lived and may disappear in about 2 weeks). Complete recovery is likely.	Disease can be avoided in most cases if immune globulins are administered within 7 days of exposure. Preventive vaccines Havrix and Vaqta are available for those traveling to areas endemic to the disease.
Hepatitis B (HBV)	Transmitted through body fluids from sexual contact or parenterally. May also be transmitted to fetus during pregnancy.	Gradual onset with incubation 6 to 24 weeks. Infection may be acute and self-limiting or may lead to persistent viremia with chronic liver disease or chronic carrier state. There is a gradual and prolonged elevation of ALT liver enzyme. HbsAg is present in early infection. Anti-HBs is present in past infections and anti-Hbe is present in chronic carriers.	Hepatitis B hyperimmune globulin (HBIG) is recommended after exposure to the hepatitis B virus. Recombivax HB and Engerix-B are used prophylactically for prevention in health workers and other high-risk populations. Liver enzymes should be monitored. Instruct clients concerning safe sexual practices and to avoid sharing of needles.
Hepatitis C (HCV)	Transmitted through sexual or parenteral routes.	Gradual onset with incubation of 5 to 12 weeks. May produce both acute and chronic hepatitis but is most often chronic. HCV has also been associated with cirrhosis and liver cancer. Causes elevation of ALT. Can be detected with serologic markers anti-HVC but is difficult to determine if infection is current or prior.	Vaccines do not currently exist for HCV. Treatment is symptomatic.
Hepatitis D (HDV)	Transmitted through blood and sexual contact.	Acute onset with incubation 3 to 13 weeks. Clinical manifestations similar to hepatitis B and those with HBV and carriers of HBV are susceptible to infection by HDV.	Vaccines do not currently exist for HDV. Treatment is symptomatic.
Hepatitis E (HEV)	Transmitted through fecal-oral route through contaminated food and water.	Rapid onset with incubation 3 to 6 weeks. Results in chronic hepatitis and cirrhosis. A serologic test for anti-HEV has been developed for detection of the virus in the stool.	

Table 13-1	Common Viral Infections (continued)		
Virus	**Transmission**	**Pathological Considerations**	**Therapeutic Management**
Herpes virus Simplex (HSV)	Transmitted through direct contact with skin and mucous membranes.	Replicates at site of entry and may pass through regional lymph nodes, enter the blood, and proliferate in the skin and mucous membranes. Most cases are subclinical. May remain latent at site of exposure and be activated by exposure to sunlight, fever, or stress. Is characterized by vesicular ulcerations on the mouth or conjunctiva with HSV 1 or in the genital area with HSV 2; recurrence is common.	Acyclovir (Zovirax) is the drug of choice as an antiviral agent. This drug reduces viral shedding, decreases local symptoms, and decreases severity and duration of acute episodes. It may be used topically, orally, or parenterally.
Varicella zoster (shingles)	Transmitted primarily through the respiratory tract, initially in form of chicken-pox. Reactivated in form of shingles.	Primarily seen in older adults and immunocompromised clients; results from reactivation of latent virus that has been dormant in sensory cells of the dorsal root ganglion. Exact mechanism is not known. Painful lesions appear to follow a specific dermatome, with lesions appearing on the trunk, chest, forehead, face and neck.	Acyclovir (Zovirax) and vidarabine (Vira-A) have been used for treatment. The vaccine ZIG (zoster immunoglobulin) may be useful for prevention in immunocompromised clients. High doses of interferon alfa (Roferon-A) have also proven useful in reducing viral replication.
Cytomegalovirus (CMV)	Transmitted through saliva, urine, semen, breast milk, and vaginal secretions.	Latent infection usually seen in immunocompromised clients. Highly necrotizing to cells. Fluorescent antibody techniques are used for diagnosis.	Antiviral agents include ganciclovir (Cytovene) and foscarnet (Foscavir). CMV immunoglobulin used in combination with an antiviral has also proven useful.
Epstein-Barr	Transmitted through respiratory droplets or saliva.	Replicates in parotid gland and disseminated through the blood. Incubation 4 to 7 weeks. Associated with mononucleosis. Signs and symptoms include lymphadenopathy, fever, chills, sore throat and often a thick tonsillar exudate. Recovery may take up to 4 weeks. WBCs are markedly elevated. Antibodies to the Epstein-Barr nuclear antigen appear during the convalescent period.	Disease is self-limiting and treatment is supportive.

Table 13-1	Common Viral Infections (continued)		
Virus	**Transmission**	**Pathological Considerations**	**Therapeutic Management**
Human immunodeficiency virus (HIV)	Transmitted through blood and body fluids.	Incubation may be 3 to 10 years in adults. CD4 protein of helper T lymphocytes is a receptor for the virus, which attaches by means of its gp120 surface protein. The virus envelope fuses with the cell membrane and the virus enters the cell. The virus makes a DNA copy of its own RNA using the reverse transcriptase enzyme and the DNA copy is inserted into the genetic material of the infected cell. Infected individuals become immuno-compromised and subject to numerous opportunistic in-fections. A positive ELISA test for presence of antibodies is confirmed through the Western Blot.	Antiviral agents used to treat HIV include nucleoside re-verse transcriptase inhibitors (NRTIs), non-nucleoside re-verse transcriptase inhibitors (NNRTIs), protease inhibitors (PIs) and a fusion inhibitor. Protease inhibitors have been associated with reduction of viral loads to undetectable levels. Compliance with drug regimens is essential and side effects often make compli-ance difficult.
Influenza	Transmitted through droplets of upper respiratory secretions.	Incubation period may be 1 to 7 days. Viral replication occurs in epithelial cells of the upper respiratory tract. The virus does not typically enter the blood. Systemic symptoms are derived from endogenous pyrogens and release of inter-feron. Symptoms include head-ache, body aches, chills, fever, and rhinitis. Complications may include bronchial pneu-monia or secondary bacterial infection. Guillain-Barré and Reye's syndromes have been associated with episodes of influenza.	Amantadine (Symmetrel) is the antiviral agent that prevents penetration of Influenza A into cells and limits replication if administered within 48 hours of onset. Vaccines are formu-lated each year that can be effective for prevention for up to 6 months. Vaccines are recommended for the elderly and high-risk clients.

2) T-lymphocytes will decrease with the HIV/AIDS virus, autoimmune disor-ders, and corticosteroids

3) Neutrophil counts will decrease in most viral infections

b. Enzyme-linked immunosorbent assay (ELISA) and Western Blot are positive in diagnosis of HIV

c. Epstein-Barr nuclear antigen (EBNA) is used to confirm infectious mononucleosis

D. Nursing management

1. Medications

    a. Antiviral agents (viruses are not sensitive to antibacterials since viruses have no cell wall or cytoplasm and the virus is typically immersed in the host cell); refer again to Table 13-1

    b. Acyclovir (Zovirax), a popular medication for treating herpes; amantidine (Symmetrel) for influenza; interferon alfacon–1 (Infergen) for hepatitis

    c. Anti-pyretic agents to reduce fever

    d. Analgesics to relieve pain and discomfort

2. Instruct client/family concerning infection control measures (good handwashing, etc.)

3. Provide quiet environment, limiting visitors as needed

4. Provide comfort measures to ensure adequate rest

5. Assist with self-care activities as needed

6. Monitor vital signs

7. Institute isolation precautions according to route of transmission

8. Document response to medication

9. Evaluate response to activity, noting weakness, fatigue, or dyspnea

10. Preventive vaccines should be encouraged when available

11. Instruct clients with genital herpes to avoid genital sexual contact during the acute phase, especially during the breakout

Practice to Pass

What are the implications of the presence of latent or recurrent viruses?

III. BACTERIAL INFECTIONS

A. Overview

1. Bacteria are single-celled organisms that use the human body as a source for nutrients and environment for growth

2. They contain a single chromosome and are capable of autonomous reproduction

3. Bacteria are classified according to shape, staining characteristics, and requirements related to oxygen

B. Pathophysiology

1. Bacterial growth depends on the body's immune system function and ability of bacteria to resist body defenses

2. Bacteria may produce substances that enhance resistance to host defenses

    a. Production of adherins allows bacteria to strongly attach to structures and penetrate underlying tissues

    b. Development of carbohydrate or protein capsule or slime layers help prevent phagocytosis

    c. Production of leukocidins help destroy phagocytes

    d. Production of enzymes that break down fibrin clots or connective tissue (i.e., streptokinase, hyalurinidase, collagenase, elastase, etc.) and allow bacteria to more easily spread into tissues; production of coagulase causes clotting of plasma and allows bacteria to form a fibrin layer of protection

3. Bacteria may produce toxins that cause damage to cells and tissues

    a. Exotoxins are proteins secreted from organisms into tissues; they have variable specificity and may cause fatal effects

        1) Exotoxins are produced by Gram-positive and Gram-negative organisms and most are denatured by extreme heat

        2) Common examples of the effects of exotoxins are found in botulism and tetanus

    b. Endotoxins are lipopolysaccharides released from bacterial cell membranes with cell division or destruction

        1) They are produced only by Gram-negative bacteria and can withstand high heat

        2) Endotoxins usually cause fever and induce production of cytokines that activate the complement cascade and may cause septic shock

        3) They are generally less toxic than exotoxins

4. Complement proteins may be activated by contact with bacterial cell wall or with release of endotoxins

    a. This activation results in opsonization of microorganisms (to enhance phagocytosis), activation of leukocytes, and destruction of bacterial cells

    b. Encapsulated bacteria are protected from phagocytosis unless coated with anticapsular antibody

    c. Antibiotics are often necessary to assist the immune system in destroying bacteria

5. Common bacteria causing infectious diseases are identified in Table 13-2

C. Nursing assessment

1. Assessment includes identifying organ system(s) affected by infection; signs and symptoms of infection (fever, malaise, and local or organ-specific indicators); VS; complaints of pain; palpation of lymph nodes

2. Diagnostic tests

    a. CBC

        1) WBC (expressed as number of WBCs per cubic mm) will be elevated ($> 10,000/mm^3$)

        2) Neutrophil count: expressed as absolute neutrophil count (ANC) or percentage of the total WBC; is elevated with most bacterial infections

            a) Both segmented neutrophils (mature) and bands (immature neutrophils) will likely be elevated with infection

            b) With severe or prolonged infection, the percentage of bands will increase to a greater extent than segmented neutrophils (often referred to as a "shift to the left")

            c) Some bacterial infections (typhoid, brucellosis, etc.) may cause neutropenia

    b. Culture and sensitivity: aids in identifying the organism and determining the antibiotic that can be most effective; collect prior to administering any antibiotics; cultures and first antibiotic administration should be done according to agency protocol in a timely manner

    c. Gram stain: allows presumptive identification of the category of bacteria

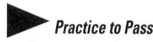

Practice to Pass

What are some examples of descriptions of bacteria in terms of shape? Staining characteristics? Requirements for oxygen?

Table 13-2 **Common Bacteria That Cause Infectious Disease**

Bacteria/ Disease Process	Type/ Morphology	Transmission	Pathological Effects	Nursing Management
Clostridium tetani (tetanus)	Gram-positive bacillus; spore-forming	Spores distributed in soil and intestinal tract of humans and animals. Infects wounds from injury.	Clinical manifestations caused by spore generation of exo-toxin with affinity for CNS. Manifestations include neck stiffness, dysphagia, muscle rigidity.	Treated with tetanus antitoxin or immune globulins. Prevention with tetanus toxoid. May require mechanical ventilation.
Clostridium botulinum (botulism)	Gram-positive bacillus; spore-forming	Inhabits soil; frequent contaminant of fruits, vegetables, and fish. Spores are highly heat resistant.	Life-threatening paralytic illness is caused by neurotoxins. Prevents release of Ach from nerve terminals of neuro-muscular junction. Damage to cranial nerves causes vision, hearing, and speech difficulties.	Treated with antitoxin from horse serum that only affects circulating toxin; has no effect on toxin bound to nerve cells. Recovery is very gradual over weeks to months.
Clostridium difficile (pseudomembranous colitis)	Gram-positive bacillus; spore-forming	Hospital acquired; acquired by antibiotic use.	Broad spectrum antibiotics are the most common cause, altering normal flora and allowing *c. difficile* colonization. Leads to abdominal cramping and severe diarrhea that is foul-smelling and can lead to de-hydration and/or electrolyte loss.	Treated with vancomycin and metronidazole (Flagyl).
Corynebacterium diphtheriae (diphtheria)	Gram-positive; nonspore-forming	Airborne droplets colonizing in upper respiratory system.	Produces toxin resulting in epi-thelial cell necrosis. Inflam-matory response causes production of pseudomem-brane that may lead to suffocation.	Antitoxin must be administered prior to cell penetration by toxin. Should test for hyper-sensitivity to horse serum pro-teins prior to administration. Prevention is through vaccine. Penicillin may be used but is rarely effective when used alone.
Coliform bacteria *Escherichia coli*	Gram-negative, nonspore-forming rod	Normal resident bacteria of intestines. May spread to urinary tract or wounds directly through fecal contamination or through the blood.	Frequent source of nosocomial infection. Manifestations in-clude fever and chills. May de-velop shock from endotoxins. Also frequently cause urinary tract infections.	Prevention through good handwashing and hygiene practices. Treated with cephalosporins, fluoro-quinolones, or aminoglyco-sides. Should monitor for nephrotoxicity and ototoxicity with aminoglycosides.

Table 13-2	Common Bacteria That Cause Infectious Disease (continued)			
Bacteria/ Disease Process	**Type/ Morphology**	**Transmission**	**Pathological Effects**	**Nursing Management**
Klebsiella pneumoniae	Gram-negative rod, heavily encapsulated	Found in soil, water, food, and intestinal tract.	Also associated with hospital acquired infections. Responsible for severe repiratory tract infections in debilitated clients. Manifestations include productive cough and weakness.	Treated with aminoglycosides that bind to ribosomes and prevent protein synthesis in bacteria and with later generation cephalosporins, which interfere with cell wall synthesis.
Pseudomonas	Gram-negative rod	Common resident of skin and mucous membranes. Spreads through direct contact.	Major threat to hospitalized and debilitated clients.	Treated with aminoglycosides and later-generation cephalosporins.
Helicobacter pylori	Gram-negative spiral or straight rod	Penetrates gastric mucosa and colonizes gastric epithelium.	Produces enzyme urease that raises pH, allowing bacteria to survive in normally acidic environment. Urea in stomach is converted to ammonia, which is cytotoxic to gastric cells. Causes depletion of gastric mucus, allowing erosion of mucosa.	Treated with macrolides (azithromycin [Zithromax] and clarithromycin [Biaxin]) and metronidazole (Flagyl). Macrolides inhibit protein synthesis while metronidazole disrupts DNA synthesis. Alcohol should be avoided with metronidazole. Macrolides have frequent interactions with drugs.
Haemophilus influenza	Gram-negative bacillus	Occurs only in humans; more common in children than adults. Transmitted person to person through respiratory route.	Virulence enhanced by polysaccharide capsule that resists action of complement. Does not produce exotoxin and endotoxin does not appear to play significant role. Results in otitis media, sinusitis, and respiratory tract infections.	Prevention is through vaccine. Drugs of choice for treatment are cephalosporins.

Table 13-2	Common Bacteria That Cause Infectious Disease (continued)			
Bacteria/ Disease Process	**Type/ Morphology**	**Transmission**	**Pathological Effects**	**Nursing Management**
Gonorrhea (*neisseria gonorrhoeae*)	Gram-negative diplococcus	Transmitted through sexual contact. Primary site of infection is the cervix. Primary site in men is the urethra.	Bacteria contain pili, which aid in attachment to mucosal surfaces in humans and inhibit phagocytosis. Most strains produce extracellular proteases that inactivate immunoglobulins. They also produce a cytotoxic factor that damages ciliated epithelial cells. May be asymptomatic in women but result in salpingitis, pelvic inflammatory disease, and infertility; men generally experience purulent discharge and dysuria and may experience urethral stricture.	Drug of choice is a cephalosporin such as ceftriaxone (Rocephin). TMP/SMX (Bactrim) and ciprofloxacin (Cipro) may also be used. Ciprofloxacin inhibits DNA replication while TMP/SMX prevents synthesis of proteins and nucleic acid. Client should be instructed to avoid unprotected sexual contact.
Staphylococcus	Gram-positive cocci that grow in clusters in short chains.	Transmitted through hair follicles into the bloodstream or through the urinary or respiratory tract.	Common resident of skin. Hardy nonspore-forming bacteria that are heat stable. Some forms of this anaerobe produce coagulase, causing clots in citrated plasma. Pathogenic staph release a number of toxins including hemolysins, leukocidin, enterotoxins, and ex-foliatin. They have also been implicated in toxic shock syndrome.	Humans have high resistance to staph due to development of high antibody titers. Penicillinase-resistant penicillins and cephalosporins are the drugs of choice, however, resistant strains have developed. Vancomycin (Vancocin) is the drug of choice for methicillin-resistant strains; it interferes with cell wall synthesis. In cases where resistance has developed to vancomycin, drugs such as quinupristin and dalfopristin (Synercid) and linezolid (Zyvox) or combination therapy using mupirocin (Bactroban) and rifampin (Rifadin) have been effective. Daptomycin (Cubicin) is a newer drug replacing vancomycin.

Table 13-2	Common Bacteria That Cause Infectious Disease (continued)			
Bacteria/ Disease Process	Type/ Morphology	Transmission	Pathological Effects	Nursing Management
Streptococcus	Gram-positive cocci that grow in chains or as diplococci.	Transmitted through respiratory droplets or direct contact with secretions.	*Group A beta-hemolytic streptococcus* produces erythrogenic toxin responsible for rash in scarlet fever. Two hemolysins are produced as well as streptokinase that promotes lysis of human blood clots. Diseases produced include pharyngitis, otitis media, peritonsillar abcesses, meningitis, and pneumonia. Glomerulonephritis and rheumatic fever are complications that can result from streptococcal infection.	Penicillin is the drug of choice, with erythromycin used for those allergic to penicillin. Clients should be instructed in the importance of completing the entire course of prescribed antibiotics.
Tuberculosis (*Mycobacterium tuberculosis*)	Acid-fast and aerobic bacillus (due to large amounts of lipids in cell wall)	Tubercle is transmitted through respiratory droplets from humans, cows, or birds. May also enter blood and lymph system and travel to other parts of the body.	Grows slowly and often results in self-limiting lesion. Initial lesion appears as area of non-specific pneumonitis. The caseous lesion heals by fibrosis and calcification, and can be reactivated with low host resistance. Exotoxins or endotoxins are not produced. Mycobacteria primarily affect the lungs but may also cause infection in the kidney, liver, and genitourinary tract.	Previous mycobacterial infection can be detected through a PPD skin test, however this does not necessarily indicate active infection. The drugs of choice for treatment of tuberculosis are the antitubercular agents isoniazid (INH) and rifampin (Rifadin), which interfere with protein synthesis or cell wall synthesis. Streptomycin and pyrazinamide (Tebrazid) are also used; It should be noted that standard antibiotics are not effective against mycobacteria. Treatment usually continues for 3 to 6 months and client compliance must be encouraged.

D. Nursing management

1. Medications include antimicrobial agents, antipyretics, and NSAIDs

!▷ 2. Teach and encourage good hand washing since this is the single most effective way to prevent the spread of infection

3. Employ appropriate protective barriers (such as gloves, mask, goggles, gowns) when caring for clients with bacterial infections

4. Instruct client and family in methods to prevent spread of infection

5. Encourage balance of rest and activity

!▷ 6. Encourage compliance with medication regimen; stress the completion of all medications even though symptoms improve to avoid bacterial resistance

7. Encourage increased fluid intake with most anticrobials

8. Document response to therapy

9. Collect lab specimens as needed to validate resolution of infection

IV. FUNGAL INFECTIONS

A. Overview

1. Fungi may be unicellular (yeasts) or multicellular (hyphae), or may alternate between the two forms

2. Fungi can cause allergic, toxic, and infectious disease in humans

3. Some fungi are part of the normal flora of the skin, mouth, intestines, and vagina

B. Pathophysiology

1. Fungi obtain nutrients by absorption and almost all are aerobic and reproduce by spores

   a. Spores germinate to produce different morphologic forms such as single-celled yeasts or multicelled molds

   b. The cell wall is rigid and composed primarily of polysaccharides external to the cell membrane

2. The plasma membrane contains ergosterol rather than cholesterol, which is useful in antifungal therapy

3. Humans have a high level of innate immunity to fungi, and most infections are mild and self-limiting

4. Factors related to resistance include the fatty acid content of skin, pH of the skin and mucous membranes, normal flora, epithelial turnover, and cilia in the respiratory tract

5. Infections are classified according to three levels

   a. Superficial: limited to outer layers of skin and hair (tinea versicolor)

   b. Cutaneous: extending deeper into keratinized layers of the epidermis (caused by dermaphytes); tinea and candida are the primary examples

   c. Subcutaneous: involves the dermis, subcutaneous tissue, muscle, and fascia

      1) Most infections of this type are chronic and visualized as skin lesions

      2) They may be initiated by trauma and may require surgical excision

6. Fungal infections can also be systemic; this form originates primarily in the lung, but may appear as a secondary infection elsewhere; histoplasmosis is a common example

7. Opportunistic mycotic infections are often seen in immunocompromised individuals (those with AIDS, receiving chemotherapy, etc.) or those on long-term antibiotic therapy; the most common forms are candidiasis, aspergillosis, and zygomycosis

8. Transmission is through direct contact with persons or inanimate objects

9. Moisture increases the risk of growth and spread of fungal infection

C. Nursing assessment

1. Assessment includes location, size, and characteristics of lesions of the skin and mucous membranes; complaints of discomfort (itching); and specific assessment (vagina, mouth, nails)

2. Diagnostic tests

   a. Cultures of skin, nails, or hair

   b. Microscopic examination of scrapings from lesions

   c. Observation under ultraviolent light (spores fluoresce blue-green)

D. Nursing management

1. Medications

   a. Superficial, cutaneous, and subcutaneous fungal infections are generally treated with topical antifungal agents

      1) These include clotrimazole (Lotrimin), ketoconazole (Nizoral), nystatin (Mycostatin), fluconazole (Diflucan), and terbinafine (Lamisil)

      2) Most commonly reported side effects include burning, pruritis, and local irritation

   b. Amphotericin B (Fungizone) remains the drug of choice for severe systemic mycoses

      1) It is often given along with flucytosine (5-FC) for a synergistic effect

      2) Amphotericin B is associated with many adverse effects including fever, chills, cardiac dysrhythmias, and nephrotoxicity

   c. Other systemic antifungal agents include flucytosine (5-Fluorocytosine), fluconazole (Diflucan), ketoconazole (Nizoral), and nystatin (Mycostatin)

2. Instruct individuals concerning method of transmission and conditions that increase risk

3. Teach clients importance of using clean articles for personal hygiene each day

4. Teach clients that antifungals often take 7 to 10 days to work

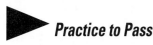

Practice to Pass

How would topical corticosteroids aggravate treatment of a fungal infection?

V. CHLAMYDIAL INFECTIONS

A. Overview

1. Chlamydial organisms are obligate nonmotile intracellular parasites associated with many sexually transmitted infections (STIs)

2. Chlamydia is the most common bacterial STI in the United States

3. Originally considered a virus, it is now recognized as a bacteria since it contains both RNA and DNA and has a cell wall similar to Gram-negative bacteria

4. Chlamydial infection can lead to pelvic inflammatory disease, infertility, ectopic pregnancy, and chronic pelvic pain

B. Pathophysiology

1. Chlamydia are unicellular organisms that reproduce asexually in the host cells of mammals and birds and transmit directly to humans

2. The cell wall of chlamydia is similar in structure to Gram-negative bacteria with a lipid cytoplasmic membrane; DNA occurs as an irregular mass in cytoplasm and cells lack flavoproteins and cytochromes

3. The cell cycle begins with a highly infectious small cell taken into a host cell by phagocytosis

   a. The cell retains its integrity and is reorganized into a large cell that multiplies by binary fission

   b. The large cells then reorganize into small cells capable of infecting new host cells

   c. The cell cycle varies between 24 to 48 hours

4. They generally become parasites of epithelial cells, mainly targeting mucous membranes of the eye or genitourinary tract; some forms of chlamydia transmitted by birds can cause infection of the lungs

5. There is generally low pathogenicity except in an immunocompromised host; compromised hosts can easily become reinfected

6. Infection can remain latent or subclinical for years

7. Chlamydia has on its surface a peptide similar to one in heart myosin; this can trigger T cells that attack both chlamydia and heart cells, causing myocarditis

8. Many clients with chlamydial infection are asymptomatic initially; some may complain of vaginal discharge within 1 to 3 weeks of infection; later signs and symptoms may include lower back pain, nausea, and fever

C. Nursing assessment

1. Assessment includes symptom analysis of pain, VS, inspection of vaginal discharge (females) or penile discharge (males)

2. Diagnostic tests

   a. Cell tissue culture is the primary diagnostic tool

   b. Enzyme immunoassay (EIA) tests may be used for high-risk clients but result in a fairly high percentage of false positive results

   c. Nucleic amplification tests (usually along with urine tests and cervical swab) have been developed and have been found effective

D. Nursing management

1. Medications

   a. Macrolides: single-dose or 7-day azithromycin (Zithromax)

   b. Tetracyclines: doxycycline (Vibramycin) for 7 days

2. Instruct clients concerning transmission through sexual contact

3. Instruct clients about need to treat sexual partners

VI. SPIROCHETAL INFECTIONS

A. Overview

1. Spirochetes are spiral-shaped bacteria with great motility that live primarily as extracellular pathogens, rarely growing within a host cell

    2. Spirochetes possess both DNA and RNA and can penetrate mucous membranes, entering the blood and lymphatic system

B. Pathophysiology

    1. Infections may remain latent for years

    2. Humoral and cell-mediated immune responses are activated and may decrease spirochete load, but generally will not eliminate disease

    3. Most common spirochetes are *Treponema pallidum* and *Borrelia burgdorferi*

    4. *Treponema pallidum* causes sexually transmitted infection (syphilis), the third most common STI in the United States

        a. First signs include indurated, circumscribed, painless ulcer at the site of infection that lasts 10 to 14 days and heals spontaneously

        b. May experience headache, low-grade fever, and lymphadenopathy

        c. Enters period of latency where a certain percentage will develop tertiary symptoms with long-term effects in the central nervous system (CNS), blood vessels, and perivascular areas

    5. *Borrelia burgdorferi* causes Lyme disease, the most common tick-transmitted disease

        a. Lesion expands uniformly from site of bite that is clear in center, with redness at the periphery

        b. Host response often leads to complications such as arthritis and neuropathies; if left untreated may lead to destruction of bone and joints

        c. Symptoms may include fever, neck stiffness, neurological complications such as Bell's palsy or Lyme disease

C. Nursing assessment

    1. Assessment includes appearance and location of lesions; VS; signs of lymphadenopathy; sexual history for suspicion of syphilis; complaints of discomfort

    2. Diagnostic tests

        a. Cultures (may take 8 to 12 weeks)

        b. Serologic testing for antibodies (may be negative in early stages) include ELISA and indirect fluorescent antibody tests (IFA)

D. Nursing management

    1. Medications include penicillins and doxycycline (as drugs of choice)

    2. Teach individuals to wear protective clothing and/or avoid tick-infested areas

    3. Encourage to seek early intervention for suspected tick bites

    4. Instruct in use of protective barriers during intercourse for prevention of syphilis

VII. RICKETTSIAL INFECTIONS

A. Overview

    1. Rickettsia are similar to Gram-negative bacteria that can only reproduce within certain susceptible cells

    2. They are transmitted to humans by arthropod vectors through bites or feces of ticks, lice, or fleas

    3. The most common diseases caused by rickettsiae are typhus and Rocky Mountain spotted fever

B. Pathophysiology

1. Rickettsiae are extremely small rod-shaped, coccoid, or pleomorphic bacteria that are intracellular parasites because of a highly permeable cytoplasmic membrane

2. They typically consist of three layers: an inner cytoplasmic membrane, a rigid cell wall, and an outer layer, and they multiply by binary fission

3. They are primarily found in the endothelium of small blood vessels, particularly the brain, skin, and heart

   a. Hyperplasia of endothelial cells and localized thrombus formation lead to obstruction of blood flow, with escape of red blood cells into surrounding tissue

   b. Inflammation of blood vessels occurs (angiitis)

4. Clinical manifestations are believed to be caused by production of endotoxin

5. Untreated cases result in a 20% to 25% fatality

6. Signs and symptoms include skin rash, headache, malaise, muscle aches, chills and nausea and vomiting; fever of sudden onset may last 2 to 3 weeks

C. Nursing assessment

1. Assessment includes VS, skin, pain, and symptom analysis of complaints

2. Diagnostic tests

   a. Complement fixation test (may be positive within 14 days)

   b. Indirect fluoroscent antibody test (detects IgM and IgG antibodies)

D. Nursing management

1. Medications include tetracycline (Doxycycline) and chloramphenicol (Chloromycetin)

2. Careful monitoring is required with chloramphenicol due to risk of possible bone marrow suppression

3. Teach individuals importance of prevention through avoidance of arthropod carriers and use of repellent in high-risk areas

4. Sulfonamides should be avoided because they may stimulate rickettsial growth

VIII. PROTOZOAL INFECTIONS

A. Overview

1. Protozoa are unicellular organisms that may be spherical-, spindle-, or cup-shaped

2. Protozoal infections are among the most common infections of humans throughout the world

3. They occur primarily as parasites of the gastrointestinal and genitourinary systems and may result in pneumonia as an opportunistic infection in immunocompromised clients

B. Pathophysiology

1. Protozoans reproduce asexually by fission, schizogony (multiple fission), or budding

   a. Some also reproduce sexually by fusion of haploid sex cells

   b. Some protozoa produce cysts that enable them to survive outside their host

2. The most common types of infections caused by protozoa are amebiasis, giardiasis, malaria, toxoplasmosis, and *Pneumocystis carinii* pneumonia

3. *Amoeba* are transmitted by the fecal-oral route
   a. Cysts are excreted in the feces of an infected individual or carrier and ingested through contaminated food, water, or objects
   b. They penetrate the walls of the large intestines causing ulceration and may enter the blood to cause damage to other organs
   c. Certain forms can also be transmitted through mucous membranes via contaminated water
   d. Many individuals serve as carriers without clinical symptoms
   e. Early clinical manifestations include diarrhea with mucus and blood, and flatulence, alternating with constipation
   f. Later manifestations of amebic disorders may include lesions of ulcerative colitis, secondary infection in other parts of the body, and amebic liver abscess

4. *Giardiasis* is the most common protozoan intestinal disease in the United States and is also transmitted through the fecal-oral route
   a. Cysts are ingested through contaminated food or water and result in gastroenteritis
   b. Clinical manifestations include epigastric pain and nausea

5. *Malaria* is caused by a particular genus of protozoa called *plasmodium* and is transmitted through the bite of an infected mosquito
   a. Once infected, a primary exoerythrocytic cycle of asexual reproduction occurs in the human liver and leads to synchronous lysis of large numbers of erythrocytes
   b. Extensive erythrolysis results in anemia and splenomegaly
   c. Since this activity occurs primarily in capillaries, small hemorrhages and ischemia from vascular plugging lead to tissue anoxia
   d. Early symptoms of malaria include headache, anorexia, nausea, vomiting, and photophobia; this may be followed by chills, high fever, and muscle pain

6. *Toxoplasmosis* is acquired through ingestion of cysts from cat feces, by ingesting uncooked meat or unpasteurized dairy products, or through blood transfusions
   a. While healthy individuals often remain asymptomatic, early symptoms may include chills, fever, headache, lymphadenitis, and extreme fatigue
   b. Reactivation toxoplasmosis has become a significant opportunistic infection in immunocompromised individuals

7. *Pneumocystis jerovici* (also known as *Pneumocystis carinii*) pneumonia results from a protozoan that produces cysts in the lungs of several animal species and is increasingly common in immunocompromised individuals
   a. The protozoa line the alveolar walls and block gas exchange
   b. Accumulations of lymphocytes, macrophages, and plasma cells, with almost no phagocytosis, results in aggregation of parasites, cellular debris, and plasma proteins that lead to interstitial plasma cell pneumonia
   c. Symptoms include a dry, nonproductive cough and absence of sputum; progressive dyspnea may lead to cyanosis

C. Nursing assessment
   1. Assessment includes gastrointestinal symptoms; risk for protozoal disorders; complaints of pain and/or nausea; VS; intolerance to light; palpation of lymph nodes; activity level; characteristics of sputum if present

2. Diagnostic tests

a. Amoeba and giardiasis: note presence and morphology of cysts in fecal smear

b. Malaria: observe erythrocytic stages on blood smears; CBC

c. Toxoplasmosis: serologic tests (indirect fluorescent antibody, indirect hemagglutination assay, enzyme-linked immunosorbent assay [ELISA])

d. Pneumocystitis: lung tissue biopsy or needle aspiration

D. Nursing management

1. Medications

a. Amebiasis and giardiasis: drug of choice is metronidazole (Flagyl); disrupts DNA synthesis and synthesis of nucleic acid

b. Malaria: drugs of choice are chloroquine (Aralen Hydrochloride) and hydroxychloroquine (Plaquenil); interfere with protein synthesis and inhibit DNA and RNA replication as well as nucleic acid synthesis

c. Toxoplasmosis: pyrimethamine (Daraprim) and pyrimethamine/sulfadoxine (Fansidar); folic acid antagonists

d. Pneumocystitis: trimethoprim/sulfamethoxazole (Bactrim), a folic acid antagonist

2. Instruct individuals to boil water prior to drinking in areas with untreated water

3. Instruct on proper handwashing after defecating

IX. HELMINTHIC INFECTIONS

A. Overview

1. Helminths (worms) are complex organisms that gain entry into humans primarily through ingestion of fertilized eggs or penetration of larvae through the skin or mucous membranes

2. Helminths are classified as

a. Cestodes (tapeworms)

b. Nematodes (roundworms)

c. Trematodes (flukes)

B. Pathophysiology

1. Cestode infections are caused by tapeworms living in the intestines

a. Tapeworms are flat, segmented worms with structures that allow attachment to the intestinal wall

b. These usually cause little pathology and begin with ingestion of eggs or cysts from infected beef, pork, or fish

c. The cyst lodges in the intestinal mucosa and can cause symptoms including diarrhea, abdominal pain, nausea, fatigue, anorexia, and paresthesias

d. The large size of the adult tapeworm results in irritation to the mucosa and infestations can result in intestinal obstruction

e. Eggs can enter the blood and migrate to various tissues (including the brain)

2. Nematodes are elongated, unsegmented, cylindrical worms

a. The eggs develop in the soil, and once ingested, they hatch and larvae undergo migration through the lungs before localizing and maturing in the small intestine

b. Migration through the walls of the alveoli causes irritation and may result in transient pneumonitis, which may be asymptomatic

c. This may result in fever, coughing, blood in the sputum, and elevated eosinophil counts

d. Intestinal nematodes may result in abdominal distention, fever, and obstruction

3. Trematodes are unsegmented, flat, leaf-shaped worms that require asexual reproduction in a snail intermediate host

a. Humans become infected by ingesting poorly cooked fish, crabs, or snails

b. They usually have suckers for attaching to the GI mucosa

c. Flukes may infect various tissues including blood vessels, intestines, the liver or lungs

d. Flukes cover themselves with host antigens to avoid antibody response in order to exist in the blood

e. Inflammatory responses from migrating eggs often lead to scarring and fibrosis in affected organs

f. Early symptoms include fever, malaise, abdominal pain, itching (rectal), and gastroenteritis

g. Untreated infections can lead to chronic disorders in affected organs

C. Nursing assessment

1. Assessment includes complaints of discomfort, weight, bowel patterns, VS, and energy level

2. Diagnostic tests

a. Examination of stool specimens for ova, cysts, and parasites

b. CT scan

c. CBC: eosinophilia

D. Nursing management

1. Medications

a. All types helminths: drug of choice is mebendazole (Vermox), which inhibits uptake of glucose and other nutrients

b. Other drugs used for cestodes

1) Albendazole (Albenza), which causes degeneration of cytoplasmic microtubules in intestinal wall of helminths, causing decreased ATP production and energy depletion

2) Praziquantel (Biltricide) causes loss of intracellular calcium and paralysis of parasites

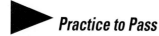

Practice to Pass

What is the most severe and life-threatening complication of infestation with worms?

c. Other drugs for nematodes

1) Diethylcarbamazine (Hetrazan) inhibits embryogenesis of nematodes

2) Ivermectin (Stomectol) inhibits CNS signals, leading to paralysis of nematode

3) Piperazine (Antepar) and pyrantel (Antiminth) block acetylcholine at neuromuscular junction, resulting in paralysis of the worm

d. Other drugs for trematodes: oxamniquine (Vansil) and praziquantel (Biltricide) cause loss of intracellular calcium and paralysis of parasites

2. Teach clients about the importance of cooking meat; freezing meat for several days can also destroy infectious eggs

X. MYCOPLASMAL INFECTIONS

A. Overview

1. Mycoplasma species are the smallest known free-living organisms
2. They are pleomorphic organisms with no cell wall (therefore resistant to cell wall–active antibiotics)
3. Mycoplasma pneumonia is also known as atypical or walking pneumonia

B. Pathophysiology

1. Mycoplasma are generally slow growing but vary widely in growth rates; they require fatty acids (sterol) and serum protein for growth and generally adhere to mucosal epithelium
2. Mycoplasma pneumonia occurs most often in children, young adults, and the elderly
   a. It is transmitted by droplets, with an incubation period of 2 to 3 weeks
   b. Individuals may be asymptomatic, however, common signs and symptoms include headache, low-grade fever, malaise, anorexia, and hacking cough

C. Nursing assessment

1. Assessment includes VS, complaints of pain or discomfort, activity level, nutritional assessment, lung sounds, and presence of cough
2. Diagnostic tests
   a. Cold agglutin antibody titer may be done but is insensitive and nonspecific
   b. Enzyme immunoassay (EIA): positive
   c. Chest x-ray (CXR) will show infiltrates

D. Nursing management

1. Medications
   a. Drug of choice: macrolides—azithromycin (Zithromax)
   b. Clarithromycin (Biaxin)
   c. Analgesics or NSAIDs for discomfort
   d. Antipyretics for fever
2. Encourage balance of rest and activity
3. Offer fluids unless contraindicated
4. Administer oxygen if needed

XI. MYCOBACTERIAL INFECTIONS

A. Overview

1. A group of acid-fast bacteria belonging to the *Mycobacteriaceae* family
2. Organisms are slender, Gram-positive rods
3. Common diseases include *M. tuberculosis* (tuberculosis); *M. leprae* (leprosy), and *M. avium-intracellulare* (an opportunistic infection)

B. Pathophysiology

1. The organisms are surrounded by a waxy capsule that is hard to penetrate
2. The organisms may form branches of a fungal nature
3. Are classified as common facultative intracellular parasites; able to survive and grow within a macrophage

4. Humans are the only natural host
5. The response to the cell includes tissue damage as a result of chronic inflammation
6. *M. tuberculosis* (tuberculosis) is an aerobic acid-fast rod
   a. Contagious by respiratory droplets
   b. Incubation is variable, 4 to 8 weeks
   c. Can be reinfected
   d. Signs and symptoms include lung involvement (can be seen on chest x-ray); fever, pleurisy; night sweats; cough; weight loss
7. *M. leprae* (leprosy)
   a. Also known as Hansen's disease; caused by an acid-fast rod-shaped bacillus
   b. Contracted by close contact or prolonged exposure
   c. Skin or nasal mucosa can be portal of entrance
   d. Incubation period is 3 to 5 years
   e. Signs and symptoms include: lesions of skin that are destructive, as well as involvement of peripheral nerves, upper respiratory passages, testes, hands, and feet; muscle weakness
   f. Erythema nodosum leprosum (ENL) reaction may develop during the end of the first year of therapy with red, painful nodules that become ulcerated and necrotic
8. *M. avium-intracellulare*
   a. An opportunistic organism; that is an acid-fast rod
   b. Contracted by respiratory transmission from soil, water, dairy products, birds, and mammals
   c. Signs and symptoms are pulmonary in nature

C. Nursing assessment
1. Assessment includes lung sounds; symptom analysis; VS; skin assessment; height and weight analysis; nutritional assessment; presence of cough
2. Diagnostic tests
   a. Sputum analysis: culture and sensitivity as well as acid-fast bacillus
   b. CXR
   c. Skin lesion biopsy
   d. Leprosy
      1) Lymphocyte transformation test
      2) Leukocyte migration inhibition test
   e. Tuberculosis: positive TB skin test (PPD or Mantoux), with induration of 10 mm or greater for clients not generally at risk, or 5mm or greater for those with frequent exposure or greater risk (immunocompromised)

D. Nursing management
1. Medications
   a. Leprosy
      1) Dapsone (DDS)
      2) Thalidomide (Thalomid): drug of choice for ENL
      3) Corticosteroids
   b. Tuberculosis
      1) Isoniazid (INH), pyrazinamide (PZA), rifampin (RMP) and others
      2) Combining INH and RMP is most effective

! ▶ **2.** Teach the client and family about exposure and proper incubation periods to avoid infecting others

! ▶ **3.** Stress the need to continue therapy even if feeling better; avoid alcohol with INH

XII. PRION INFECTIONS

A. Overview

1. Prions are mutant forms of protein on the surface of some animal cells that are similar to viruses in ability to cause infection, although smaller in size
2. Prions lack nucleic acid found in viruses
3. They have been linked to chronic degenerative diseases of the central nervous system

B. Pathophysiology

1. Although little is known about the exact mechanism of action, characteristics of the disorders have been identified
2. The disorders are characterized by long incubation periods with a protracted course that usually results in death
3. Pathologic lesions are usually limited to a single organ or tissue system
4. Examples of prion disorders include spongiform encephalopathies such as Creutzfeldt-Jacob disease
   a. This disorder begins with personality changes, memory loss, and altered visual acuity and results in progressive dementia, ataxia, and somnolence and eventually leads to death within 1 to 2 years after onset of symptoms
   b. It is thought to have been transmitted through corneal transplants and contaminated growth hormone
   c. The CNS alterations occur primarily in the cerebral cortex and cerebellum

C. Nursing assessment and management

1. Assess history and pattern of memory loss or changes in personality
2. Document progressive physical and behavioral changes

Case Study

A client has been hospitalized with an intestinal obstruction and undergoes surgery. While recovering from the surgery she develops chills, fever, and malaise and the surgical site is noted as red with purulent drainage. Because of a recent increase in the incidence of methicillin-resistant Staphylococcus aureus *(MRSA) within the hospital unit, the physician suspects MRSA as the source of the wound infection.*

1. What type of infection is this considered, and what is the most important nursing intervention concerning prevention?

2. What is the most appropriate diagnostic test to determine the causative organism?

3. What other relevant laboratory findings should be observed?

4. What is the drug of choice for treating MRSA and what adverse effects should the nurse consider?

5. If the culture reveals vancomycin-resistant *Staphylococcus aureus* (VRSA), what medications are effective?

For suggested responses, see page 537.

POSTTEST

1 A client diagnosed with a bacterial infection that is resistant to penicillin asks the nurse, "Why can't penicillin be used to treat this infection?" The nurse's reply incorporates what pertinent information about the role of the bacterial capsule?

1. Protects the pathogenic bacteria from host defenses
2. Plays a major role in adherence of bacteria
3. Does not protect the organism from phagocytosis
4. Always composed of glutamic acid

2 The nurse reviews which of the following client laboratory test results that is expected to be elevated with nematode infestation?

1. Neutrophils
2. Liver enzymes
3. Red blood cells
4. Eosinophils

3 A nurse researcher is interested in the epidemiology of human immunodeficiency virus (HIV), and a nursing student is assisting with the research. The student will expect to collect data related to the:

1. Retroviral genotypes found in that community.
2. Transmittal of the disease in the community.
3. Most effective treatment regimens and the CD4 cell counts of the study population.
4. Distribution of the disease in the population being studied.

4 A young male college student comes to the clinic after contracting genital herpes. Which of the following interventions by the nurse would be most appropriate?

1. Encourage him to maintain bedrest for several days
2. Monitor his temperature every four hours
3. Instruct him to avoid sexual contact during acute phases of illness
4. Encourage him to use antifungal agents regularly

5 A client has been diagnosed with genital herpes and wants to reduce the length and severity of the outbreak. About which of the following drugs will the nurse plan to teach the client?

1. Penicillin (Bicillin)
2. Rifampin (Rifadin)
3. Acyclovir (Zovirax)
4. Podophyllin (Condylox)

6 A young adult male relates to the nurse that he has recently experienced signs and symptoms of infection. His neutrophil count is lower than normal. The nurse concludes that most likely he:

1. Has a bacterial infection.
2. Has a viral infection.
3. Has an immune deficiency disorder.
4. Is recovering from the illness.

7 A young girl presents with fever and abdominal distention. Her mother states that she has also "coughed up blood" in recent days. The nurse considers that which of the following health problems is compatible with these symptoms?

1. Mycoplasma pneumonia
2. Rickettsial infection
3. Infection with nematodes
4. Infection with spirochetes

8 The nurse is teaching a client recently diagnosed with Creutzfeldt-Jakob disease about the disease process. The nurse will base the teaching on what knowledge of the disease?

1. Prions are opportunistic organisms frequently seen in clients with human immunodeficiency virus (HIV)
2. Prions have been linked to chronic degenerative central nervous system disorders, called transmissible neurodegenerative diseases
3. Lesions caused by the microorganisms associated with this disease are usually distributed throughout the body
4. Prions are similar to viruses in their nucleic acid structure but there is no drug to treat the infection

9 A client has a white blood cell count (WBC) of 15,000, of which 60% are segmented neutrophils (segs) and 3% are bands. An antibiotic is prescribed. Three days later the WBC remains at 15,000, with 62% segs and 10% bands. The nurse concludes that this most likely indicates:

1. The infection is resolving.
2. The client is immunocompromised.
3. The infection is severe or prolonged and not responding to antimicrobial agents.
4. There is a shift to the right in the differential.

10 A client in the clinic asks why an antibiotic is needed to treat "a tick bite with a funny-looking ring around it." The nurse will base the response on what conclusions? Select all that apply.

1. Disease is caused by rickettsial pathogens
2. Humoral and cell-mediated responses by the body will not generally be sufficient to eliminate the disease
3. Disease is transmitted by ticks
4. If untreated, it may lead to complications of arthritis and destruction of joints
5. The most frequent time of onset is in the summer months

➤ *See pages 401–403 for Answers & Rationales.*

ANSWERS & RATIONALES

Pretest

1 **Answer: 3** An opportunistic infection is one in which an individual develops an infection from an organism that does not cause disease in healthy individuals. This occurs with compromised immunity. Options 1, 2, and 4 describe an etiology that is environmental in origin. **Cognitive Level:** Application **Client Need:** Physiological Integrity: Physiological Adaptation **Integrated Process:** Nursing Process: Analysis **Content Area:** Adult Health: Immunological **Strategy:** The critical word in the question is *opportunistic.* Review medical terminology if needed. **Reference:** LeMone, P., & Burke, K. (2008). *Medical-surgical nursing: Critical thinking in client care* (4th ed.). Upper Saddle River, NJ: Pearson/Prentice Hall, p. 353.

2 **Answer: 2** Antibiotics may affect the outcome of the culture. The culture should be taken before the antibiotic is started. Fever will continue to be present until the bacteria are eliminated, making administration of the antibiotic a priority. All the other actions are appropriate but not the *first* action to take. **Cognitive Level:** Analysis **Client Need:** Physiological Integrity: Physiological Adaptation **Integrated Process:** Nursing Process: Implementation **Content Area:** Adult Health: Immunological **Strategy:** All options are correct actions but the question asks what to do *first.* Consider the importance of an accurate culture and sensitivity on the client's outcome to make your selection. **Reference:** Kee, J. (2005). *Laboratory and diagnostic tests with nursing implications* (7th ed.). Upper Saddle River, NJ: Pearson/Prentice Hall, p. 152.

3 **Answers: 1, 3, 4, 5** Options 1, 3, 4, and 5 are correct mechanisms of bacterial resistance. Leukocytosis is a positive host defense increasing the white blood cells to

fight infection. The prevalence of bacterial resistance is a great concern in the treatment of infectious diseases. **Cognitive Level:** Application **Client Need:** Physiological Integrity: Pharmacological and Parenteral Therapies **Integrated Process:** Nursing Process: Implementation **Content Area:** Adult Health: Immunological **Strategy:** Differentiate between leukocytosis and leukopenia and read carefully. Recall that mechanisms of bacterial resistance are numerous. **Reference:** Porth, C. M. (2005). *Pathophysiology: Concepts of altered health states* (7th ed.). Philadelphia, PA: Lippincott Williams & Wilkins, p. 360.

4 **Answer: 2** A pathogen is any organism capable of causing disease. Pathogenicity refers to the ability of the organism to cause pathologic changes. Communicability is the ability to be transmitted from one person or organism to another. Toxigenicity is the ability of a microorganism to produce endotoxins or exotoxins. Latency is a period during which an organism has infected an individual but has not yet caused symptoms. **Cognitive Level:** Application **Client Need:** Physiological Integrity: Physiological Adaptation **Integrated Process:** Teaching/Learning **Content Area:** Adult Health: Immunological **Strategy:** If the terms are unfamiliar, try decoding them for root word, suffix, and prefix. **Reference:** Porth, C. M. (2005). *Pathophysiology: Concepts of altered health states* (7th ed.). Philadelphia, PA: Lippincott Williams & Wilkins, pp. 341–342.

5 **Answer: 1** Bacterial infections are characterized by fever, body aches, possible regional lymph node involvement, and local signs of infection. Fungal infections are characterized by itching or rashes on skin, or thrush in mouth or vaginal discharge. Protozoal infections have skin manifestation such as itching or rash, diarrhea, and possibly fever if of malarial origin. Rickettsial infections are accompanied by skin rashes, muscle aches, headache, and possibly fever and chills. **Cognitive Level:** Application **Client Need:** Physiological Integrity: Physiological Adaptation **Integrated Process:** Nursing Process: Analysis **Content Area:** Adult Health: Immunological **Strategy:** Familiarity with the types of infections caused by the different microorganisms is helpful in answering this question. Recall that the question is asking about the presence of both fever and regional lymph node involvement in making a selection. **Reference:** Porth, C. M. (2005). *Pathophysiology: Concepts of altered health states* (7th ed.). Philadelphia, PA: Lippincott Williams & Wilkins, p. 359.

6 **Answer: 1** Influenza virus is transmitted through respiratory droplets. Herpes virus is transmitted by direct contact and HIV through blood and body fluids. Cytomegalovirus is an opportunistic infection. **Cognitive Level:** Analysis **Client Need:** Safe, Effective Care Environment: Safety and Infection Control **Integrated Process:** Nursing Process: Assessment **Content Area:** Adult Health: Immunological **Strategy:** The critical words in the question are *casual contact.* Visualize each of the infections and recall the mode of transmission to make a selection. **Reference:** Porth, C. M. (2005). *Pathophysiology: Concepts of altered health states* (7th ed.). Philadelphia, PA: Lippincott Williams & Wilkins, p. 352.

7 **Answers: 2, 3** Epidemiological studies indicate chlamydia as the most prevalent sexually transmitted infection (STI) in the United States. Cultures and sensitivity testing will be done for both chlamydia and gonorrhea. Syphilis is diagnosed by tissue scraping and microscopic analysis or by blood testing. Viruses can be cultured but do not undergo sensitivity testing, since this applies to antibiotics, which are utilized for bacterial infections. **Cognitive Level:** Analysis **Client Need:** Physiological Integrity: Physiological Adaptation **Integrated Process:** Nursing Process: Assessment **Content Area:** Adult Health: Immunological **Strategy:** Note that two of the options are bacteria that cause STIs. Note that both will need to be cultured and undergo sensitivity testing. **Reference:** LeMone, P., & Burke, K. (2008). *Medical-surgical nursing: Critical thinking in client care* (4th ed.). Upper Saddle River, NJ: Pearson/Prentice Hall, pp. 1844–1845.

8 **Answer: 3** Foods such as undercooked ground meat or unpasteurized fruit juices may be contaminated with *E. coli,* the organism that produces the toxin and disease. Option 1 describes botulism; option 4 describes a *Staphylococcus aureus* infection. The disease is not spread from kissing (option 2). **Cognitive Level:** Application **Client Need:** Health Promotion and Maintenance **Integrated Process:** Nursing Process: Implementation **Content Area:** Adult Health: Im-

munological **Strategy:** Recall that this bacterial exotoxin is one that has received media attention, and nurses should be aware of the problem. **Reference:** Porth, C. M. (2005). *Pathophysiology: Concepts of altered health states* (7th ed.). Philadelphia, PA: Lippincott Williams & Wilkins, p. 354.

9 **Answer: 3** Rickettsia are parasites of ticks, fleas, and lice. Influenza is an example of transmission by respiratory droplets, encephalitis is transmitted by mosquitoes; lice and scabies are transmitted by direct contact. **Cognitive Level:** Application **Client Need:** Safe, Effective Care Environment: Safety and Infection Control **Integrated Process:** Nursing Process: Analysis **Content Area:** Adult Health: Immunological **Strategy:** Recall that a vector is needed to transmit this infection. Knowing that narrows the answer choices to two options. **Reference:** Porth, C. M. (2005). *Pathophysiology: Concepts of altered health states* (7th ed.). Philadelphia, PA: Lippincott Williams & Wilkins, p. 347.

10 **Answer: 2** Infection occurs in a predictable sequence commonly known as the steps in the chain of infection. The chain requires virulence of the organism, a reservoir or source, movement from a reservoir via a portal of exit, a method of transmission and entry into a susceptible host. Infection does not relay on linkages among different form of organisms (option 1) or clustering of bacteria in a pattern (option 3). Increasing virulence patterns among microorganisms (option 4) may lead to drug resistance, but not to transmission of infection. **Cognitive Level:** Comprehension **Client Need:** Physiological Integrity: Physiological Adaptation **Integrated Process:** Nursing Process: Analysis **Content Area:** Adult Health: Immunological **Strategy:** The critical words in the question are *chain of infection.* Eliminate the options that are not applicable to the chain. Read the question again if needed—it is asking about the development of an infectious disease in the community. **Reference:** LeMone, P., & Burke, K. (2008). *Medical-surgical nursing: Critical thinking in client care* (4th ed.). Upper Saddle River, NJ: Pearson/Prentice Hall, pp. 311–312.

Posttest

1 **Answer: 1** The development of resistant strains of bacteria is the reason penicillin will not treat this client's infection. The capsule contributes to the invasiveness of pathogenic bacteria. Encapsulated bacteria are protected from phagocytosis unless coated with anticapsular antibody. **Cognitive Level:** Application **Client Need:** Physiological Integrity: Physiological Adaptation **Integrated Process:** Nursing Process: Analysis **Content Area:** Adult Health: Immunological **Strategy:** Beware of critical words such as *always.* Look for opposite options as a strategy and eliminate one of them using baseline nursing knowledge of how bacterial resistance occurs. **Reference:** Porth, C. M. (2005). *Pathophysiology: Concepts of altered health states* (7th ed.). Philadelphia, PA: Lippincott Williams & Wilkins, p. 350.

2 Answer: 4 Eosinophilia is present with allergies and infestation with parasites such as nematode infestation. Neutrophils (option 1) are elevated with acute infections and bacterial organisms. Liver enzymes (option 2) and red blood cells (option 3) are irrelevant.

Cognitive Level: Application **Client Need:** Physiological Integrity: Physiological Adaptation **Integrated Process:** Nursing Process: Assessment **Content Area:** Adult Health: Immunological **Strategy:** First recall that white blood cells help to fight infection to eliminate options 2 and 3. Next recall the role of neutrophils with acute infection and bacterial infections to eliminate option 1. **Reference:** Kee, J. L. (2005). *Laboratory and diagnostic tests with nursing implications* (7th ed.). Upper Saddle River, NJ: Pearson/Prentice Hall, p. 456.

3 Answer: 4 Epidemiology is the study of how various states of health are distributed in the population. This study applies to HIV studies or any other epidemiological study. Option 1 is not studied. Option 2 relates to mode of transmission. Option 3 is in the arena of medical research, not nursing research.

Cognitive Level: Application **Client Need:** Health Promotion and Maintenance **Integrated Process:** Nursing Process: Assessment **Content Area:** Adult Health: Immunological **Strategy:** Apply the definition of epidemiology to this study of disease in a population. **Reference:** LeMone, P., & Burke, K. (2008). *Medical-surgical nursing: Critical thinking in client care* (4th ed.). Upper Saddle River, NJ: Pearson/Prentice Hall, pp. 309–310.

4 Answer: 3 Herpes is a virus spread through direct contact. Therefore the client should avoid sexual contact during the acute phases of illness and should use protection against transmitting the infection thereafter. An antifungal would not be useful; bedrest and temperature measurement are usually not necessary.

Cognitive Level: Application **Client Need:** Safe, Effective Care Environment: Safety and Infection Control **Integrated Process:** Nursing Process: Implementation **Content Area:** Adult Health: Immunological **Strategy:** Consider what instructions are needed to prevent the spread of the infection while it is active in this first outbreak. **Reference:** LeMone, P., & Burke, K. (2008). *Medical-surgical nursing: Critical thinking in client care* (4th ed.). Upper Saddle River, NJ: Pearson/Prentice Hall, pp. 452–455.

5 Answer: 3 Acyclovir is the antiviral drug of choice for treating herpes virus. Penicillin products are used for a wide variety of bacterial infections. Rifampin is used for tuberculosis and podophyllin is used to treat genital warts.

Cognitive Level: Application **Client Need:** Physiological Integrity: Pharmacological and Parenteral Therapies **Integrated Process:** Nursing Process: Implementation **Content Area:** Adult Health: Immunological **Strategy:** Note that only one of the options is an antiviral. The name is a clue. **Reference:** LeMone, P., & Burke, K. (2008). *Medical-surgical nursing: Critical thinking in client care* (4th ed.). Upper Saddle River, NJ: Pearson/Prentice Hall, pp. 453–454.

6 Answer: 2 Neutrophil counts are often decreased in viral infections and elevated in bacterial infections. Neutropenia can also occur because of chemotherapy and immunosuppression. However, with immunosuppression the client's illness would not resolve untreated. The client's neutrophil count should be returning to normal if the infection has resolved, but more than one laboratory measurement of the neutrophil count would be needed to make this determination.

Cognitive Level: Application **Client Need:** Physiological Integrity: Reduction of Risk Potential **Integrated Process:** Nursing Process: Analysis **Content Area:** Adult Health: Immunological **Strategy:** Specific knowledge is needed to answer the question. Learn the CBC differential values and what causes the various changes in values. Nurses must be able to interpret them. **Reference:** Kee, J. L. (2005). *Laboratory and diagnostic tests with nursing implications* (7th ed.). Upper Saddle River, NJ: Pearson/Prentice Hall, p. 456.

7 Answer: 3 Abdominal distention is caused from infestation of worms. Blood in sputum often results from migration of worms through alveoli. Mycoplasma pneumonia has similar side effects as bacterial pneumonia (cough, fatigue, crackles, and fever). Spirochetes cause fever, neck stiffness, and lymphadenopathy; rickettsial infections cause headaches, nausea, vomiting, and muscle aches.

Cognitive Level: Analysis **Client Need:** Physiological Integrity: Physiological Adaptation **Integrated Process:** Nursing Process: Assessment **Content Area:** Adult Health: Immunological **Strategy:** Consider both the gastrointestinal and the pulmonary symptoms when selecting the answer. **Reference:** LeMone, P., & Burke, K. (2008). *Medical-surgical nursing: Critical thinking in client care* (4th ed.). Upper Saddle River, NJ: Pearson/Prentice Hall, p. 779–781.

8 Answer: 2 Prions, related to the agent causing bovine spongiform encephalopathy or mad cow disease, are associated with degenerative encephalopathies. While similar to viruses, they are protein particles lacking nucleic acid. Lesions are usually limited to a single organ such as the brain. **Cognitive Level:** Application **Client Need:** Physiological Integrity: Physiological Adaptation **Integrated Process:** Teaching/Learning **Content Area:** Adult Health: Immunological **Strategy:** First identify the agent causing the disease. Next determine the pathology. **Reference:** Porth, C. M. (2005). *Pathophysiology: Concepts of altered health states* (7th ed.). Philadelphia, PA: Lippincott Williams & Wilkins, p. 343.

9 **Answer: 3** With bacterial infection there is an increased need for neutrophils. When the percentage of immature neutrophils (bands) increases at a greater rate than mature neutrophils (segs), it is an indication that the infection is severe or prolonged. This is often referred to as a shift to the left. **Cognitive Level:** Analysis **Client Need:** Physiological Integrity: Physiological Adaptation **Integrated Process:** Nursing Process: Analysis **Content Area:** Adult Health: Immunological **Strategy:** Learn the CBC differential values and the implications of abnormal values or changes. In

this question, evaluate the trend of increasing bands. **Reference:** Kee, J. L. (2005). *Laboratory and diagnostic tests with nursing implications* (7th ed.). Upper Saddle River, NJ: Pearson/Prentice Hall, p. 456–457.

10 **Answers: 2, 3, 4, 5** The lesion described is typical for Lyme disease. Lyme disease is a spirochete infection caused by *Borrelia burdorferi*. Lyme disease is carried by mice or deer and ticks are vectors. Examples of rickettsial infections are typhus and Rocky Mountain spotted fever. **Cognitive Level:** Analysis **Client Need:** Physiological Integrity: Physiological Adaptation **Integrated Process:** Nursing Process: Planning **Content Area:** Adult Health: Immunological **Strategy:** First determine what the client's problem is. Then apply knowledge of that disease to select the correct options. **Reference:** Porth, C. M. (2005). *Pathophysiology: Concepts of altered health states* (7th ed.). Philadelphia, PA: Lippincott Williams & Wilkins, p.1266.

References

Corbett, J. V. (2004). *Laboratory tests and diagnostic procedures with nursing diagnoses* (6th ed.). Upper Saddle River, NJ: Prentice Hall.

Kee, J. L. (2005). *Laboratory and diagnostic tests with nursing implications* (7th ed.). Upper Saddle River, NJ: Prentice Hall.

LeMone, P., & Burke, K. M. (2008). *Medical-surgical nursing: Critical thinking in client care* (4th ed.). Upper Saddle River, NJ: Prentice Hall.

Lilley, L. L., Harrington, S., & Snyder, J. (2005). *Pharmacology and the nursing process* (4th ed.). St. Louis: Mosby.

Porth, C. (2005). *Pathophysiology: Concepts of altered health states* (7th ed.). Philadelphia, PA: Lippincott Williams & Wilkins, pp. 339–364.

Wilkinson, J. M. (2006). *Nursing diagnosis handbook with NIC interventions and NOC outcomes* (8th ed.). Upper Saddle River, NJ: Prentice Hall.

Wilson, B. A., Shannon, M. T., & Stang, C. L. (2006). *Nursing drug guide 2006*. Upper Saddle River, NJ: Prentice Hall.

14 Integumentary Health Problems

Chapter Outline

Risk Factors Associated with Integumentary Health Problems

Malignant Conditions of the Skin

Benign Conditions of the Skin

Bacterial Infections of the Skin

Viral Infections of the Skin

Fungal Infections of the Skin

Infestations and Insect Bites

Allergic Conditions of the Skin

Burns

 NCLEX-RN® Test Prep

Use the CD-ROM enclosed with this book to access additional practice opportunities.

Objectives

➤ Define key terms associated with integumentary health problems.

➤ Identify risk factors associated with integumentary health problems.

➤ Explain common etiologies of integumentary health problems.

➤ Describe the pathophysiological processes associated with integumentary health problems.

➤ Distinguish between normal and abnormal integumentary findings obtained from nursing assessment.

➤ Prioritize nursing interventions associated with integumentary health problems.

Review at a Glance

acne an androgenically stimulated, inflammatory disorder of the sebaceous glands, resulting in comedomes, papules, inflamed pustules, and occasionally scarring

atopic dermatitis an inflammation of the skin from an unknown source in an individual with irritable skin; also known as eczema

basal cell carcinoma malignant tumor of the skin originating from the basal cells of the epidermis

burn tissue injuries caused by the application of heat, chemicals, electricity, or radiation to the tissue

candidiasis a fungal infection caused by Candida albicans, a yeast-like fungus that most often causes superficial cutaneous infections

carbuncle (carbunculosis) aggregates of infected follicles coalesced together to form one large lesion

cellulitis a diffuse inflammation of the skin and subcutaneous layers with various presenting lesions including vesicles (small sacs of fluid), bullae (large blisters), abscesses, and plaques

contact dermatitis an eruption of the skin related to contact with an irritating substance or allergen

dermatophyte a group of fungi that have the ability to infect and survive only on keratin, classified as tinea infections

exfoliative dermatitis an inflammation of the skin characterized by erythema involving loss of exfoliated (peeling) skin

folliculitis an inflammation of the hair follicle usually caused by the organism Staphylococcus aureus or Pseudomonas aeruginosa

furuncle (furunculosis) also known as an abscess or boil, a deep folliculitis consisting of a pus-filled mass that is painful and firm

herpes simplex a viral infection that occurs within the keratinolytics and manifests as painful vesicles that often occur in clusters on the skin

herpes zoster a viral infection (also known as shingles) that manifests as a cluster of vesicles on the skin; a reactivation of the varicella virus in the dorsal root ganglia that remained in the latent form after the primary infection

impetigo a superficial skin infection initially seen as an erythemic vesicle, later changing to a honey-colored crusted lesion

lentigo a brown macule resembling a freckle except the border is usually regular

malignant melanoma a skin cancer arising from the melanocytes

molluscum contagiosum a benign, viral infection of the skin caused

by the poxvirus inducing epidermal cell proliferation

pediculosis an infestation of the skin or hair by the species of blood-sucking lice capable of living as external parasites on the human host

psoriasis a genetically determined, chronic epidermal proliferative disease characterized by erythematous, dry scaling patches, usually with a heavy, silvery surface

seborrheic dermatitis an acute inflammation of the skin from an unknown cause that usually begins on the scalp and has rounded, irregular lesions and yellow scales

seborrheic keratosis benign plaques, beige to brown or maybe black in color, ranging in size from 3 to 20 mm with a velvety or warty surface

squamous cell carcinoma a slow-growing cancer of atypical squamous cells that originates in the epidermis and may metastasize

tinea versicolor common noninflammatory fungal infection caused by lipophilic yeast

urticaria an itchy rash (hives)

warts virus-induced epidermal tumors

PRETEST

1 The nurse is teaching self-care to a client with psoriasis. The nurse should encourage which of the following for his scaled lesions?

1. Petroleum-based emollients and moisturizers to soften the scales
2. Importance of follow-up appointments
3. Use of a clean razor blade each time he shaves
4. Keep occlusive dressings on the lesions 24 hours a day

2 The nurse teaches a client that the first step in self-management of contact/irritant dermatitis is to do which of the following?

1. Take antihistamines to control the itch
2. Identify and remove the causative agent
3. Use over-the-counter (OTC) hydrocortisone cream
4. Seek allergy testing

3 A mother asks how her 2nd-grade child got head lice. The nurse responds by telling the mother that lice:

1. Only occur in socioeconomically deprived people.
2. Were probably spread by person-to-person contact in the classroom.
3. Are an airborne infestation.
4. Are due to improper washing of her hair.

4 The nurse conducting a health fair teaches attendees that which of the following groups of people are most at risk for developing malignant melanoma?

1. Light-skinned people who work indoors and vacation in sunny climates
2. Dark-skinned people who work indoors and have intermittent sun exposure
3. Light-skinned people working outdoors with regular sun exposure
4. Dark-skinned people who work outdoors getting regular sun exposure

5 A client is admitted to the Emergency Department with 50% burns to the chest and arms. The skin is white, dry, and there is no pain. The nurse assesses the type of burn the client has as which of the following?

1. Superficial thickness
2. Superficial partial thickness
3. Deep partial thickness
4. Full thickness

6 A young boy is brought to the trauma unit with a chemical burn to the face. The nurse's priority assessment would be which of the following?

1. Skin integrity of the face
2. Blood pressure and pulse
3. Adequacy of respirations
4. Amount of pain

7 The mother of 10-year-old girl tells the pediatric office nurse that her child has dandruff. On examination, the nurse notices the whitish flakes don't brush off the hair, and there is a papular rash on the child's neck. The nurse suspects which of the following disorders?

1. Tinea capitis
2. Dandruff
3. Seborrheic dermatitis
4. Pediculosis capitis

8 The nurse is most concerned about a wasp sting for a client who:

1. Has never been stung before.
2. Has a history of fever or chills when bitten.
3. Had hives and shortness of breath with the last sting.
4. Had a rise in blood pressure to 140/90 when stung.

9 A client who has been on two antibiotics complains of burning on the tongue and not wanting to eat. Inspection of the tongue reveals a white, milky plaque that does not come off with rubbing. The nurse suspects which condition?

1. Impetigo
2. Candidiasis
3. Burns
4. Herpes

10 The nurse would include which of the following pieces of information in health teaching for a client with warts on the fingers? Select all that apply.

1. Common warts grow above the skin with a rough surface and ragged borders
2. Warts resolve spontaneously when immunity to the virus develops but this may take up to five years
3. Warts can be transmitted through skin contact
4. Warts only appear in childhood
5. The causative agent is a virus

➤ *See pages 430–432 for Answers & Rationales.*

I. RISK FACTORS ASSOCIATED WITH INTEGUMENTARY HEALTH PROBLEMS

A. Malignant conditions

1. Skin pigmentation
2. Preexisting lesions
3. Exposure to chemicals
4. Radiation or excessive sun
5. Trauma
6. Viruses
7. Ethnicity (Caucasian)
8. Fair-skinned complexions

B. Individuals with fair skin and light-colored hair and those with heavy (even intermittent) sun exposure are more at risk for malignant melanoma

C. Benign conditions: exposure to sun, local trauma, infections, stress, physical disorders, and drugs

D. Bacterial conditions: individuals with a compromised immune system, other disorders such as diabetes mellitus, or lack of proper hygiene and nutrition

E. Viral infections: depressed immune system, infection with human immunodeficiency virus (HIV), individuals with radiation, chemotherapy, or major organ transplants

F. Fungal infections: debilitating disease, poor nutrition, poor hygiene, tropical climates, contact with infected persons or animals, communal showers and pools, occlusive footwear, excessive sweating, sharing of footwear, excessive moisture from clothing, or use of incontinence undergarments with the elderly

G. Bites and infestations: living in overcrowded conditions or developing countries, unsanitary conditions, and certain geographic regions

H. Allergic conditions: immunosuppressed states (such as acquired immunodeficiency syndrome [AIDS]), drug therapy, and heredity

I. Burns: small children and elderly, high-risk occupations, individuals with decreased sensation to extremities or certain parts of the body

II. MALIGNANT CONDITIONS OF THE SKIN

A. Overview

1. Defined as skin cancer from a malignant tumor or neoplasm of the skin
2. There are three types of malignant conditions: basal cell carcinoma, melanoma, and squamous cell carcinoma
3. Causes include ultraviolet exposure, extremes in weather, radiological treatment, chemicals, trauma, burns, or chronic infections; fair-skinned people, older adults, and those who live in warm climates are at increased risk

B. Pathophysiology

1. **Basal cell carcinoma** is an abnormal growth of cells in the basal layer of the epidermal skin; it is the least aggressive type and rarely metastasizes to other

organs; it is the most common form of skin cancer and may invade surrounding tissue, destroying parts of the body; the tumor takes many forms

    a. Nodular basal cell carcinoma is the most common and appears on the neck, face, and head; it is a pearly colored nodule with well-defined margins and a depressed center or rolled edge

    b. Superficial basal cell carcinoma is the second most common tumor that is located on the trunk and extremities

    c. Other forms include pigmented basal cell (head, neck, and face), rare morpheaform basal cell (head and neck), and keratotic basal cell (pre- and postauricular groove)

2. **Squamous cell carcinoma** is a more aggressive, slow-growing cancer of atypical squamous cells that originate in the epidermis and may metastasize via the lymphatic system

    a. Proliferation of keratinizing cells of the epithelium causes the tumor, forming keratin "pearls"

    b. It is most common on sun-exposed areas such as the nose, lips, and hands

    c. The lower lip is a frequent location, especially in smokers

    d. It appears as a firm, irregular, flesh-colored papule with a scaly, keratotic surface

    e. It may be erythemic, sore, and/or bleed if touched

3. **Malignant melanoma** is a cancerous tumor arising from the melanocytes (melanin-producing cells in the deepest epithelial layer), which has the ability to metastasize to any organ

    a. The melanoma initially grows superficially and laterally continuing to the epidermis and dermis

    b. It then grows vertically with penetration of the reticular dermis and subcutaneous fat

    c. This type of melanoma frequently affects young people with common sites being the back and legs

    d. Melanomas tend to have asymmetry, border irregularity, color variation, and diameter greater than 6 mm (see Box 14-1); key signs include irregular, circular-bordered lesion with hues of tan, black, or blue

    e. Precursor lesions of a malignant melanoma include dysplastic nevi (atypical mole), congenital nevi (present at birth), and lentigo maligna (tan or black patch that has the appearance of a freckle)

    f. Classification of tumors includes superficial-spreading melanoma (about 70%) that arises from preexisting nevus, lentigo maligna melanoma, nodular melanoma, and acral lentiginous melanoma

C. Nursing assessment

1. Assessment

    a. A symptom analysis about any skin changes or new growths and a history of the amount of sun exposure or sunburn

    b. Assessing any family history of skin disorders, and past history of burns, injury, trauma, or cigarette smoking

Box 14-1	**A**symmetry
ABCDs of Malignant Melanoma	**B**order irregularity **C**olor variegation **D**iameter greater than 6 mm

c. Assessing any area/preexisting lesion for change in color, size, or shape, noting any local soreness, oozing or bleeding lesions, pruritis, lymph node enlargement, liver, and spleen

2. Diagnostic tests: shave biopsy (for diagnosis), punch biopsy, incisional biopsy (remove part of tumor), or excisional biopsy (remove all of tumor); for malignant melanoma, a liver profile, complete blood count (CBC), electrolytes, CT scan of liver and brain, chest x-ray (CXR), bone scan, magnetic resonance imaging (MRI) of liver, and biopsy of lymph nodes

D. Nursing management

1. Assess all lesions over the entire body; encourage yearly examinations for a client with excessive moles

 2. Teach self-monitoring and examination of existing skin lesions and for any new lesions; early diagnosis and intervention are crucial

3. Instruct the client to avoid contact with chemical irritants

4. Teach the client about the importance of sun exposure protection, wearing layered clothing while outdoors, avoiding midday sun (between 10 a.m. and 2 p.m), and using sunscreen with a sun protection factor (SPF) over 15

5. Encourage verbalization of client concerns and changes in body image

6. Educate clients about the harmful effects of tanning beds

III. BENIGN CONDITIONS OF THE SKIN

A. Overview

1. Defined as conditions of the integumentary system that are cutaneous growths with no malignant potential

2. Benign conditions include acne, lentigo, psoriasis, and seborrheic keratosis

3. Causes

   a. Acne: oversecretion of sebum and dysfunction of hormones

   b. Lentigo: prolonged exposure to the sun

   c. Psoriasis and seborrheic keratosis: genetics

B. Pathophysiology

1. **Acne** is an androgen-stimulated, inflammatory disorder of the sebaceous glands resulting in comedones (open form—blackhead; closed form—whitehead), papules (pimples), inflammatory pustules, cysts, and occasional scarring

   a. There are three stages of acne

      1) Mild: few to several papules, no nodules, and occurring on the face/neck only

      2) Moderate: several to many papules or pustules and few to several nodules on the face, back, chest, or upper arms

      3) Severe: numerous and/or extensive papules or pustules, many nodules with acne-induced atrophic scarring

   b. Acne involves several factors including increased sebum production, abnormal keratinization of the follicular epithelium, proliferation of propriobacterium acnes, and inflammation

   c. The rate of sebum production is determined genetically; it is increased by the presence of androgens with the earliest changes occurring in the prepubescent years

   d. There are three types of acne: *acne vulgaris* (common adolescent type), *acne conglobata* (causes scarring), and *acne rosacea* (chronic form)

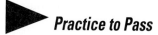

       e. Acne is graded as follows: *Grade 1*—comedonal (open or closed); *Grade 2*—papular with over 25 lesions on the face and trunk; *Grade 3*—pustular with over 25 lesions, mild scarring; and *Grade 4*—nodulocystic, inflammatory nodules, and cysts with extensive scarring

  2. **Lentigo** is a brown macule resembling a freckle except the border is usually regular

       a. There are three types of lentigo: benign lentigo, lentigo maligna, and senile lentigo

       b. *Benign lentigo* may first appear on young children with ultraviolet light exposure and fade in color during the winter months

       c. *Lentigo maligna* is a brown- or black-mottled, irregular bordered, slowly enlarging lesion with an increased number of melanocytes; it is considered pre-malignant in that one-third may progress to a melanoma, usually 10 to 15 years later

       d. *Senile lentigo,* also known as liver spots, occurs on skin exposed to ultraviolet light, especially in older Caucasians

  3. **Psoriasis** is a genetically determined, chronic epidermal proliferative disease that is characterized by erythematous, dry scaling patches and a heavy, silvery surface; there are often recurring remissions and exacerbations

       a. Psoriasis is principally caused by an alteration in cell kinetics of the keratinocytes where the cell cycle is shortened from 311 hours to 36 hours with an increase in epidermal cells

       b. It is often triggered by an infection, most often a streptococcal pharyngitis or a viral upper respiratory infection

       c. There are two types: *Type 1,* which affects the young person who has a strong family history of the disease and is the more aggressive type, and *Type 2,* which affects the older person who generally has no family history of the disease

       d. Type 2 is a more stable type of disease

       e. It is a lifelong process without a cure

  4. **Seborrheic keratosis** is characterized by benign plaques, beige, brown, or maybe black in color, ranging in size from 3 to 20 mm with a velvety or warty surface

       a. Seborrheic keratosis is caused by a proliferation of immature keratinocytes and melanocytes occurring totally within the dermis that is generally seen beginning in middle age

       b. They appear as "stuck on" spots usually present on the face, neck, scalp, back, and upper chest and may bleed when irritated by clothing or picked

C. Nursing assessment

  1. Acne

       a. Assessment

           1) Conduct a symptom analysis regarding onset, type of lesions, and distribution

           2) Inquire about types of cleansers, lubricants/moisturizers, and previous treatments and results

           3) In females, question about flare-ups of acne around menstrual cycle and the use of oral contraceptives

           4) Examine the skin to determine the type of acne (mild, moderate, or severe) and document areas of involvement

           5) Determine the grade of acne present

      b. Diagnostic tests: there are no diagnostic tests for acne; a culture may be taken to differentiate acne from other conditions if pustules are present

  2. Lentigo

      a. Assessment includes symptom analysis regarding onset, location, duration, color changes, and enlargement; ask the client about sun exposure and use of sunscreens

      b. Diagnostic tests: may not require any tests, but a biopsy is suggested for any suspicious lesion

  3. Psoriasis

      a. Assessment includes determining the location, onset, and duration of the plaques; inquire about previous treatments and results obtained; assess for any triggering factors such as emotional stress, trauma, or seasonal changes

      b. Diagnostic tests: skin biopsy may be needed to differentiate psoriasis from other conditions, or ultrasonography to measure skin thickness

  4. Seborrheic keratosis

      a. Assessment includes determining the location, onset, and duration of the plaques; inquire about any changes in the lesion, erythema, or bleeding at the site; assess the client's sun exposure history and any treatments or interventions used in the past

      b. Diagnostic tests: none specific

D. Nursing management

  1. Acne

      a. Medications

          1) Benzoyl peroxide preparations (over-the-counter), which have an antibacterial, keratolytic, and drying effect

          2) Topical solutions such as clindamycin (Cleocin T solution), erythromycin (A/T/S or EryDerm), tetracycline (Topicycline), isotretinoin (Accutane), azelaic acid (Azelex), and tretinoin (Retinoic acid, Vitamin A, Retin-A)

          3) Topical antibiotics may assist in decreasing the formation of new lesions even though it is not an infection

          4) Many of these topical solutions are drying to the skin; a small amount should be tested on a hidden area of the skin first, before applying to the entire face

          5) Most of these agents have the side effect of photosensitivity; sun protection should be used

      b. Management is aimed at controlling the disease and is not curative

      c. Instruct the client to use a mild antibacterial soap, avoid cosmetics containing oil, and confine moisturizing lotions to dry patches of skin only

      d. Instruct client not to pick at lesions, which could cause scarring

      e. Educate the client that improvement may not be seen until treatment is used for 6 to 8 weeks

      f. Dietary factors have not been shown to effect sebum production, but the client should be counseled on a well-balanced diet

  2. Lentigo

      a. Medications include tretinoin (Retinoic acid, Retin-A); however, no meds are necessarily required; cosmetics or bleaching solutions may be preferred by clients

!   **b.** Instruct the client on the ABCD method of assessing skin lesions: asymmetry, border, color, and diameter

    c. Teach the client to inspect the skin regularly and to seek medical advice for any noted changes

!   **d.** Instruct to use layered clothing while in sunlight and to use sunscreens with a sun protection factor (SPF) over 15

3. Psoriasis

!   **a.** Medications include topical corticosteroids and tar preparations to decrease inflammation and suppress mitotic activity of psoriasis, anthralin (Dithranol), and calcipotriene (Dovonex)

    b. Photochemotherapy that involves the drug methoxsalen and exposure to ultraviolet-A (UVA) rays has been effective in severe forms and promoting remission; hyperkeratosis is decreased with exposure to UVA and ultraviolet-B (UVB) light

    c. Aveeno baths, tar shampoos, and wet dressings may help alleviate itching

!   **d.** Instruct the client on the use of moisturizing soaps, emollients, and scalp oils to soften scales followed by soft brushing while bathing

    e. Instruct the client about medication treatments and side effects

    f. Emphasize that the disorder is not contagious

    g. Provide the client the opportunity to discuss feelings regarding the disorders impact on the individual's life

    h. Counsel the client on the importance of maintaining a healthy lifestyle, which includes a well-balanced diet, exercise, moderate alcohol intake, and avoidance of tobacco products

    i. Discuss the role of stress in relation to flare-ups of the lesions

4. Seborrheic keratosis

    a. Medication treatment is usually not required; treatment is at the preference of the client for cosmetic purposes

    b. Educate the client to use sunscreens with a SPF over 15, decrease sun exposure, and avoid tanning; instruct client to wear hats and protective clothing while in the sun

    c. Provide assurance that the lesions are benign in nature

    d. Teach the client the ABCD of skin lesions; assure client that treatment is not necessary unless requested for cosmetic purposes

> **Practice to Pass**
>
> A client has been diagnosed with acne. What self-care strategies should the nurse explain?

IV. BACTERIAL INFECTIONS OF THE SKIN

A. Overview

    1. Defined as a break in the skin integrity and invasion of a pathogenic organism

    2. Disorders include impetigo, cellulitis, folliculitis; other lesions are the furuncle (furunculosis) and carbuncle (carbunculosis)

    3. May be primary (caused by one organism) or secondary (caused by disease process or trauma to the skin)

    4. Causes include poor hygiene, deficient nutrition, skin trauma, and excess moisture to the skin; systemic diseases such as diabetes mellitus and malignancies may contribute to furuncles

B. Pathophysiology

1. **Impetigo** is a superficial skin infection initially seen as an erythemic vesicle and later changes to a honey-colored crusted lesion

   a. It is most commonly seen in 2- to 6-year-olds and may be enhanced by crowded living conditions, poor hygiene, and warm climates

   b. *Staphylococcus aureus* and *Streptococcus pyogenes* (beta-hemolytic) are the most common organisms causing the infection

   c. Impetigo is most often found on the face, arms, legs, and buttocks

   d. Signs and symptoms include extreme itching and red, macular lesions

   e. Impetigo spreads quickly, therefore treatment should be started early

2. **Cellulitis** is a diffuse inflammation of the skin and subcutaneous layers with various presenting lesions including vesicles (small sacs of fluid), bullae (large blisters), abscesses, and plaques

   a. Involved organisms usually are *Streptococcus, Haemophilus influenzae,* or *Staphylococcus aureus* (including methicillan-resistant strain called MRSA)

   b. There is usually a preceding wound or trauma to the skin, even a minor skin scrape, and it is most common in adults

   c. Signs and symptoms include erythema, warmth, edema, and pain; also frequently present are fever, chills, malaise, and lymphadenopathy

3. **Folliculitis** is an inflammation of the hair follicle usually caused by the organism *Staphylococcus aureus* or *Pseudomonas aeruginosa*

   a. It can occur at any age, occurs more in males, and is aggravated by shaving

   b. A stye is a folliculitis on the eyelid

   c. Signs and symptoms include red lesions or erythemic pustules that can be painful

4. **Furuncles (furunculosis):** a furuncle (abscess or boil) is a deep folliculitis consisting of a pus-filled mass that is painful and firm

   a. It is common in children, teens, and young adults

   b. It is caused by *Staphylococcus aureus* (including MRSA), and common sites of infection are the nares, neck, axilla, and genital area

   c. Furunculosis is the condition resulting from multiple boils

   d. Signs and symptoms are deep, firm, red nodules that are painful and usually drain purulent secretions

5. **Carbuncles (carbunculosis)** are aggregates of infected follicles convalesced together to form one large lesion

   a. Carbunculosis is a condition of several carbuncles

   b. Signs and symptoms include painful nodes with pus, chills, fever, and leukocytosis

C. Nursing assessment

1. Assessment includes location, appearance (erythema, swelling, drainage), onset, and duration of lesions; symptom analysis of associated symptoms of fever, chills, and previous outbreaks; vital signs (VS); palpate surface of lesion and adjacent lymph nodes for fluctuance (fluid-filled); assess tetanus prophylaxis status

2. Diagnostic tests: wound culture and sensitivity (C&S) to identify organism and verify antibiotic choice

▶ *Practice to Pass*

A client is being discharged home after hospitalization for cellulitis. What specific discharge instructions should be given?

!▷

D. Nursing management

1. Medications include topical antibiotic ointments or oral antibiotics for 10 to 14 days; instruct on the frequent use of antibacterial soaps for preventive therapy

2. Cleanse the site with warm soapy water 2 to 3 times per day; avoid irritating lotions/creams

3. Use warm compresses for comfort

4. Instruct client to use a clean razor each time he or she shaves

5. Incision and drainage of lesion may be necessary

V. VIRAL INFECTIONS OF THE SKIN

A. Overview

1. Defined as conditions of the skin resulting in a break in the integrity of the skin and the invasion of a virus or intracellular pathogen

2. Disorders include herpes simplex type I (HSV I), type II (HSV II), herpes zoster, molluscum contagiosum, and warts

3. Causes include drugs with immunosuppressive action such as corticosteroids, birth control pills, and antibiotics; stress and sunlight have been attributed to herpes simplex

B. Pathophysiology

1. **Herpes simplex** is a viral infection that occurs within the keratinolytics and is manifested by painful vesicles that occur in clusters on the skin (HSV I), also known as fever blister, or genital mucosa (HSV II)

   a. The virus transverses the afferent nerves to the host ganglion: the trigeminal ganglia are the target of HSV I and usually affect the lips, face, buccal mucosa, and throat

   b. The sacral ganglia is the target for HSV II; it affects the genital area and is considered a sexually transmitted infection (STI)

   c. The herpes simplex virus occurs in three stages: *primary*—initial outbreak of the virus occurs as blisters; *latency*—virus remains dormant in the ganglia; and *recurrent stage*—the virus is reactivated, travels along the peripheral nerves to the site of the initial infection causing characteristic symptoms

   d. Transmission is by direct contact with the active lesions or by virus containing fluid such as saliva or cervical secretions with no evidence of active disease; the incubation period ranges from 2 to 14 days; recurrent infections may be triggered by skin trauma, stress, or illness

!▷   e. Signs and symptoms include erythema, vesicles, discomfort (burning, tingling, or pain), fever, and sore throat; there may be associated tenderness, pain, and burning prior to eruption of the lesions and may be associated with fever, myalgia, malaise, or cervical lymphadenopathy; HSV I infections in infants and children usually appear as a gingivostomatitis with symptoms of pain in the mouth and/or throat and may be accompanied by fever and malaise

2. **Herpes zoster** is a viral infection (also known as shingles) that is manifested as a cluster of vesicles on the skin that usually follows along a dermatome and is unilateral; the vesicles may have purulent fluid in 3 to 4 days, then form crusts that fall off in 2 to 3 weeks

   a. It is a reactivation of the varicella virus in the dorsal root ganglia that remained in the latent form after the primary infection of chickenpox

       b. Signs and symptoms include erythematous lesions, itching, burning, and pain (may be severe); a complication is visual loss and severe pain along one of the nerves; fever, headache, and malaise may precede the rash

       c. It is commonly seen in older adults but can also affect children

  3. **Molluscum contagiosum** is a benign viral infection of the skin characterized by white to flesh-colored, shiny dome-shaped papules with a firm, waxy appearance

       a. It is caused by the poxvirus inducing epidermal cell proliferation; it spreads by direct contact and has an incubation period from 2 to 7 weeks and lasts as long as 6 months

       b. It is a common cutaneous manifestation in human immunodeficiency virus (HIV) infection

       c. Humans are the only known source; the lesions occur in groups and are more common in children and adolescents but may affect all age groups

       d. Signs and symptoms include small, waxy, epithelial tumors that may be solid or semiliquid

  4. **Warts** are virus-induced epidermal tumors and are commonly seen in children and young adults

       a. The wart virus is located within the epidermal layer proliferating from a mass

       b. They are transmitted by touch and often appear on the hands, periungual regions, and plantar surfaces

       c. Most warts resolve in 12 to 24 months without treatment and are asymptomatic except for plantar warts, which may be very painful

       d. There are several types of warts: common (dome-shaped, above the skin, scaly, irregular surface), filiform (thin projections on a narrow stalk usually on the face), flat (flat-topped, skin-colored papules located on the face and extremities), plantar (occur on weight-bearing surfaces of the feet), and genital (considered an STI on glans of penis, anal region, and vulva)

       e. Signs and symptoms include lesions, which are round, raised, rough, and gray; genital warts are cauliflower in appearance

C. Nursing assessment

  1. Herpes simplex virus

       a. Assessment includes identifying the clinical stage of the disease; the primary stage usually occurs 2 to 14 days following inoculation; lesions are usually grouped vesicles that may rupture, leaving erosions that form crusts; the crusts signal the end of the viral shedding; ask about previous occurrences and exposures to infected persons

       b. Diagnostic tests: viral culture for the most definitive diagnosis

  2. Herpes zoster

       a. Assessment includes inquiring about prior varicella infection and immunocompromised status, examining the skin for presence and distribution of characteristic lesions, and determining if there is ophthalmic involvement

       b. Diagnostic tests: Tzanck smear to identify herpes virus, culture of vesicles, and immunofluorescence to identify varicella

3. Molluscum contagiosum

    a. Assessment includes inquiring about location, appearance, onset, and duration of lesion, past medical history including HIV infection, examination of the skin for lesions, and palpating the lesions for firm or fluid-filled consistency

    b. No diagnostic tests are recommended

4. Warts

    a. Assessment includes identifying the type of wart, onset, location, and duration of lesion, and about any previous treatments used

    b. No diagnostic tests are recommended

D. Nursing management

1. Herpes simplex

    a. Medications during the primary stage of HSV I include oral viscous xylocaine, Orabase, use of over-the-counter (OTC) products such as Blistex to prevent drying and acetaminophen (Tylenol) for pain; applying ice may help to reduce the swelling

    b. Medications during the recurrent stage of HSV I or II include topical antiviral agents such as penciclovir (Denavir), which is not recommended for children, or acyclovir (Zovirax) ointment applied every 2 hours to speed healing and relieve pain; oral antivirals, such as acyclovir (Zovirax), valacyclovir (Valtrex), or famciclovir (Famvir), may be used in severe cases or for the immunocompromised client with persistent lesions

    c. Instruct client to use sunscreen as a measure to reduce number of outbreaks

    d. Instruct client about how to decrease the spread of HSV to others

    e. Educate client to avoid sexual activity when active lesions are present and to use condoms with each sexual contact

2. Herpes zoster

    a. Medications include nonsteroidal antiinflammatory drugs (NSAIDs) or acetaminophen (Tylenol) for pain and fever; wet compresses of Burow's solution or tap water may be used for comfort measures; systemic therapy with acyclovir (Zovirax), vidarabine (Vira-A), and corticosteroids are indicated for clients when the outbreak is less than 72 hours old or when over 72 hours old with newly developing lesions, when clients are over age 50, and for immunocompromised clients

    b. Suppression of pain, inflammation, and infection is the goal of therapy

    c. Teach client about the possibility of post-herpetic pain (pain that persists more than one month after lesions have healed)

    d. Instruct on signs and symptoms of secondary bacterial infections, usually caused from scratching the lesions, which are itchy

    e. Ophthalmic involvement requires emergency referral to an ophthamologist

    f. Instruct to avoid clients who may be at risk for infection; such as neonates, pregnant women, and immunosuppressed persons, as well as those who have not previously had chickenpox

    g. Stress that follow-up in 1 to 3 days and then again in 7 to 10 days is necessary

    h. Educate the client about the disease and measures to maintain health

    i. Inform the client that scarring at the site of the infection may occur

3. Molluscum contagiosum

    a. Medications include liquid nitrogen therapy (client preference), and Duofilm or tretinoin (Retin-A, Avita) for removal of the lesions

    b. Instruct the client that these medications are to be used at bedtime; the area should be exfoliated before reapplication and petroleum jelly applied to the surrounding skin

    c. For a small number of asymptomatic lesions of molluscum contagiosum, observation for several months is indicated

4. Warts

    a. Medications include liquid nitrogen and topical preparations (acid therapy) to be used nightly for 6 to 8 weeks; instruct to apply petroleum ointment on surrounding skin to prevent irritation; OTC products for freezing warts are now available

    b. Most clients request treatment/removal of the wart lesion; the filiform wart is usually removed by curettage, cryotherapy, or electrodessication

    c. Instruct the client about signs and symptoms of infection after removal and pain relief measures if applicable

    d. Educate the client that warts (because they are viral) may reappear in the same site or on other areas of the skin

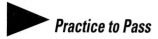

Practice to Pass

A client has been diagnosed with herpes simplex type II (HSV II). What explanation should be given about this disease?

VI. FUNGAL INFECTIONS OF THE SKIN

A. Overview

1. Defined as infections caused by fungi (dermatophytes), which are living organisms found on the stratum corneum, hair, and nails

2. Include candidiasis, tinea versicolor, and dermatophyte infections are named for the area of the body involved, including tinea capitis, tinea corporis, tinea cruris, tinea pedis, and tinea unguium

3. Causes include excess moisture, contact with an infected person or animal, use of broad-spectrum antibiotics, disorders such as diabetes mellitus, malnutrition, iron deficiency anemia, immunosuppressed states, pregnancy, and aging process

B. Pathophysiology

1. **Candidiasis** is an infection caused by *Candida albicans,* a yeast-like fungus that most often causes superficial cutaneous infections

    a. *Candida albicans* fungi are part of the normal flora of the skin and mucous membranes; overgrowth is caused when conditions such as moisture, warmth, and breaks in the epidermal barrier occur

    b. Includes oral (thrush), vagina (vulvovaginitis), diaper area (perineal), glans and prepuce of the penis (balantitis), nail folds (paronychia), perineal area, the axilla, umbilical area, and under the breasts

    c. Candida organisms may also be a causative agent in otitis externa and scalp disorders

    d. The fungus needs a host and certain conditions in order to become pathogenic, such as a depressed immune state, debilitation, poor nutrition, moisture, use of antibiotics or steroids (see causes)

    e. Signs and symptoms include lesions that are bright red, smooth macules with a macerated appearance and a scaling, elevated border

> **f.** Characteristic "satellite" lesions are small, similar-appearing macules outside the main lesion; specific areas of the body manifest as:
> > **1)** Oral thrush: white, milky, nonremovable plaques on the oral mucosa that may be associated with a burning sensation or decreased taste
> > **2)** Vagina (vulvovaginitis): excessive itching and a thick, white, curdy vaginal discharge
> > **3)** Perineal area (or diaper in an infant or young toddler): erythema, papules, pustules, and a scaling border
> > **4)** Balanitis: flattened pustules, edema, scaling, erosion, burning, and tenderness on the penis
> > **5)** Paronychia: erythema, edema and tenderness with possible creamy, purulent discharge with pressure on the nail bed; the nails usually become discolored and have ridging

  2. Tinea versicolor is a common noninflammatory fungal infection caused by lipophilic yeast and *Pityrosporum orbiculare,* which is part of the normal flora of the skin

    a. Overgrowth occurs for unknown reasons and the infection is not contagious

    b. Signs and symptoms include multiple small, circular macules of various colors (white, pink, or brown) usually on the upper trunk, which are usually asymptomatic

  3. Dermatophyte infections are caused by a group of fungi that have the ability to infect and survive only on keratin; they can affect all age groups

    a. These infections include tinea capitis (ringworm of the scalp), tinea corporis (ringworm of the body), tinea cruris (ringworm of the groin and upper thighs), tinea pedis (ringworm of the foot or athlete's foot), and tinea unguium (ringworm of the nails or onychomycosis)

    b. Dermatophyte infections (tineas) have three causative agents: *Microsporum, Trichophyton,* or *Epidermophyton*

    c. Signs and symptoms
> **1)** Tinea capitis: erythema and scaling of the scalp with patchy hair loss
> **2)** Tinea corporis: lesions are generally circular, erythematous, well-marginated with a raised, scaly vesicular border
> **3)** Tinea cruris: lesions are sharply demarcated, scaling patches and usually extremely pruritic
> **4)** Tinea pedis: lesions are fine, vesiculopustular, or scaly areas that are usually itchy
> **5)** Tinea unguium: usually involves only 1 to 2 nails; toenails are affected more often than fingernails; characteristic features include distal thickening and yellowing of the nail plate

C. Nursing assessment

  1. Assessment

    a. Symptom analysis about onset, duration, distribution, and presence of symptoms

    b. Possible contact with others (including animals) with similar lesions

    c. Previous treatments used and results

    d. Any underlying chronic conditions and past or present medications

    e. Examination of skin to determine type and distribution of lesions and associated symptoms

2. Diagnostic tests: a culture of scraping (skin, hair, or nails) or microscopic examination of scaling using a 10% potassium hydrogen (KOH) preparation; a Wood's lamp, which uses ultraviolet (UV) light; area fluoresces blue-green in the presence of a fungal infection

D. Nursing management

1. Medications

   a. Antifungals that are available in various forms (creams, powders, shampoos, vaginal suppositories, and oral tablets) containing the following drugs: clotrimazole (Mycelex), nystatin (Mycostatin, Nilstat), miconazole (Monistat), undecylenic acid (Desenex), ketoconazole (Nizoral), fluconazole (Diflucan), and amphotericin B (Fungizone)

   b. Topical treatment is preferred, but some cases require oral medications such as miconazole (Monistat), nystatin (Nilstat), ketoconazole (Nizoral), and fluconazole (Diflucan)

   c. Systemic therapy is necessary for moderate to severe infection that occurs in immunocompromised persons

2. Instruct clients to avoid sharing linens or personal items

3. Instruct clients to dry all skin folds and use a clean towel and washcloth daily

4. For tinea pedis, put socks on before underwear to prevent spread of infection from feet; wear light cotton socks and change frequently; wear sandals or open-toed shoes when possible but avoid plastic footwear and occlusive shoes

5. Apply drying or dusting powders and topical antiperspirants to decrease moisture

6. For vaginal candida, avoid tight clothing and pantyhose, bathe frequently and dry genital area thoroughly; treatment of the sexual partner may be necessary to avoid reinfection or have partner use condoms until resolved; avoid douching and change perineal pads frequently

7. Reducing the risk of fungal infections can occur with weight loss by obese clients and maintenance of normal serum glucose levels in diabetic clients to decrease risk of infection

8. Instruct clients that relief of symptoms may occur quickly with topical medication but stress the need to use topical applications for 7 to 10 days

9. Follow-up visits should be scheduled every 2 to 4 weeks for clients receiving long-term oral antifungal treatment to monitor liver function profile and complete blood count (CBC)

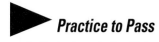

Practice to Pass

A client returns to the clinic with recurrent tinea pedis. What should the client be told regarding preventive measures?

VII. INFESTATIONS AND INSECT BITES

A. Overview

1. Defined as an invasion of the skin by an insect or parasite

2. Disorders include common insect bites (stings) and pediculosis

3. Causes include living in infested areas and contact with an infected person or clothing/material

B. Pathophysiology

1. An insect sting or bite occurs when there is secretion of venom into the skin by an insect or spider; arthropods affect many by being pests, inoculating poison, invading tissues, or transmitting disease

    a. Honeybees, wasps, hornets, and yellow-jackets embed a firm, sharp stinger in the skin that injects venom, a protein with enzyme activity that causes local or general reactions classified as toxic or allergic (0.4% of reactions are allergic)

    b. There are many species of spiders, but the brown recluse spider and the black widow are the two species capable of producing severe reactions

        1) The brown recluse spider is small, light brown, and lives in dark areas such as closets, basements, and under porches; the bite can cause local or general reactions, even death; the venom is equivalent to that of a rattlesnake

        2) The black widow bite resembles a pinprick, injecting a neurotoxin that causes an ascending motor paralysis; the potent toxin is rapidly absorbed, causing necrosis at the site

    c. IgE-mediated hypersensitivity to the insect venom may be confirmed by skin testing with suitable dilutions of available venom—usually done by an allergist

    d. Signs and symptoms

        1) Brown recluse spider: a large area of necrosis at the site, pain, itching and swelling; after a week, the area has extreme swelling with a raised white or black center (volcano appearing)

        2) Black widow spider: pain at the site, which lasts only briefly, rigid abdominal muscles with extreme abdominal pain, and motor paralysis

        3) General reactions to insect bites: redness, itching, swelling, warmth, and extreme pain

        4) Systemic symptoms such as fever, chills, nausea, vomiting, and weakness may occur

        5) Anaphylactic reactions such as shortness of breath and wheezing may appear if the client is allergic to the sting

2. Pediculosis is an infestation of the skin or hair by the species of blood-sucking lice capable of living as external parasites on the human host

    a. Pediculosis capitis is the head louse, the size of a sesame seed ranging in color from clear to red/brown

    b. Pediculosis pubis ("crabs") infests the genital area and is one of the most common sexually transmitted diseases; pubic lice can be spread by sexual contact

    c. Head lice are common among schoolchildren of all socioeconomic backgrounds and are spread by close contact as well as sharing combs, hats, and scarves

    d. *Scabies* is the infestation of the skin by the mite Sarcoptes scabier hominis

        1) In scabies, the fertilized female mite burrows into the skin and remains there, laying 2 to 3 eggs per day

        2) The eggs hatch in 3–4 days, reach maturity in 4 days, migrate to the skin surface, mate, and repeat the cycle

        3) Scabies is more common among people who don't have access to bathing or laundry facilities; lice can live in clothing and be transmitted also by contact with infected clothing or bed linens

    e. Signs and symptoms

        1) Pediculosis corporis: macules, wheals, and papules, pruritus, excoriation from scratching; lines in the skin folds are common, representing the burrowing of the mite; the lesions may be erythematous papules or purplish nodules accompanied by raised burrows (thread-like linear ridges with a tiny black dot at one end)

2) Pediculosis pubis: pruritus, irritation of genital area, and blue- or slate-colored macules

3) Pediculosis capitis: itching, eczematous dermatitis, inflammation caused by scratching, pustules, crusts, matted, odorous hair

C. Nursing assessment

1. Insect stings and bites

  a. Assessment includes symptom analysis regarding type of bite or sting, when it occurred, and location of bite or sting; assess for anaphylactic reactions and refer for immediate treatment; assess the site for symptoms specific to the type of bite

  b. Diagnostic tests: there are no tests indicated unless a severe allergic reaction is noted; a CBC and IgE may be performed if necessary

2. Pediculosis

  a. Assessment

    1) Questions about intense pruritis—the most common symptom in pediculosis

    2) Appearance: head lice may resemble dandruff flakes; however, they are not easily brushed off because nits cling to hair shafts

    3) A papular urticaria, which may be present at the neck or pubic area

    4) Severity of itching: nocturnal itching, which is a classic symptom of scabies, as well as itching during exposure to hot water or steam

    5) Inquire about onset of symptoms; client becomes itchy approximately 10 to 14 days after exposure

  b. Diagnostic tests: skin scraping of the scabies nodule may be recommended to reveal portions of the mite but clinical diagnosis is usually made by presentation

D. Nursing management

1. Insect stings and bites

  a. Medications include local analgesics such as ibuprofen and antihistamines such as diphenhydramine (Benadryl) that are used for mild reactions; epinephrine 1:1000 or an Epi–pen may be used for mild symptoms also

  b. Outpatient or inpatient treatment for stings and bites depends on the individual response

    1) First aid treatment may include removal of the stinger by scraping; do not squeeze or use a tweezer; then clean the wound

    2) Apply ice packs to the bite, 10 minutes on/10 minutes off

    3) Elevate the affected part, maintain adequate airway, and transport to emergency facility if warranted

    4) The wound from a brown recluse spider should not be opened but cleansed daily and allowed to erupt on its own

  c. If the history suggests a severe anaphylactic reaction, initiate emergency treatment immediately and transport to the local emergency department; if the client is stable, assess the client's vital signs and examine the site for erythema and edema

  d. Educate the client to prevent re-exposure and about the risks of increasing severity of responses in the future

  e. Instruct the client to use insect repellants when outdoors or in infected areas

  f. For clients allergic to insect bites, an Epi-pen should be available at all times; educate on its proper use if prescribed

    g. Client may need referral for allergy testing if a mild to severe anaphylactic reaction occurs

    h. For sensitive individuals, a medical alert tag should be obtained and worn at all times

2. Pediculosis

    a. Medications to kill the nits include lindane (Kwell), which comes in a lotion or shampoo; gamma benzene hexachloride, malathion (Prioderm lotion) or permithrin (NIX), corticosteroids for itching, and antibiotics as needed for infections

    b. Nits on the hair must be mechanically removed

    c. Instruct the client as to the proper way to treat the condition; some medications such as NIX take only one treatment, while others (Lindane) take two treatments, 7 days apart, in order to kill the eggs; advise that olive oil or a solution of 50 parts white vinegar to 50 parts water may loosen nits

    d. Educate clients about mode of transmission (person to person) and preventive measures such as not sharing personal items

    e. Instruct the client/family to machine wash all washable clothing and dry in a hot dryer at least 20 minutes; upholstered furniture, pillows, and stuffed animals may be ironed with a hot iron or vacuumed

    f. Stress importance that all family members must be treated at the same time

VIII. ALLERGIC CONDITIONS OF THE SKIN

A. Overview

1. Allergic conditions are those that cause inflammation (dermatitis) as a result of contact with an allergen, infection, or disease; these can be acute or chronic

2. Disorders include contact dermatitis, atopic dermatitis, seborrheic dermatitis, exfoliative dermatitis, and urticaria

3. Causes include plants such as poison oak, poison sumac, or poison ivy; harsh chemicals; dyes; perfumes; latex gloves; metals; insecticides; soaps; detergents; foods; drugs such as methyldopa for hypertension, diseases such as AIDS, leukemia, and lymphoma; transfusion reactions; insect bites or stings; heat; cold; stress; sunlight; and serum sickness

B. Pathophysiology

1. **Contact dermatitis** is an eruption of the skin related to contact with an irritating substance or allergen (see Box 14-2)

    a. *Irritant contact dermatitis* affects individuals exposed to specific irritants producing an immediate response

    b. *Allergic contact dermatitis* is an allergic reaction mediated by IgE and affects only individuals previously sensitized to the irritant, thus it is a delayed hypersensitivity reaction; a sensitizing antigen is formed on initial contact, which is taken to the T cells; these T cells become sensitized and this creates the initial sensitizing effect; upon subsequent exposures, skin reactions will occur (see Figure 14-1)

    c. The location of the rash helps provide clues about the offending agent

    d. Signs and symptoms include acute contact dermatitis and presents as papules, vesicles, bullae with surrounding erythema; crusting, oozing, and pruritis may

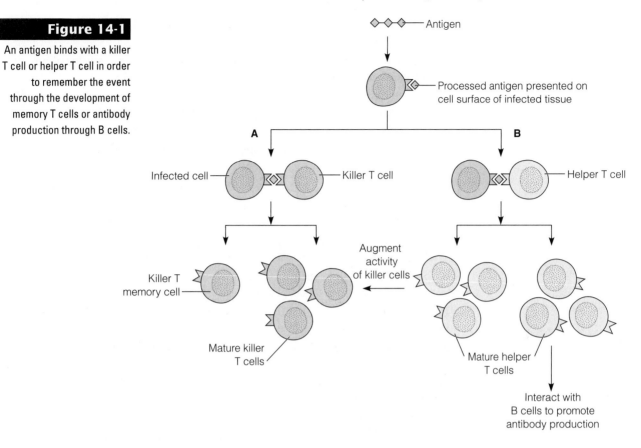

Figure 14-1

An antigen binds with a killer T cell or helper T cell in order to remember the event through the development of memory T cells or antibody production through B cells.

Box 14-2

Common Causes of Contact Dermatitis

➤ Acids

➤ Alkalis: soaps, detergents, household ammonia, lye, cleaners

➤ Bromide

➤ Chlorine

➤ Coloring agents

➤ Cosmetics: perfumes, dyes, oils

➤ Dusts of lime, arsenic, wood

➤ Hydrocarbons: crude petroleum, lubricating oil, mineral oil, paraffin, asphalt, tar

➤ Iodine

➤ Insecticides

➤ Fabrics: wool, polyester, dyes, sizing

➤ Metal salts: calcium chloride, zinc chloride, copper, mercury, nickel, silver

➤ Plants: ragweed, poison oak, poison ivy, poison sumac, pine

➤ Rubber products

➤ Soot

Source: LeMone, P., & Burke, K. (2004). *Medical-surgical nursing: Critical thinking in client care* (3rd ed.). Upper Saddle River, NJ: Prentice Hall, p. 380.

be present; chronic contact dermatitis may present with an erythematous base, thickening of the skin, scaling, and fissuring

2. **Atopic dermatitis** (eczema) is a common inflammatory skin disorder of unknown cause and is seen frequently with children and adults
   a. Although the cause is unknown, a cell-mediated immunity, excess sensitivity to histamine, and increased levels of IgE are related to the disorder
   b. The condition has allergic, heredity, and/or psychological components
   c. The initiation of the immune response triggers an inflammatory reaction
   d. A complication is secondary infection
   e. Signs and symptoms include erythema, scaling, pruritis, and lesions on the hands, feet, arms, and legs

3. **Seborrheic dermatitis** is an acute inflammatory condition with an unknown cause
   a. It affects the scalp (cradle cap), forehead, postauricular regions, eyebrows, eyelashes, nasolabial folds, axillary, and genital areas; all ages can be affected
   b. Signs and symptoms include yellow or white plaques that may scale, crusts with a greasy appearance, pruritus, oozing, and loss of hair

4. **Exfoliative dermatitis** is an inflammation of the skin characterized by erythema involving loss of exfoliated (peeling) skin
   a. Local and systemic effects may occur and have either an unknown cause or may be associated with other diseases or causes
   b. A complication of the generalized form is debilitation, dehydration, and secondary infection
   c. Signs and symptoms
      1) Local effects: scaling, erythema, pruritus, loss of hair and nails
      2) Systemic effects: weakness, malaise, hypothermia or fever, lymphadenopathy, hepatomegaly, eosinophilia, and depression

5. **Urticaria** (hives) is described as an itchy rash that may be recurrent
   a. *Acute urticaria* usually subsides over several hours; examples include solar urticaria (exposure to sun), delayed pressure urticaria (produced by pressure, occurs after delay of 1 to 4 hours), aquagenic urticaria (ordinary water), and occurs because of an allergic reaction
   b. *Chronic urticaria* persists over 6 weeks; examples include cold urticaria (from cooling to rewarming), cholinergic urticaria (heat urticaria), and induced urticaria (extreme exercise)
   c. Urticaria is caused by a massive release from mast cells in the superficial layers of the skin and is a vascular reaction of the skin
   d. True urticaria lesions do not remain in the same area over 24 hours; if present longer than 72 hours, cutaneous vasculitis must be considered a possible cause
   e. Signs and symptoms include single or multiple areas of raised, blanched central wheals surrounded by a red flare that is highly pruritic; it may occur anywhere on the body with size ranging from 1–2 mm to 15–20 cm

C. Nursing assessment
   1. Assessment for dermatitis conditions
      a. A symptom analysis regarding location, duration, and associated symptoms
      b. Ask about occupation or recreational activities
      c. Review exposures to any irritants or allergens and previous treatments
      d. Examine the skin to determine location and distribution

    2. Assessment for urticaria includes a symptom analysis of the onset, duration, and possible causes and skin examination to determine distribution

    3. Diagnostic test: scratch or intradermal tests for allergy testing, IgE level, eosinophil level, and skin biopsy for diagnostic purposes

D. Nursing management

    1. Contact/irritant dermatitis

        a. Medications include aluminum acetate for drying, antihistamines or calamine lotion for pruritus, cortisone if needed, and topical emollients

        b. The first step in managing contact/irritant dermatitis is to identify and remove the causative agent

        c. Wet dressings and oatmeal baths may aid in alleviating oozing and pruritic lesions

        d. Instruct the client on signs and symptoms of secondary bacterial infections

    2. Atopic dermatitis

        a. Medications include antihistamines, softening lotions, cortisone lotion, and oral antibiotics if needed

        b. Instruct client to avoid soaps and ointment, keep bathing to a minimum; bath oils may help soften skin

        c. Clothing should be of a soft texture and wool should be avoided

        d. Clip fingernails to decrease damage while scratching

    3. Seborrheic dermatitis

        a. Medications include selenium containing shampoos, keratolytic agents, topical and systemic cortisone lotions

        b. Frequent shampooing is suggested if on the scalp

        c. Scrupulous skin hygiene and keeping the skin dry is imperative

    4. Exfoliative dermatitis

        a. Medications include corticosteroids, emollients, and antihistamines

        b. Treatment is the same as contact dermatitis

    5. Urticaria

        a. Medications include antihistamines to reduce itching and prevent prolonged symptoms; corticosteroids may be used for pressure urticaria and topical sunscreens are recommended for solar urticaria

        b. If urticaria occurred as a result of an allergic reaction, stress that possible life-threatening reactions may occur on reexposure

        c. Recommend cool moist compresses to help control itching, increasing fluids and use of skin lubricants, and avoidance of harsh soaps, frequent bathing, and products with alcohol

        d. Referrals to an allergist or dermatologist should be considered for unresolved itching

IX. BURNS

A. Overview

    1. **Burns** are defined as interruptions in skin integrity resulting in tissue loss or injury caused by heat, chemicals, electricity, or radiation

2. A superficial thickness burn (first degree) involves a minimal depth of the skin and is limited to the outer skin layer (epidermis)

3. Superficial and deep partial thickness burns (second degree) involves damage extending through the epidermis and into dermis; regeneration of the epidermis is not impaired

4. A full thickness burn (third degree) involves the epidermis and dermis with damage into the underlying tissue

5. Causes include thermal, chemical, electrical, and radiation

    a. *Thermal burns* are the result of dry heat (flames) or moist heat (steam or hot liquids) and are the most common type of burn; they cause cellular destruction that results in vascular, bony, muscle, or nerve complications

    b. *Chemical burns* are caused by direct contact with either acidic or alkaline agents; they destroy tissue perfusion, leading to necrosis

    c. *Electrical burns* follow the path of least resistance (muscles-bones-blood vessels-nerves); the severity of the burn depends on the type and duration of current and amount of voltage; electrical burns include sources such as direct current, alternating current, and lightning

    d. A *radiation burn* is usually associated with sunburn or radiation treatment for cancer; it is usually superficial; extensive exposure may lead to tissue damage and multisystem involvement

B. Pathophysiology

1. A burn from any source is a major insult to the entire body, interrupting skin integrity (which could lead to infection) as well as causing many systemic effects

2. Within several hours, capillary integrity is lost due to the release of several mediators of inflammation, primarily histamine and prostaglandin, which are vasodilators

3. Fluid passes from the intravascular system (causing hypotension) to the interstitial system (causing massive edema)

4. This fluid begins to shift back within 24 to 48 hours and intravascular overload then becomes a concern

5. The loss of intravascular volume causes an increased blood viscosity (with a risk for clots), decreased cardiac output (possibly leading to shock or pulmonary congestion), decreased renal blood flow (causing hypoxia and decreased urinary output), and renin-angiotension-aldosterone (RAA) system activation to increase volume, which leads to retention of sodium and water and further edema

6. Cells cannot maintain adequate electrolyte shifts and results in the following: excess sodium intracellularly, excess potassium extracellularly; these effects as well as shifts in magnesium and phosphorus can lead to cardiac dysrhythmias and altered central nervous system function

7. Cortisol is released because of the stress and depresses the immune system, which intensifies the risk for infection

8. The sympathetic nervous system is activated, along with the stress factor, increasing metabolic rate and oxygen demands; this hypermetabolism, the increased energy needed for healing, and the release of cortisol and epinephrine lead to a breakdown of tissue, protein metabolism, and fat wasting

9. Glucose is released as a result of the stress and causes hyperglycemia

	System	Major Complication
Table 14-1		
Complications of Burns	Immune	Infection with *Staphylococcus aureus* or methicillin resistant *staphylococcus aureus* (MRSA), septic shock
	Cardiovascular	Blood clots leading to stroke or myocardial infarction, heart failure, cardiac arrest, pulmonary edema
	Gastrointestinal	Peptic ulcer (decreased blood flow to gut), impaction
	Respiratory	Acute respiratory distress syndrome (ARDS), lung damage if inhalation, hypoxia
	Hematological	Burn shock, disseminated intravascular coagulopathy (DIC), anemia
	Renal	Oliguria, renal failure
	Fluids and electrolytes	First 24 to 48 hours: hyponatremia, hypokalemia, hypoproteinemia, hypochloremia
		After 24 to 48 hours: hypernatremia, hyperkalemia, hypovolemic shock, and dehydration

10. Complications are numerous (see Table 14-1)

11. Signs and symptoms

    a. Superficial thickness burn: erythema of the tissue; the skin may be tender and blanches under pressure

    b. Partial thickness burn: the skin is red and blistered and very tender or painful; appearance may vary depending on whether burn is superficial partial thickness or deep partial thickness; the deeper the burn, the more it begins to resemble full thickness

    c. Full thickness burn: skin is tough and leathery but not tender; may also appear waxy or pearly white

C. Nursing assessment

    1. Assessment

        a. A symptom analysis of the cause of the burn, time occurred, past medical history, and present medications and allergies

        b. Overall general appearance for distress and amount of pain

        c. Depth of the burn

        d. Extent of the burn (% total body surface area or TBSA) using the Rule of Nines (see Figure 14-2)

        e. Cardiac status, respiratory status, airway patency, and hydration status; airway status is essential whenever the burn has the capability of compromising the airway because of edema (note singed eyebrows, nasal hair, or eyelashes; note soot; edema will peak 24 to 48 hours post–injury)

        f. Keep in mind possibilities of abuse and neglect; inquire about past injuries and burns

    2. Diagnostic tests: Rule of Nines to estimate burn size; blood urea nitrogen (BUN), creatinine clearance, urine output, urinalysis to avoid shock; CBC, electrolytes, albumin, bilirubin, alkaline phosphatase, arterial blood gases (ABGs), type and crossmatch (TXM), chest x-ray (CXR), electrocardiogram (ECG); C & S (if indicated); pulmonary function tests

D. Nursing management

    1. Medications include opioid and/or nonopioid analgesics for pain, sedatives, tetanus (if not current), antibiotics, antacids or H_2 receptor blockers, topical antimicrobials such as silver nitrate, silver sulfadiazine, polysporin, etc.

Figure 14-2 The "Rule of Nines" is a method of quickly estimating the percentage of total body surface area of the burn injury.

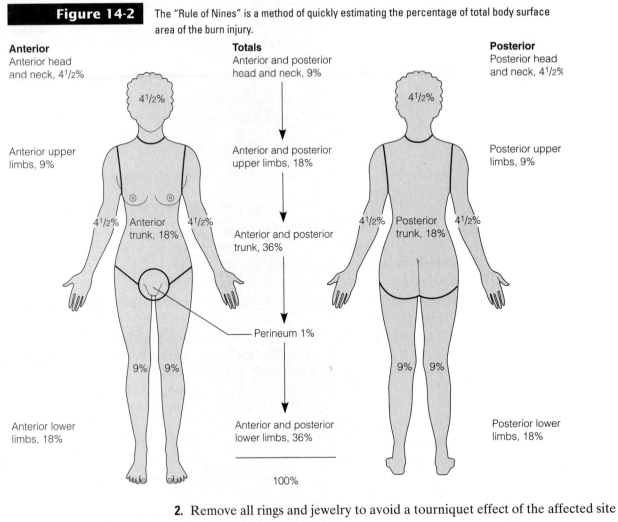

Anterior
Anterior head and neck, 4¹/2%

Anterior upper limbs, 9%

Anterior trunk, 18%

4¹/2% 4¹/2%

9% 9%

Anterior lower limbs, 18%

Totals
Anterior and posterior head and neck, 9%

Anterior and posterior upper limbs, 18%

Anterior and posterior trunk, 36%

Perineum 1%

Anterior and posterior lower limbs, 36%

100%

Posterior
Posterior head and neck, 4¹/2%

Posterior upper limbs, 9%

Posterior trunk, 18%

4¹/2% 4¹/2%

9% 9%

Posterior lower limbs, 18%

2. Remove all rings and jewelry to avoid a tourniquet effect of the affected site

3. Flush a chemical burn copiously with water and apply cool compresses; remove affected clothing and cover the area with a dry sheet

4. Administer oxygen if necessary for any type of burn

5. Maintain proper hydration and encourage high-protein, high-calorie diet; monitor intake and output (I&O)

6. For superficial thickness burns, topical anesthetic creams or spray may be used several times a day to relieve pain and no dressings are needed

7. For partial thickness burns, leave blisters intact

8. Small burns may be covered with antibiotic ointment and a nonadherent dressing to absorb drainage

9. For larger burns, cover the area with silver sulfadiazine 1% as prescribed, and apply a nonadherent dressing covered by a bulky dressing to absorb any drainage

10. Full thickness burns will not heal on their own and require skin grafting

11. Use meticulous sterile technique (and possibly protective isolation) to decrease the risk of infection

12. Monitor pain management needs and treat pain before debriding episodes and around the clock if needed

13. Administer tetanus toxoid if tetanus prophylaxis is not up to date

14. Educate the client on use of sunscreens, accessing electrical cords/outlets, isolating household chemicals, use of low temperature setting for hot water heater, use and proper maintenance of household smoke detectors, risks of smoking in bed, and proper storage and use of flammable substances

15. Instruct the client and family regarding care of the burn at home, and signs and symptoms of infection

16. Evaluate need for counseling and family support, physical, vocational, or occupational rehabilitation

17. Encourage the client to verbalize feelings of despair or depression if disfigurement has occurred

Case Study

The client is an 80-year-old female who has noticed a blistery rash on her abdomen for the past several days. The health care provider informs her that she has herpes zoster.

1. What history should the nurse obtain from the client?

2. What assessment should the nurse perform?

3. How should the nurse explain the disease?

4. What medication instructions are necessary?

5. What home instructions should be given to the client regarding her disease?

For suggested responses, see pages 537–538.

POSTTEST

1 A 19-year-old female has been complaining for several days of severe itching under her waistband and in her axillae. She thinks she has been bitten by something because she can feel a line of small bumps at the sites. The nurse suspects which of the following conditions based on this assessment data?

1. Insect bites
2. Herpes zoster
3. Scabies
4. Pediculosis capitis

2 A 23-year-old male presents with a pustular inflammation of his anterior neck and under his chin. Which of the following would the nurse recommend as an important management strategy?

1. Squeeze the pustules periodically
2. Keep the area moist
3. Changing razors each time he shaves
4. Decrease fat in the diet

3 A client asks the nurse in the dermatologist's office about what characteristics folliculitis, furunculosis, and carbunculosis all have in common. The nurse replies that all three disorders are:

1. Viral infections involving the epidermal layer of the skin.
2. Fungal infections caused by poor hygiene.
3. Bacterial infections that are highly contagious.
4. Bacterial infections involving the hair follicles.

4 A 2-year-old child developed crusted lesions on her chin within the past three days. They started as a single blister that broke, discharging a honey-colored liquid that became a "stuck-on" crust. New blisters and crusts have been forming in the adjacent skin area. The nurse determines that this clinical picture is consistent with which of the following?

1. Impetigo
2. Scabies
3. Herpes simplex
4. Contact dermatitis

5 The nurse would include which of the following in the nursing management and teaching of the client with psoriasis? Select all that apply.

1. Emphasize that the disease cannot be transmitted by skin-to-skin contact
2. Emphasize the importance of keeping the areas dry
3. Medications can be tried but none bring about any improvement
4. Topical emollients, coal tar products, and corticosteroids soften and help remove the plaques
5. There is no cure for psoriasis; goal of treatment is to suppress the symptoms

6 A client presents to the clinic with thick, silver-white scaly patches over reddened skin. The client expresses fear of skin cancer since it appears as skin sores that do not heal. The nurse's response best response to the client is:

1. "You can stop worrying right away. You just have psoriasis."
2. "You do not have cancer. You have herpes zoster, also called shingles, which can be treated with medications."
3. "Impetigo can look like that. Try to manage your anxiety until the biopsy and cultures confirm a diagnosis."
4. "It looks more like psoriasis. What do you know about psoriasis?"

7 The nurse is staffing a booth on skin assessment at a community health fair and has provided a handout with the ABCD acronym for early diagnosis of malignant melanoma. The nurse concludes that an attendee is not reading the handout correctly after the attendee states which acronym?

1. A — Area of sun-exposed skin — check the face, hands, arms, and back
2. B — Border irregular — not round
3. C — Color variegated — black and brown
4. D — Diameter greater than 6 mm — ¼ inch

8 A man sustained burns to the arms and chest when a fire got out of control in a campground. A fellow nurse camper immediately removes jewelry from the affected burn site to accomplish which priority objective?

1. Be able to assess the fingers more accurately
2. Prevent a tourniquet effect at the site
3. Prevent infection
4. Avoid interference with first aid treatment of the burn

9 The nurse working at a summer camp on a hot, humid day notes that a group of 9- and 10-year-old children are playing a baseball game. The nurse determines that the children are at immediate risk for dehydration and which of the following conditions?

1. Skin cancer
2. Formation of nevi
3. Full thickness skin burns
4. Superficial thickness skin burns

10 When evaluating a client with a new pigmented skin lesion, the nurse would place highest priority on asking the client about which of the following?

1. Whether any new foods have been introduced into the diet
2. What cosmetics or skin products are being used
3. Sun tanning habits
4. History of food or environmental allergies

➤ *See pages 432–433 for Answers & Rationales.*

ANSWERS & RATIONALES

Pretest

1 **Answer: 1** Emollients will ease the problem of dry skin that increases pruritus and causes the psoriasis to be worse. Washing and drying the skin with rough linens or pressure may cause excoriation. Constant occlusion may increase the effects of the medication and increase the risk of infection.

Cognitive Level: Application **Client Need:** Health Promotion and Maintenance **Integrated Process:** Nursing Process: Implementation **Content Area:** Adult Health: Integumentary **Strategy:** This is not a life threatening problem needing close medical supervision. Choose the option that best strengthens the self care – what the question is asking. **Reference:** Porth, C. M. (2005). *Pathophysiology: Concepts* *of altered health states* (7th ed.). Philadelphia, PA: Lippincott Williams & Wilkins, p. 1473.

2 **Answer: 2** In order to plan the appropriate management of contact/irritant dermatitis, the cause of the inflammation should be identified. Removal of the cause may be all the treatment needed. Antihistamines and hydrocortisone creams are treatment options. Skin testing may be helpful to determine the allergen if not evident in the history.
Cognitive Level: Application **Client Need:** Physiological Integrity: Physiological Adaptation **Integrated Process:** Teaching/Learning **Content Area:** Adult Health: Integumentary **Strategy:** The critical word in the question is *first step*. This is an allergic condition and the problem is contact with the skin. The answer is almost common sense. **Reference:** LeMone, P., & Burke, K. (2008). *Medical-surgical nursing: Critical thinking in client care* (4th ed.). Upper Saddle River, NJ: Pearson/Prentice Hall, p. 339.

3 **Answer: 2** Lice are transmitted by direct contact with infested persons or by sharing hats, brushes, or combs of infected persons. Classrooms are excellent areas for close contact, and children often do not know when other classmates have lice. Options 1, 3, and 4 are factually inaccurate statements.
Cognitive Level: Application **Client Need:** Safe, Effective Care Environment: Safety and Infection Control **Integrated Process:** Nursing Process: Assessment **Content Area:** Adult Health: Integumentary **Strategy:** Apply knowledge of the spread and incidence of pediculosis by recalling that direct contact is needed or through fomites such as inanimate objects. **Reference:** LeMone, P., & Burke, K. (2008). *Medical-surgical nursing: Critical thinking in client care* (4th ed.). Upper Saddle River, NJ: Pearson/Prentice Hall, p. 451.

4 **Answer: 1** Melanoma is more common in fair-skinned persons who work indoors and have sun exposure on weekends and vacations. Severe blistering sunburn as a child and intermittent sun exposure increases the susceptibility as adults. Sun exposure is a significant risk, but other risk factors such as atypical moles, immunosuppression, and tanning salons contribute to the problem. Episodic intense sun exposure is more damaging than constant exposure.
Cognitive Level: Application **Client Need:** Health Promotion and Maintenance **Integrated Process:** Teaching/Learning **Content Area:** Adult Health: Integumentary **Strategy:** The choices are between light- and dark-skinned persons and regular or intermittent sun exposure. With options that contain two or more parts, both parts must be correct for the answer to be right. **Reference:** Porth, C. M. (2005). *Pathophysiology: Concepts of altered health*

states (7th ed.). Philadelphia, PA: Lippincott Williams & Wilkins, pp. 1478–1479.

5 **Answer: 4** There is no sensation of pain to light touch in full thickness (formerly third degree) burns because the pain and touch receptors have been destroyed. There may not be pain with some deep partial thickness degree burns (option 3), but the appearance described is characteristic of full thickness. Superficial thickness burns (option 1) resemble a sunburn and are painful, while superficial partial thickness burns (option 2) are likely to be reddened and accompanied by blistering and pain.
Cognitive Level: Application **Client Need:** Physiological Integrity: Physiological Adaptation **Integrated Process:** Nursing Process: Assessment **Content Area:** Adult Health: Integumentary **Strategy:** Determine the classification of the burn from the assessment data given. Specific nursing knowledge is needed to answer the question, so review this material if the question was difficult. **Reference:** Porth, C. M. (2005). *Pathophysiology: Concepts of altered health states* (7th ed.). Philadelphia, PA: Lippincott Williams & Wilkins, pp. 1482–1483.

6 **Answer: 3** A burn involving the face, neck, or chest may cause airway closure because of the edema that occurs within hours. For this reason the nurse needs to assess the adequacy of the client's respirations. The nurse will also assess skin integrity (option 1), blood pressure and pulse (option 2), and pain (option 4), but these are not the highest priority assessments.
Cognitive Level: Analysis **Client Need:** Physiological Integrity: Physiological Adaptation **Integrated Process:** Nursing Process: Assessment **Content Area:** Child Health **Strategy:** Prioritize and assess for the most life threatening problem first. Remember the ABCs: airway, breathing, and circulation. Airway always comes first, even before pain. **Reference:** Porth, C. M. (2005). *Pathophysiology: Concepts of altered health states* (7th ed.). Philadelphia, PA: Lippincott Williams & Wilkins, p. 1483.

7 **Answer: 4** Pediculosis capitis is head lice, and nits are cemented to the hair shaft. They are most commonly seen on hair on the back of the head near the nape of the neck. A papular excoriation may be present at the nape of the neck secondary to scratching.
Cognitive Level: Application **Client Need:** Physiological Integrity: Physiological Adaptation **Integrated Process:** Nursing Process: Analysis **Content Area:** Child Health **Strategy:** The data described is characteristic of a common parasitic infestation. Read the question again carefully for clues. **Reference:** LeMone, P., & Burke, K. (2008). *Medical-surgical nursing: Critical thinking in client care* (4th ed.). Upper Saddle River, NJ: Pearson/Prentice Hall, p. 451.

ANSWERS & RATIONALES

8 Answer: 3 If the client previously had a reaction to a wasp sting, immediate treatment must be administered. If a reaction is anticipated, do not complete the exam or wait for symptoms to develop, be proactive. Pain often causes the blood pressure to rise. The client who has never been stung should be monitored closely.
Cognitive Level: Analysis **Client Need:** Physiological Integrity: Physiological Adaptation **Integrated Process:** Nursing Process: Analysis **Content Area:** Adult Health: Integumentary **Strategy:** Remember that insect venom can cause a type I hypersensitivity reaction. Sometimes these are life threatening. Look for an option with this potential. **Reference:** Porth, C. M. (2005). *Pathophysiology: Concepts of altered health states* (7th ed.). Philadelphia, PA: Lippincott Williams & Wilkins, p. 235.

9 Answer: 2 Candidiasis (oral thrush) often develops as a result of the overgrowth of fungal organisms after a client has been on an antibiotic. This side effect is a "superinfection" growth of nonsusceptible organisms.
Cognitive Level: Application **Client Need:** Physiologic Integrity: Physiological Adaptation **Integrated Process:** Nursing Process: Assessment **Content Area:** Adult Health: Integumentary **Strategy:** The history of two antibiotics is a clue to the new problem. **Reference:** LeMone, P., & Burke, K. (2008). *Medical-surgical nursing: Critical thinking in client care* (4th ed.). Upper Saddle River, NJ: Pearson/Prentice Hall, p. 449.

10 Answers: 1, 2, 3, 5 Viral infections cause warts, which appear in many types. The common wart fits the description in options 1 and 2. Warts can be transmitted through skin contact and any age person can get them.
Cognitive Level: Application **Client Need:** Physiologic Integrity: Physiological Adaptation **Integrated Process:** Teaching/Learning **Content Area:** Adult Health: Integumentary **Strategy:** Read the options carefully. An absolute word (*only*) makes one option incorrect. **Reference:** LeMone, P., & Burke, K. (2008). *Medical-surgical nursing: Critical thinking in client care* (4th ed.). Upper Saddle River, NJ: Pearson/Prentice Hall, p. 451.

Posttest

1 Answer: 3 Scabies, a parasitic infection caused by a mite, presents with small red-brown burrows (bumps in a line) that produce intense itching. Options 1, 2, and 4 would not cause lines of bumps, although pediculosis can cause intense itching. Zoster may cause linear bumps but in a pattern following a dermatome, not in the body areas for this client.
Cognitive Level: Analysis **Client Need:** Physiological Integrity: Physiological Adaptation **Integrated Process:** Nursing Process: Analysis **Content Area:** Adult Health: Integumentary **Strategy:** Analyze all the data given and consider the expected manifestations with each of the options. One infestation fits the description. **Reference:** LeMone, P., & Burke, K. (2008). *Medical-surgical nursing: Critical thinking in client care* (4th ed.). Upper Saddle River, NJ: Pearson/Prentice Hall, p. 451.

2 Answer: 3 Folliculitis is an inflammation of the hair follicle caused by infection, chemical irritants, or injury, including shaving. It is most commonly caused by *Staphylococcus aureus.* Using a clean razor each time he shaves will decrease the risk of reinfection. Keeping it moist and making dietary changes will not be effective. Pustules should not be squeezed.
Cognitive Level: Application **Client Need:** Health Promotion and Maintenance **Integrated Process:** Nursing Process: Implementation **Content Area:** Adult Health: Integumentary **Strategy:** Pustules indicate infection. Choose an option that fits the gender given in the question. **Reference:** LeMone, P., & Burke, K. (2008). *Medical-surgical nursing: Critical thinking in client care* (4th ed.). Upper Saddle River, NJ: Pearson/Prentice Hall, p. 446.

3 Answer: 4 All three diagnoses are a bacterial infection of the skin arising from the hair follicle, where bacteria can accumulate, grow, and cause a localized infection. They are not highly contagious (option 3), and they are not associated with viral or fungal infections (option 1 and 2).
Cognitive Level: Application **Client Need:** Physiological Integrity: Physiological Adaptation **Integrated Process:** Teaching/Learning **Content Area:** Adult Health: Integumentary **Strategy:** Determine the causative agent and eliminate the options that have the incorrect etiology. **Reference:** LeMone, P., & Burke, K. (2008). *Medical-surgical nursing: Critical thinking in client care* (4th ed.). Upper Saddle River, NJ: Pearson/Prentice Hall, pp. 446–447.

4 Answer: 1 Impetigo is an infection of the skin typically beginning with a vesicle or pustule. The lesion ruptures, leaving an open area that discharges a honey-colored serous liquid that hardens into a crust. Impetigo spreads quickly if not treated. Scabies and herpes simplex are other types of infections that have manifestations on the skin. Contact dermatitis is triggered by an allergen.
Cognitive Level: Application **Client Need:** Physiological Integrity: Physiological Adaptation **Integrated Process:** Nursing Process: Analysis **Content Area:** Child Health **Strategy:** Recall the definitions of the various disorders listed. Note that the data given is a classic description of a common, superficial problem seen mostly in infants and young children. **Reference:** LeMone, P., & Burke, K. (2008). *Medical-surgical nursing: Critical thinking in client care* (4th ed.). Upper Saddle River, NJ: Pearson/Prentice Hall, pp. 432.

5 **Answers: 1, 4, 5** Psoriasis is a chronic disease with factors such as stress precipitating an exacerbation. The disease cannot be transferred to another person. Keeping the skin moist with an emollient lotion relieves the itching, and medications can be effective. Although there is no cure, treatment can suppress the hyperkeratosis and inflammation.
Cognitive Level: Application **Client Need:** Physiological Integrity: Physiological Adaptation **Integrated Process:** Nursing Process: Implementation **Content Area:** Adult Health: Integumentary **Strategy:** Note that some of the options contradict each other. Eliminate one of the opposing pairs. **Reference:** LeMone, P., & Burke, K. (2008). *Medical-surgical nursing: Critical thinking in client care* (4th ed.). Upper Saddle River, NJ: Pearson/Prentice Hall, pp. 443–446.

6 **Answer: 4** The description of the lesions matches psoriasis, a common disease of T-cell-mediated autoimmune response that occurs worldwide. The best nurse's response is one that reassures, gives correct information, and allows the client to express feelings or concerns. It also begins assessing the client's existing knowledge of the disease to begin planning for teaching and management.
Cognitive Level: Analysis **Client Need:** Physiological Integrity: Physiological Adaptation **Integrated Process:** Communication and Documentation **Content Area:** Adult Health: Integumentary **Strategy:** Look for the option that assures the client and encourages expression of fears and concerns. **Reference:** Porth, C. M. (2005). *Pathophysiology: Concepts of altered health states* (7th ed.). Philadelphia, PA: Lippincott Williams & Wilkins, p. 1472.

7 **Answer: 1** Melanomas tend to have asymmetry (A), border irregularity (B), color variegation (C), and diameter (D) greater than 6 mm. The ABCD rule can be applied to any skin condition, but malignant melanoma is the most severe and has changes in all four of the rules. Although sun-exposed areas are the site in 90% of Caucasians, non-sun-exposed areas are often the site in darker-skinned clients.
Cognitive Level: Application **Client Need:** Physiological Integrity: Physiological Adaptation **Integrated Process:** Nursing Process: Assessment **Content Area:** Adult Health: Integumentary **Strategy:** Acronyms can help in remembering concepts. Recall the critical words in the ABCD rule of asymmetry, border, color, and diameter. This will help to evaluate the options. **Reference:** Porth, C. M. (2005). *Pathophysiology: Concepts of altered health states* (7th ed.). Philadelphia, PA: Lippincott Williams & Wilkins, p. 1480.

8 **Answer: 2** Restrictive jewelry and clothing are removed immediately from the burn victim to prevent circumferential constriction of the torso and extremities when edema formation begins. Assessment of the fingers and interference with treatment may require removal of jewelry, but the primary reason is option 2.
Cognitive Level: Application **Client Need:** Physiological Integrity: Physiological Adaptation **Integrated Process:** Nursing Process: Implementation **Content Area:** Adult Health: Integumentary **Strategy:** Note the critical word in the question is *priority*. Meaning that the correct action is more important than the others, even if all would be technically correct. To help make a selection, recall what nursing actions are needed to prevent complications from an expected physiological response to burns. **Reference:** Porth, C. M. (2005). *Pathophysiology: Concepts of altered health states* (7th ed.). Philadelphia, PA: Lippincott Williams & Wilkins, p. 1484.

9 **Answer: 4** A superficial thickness burn such as a sunburn involves only the epidermal layer of the skin. The color ranges from pink to bright red and usually no blisters form. This is the greatest risk besides dehydration unless the children are wearing sunscreen. The next action that the nurse should take is to determine whether the children are wearing sunscreen. Skin cancer can develop later in life because of sunburns. Nevi are one type of skin lesion. Sunlight would not cause full thickness burns.
Cognitive Level: Application **Client Need:** Health Promotion and Maintenance **Integrated Process:** Nursing Process: Assessment **Content Area:** Child Health **Strategy:** Visualize the scenario presented in the question and use the process of elimination to choose the most likely answer that represents an ordinary sunburn. **Reference:** Porth, C. M. (2005). *Pathophysiology: Concepts of altered health states* (7th ed.). Philadelphia, PA: Lippincott Williams & Wilkins, pp. 1482–1483.

10 **Answer: 3** Tanning and sun exposure can increase susceptibility to skin cancer, and not all individuals use a sunscreen or consider tanning as having serious consequences. Assessment of foods, cosmetics, and environmental factors are all aimed at assessing for allergies, which have a greater tendency to be characterized by a rash than a new and pigmented lesion.
Cognitive Level: Analysis **Client Need:** Health Promotion and Maintenance **Integrated Process:** Nursing Process: Assessment **Content Area:** Adult Health: Integumentary **Strategy:** Consider what problem the nurse is assessing for. Choose the option that gathers data related to risk factors, and eliminate each of the incorrect options because they all focus on allergies. **Reference:** Porth, C. M. (2005). *Pathophysiology: Concepts of altered health states* (7th ed.). Philadelphia, PA: Lippincott Williams & Wilkins, pp. 1478–1481.

ANSWERS & RATIONALES

References

Dambro, M. (2005). *Griffith's five minute clinical consult 2005 for PDA*. Philadelphia, PA: Lippincott Williams & Wilkins.

Kasper, D., Braunwald, E., Fauci, A., Hauser, S., Longo, D. & Jameson, J. (2004). *Harrison's principles of internal medicine* (16th ed.). New York: McGraw-Hill.

Kee, J. L. (2005). *Laboratory and diagnostic tests with nursing implications* (7th ed.). Upper Saddle River, NJ: Prentice Hall.

LeMone, P., & Burke, K. (2008). *Medical-surgical nursing: Critical thinking in client care* (4th ed.). Upper Saddle River, NJ: Prentice Hall.

Weber, J. (2004). *Nurse's handbook of health assessment* (5th ed.). Philadelphia, PA: Lippincott, Williams & Wilkins.

Porth, C. (2005). Pathophysiology: *Concepts of altered health* states (7th ed.). Philadelphia, PA: Lippincott Williams & Wilkins, pp. 1449–1494.

Hematological and Oncological Health Problems

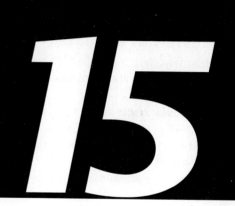

Chapter Outline

Risk Factors for Hematological and Oncological Health Problems

Leukemia

Lymphoma

Multiple Myeloma

Thrombocytopenia

Hemophilia

Anemia

Sickle Cell Anemia

Polycythemia (Polycythemia Vera)

Objectives

➤ Define key terms associated with hematological and oncological health problems.

➤ Identify risk factors associated with the development of hematological and oncological health problems.

➤ Explain the common etiologies of hematological and oncological health problems.

➤ Describe pathophysiological processes associated with specific hematological and oncological health problems.

➤ Distinguish between normal and abnormal hematological and oncological health findings obtained from nursing assessment.

➤ Prioritize nursing interventions associated with specific hematological and oncological health problems.

NCLEX-RN® Test Prep

Use the CD-ROM enclosed with this book to access additional practice opportunities.

Review at a Glance

achlorhydria the absence of free hydrochloric acid in a pH maintained at 3.5

cheilosis cracks in the corners of the mouth

factor VIII an alpha globulin that stabilizes fibrin clots

factor IX a vitamin-dependent beta globulin essential in stage 1 of the intrinsic coagulation system as an influence on the amount of thromboplastin available

ferritin an iron-phosphorus-protein complex that contains about 23% iron

hemoglobin electrophoresis a blood test that causes the hemoglobin molecule to migrate in solution in response to electric currents to determine the presence and percentage of hemoglobin S

intrinsic factor a substance secreted by the parietal cells of the gastric mucosa that promotes absorption of vitamin B_{12}

mean corpuscular hemoglobin (MCH) a measurement of the average weight (concentration) of hemoglobin in red blood cells (RBCs)

mean corpuscular hemoglobin concentration (MCHC) the ratio of the weight of hemoglobin to the volume of erythrocytes

mean corpuscular volume (MCV) a measurement of the size (volume) of the red blood cells (RBCs)

neutropenia a decrease in neutrophils

nadir the lowest point of bone marrow suppression following chemotherapy

paresthesias altered sensations such as numbness or tingling in the extremities

pernicious anemia the body's inability to absorb vitamin B_{12} because of a lack of intrinsic factor, a substance secreted by the parietal cells of the gastric mucosa

petechiae small, flat, purple or red spots on the skin or mucous membranes caused by minute hemorrhage in the dermis or submucous layer

Philadelphia chromosome characteristic chromosomal abnormality present in chronic myelogenous leukemia (CML)

pica craving to eat unusual substances such as clay or starch

plethora engorged or distended blood vessels causing a ruddy color of the face, hands, feet, ears, and mucous membranes

proprioception ability to identify one's position in space; problems may include difficulty with balance and spinal cord damage

purpura hemorrhage into the tissues as evidenced by bruising

Schilling test a vitamin B_{12} absorption test that indicates lacks of intrinsic factor by measuring excretion of orally administered radionuclide labeled B_{12}

PRETEST

1 A client with anemia has a hemoglobin of 6.5 grams/dL. The client is experiencing symptoms of cerebral tissue hypoxia. Which of the following nursing interventions would be the most important in providing care?

1. Provide rest periods throughout the day
2. Institute energy conservation techniques
3. Assist in ambulation to the bathroom
4. Check temperature of water prior to bathing

2 The nurse is caring for a client experiencing heart failure as a complication from multiple myeloma. A family member asks what is causing the problem. The nurse's best response includes that:

1. Proteins secreted by the abnormal plasma cells have caused the blood to thicken, resulting in heart failure.
2. Increased white blood cells and platelets have caused blood clots to form in the heart and blood vessels.
3. Healthy infection-fighting immunoglobulins are being produced in response to the myeloma progression.
4. The complications mean HIV is an additional worry but the medications should prevent the cell counts from dropping.

3 A client has a platelet count of 60,000/mL. What precautions does the nurse need to include in the plan of care?

1. Not allowing visitors or staff with infections to have direct contact
2. Removing clutter and objects that could contribute to a fall
3. Checking for a positive Homan's sign or calf tenderness
4. Encouraging foods like green, leafy vegetables

4 A 40-year-old client is referred to a hematologist with a tentative diagnosis of acute myelogenous leukemia (AML). The client's only symptom is fatigue. Which of the following laboratory or diagnostic tests would the nurse expect to be ordered first?

1. Liver function studies
2. Uric acid
3. Lumbar puncture
4. Bone marrow biopsy

5 Which of the following dietary recommendations should the nurse make to increase the intake of nutrients needed for erythropoiesis?

1. Milk, eggs, liver, and green, leafy vegetables
2. Apples, peanuts, oats, and cottage cheese
3. Cantaloupe, lima beans, and sweet potatoes
4. Dry yeast, grapefruit, and tuna fish

6 A client has an order for an iron preparation to be given by injection because the intravenous (IV) route is not possible for this client. The nurse expects the medication order to be written for which of the following routes?

1. Subcutaneous (SubQ) alternating with intramuscular (IM)
2. Deep gluteal intramuscular (IM) injection, using the Z-track method
3. Intramuscular in the deltoid to promote medication dissipation through muscle contraction
4. Subcutaneous injection with weekly site rotation

7 The nurse is applying pressure to a small bleeding laceration. Because the client has normal blood clotting, the nurse plans to safely release the pressure:

1. During the platelet phase, which occurs seconds after the injury.
2. During the clot retraction phase in three to four minutes.
3. When fibrin reinforces the platelet plug in the coagulation cascade within one to two minutes.
4. When the plasmin system produces fibrinolysis in clot dissolution in five to seven minutes.

8 A client has megaloblastic anemia along with some neurological symptoms. The nurse prepares to collect what specimen to verify the diagnosis of pernicious anemia?

1. Blood for storage of vitamin B_{12}
2. Gastric contents to test for pH
3. Urine for a 24-hour collection
4. Blood for detection of parietal cell and intrinsic factor antibodies

9 A client with a history of sickle cell anemia has recovered from an episode of sickling. At this time, the nurse plans to teach the client to avoid which conditions that may trigger another episode? Select all that apply.

1. Hypothermia
2. Dehydration
3. Bedrest
4. Excessive exercise
5. Infections

10 The nurse diligently assesses a client diagnosed with leukemia and who also has neutropenia for signs of infection. When questioned by a family member, the nurse uses which of the following as the best explanation as to why signs of infection may be absent or muted in this client?

1. Most infections are caused by organisms that are part of the body's normal flora
2. The white blood cells (WBCs) drop rapidly and recovery time is slow
3. Neutrophils necessary to produce an inflammatory response are inadequate in number or immature.
4. The immunoglobulins are reduced.

➤ *See pages 455–456 for Answers & Rationales.*

I. RISK FACTORS FOR HEMATOLOGICAL AND ONCOLOGICAL HEALTH PROBLEMS

A. **Lifestyle factors** such as smoking and alcohol consumption

B. **Dietary and nutritional factors** such as decreased intake of B vitamins and iron

C. **Leukemia:** occupational and physical environment risk factors such as exposure to chemicals (such as benzene and arsenic) or to large amounts of radiation, genetic factors, Down syndrome, viral etiology, and chemotherapeutic agents

D. **Lymphoma:** viral exposure, genetics, ethnicity, and/or immune system compromise

E. **Hematological cancers:** iatrogenic agents such as immunosuppressive agents as well as chemotherapy

F. **Anemia:** socioeconomic factors, such as poverty and inadequate nutrition

II. LEUKEMIA

A. **Overview**

1. Defined as a malignant neoplasm of the blood-forming tissues of the bone marrow, spleen, and lymph system

2. Characterized by an abnormal proliferation and accumulation of immature white blood cells (WBCs or leukocytes) and their precursors that infiltrate the bone marrow and peripheral blood as well as body organs and tissues

3. Types: categorized by the type of WBC affected (granulocytic, lymphocytic, monocytic) and the course and duration of the disease (acute or chronic)

   a. Acute lymphocytic/lymphoblastic leukemia (ALL)

      1) Immature lymphocytes proliferate in the marrow

      2) Abnormal leukemic cells resemble immature lymphocytes or lymphoblasts

      3) Most common in children between the ages of 2 and 10

      4) A second rise in incidence occurs in middle age and in older adults

   b. Acute myelogenous/myelocytic leukemia (AML) or acute granulocytic leukemia (AGL)

      1) Immature granulocytes proliferate and accumulate in the marrow

      2) Rate of incidence increases with age (especially over 50 years)

      3) Auer rods may be present in the cytoplasm of the myeloblasts; a standard diagnostic criterion for AML is that over 30% of hematopoietic cells must be myeloblasts

      4) Myelodysplastic syndrome, a hematological disorder of the bone marrow, is referred to as pre-leukemia and may progress to AML; this syndrome has abnormal hematologic cell production and low peripheral blood counts

   c. Chronic lymphocytic leukemia (CLL)

      1) Abnormal incompetent lymphocytes proliferate, accumulate, and spread to other lymphatic tissue

      2) More common in men

      3) Occurs most frequently between the ages of 50 and 70; more gradual onset

   d. Chronic myelogenous leukemia (CML)

      1) Abnormal stem cells lead to an uncontrolled proliferation of granulocyte cells resulting in a marked increased in circulating blast cells, which can then lead to leukostasis and intracerebral hemorrhage

2) In most cases, the characteristic chromosomal abnormality is present; referred to as the **Philadelphia chromosome** (an abnormal chromosome 22)

3) Occurs primarily between the ages of 30 to 50, incidence is slightly higher in men; more gradual onset

4. Cause is usually unknown, but may be related to risk factors (identified in previous section)

B. Pathophysiology

1. Abnormal or immature WBCs form and do not function properly; because of the massive proliferation of abnormal immature cells, fewer normal WBCs are produced; the abnormal cells continue to multiply and infiltrate, causing damage to the bone marrow, spleen, lymph nodes, liver, kidneys, lungs, gonads, skin, and central nervous system (CNS)

2. Normal bone marrow becomes diffusely replaced with abnormal or immature WBCs, interfering with the bone marrow's ability to produce other types of cells such as erythrocytes and thrombocytes; bone marrow becomes functionally incompetent with resulting bone marrow suppression

3. Acute leukemia has a rapid onset, progresses rapidly, with a short clinical course; left untreated, death will result in days or months; symptoms relate to a depressed bone marrow, infiltration of leukemic cells into other organ systems, and hypermetabolism of leukemia cells

4. Chronic leukemia has a more insidious onset with a more prolonged clinical course; asymptomatic early in the disease; life expectancy may be more than 5 years; symptoms relate to hypermetabolism of leukemia cells infiltrating other organ systems; cells are more mature and function more effectively

5. Signs and symptoms include anemia, infection from inadequate functional WBCs to defend against pathogens, hemorrhage from thrombocytopenia, shortness of breath, fatigue, malaise, weakness, weight loss, decreased activity tolerance, bone or joint pain, headaches, visual disturbances, anorexia, fever, anemia, petechiae or other ecchymosis, gingival bleeding, epistaxis, pallor, generalized lymphadenopathy, hyperuricemia, splenomegaly, increased WBCs, hepatomegaly

C. Nursing assessment

1. Assessment includes breath sounds, activity tolerance, pain, nutrition, vital signs, oral mucosa, signs of bleeding or infection, and enlargement of spleen, liver, or lymph nodes

2. Infection is a common presenting factor in acute leukemia, but signs and symptoms may be absent because of **neutropenia** (a decrease in neutrophils); CNS manifestations are most common in lymphocytic leukemia

3. Hemoglobin, hematocrit, platelet count, and granulocyte count will drop consistently during chemotherapy administration, reaching its lowest point 5 to 7 days after the initiation of therapy; counts will remain low for 7 to 10 days and will slowing begin rebounding, platelets first, then WBCs, then red blood cells (RBCs)

4. Diagnostic tests: bone marrow biopsy and aspirate is the only definitive diagnostic test, complete blood count (CBC), electrolytes, cultures (if infection present)

D. Nursing management

1. Medications include analgesics to control pain, antiemetics for nausea, and chemotherapeutic regimens including radioactive drugs such as sodium radio-iodine (Iodotope)

2. Massive amounts of chemotherapy are often given at one time (called induction therapy) for certain types of leukemia such as AML

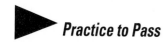

Practice to Pass

A client is being discharged following induction therapy for acute myelogenous leukemia (AML). He is in his nadir period. What type of education will he needed? What type of clinical follow-up should be expected over the next 7 to 10 days?

3. Other types of treatment: bone marrow transplant, biological therapies such as interferons and interleukins, and alternative treatments

4. Bone marrow biopsy

   a. Assess coagulation factors before procedure

   b. Posterior iliac crest, anterior iliac crest, and sternum are preferred locations

   c. After procedure, apply firm pressure for 5 minutes and observe puncture site for hemorrhage hourly for at least 4 hours

5. Protect from infection (see Box 15-1 for neutropenic precautions), especially in **nadir** period (lowest level of bone marrow function from suppression following chemotherapy); identify risk of infection by calculating the client's absolute neutrophil count (ANC): WBC (% bands + % segs) = ANC (needs to be 1,000 or greater)

6. Prevent bleeding (soft tootbrush, fall prevention, safety with razors)

7. Prevent fatigue secondary to anemia, plan adequate rest periods, limit visitors if necessary

8. Maintain hydration and nutrition, evaluate weight loss

9. Stomatitis (inflammation of mouth) is common, therefore oral assessments and good oral hygiene should be initiated daily or more frequently as needed

10. Encourage and assist client and family to discuss concerns and fears

11. Discuss hair options early in the event alopecia occurs from chemotherapy

III. LYMPHOMA

A. Overview

1. Defined as a group of malignant neoplasms that affect the lymphatic system

2. Hodgkin's disease is a malignant disorder of the lymph nodes that is characterized by the presence of the Reed-Sternberg cell

3. Non-Hodgkin's lymphomas are a broad group of neoplastic disorders that affect the lymphatic system and include all lymphomas except Hodgkin's disease

4. Cause is unknown or associated with predisposing factors

Box 15-1	➤ Use meticulous handwashing.
Neutropenic Precautions	➤ Provide oral hygiene after meals and at bedtime.
	➤ Screen all visitors and staff for colds or infections.
	➤ Monitor vital signs every four hours.
	➤ Prohibit fresh fruit or flowers, plants, and standing water.
	➤ Change intravenous (IV) tubing every 24 hours.
	➤ Avoid certain medications that may mask fever, such as acetaminophen (Tylenol) and ibuprofen (Advil).
	➤ Avoid rectal temperatures and suppositories.
	➤ Administer antibacterial/antifungal/antiviral therapy as prescribed.

B. Pathophysiology

1. *Hodgkin's disease (HD)*

    a. Reed-Sternberg cells (malignant cells) replace normal cellular structure; these are giant cell mutations of the T-lymphocyte that are present in the lymph node when diagnosed with HD

    b. Originates in one lymph node and then spreads to adjacent structures through the lymph system

    c. Eventually infiltrates other tissues including the liver, spleen, lungs, bone marrow, and ureters

    d. Peaks in two age groups: 15 to 35 years of age, and then again from 55 to 75 years of age; occurs twice as often in men than women

2. *Non-Hodgkin's lymphoma*

    a. Cells that make up lymphoid tissue become abnormal and eventually crowd out normal cells within specific regions of the lymph nodes; there are no Reed-Sternberg cells

    b. Lymphoma usually originates outside lymph nodes and becomes disseminated rapidly

    c. Incidence increases between the ages of 50 and 70; men are more frequently affected than women

3. Insidious onset, diagnosis usually occurs from pressure exerted by large nodes on surrounding tissues and/or obstruction/infiltration of lymphoma into vital organs such as the kidney, lung, or spleen

4. Staging based on Cottswold Staging Classification System

    a. Stage I: limited to a single lymph node region, lymphoid structure, or extra-lymphatic site

    b. Stage II: involvement of two or more lymph node regions on the same side of the diaphragm or localized extra-lymphatic involvement

    c. Stage III: involvement of lymph node regions or structures on both sides of the diaphragm; may involve spleen or localized extranodal disease

    d. Stage IV: diffuse or disseminated extra-lymphatic disease

5. Signs and symptoms include painless unilateral or bilateral lymph node enlargement; cervical generally involved first, then axillary and inguinal (most easily assessed since they are more superficial); clients with more advanced disease often present with: weight loss, night sweats, malaise, chills, pruritus, anorexia, nonproductive cough, dyspnea, and renal failure

C. Nursing assessment

1. Assessment includes lymph nodes, presence or absence of pain, nutritional status, weight, activity level and tolerance, respiratory status, and kidney function

2. Diagnostic tests: CBC, blood urea nitrogen (BUN), creatinine, lymph node biopsy is the only definitive diagnosis of either Hodgkin's or non-Hodgkin's lymphoma (via surgical incision or needle aspirate); lymphangiogram (radiologic examination after infusion of a blue oil–based dye into the lymphatic system to determine the extent of involvement)

D. Nursing management

1. Medications include combination chemotherapy for both Hodgkins and non-Hodgkins disease, depending on the stage

▶ **Practice to Pass**

Discuss the similarities and the differences between Hodgkin's (HD) and non-Hodgkin's lymphoma. How is the care of the client with HD the same or different from the care of the client with non-Hodgkin's lymphoma?

2. Radiation therapy
3. Post-procedure care following lymphangiogram
   a. Instruct client that urine, veins of the lower extremities, and dorsal skin of the feet may have a blue-green discoloration from dye excretion for 2 to 5 days
   b. Monitor for signs of dye-based complications: cough, dyspnea, pleuritic pain, hemoptysis
4. Protect from infection
5. Maintain normal body temperature
6. Prevent/decrease pain
7. Maintain adequate nutrition and hydration

IV. MULTIPLE MYELOMA

A. Overview

1. Defined as plasma cell neoplasms or related disorders comparable with proliferation and collection of immunoglobulin or plasma cells
2. Affects mostly men 50 to 69 years of age; more prominent in African Americans
3. Cause is unknown; however, some studies suggest that multiple myeloma reflects an inappropriate response to an antigen or a virus-like particle; genetics may be involved

B. Pathophysiology

1. Malignant plasma cells arise from one clone of B cells, proliferate within the hematopoietic tissue, and then infiltrate the rest of the bone to produce osteolytic lesions; substances secreted by the malignant plasma cells produce systemic effects and involve the bone marrow causing major complications
2. Subsequent bone destruction leads to hypercalcemia and pathologic fractures
3. Proliferation of plasma cells crowds the marrow space, usually inhibiting the production of RBCs
4. Plasma cells also synthesize and secrete an abnormally small number of immunoglobulins, increasing the risk of infection
5. In some cases, a marked increase in IgG or occasionally IgA increases the blood's viscosity, leading to occlusion of small blood vessels
6. The hallmark of multiple myeloma is the production of an abnormal immunoglobulin (the M component) indicated by elevated blood levels and the presence of Bence Jones protein in the urine
7. Signs and symptoms
   a. Gradual, insidious onset with clients suffering from recurrent infections, especially pneumonia
   b. Pain is a major problem for these clients as bony destruction begins to occur and lytic bone lesions occur
   c. Cord compression may occur from vertebral collapse
   d. Diffuse osteoporosis with a negative calcium balance may also be seen
   e. Renal stones occur with demineralization
   f. Hypercalcemia can also cause neurological disturbances (confusion, depression), gastrointestinal (GI) distress, altered musculoskeletal status, fluid and electrolyte imbalance, and altered cardiopulmonary function

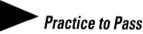

g. Renal disease may develop as a result of renal calculi and the toxic effect of Bence Jones protein on the renal epithelial cells

C. Nursing assessment

1. Assessment includes symptom analysis of pain, history of fractures, recurring pneumonia, kidney problems, musculoskeletal problems, or cardiovascular complications

2. Diagnostic tests: electrolytes, chest x-ray (CXR), CBC, BUN, creatinine, computerized tomography (CT) scan, IgE, urinalysis

D. Nursing management

1. Medications

a. Analgesics to manage pain

b. Antimicrobial therapy in the presence of positive blood cultures

c. Melphalan (Alkeran) and cyclophosphamide (Cytoxan), the most common chemotherapeutic agents used to manage the condition

d. Management of hypercalcemia through the use of steroids, IV hydration, diuretics, and medications, calcitonin (Calcimar), etidronate disodium (Didronel), gallium nitrate (Ganite), and pamidronate disodium (Aredia)

2. There is no cure for multiple myeloma, so the treatment is palliative

3. Maintaining adequate hydration is of primary concern; fluids are administered to attain a urinary output of 1.5 to 2 L/day

4. Weight-bearing, range of motion (ROM), and ambulation helps the bone reabsorb calcium; ambulation is most significant in lowering the calcium level

5. Radiation therapy is usually limited to clients with disabling pain or those with spinal cord compression

6. Blood transfusions are often indicated to manage the resultant anemia

7. Autologous and allogenic bone marrow transplants are also an option

8. Gallium nitrate (Ganite) is contraindicated with renal insufficiency (creatinine greater than 2.5 mg/dL)

9. Manage pain if metastasis occurs, instructing the client on how to take medication prior to severe pain and possible side effects

Practice to Pass

A hospitalized client with multiple myeloma who has bone metastasis was just started on long-acting morphine sulfate (MS Contin) tablets. In preparation for discharge, what important information should the nurse review with the client and significant other?

V. THROMBOCYTOPENIA

A. Overview

1. Defined as a platelet count less than 100,000/mm^3

2. Is the most common cause of abnormal bleeding

3. Hemorrhage from minor trauma and spontaneous bleeding can occur when platelet count falls below 20,000/mm^3

4. Fatal GI, cerebral, and pulmonary hemorrhage can occur if the count drops below 10,000/mm^3

5. Causes include unknown reasons, diseases (anemias, systemic lupus erythematosus, acquired immunodeficiency syndrome [AIDS]), sequelae to viral infections, chemotherapy or radiation, hypersplenism or splenomegaly, coronary bypass or autotransfusion, heparin therapy

B. Pathophysiology

1. Related to three basic mechanisms: accelerated platelet destruction or consumption, defective platelet production, or disordered platelet distribution

2. *Immune (or idiopathic) thrombocytopenia purpura* (ITP) occurs when the destruction of platelets is greatly accelerated

   a. The destruction is believed to be caused by the body's immune system and is therefore categorized as an autoimmune disorder

   b. Acute ITP is more common in children, while chronic ITP is more common in adults

   c. Platelets become coated with antibodies as a result of the autoimmune response mediated by the B lymphocytes; although the platelets function normally, the spleen sees them as foreign, and destroys them

   d. Platelet circulation time is decreased to 1 to 3 days

3. *Secondary thrombocytopenia* is a condition in which there is a defect in platelet production; this defect may occur as a result of:

   a. Medications such as thiazide diuretics, acetylsalicylic acid (ASA), ibuprofen (Advil), indomethacin (Indocin), naproxen sodium (Anaprox), sulfonamides, quinidine sulfate (Quinidex), cimetidine (Tagamet), digoxin (Lanoxin), furosemide (Lasix), heparin sodium, morphine sulfate, vitamins C and E

   b. Spices: ginger, cumin, turmeric, cloves, garlic

   c. Viral or bacterial infections

   d. Bone marrow disorders

   e. Chemotherapy and radiation therapy

4. *Disordered platelet distribution* occurs when large numbers of platelets are sequestered in the spleen; occurs as a result of lymphoma, portal hypertension, and hypothermia during heart surgery

5. Signs and symptoms include decreased platelet count; prolonged bleeding time; **purpura** (hemorrhage into the tissues as evidenced by bruising); ecchymosis (flat or raised areas of discoloration of the skin or mucous membranes caused by subcutaneous bleeding); **petechiae** (small, flat, purple or red spots on the skin or mucous membranes caused by minute hemorrhage in the dermis or submucous layer); weakness and fatigue

C. Nursing assessment

1. Assessment

   a. Evaluation of skin for signs of hemorrhage and symptom analysis of any bleeding episodes; look for petechiae and purpura on the most common areas (anterior thorax, arms, and neck); other common types of bleeding are epistaxis, menorrhagia, hematuria, and GI bleeding

   b. Activity tolerance (may be reduced from a secondary anemia)

   c. Home medications used, including herbal products

   d. Recent infections

2. Diagnostic tests: CBC, platelet count, coagulation studies including prothrombin time (PT) and partial thromboplastin time (PTT), bone marrow exam

D. Nursing management

1. Medications include steroids to suppress the immune response in ITP; immunoglobulin has been shown to have a temporary therapeutic effect in immune response disorders

Box 15-2	➤ Avoid intramuscular (IM) or subcutaneous injections.
Thrombocytopenic Precautions	➤ Avoid use of acetylsalicylic acid (aspirin) or aspirin-containing products.
	➤ Avoid use of toothbrushes and razors.
	➤ Avoid invasive or traumatic procedures.
	➤ Assess for signs of bleeding (skin, mouth, nose, feces, urine).
	➤ Guaiac all stool, urine, and emesis.
	➤ Pad side rails if necessary.
	➤ Avoid venipuncture (clients usually have a triple-lumen central line in place for blood sampling, medication administration, and blood product transfusion).
	➤ Administer stool softeners as necessary.

2. Initiate thrombocytopenic precautions (see Box 15-2)
3. Focus client education primarily on the risk for bleeding
4. Platelet transfusions may be given when platelet counts fall below 20,000/mm³, but are of little benefit in ITP
5. Educate clients about the Cushingoid side effects of steroid therapy, such as adiposity, edema, capillary fragility, and excessive hair growth
6. Treatment may consist of a splenectomy, especially in ITP

VI. HEMOPHILIA

A. Overview

1. Defined as a group of hereditary clotting factor disorders characterized by prolonged coagulation time that results in prolonged and sometime excessive bleeding

2. Hemophilia A and B are X-linked recessive disorders transmitted by female carriers, displayed almost exclusively in males (see Figure 15-1)

B. Pathophysiology

1. *Hemophilia A* (classic hemophilia) is a deficiency in **factor VIII** (an alpha globulin that stabilizes fibrin clots); deficiency is determined by first performing a PTT on the client's plasma; a factor VIII deficient plasma substrate is then mixed with the client's plasma and the degree of correction in the PTT is determined and compared to the degree of correction obtained by normal plasma
2. *Hemophilia B* (Christmas disease) is a deficiency in **factor IX** (a vitamin-dependent beta globulin essential in stage 1 of the intrinsic coagulation system as an

Figure 15-1	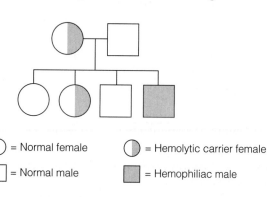
Genogram illustrating inheritance pattern for hemophilia A and B, which are X-linked recessive characteristics. Females carry the gene, but males express the gene and develop the disorder.	

influence on the amount of thromboplastin available); deficiency is determined by first performing a PTT on the client's plasma; a factor IX deficient plasma substrate is then mixed with the client's plasma and the degree of correction in the PTT is determined and compared to the degree of correction obtained by normal plasma

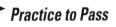

   a. Despite the difference in factor deficiency, hemophilia A and B are clinically identical

   b. Clients with hemophilia A and B form platelet plugs at the site of bleeding, but the clotting factor deficiency impairs the coagulation response and the capacity to form a stable clot

   c. With a factor level greater than or equal to 5%, bleeding is the result of trauma or surgery

   d. Spontaneous bleeding can occur with factor level activity below 1% resulting in hemoarthrosis with joint deformity and potential disability

3. *Von Willebrand's disease* is a deficiency of the von Willebrand factor (vWF) and platelet dysfunction

   a. Factor VIII has three properties, pre-coagulant activity, antigenic activity, and von Willenbrand factor activity

   b. It is classified as an autosomal dominant trait factor VIII defect; in hemophilia A, vWF is normal, but in von Willebrand's disease, vWF is characteristically low (less than 40% of control sample activity)

   c. This disorder is seen in both genders

4. Signs and symptoms

   a. Prolonged clotting times

   b. Subcutaneous ecchymosis and hematomas

   c. Bleeding from the gums

   d. GI bleeding, evidenced by hematemesis (vomiting blood), occult blood in the stools, gastric pain, or abdominal pain

   e. Urinary tract bleeding evidenced by hematuria

   f. Pain or paralysis resulting from pressure of the hematomas on nerves

   g. Hemarthrosis (joint bleeding, swelling, and damage)

   h. Slow oozing of blood from minor cuts, with the onset of bleeding being delayed for several hours, or even days after the injury

C. Nursing assessment

1. Includes assessment of bleeding, pain, skin, and oral mucosa; perform a symptom analysis of any bleeding episodes, infections, or difficulty in controlling bleeding; question use of over–the–counter medications and use of herbal products

2. Diagnostic tests: PT is normal; PTT or international normalized ratio (INR) are prolonged; fibrinogen is normal; platelet count is normal; bleeding time is prolonged in von Willebrand's disease; CBC, guaiac stool, and urinalysis (UA) may be ordered

D. Nursing management

1. Medications include replacement of deficient factor

   a. Hemophilia A: cryoprecipitate containing 8 to 100 units of factor VIII per bag at 12-hour intervals until bleeding ceases

   b. Hemophilia B: plasma or factor IX concentrate given every 24 hours or until bleeding ceases

---

► **Practice to Pass**

Both the client with hemophilia and the client with thrombocytopenia have a nursing diagnosis of Risk for injury: hemorrhage. How do these two medical diagnoses differ in their nursing interventions? How are they similar?

    c. Von Willebrand's disease: cryoprecipitate containing 8 to 100 units of factor VIII per bag at 12-hour intervals until bleeding ceases

2. Referral for genetic counseling is essential
3. Never give acetylsalicylic acid (aspirin) to a client with hemophilia
4. Stop topical bleeding as quickly as possible by applying direct pressure or ice, packing the area with gel foam or fibrin foam, and applying topical hemostatic agents such as fibrin
5. When joint bleeding occurs, totally rest the joint, apply ice, and administer hemophilia factors
6. Treatment may consist of plasmapheresis and/or prothrombin complexes for the development of antibody inhibitors against the specific coagulation factor

VII. ANEMIA

A. Overview

1. Defined as a condition where the hemoglobin content of the blood is insufficient to satisfy bodily needs
2. Caused by decrease in circulating RBCs, but may also be caused by accelerated hemolysis, decreased production, or high numbers of reticulocytes; other causes include side effects of medications, menstruation, GI bleeding

B. Pathophysiology

1. Anemia reduces the oxygen-carrying capacity of the blood, producing tissue hypoxia
2. Basic classifications of anemia are nutritional, hemolytic, and bone marrow depression; see Box 15-3 for types of anemias within each classification
3. Nutritional anemia results from nutrient deficiencies that disrupt erythropoiesis or hemoglobin synthesis

    a. *Iron-deficiency anemia*

        1) Supply of iron is inadequate for optimal formation of RBCs related to excessive iron loss caused by bleeding, decreased dietary intake, or malabsorption

---

Box 15-3	**Nutritional Anemias**
Classification of Selected Anemias	➤ Iron-deficiency anemia
	➤ Vitamin B_{12} anemia
	➤ Folic acid anemia

Hemolytic Anemias

➤ Sickle cell anemia

➤ Thalassemia

➤ Acquired hemolytic anemia

➤ Glucose-6-phosphate dehydrogenase anemia

Bone Marrow Depression Anemia

➤ Aplastic anemia

    2) Adequate iron in the RBC is essential since the oxygen molecule attaches to it

    3) Erythrocytes are small (microcytic with RBC diameter less than 6) and pale (hypochromic); **mean corpuscular volume (MCV;** measures size) is decreased and **mean corpuscular hemoglobin (MCH)** or **mean corpuscular hemoglobin concentration** or **MCHC** (calculated value of the hemoglobin present in the RBC compared to its size), will be decreased; the MCV, MCH, and MCHC should be analyzed only when the hemoglobin is low

    4) An average diet supplies the body with 12 to 15 mg/day of iron, of which only 5 to 10% is absorbed

    5) Iron is stored in the body as **ferritin,** an iron-phosphorus-protein complex that contains about 23% iron; it is formed in the intestinal mucosa, when ferritin iron joins with the protein apoferritin; ferritin is stored primarily in the reticuloendothelial cells of the liver, spleen, and bone marrow

    6) Normal iron excretion is less than 1 mg/day through the urine, sweat, bile, feces, and from desquamated skin cells; the average woman loses 0.5 mg of iron daily or 15 mg monthly during menstruation; menstruation is the most common cause of iron deficiency in women while GI bleeding is the most common cause in men

    7) Develops slowly through three phases: body's stores of iron used for erythropoiesis are depleted; insufficient iron is transported to the bone marrow; and iron deficient erythopoiesis begins, allowing small hemoglobin deficient cells to enter the peripheral circulation in large numbers; iron is needed on the hemoglobin so the oxygen molecule will attach

    8) Signs and symptoms develop gradually with the client not seeking attention until the hemoglobin drops to 7 to 8 grams/dL; manifestations include fatigue, weakness, shortness of breath, pallor (ear lobes, palms, and conjunctiva), brittle spoon-like nails; **cheilosis** (cracks in the corners of the mouth); smooth sore tongue; dizziness, hypoxia, and **pica** (craving to eat unusual substances such as clay or starch)

  b. *Vitamin B$_{12}$ deficiency anemia*

    1) Impairs cellular division and maturation especially in rapidly proliferating RBCs

    2) Macrocytic (megaloblastic) anemia (RBC diameter greater than 8)

    3) **Pernicious anemia** is the body's inability to absorb vitamin B$_{12}$ because of a lack of **intrinsic factor,** a substance secreted by the parietal cells of the gastric mucosa

    4) Laboratory examination shows an increase in the MCV and MCHC

    5) Gastric secretion analysis reveals **achlorhydria:** the absence of free hydrochloric acid in a pH maintained at 3.5

    6) Inevitably develops after total gastrectomy, with 15% of clients developing pernicious anemia after partial gastrectomy or gastrojejunostomy and increased incidence following gastric bypass surgery

    7) Lack of vitamin B$_{12}$ alters the structure and disrupts the function of the peripheral nerves, spinal cord, and brain

    8) Clients with this anemia tend to have fair hair coloring or become prematurely gray

    9) Signs and symptoms include pallor or slight jaundice with a complaint of weakness, smooth sore beefy red tongue, diarrhea, **paresthesias** such as numbness or tingling in the extremities), impaired **proprioception** (ability to identify one's position in space) which may progress to difficulty with balance and spinal cord damage)

c. *Folic acid deficiency anemia*

1) Required for DNA synthesis and the normal maturation of RBCs

2) Macrocytic (megaloblastic) anemia (RBC diameter > 8); MCV high with low hemoglobin

3) Causative etiology: poor nutrition, malabsorption syndrome, medications that impede absorption (oral contraceptives, anticonvulsants, methotrexate [MTX]), alcohol abuse, and anorexia

4) Signs and symptoms include pallor, progressive weakness, fatigue, shortness of breath, and palpitations; GI symptoms are similar to B_{12} deficiency, but usually more severe (anemia, glossitis, cheilosis, and diarrhea); neurological symptoms seen in B_{12} deficiency are not seen in folic acid deficiency and therefore assist in differentiation

C. Nursing assessment

1. Assessment includes symptom analysis of activity tolerance, skin color, nails, oral assessment, GI and nutritional assessment; neurological assessment is indicated in Vitamin B_{12} anemia

2. Diagnostic tests: CBC, MCV, MCH, MCHC; parietal cell and intrinsic factor antibodies

3. 24-hour urine for **Schilling test;** indicates if a client lacks intrinsic factor by measuring excretion of orally administered radionuclide labeled B_{12}

D. Nursing management

1. Iron-deficiency anemia

a. Medications include oral iron preparations before meals if tolerated and nausea does not occur; vitamin C enhances absorption, while antacids inhibit absorption; intramuscular (IM) iron dextran (Imferen) should be administered using the Z-track technique to prevent tattooing of the skin

1) Parenteral iron is given to clients who have an intolerance to iron preparations, habitually forget their medications, or continue to suffer blood loss

2) Because of the high risk of allergic reaction, the first dose should be infused slowly with concurrent and careful client assessment

b. Increase the number and amount of iron-rich foods, such as beef, chicken, egg yolk, pork loin, turkey, and whole-grain breads and cereals

c. Monitor for safety and injury if severe anemia occurs because of tissue and cerebral hypoxia

2. Vitamin B_{12} deficiency anemia

a. Medications include parenteral replacement of vitamin B_{12} IM; required for life for clients lacking the intrinsic factor

b. Teach clients with insufficient dietary intake to increase intake of foods such as eggs, meats, and dairy products

3. Folic acid deficiency anemia

a. Medications include oral folic acid supplements indefinitely with malabsorption or impaired folic acid metabolism

b. In malnourishment, foods containing folic acid should be added, such as green, leafy vegetables, broccoli, organ meats, eggs, and milk

Practice to Pass

What is the primary difference between pernicious anemia and anemia caused by a folic acid deficiency? How are the two similar?

VIII. SICKLE CELL ANEMIA

A. Overview

1. Defined as a hereditary, chronic form of hemolytic anemia

2. Eight percent of African Americans are heterozygous (carriers) for sickle cell anemia thereby inheriting one affected gene (or the sickle cell trait)

3. One percent of African Americans are homozygous for the disorder, thereby inheriting a defective gene from each parent, these clients have sickle cell anemia and are likely to experience sickle cell crisis

4. Caused by an autosomal genetic defect (one gene affected) that results in the synthesis of hemoglobin S (see Figure 15-2)

B. Pathophysiology

1. Produced by a mutation in the beta chain of the hemoglobin molecule though a substitution of the amino acid valine for glutamine in both beta chains

2. When there is decreased plasma oxygen tension, hemoglobin S causes RBCs to elongate, become rigid, and assume a crescent sickled shape, causing the cells to clump together and obstruct capillary blood flow, causing ischemia and possible tissue infarction

   a. Conditions likely to trigger a sickle cell crisis include hypoxia, low environmental and/or body temperature, excessive exercise, high altitudes, or inadequate oxygen during anesthesia

   b. Other causes include elevated blood viscosity or decreased plasma volume, infection, dehydration, and/or increased hydrogen ion concentration (acidosis)

3. With normal oxygenation, the sickled RBCs resume their normal shape

4. Repeated episodes of sickling and unsickling weaken the cell membranes, causing them to hemolyze and be removed

5. A vasoocclusive crisis begins with sickling in the microcirculation and leads to the following cascade:

   a. Vasospasm creates a logjam effect, which brings blood flow through the vessels to a stop

Figure 15-2

Inheritance pattern for sickle cell anemia.

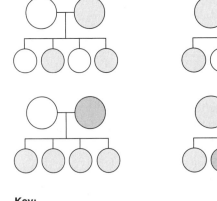

Key:

◯ Normal

◯ Sickle cell trait: heterozygous defective genes

● Sickle cell anemia: homozygous defective genes

Practice to Pass

The nurse sees a child with sickle cell anemia in the outpatient clinic who is planning to fly to Florida during spring vacation. What should the nurse teach the client and his parents to prevent the client from experiencing a crisis while away?

b. Thrombosis and infarction of local tissue occur

c. Crisis results, which is extremely painful and can last from 4 to 6 days

6. Sickle cell trait is a generally mild condition that produces few, if any, manifestations

7. Signs and symptoms include anemia with sickled cells noted on a peripheral smear; general manifestations similar to those of hemolytic anemia (pallor, jaundice, fatigue, and irritability); large joints and surrounding tissue may become swollen during crisis; priapism (abnormal, painful continuous erection of the penis) may occur if penile veins are obstructed

C. Nursing assessment

1. Assessment includes symptom analysis of activity tolerance, skin color, swelling of joints, and degree of pain if any

2. Diagnostic tests: **hemoglobin electrophoresis,** a blood test that causes the hemoglobin molecule to migrate in solution in response to electric currents, determines the presence and percentage of hemoglobin S and is used for a definitive diagnosis; CBC

D. Nursing management

1. Medications include folic acid supplements (to meet the increased metabolic demands of the bone marrow) and analgesics

2. Hydration therapy as well as scheduled transfusions will decrease number of painful crisis episodes

3. During a crisis, hydration therapy is essential to improve blood flow, reduce pain, and prevent renal damage

4. For clients experiencing a pain crisis, treatment includes rest, oxygen, use of IV opioids, and hydration

IX. POLYCYTHEMIA (POLYCYTHEMIA VERA)

A. Overview

1. Defined as an increase in the number of circulating RBCs and the concentration of hemoglobin in the blood; also known as polycythemia vera, PV, or myeloproliferative red cell disorder

2. Bone marrow stimulates an overproduction of RBCs, WBCs, and platelets thereby increasing blood viscosity, blood volume, and congestion of tissues and organs with blood

3. Can be a primary or secondary disorder

4. Causes include primary—unknown; secondary—erythropoietin-secreting tumors, Cushing's syndrome, end-stage renal disease, hypoxemia, and long-term dialysis

B. Pathophysiology

1. *Primary polycythemia*

a. Most common in Caucasian men of European Jewish ancestry

b. Is a neoplastic stem cell disorder characterized by the overproduction of RBCs, certain WBCs, and platelets

c. Erythrocytosis causes increased blood volume and viscosity with liver and spleen congestion

d. Thick, slow-moving blood becomes an ideal environment for acidosis and clotting, with resultant tissue and organ infarction secondary to thrombi

   2. *Secondary polycythemia*

   a. Most common form of PV

   b. Excess of erythropoiesis that arises as a response to an abnormal increase in erythropoietin

   c. Abnormally high levels of erythropoietin may also be produced because of hypoxemia, in turn caused by:

   1) Prolonged exposure to high altitudes

   2) Systemic disorders that affect oxygenation (chronic obstructive pulmonary disease [COPD], congestive heart failure [CHF])

   3) Hypoventilation secondary to morbid obesity

   4) Long-term smokers: "smokers' erythrocytosis"

   3. Signs and symptoms

   a. **Plethora** (engorged or distended blood vessels causing a ruddy color of the face, hands, feet, ears, and mucous membranes)

   b. Engorgement of the retinal veins (bloodshot eyes) and sublingual veins

   c. Splenomegaly (primary PV only)

   d. Hepatomegaly; headache, a feeling of fullness in the head, dizziness, weakness, fatigue on exertion, visual disturbances, hypertension, hypermetabolism, epigastric distress, and backache

   e. Pruritis that does not respond to antihistamines

   f. Manifestations of vascular disease (angina, intermittent claudication, cerebral insufficiency)

C. Nursing assessment

   1. Includes symptom analysis of pain, itching, skin color, and palpation of spleen or liver

   2. Diagnostic tests: high erythrocyte count (8 to 12 million/mm^3); decreased MCHC; increased leukocytes, thrombocytes, and total blood volume

D. Nursing management

   1. Medications include antineoplastic agents (but their side effects are often worse than the disease); radioactive phosphorus (may cause generalized suppression of hematopoiesis with resultant anemia, leukopenia, or thrombocytopenia)

   2. Encourage smoking cessation in clients who smoke

   3. Manage underlying chronic condition (COPD, CHF) with supportive measures and appropriate drug therapy

Case Study

The client is a 62-year-old female married retired schoolteacher with three grown children who live in various parts of the United States. Her husband is a pharmaceutical representative who travels frequently. The client has been a diabetic since age 25 and takes insulin twice daily. Over the last 2 months, the client has had difficulty recovering from a cold, experiences periods of extreme fatigue, lost 10 pounds, and has a low-grade temperature of 100°F. Blood studies and a bone marrow biopsy and aspirate led to the diagnosis of acute lymphocytic leukemia (ALL). Currently the client is hospitalized with a triple-lumen Hickman catheter in place and is undergoing chemotherapy with vincristine (Oncovin), daunorubicin (Cerubidine), and prednisone.

Assessment finds the client oriented to person, place, and time; reporting headache and dizziness upon standing; slight numbness, tingling of her lower extremities; petechiae cover her arms, chest, and upper thighs; skin color pale; recoil is less than 6 seconds, with dry mucous membranes. Small ulcerated area is present on outer aspect of right ankle; Hickman site is clean and dry but slightly red; no obvious dyspnea but complains of shortness of breath upon exertion; lung sounds clear; sputum slightly yellow in color; vital signs: pulse 90; blood pressure 140/84 lying and 128/72 standing; respirations 20 and regular; lab work: white blood count (WBC) 9,000/mm^3; red blood count (RBC) 2.23/mm^3; hemoglobin 8.8 grams/dL; hematocrit 26%; platelets 12,000/mm^3; WBC differential: segs 10%; bands 1%; lymphocytes 60%; glucose: 250 mg/dL; albumin 2.4 grams/dL; calcium 8.0 mEq/L.

1. What are the most important nursing diagnoses, and how should they be prioritized?

2. What is the relationship between the client's absolute neutrophil count (ANC) and the risk for infection?

3. How will the nurse know the client is developing infection?

4. What effect will the client's diabetes have on her treatment course?

5. How should the nurse prepare the client for discharge from the hospital?

For suggested responses, see pages 538-539.

POSTTEST

1 A client with anemia due to chemotherapy has a hemoglobin level of 7.0 grams/dL. Which of the following client complaints would indicate to the nurse that the client has tissue hypoxia related to anemia? Select all that apply.

1. Dizziness
2. Thirst and polyuria
3. Skin that is warm and dry to the touch
4. Fatigue and weakness
5. Dyspnea

2 A medical record indicates that a client has a positive Philadelphia chromosome. The nurse plans care for the client considering the needs of the client with which disorder?

1. Acute myelocytic leukemia (AML)
2. Hairy cell leukemia
3. Chronic myelogenous leukemia (CML)
4. Chronic lymphocytic leukemia (CLL)

3 A nurse caring for a client who has experienced a bone marrow biopsy and aspiration should assess for which of the following as the most serious complication?

1. Bleeding
2. Infection
3. Shock
4. Splintering of bone marrow fragments

4 For the client diagnosed with iron-deficiency anemia, the nurse should recommend an increased intake of which of the following foods?

1. Fresh citrus fruits
2. Milk and cheese
3. Organ meats
4. Whole-grain breads

5 The nurse would interpret that a client is most severely at risk for bleeding when which of the following is noted on laboratory test results?

1. Neutrophils are 50%
2. Lymphocytes are 30%
3. Platelets are less than 20,000/mm^3
4. Basophils are 0

6 The nurse conducting an in-service on the hematology unit is comparing the pathophysiology of acute and chronic leukemias. The nurse reminds coworkers that which of the following is a feature common to both types?

1. Compensatory polycythemia stimulated by thrombocytopenia
2. Unregulated accumulation of white blood cells in the bone marrow
3. Increased blood viscosity resulting from an overproduction of white cells
4. Reduced plasma volume in response to a reduced production of cellular components

7 The nurse would teach a client with sickle cell trait that he or she:

1. Should avoid fluid loss or overhydration.
2. Is at great risk of sickle cell crisis under triggering conditions.
3. Can expect to experience chronic anemia.
4. Should receive genetic counseling before starting a family.

8 A client with pancytopenia enters the clinic with large areas of ecchymosis on the skin. The nurse should caution the client to avoid using which of the following medications that can alter platelet function?

1. Acetylsalicylic acid (aspirin), dipyridamole (Persantine), and naproxen (Aleve)
2. Milk of magnesia (MOM), heparin (Liquaemin), and quinidine sulfate (Quinidex)
3. Senna (Senokot), furosemide (Lasix), and phenytoin (Dilantin)
4. Acetaminophen (Tylenol), sulfonamides, and penicillins

9 A male client, newly diagnosed with hemophilia, asks the nurse what problems he can expect to develop because of the disease. The nurse's best response is:

1. "Try not to worry excessively. The disease usually affects females and males only get mild cases."
2. "You may have joint bleeding, swelling, and damage because the bleeding causes inflammation in the joints and tissues."
3. "Since you have excess von Willebrand factor, you may bleed more than normal for dental extractions or surgery."
4. "Don't worry about future complications yet. If you take extra vitamin K and vitamin B$_{12}$, your problems will be postponed."

10 A client enters the clinic reporting a sore mouth. Physical assessment reveals a beefy red tongue. The nurse would next assess for what other manifestations, suspecting the client may have pernicious anemia? Select all that apply.

1. Pallor or slight jaundice
2. Weakness and trouble with proprioception
3. Diminished short term memory
4. Paresthesias such as numbness or tingling
5. Diet deficient in green, leafy vegetables

➤ *See pages 456–458 for Answers & Rationales.*

ANSWERS & RATIONALES

Pretest

1 **Answer: 3** Cerebral tissue hypoxia is commonly associated with dizziness. The greatest potential risk to the client with dizziness is injury, especially with changes in position. Planning for periods of rest and consuming energy are important for someone with anemia because of his or her fatigue level, but most important is safety. **Cognitive Level:** Analysis **Client Need:** Physiological Integrity: Physiological Adaptation **Integrated Process:** Nursing Process: Implementation **Content Area:** Adult Health: Hematological **Strategy:** Review the problems associated with cerebral hypoxia. Prioritize the nursing actions needed for a safe and effective care environment. **Reference:** Porth, C. M. (2005). *Pathophysiology: Concepts of altered health states* (7th ed.). Philadelphia, PA: Lippincott Williams & Wilkins, p. 304.

2 **Answer: 1** Major complications of multiple myeloma include bone pain, hypercalcemia, renal failure, anemia, and impaired immune responses that are a result of bone marrow involvement. The systemic effects of paraproteins secreted by the malignant plasma cells may cause a hyperviscosity of body fluids, causing heart failure. **Cognitive Level:** Application **Client Need:** Physiological Integrity: Physiological Adaptation **Integrated Process:** Nursing Process: Implementation **Content Area:** Adult Health: Hematological **Strategy:** If the answer is not known, begin by eliminating the options that are not correct for multiple myeloma. **Reference:** Porth, C. M. (2005). *Pathophysiology: Concepts of altered health states* (7th ed.). Philadelphia, PA: Lippincott Williams & Wilkins, pp. 334–335.

3 **Answer: 2** Thrombocytopenia is a platelet count less than 100,000/mL. This client is at risk of spontaneous bleeding and easy bruising, although the client is not at the severe level of below 20,000/mL. The client needs to be protected from trauma such as with the actions in option 2. Option 1 would be helpful if the client has neutropenia. Option 3 will detect deep vein thrombosis, but clotting is the opposite problem of the risk to this client. Option 4 is a generally healthy measure, although

green, leafy vegetables also are high in vitamin K and interfere with the actions of oral anticoagulants. **Cognitive Level:** Analysis **Client Need:** Physiological Integrity: Reduction of Risk Potential **Integrated Process:** Nursing Process: Planning **Content Area:** Adult Health: Hematological **Strategy:** First determine what the platelet count indicates. Then decide what nursing order is appropriate. **Reference:** Porth, C. M. (2005). *Pathophysiology: Concepts of altered health states* (7th ed.). Philadelphia, PA: Lippincott Williams & Wilkins, pp. 293.

4 **Answer: 4** Bone marrow biopsy and aspirate is the only definitive diagnosis of AML. The presence of Auer rods is diagnostic for AML. The presence of leukemic cells in the spinal fluid is more common in acute lymphocytic leukemia (ALL). Uric acid and lactic dehydrogenase levels may be elevated in AML, but this is not diagnostic for the disease. **Cognitive Level:** Application **Client Need:** Physiological Integrity: Reduction of Risk Potential **Integrated Process:** Nursing Process: Assessment **Content Area:** Adult Health: Hematological **Strategy:** Consider what body system is affected by the AML. What diagnostic test is most applicable? **Reference:** LeMone, P., & Burke, K. (2008). *Medical-surgical nursing: Critical thinking in client care* (4th ed.). Upper Saddle River, NJ: Pearson/Prentice Hall, pp. 1121–1122.

5 **Answer: 1** Option 1 contains foods high in protein, folic acid, iron, and vitamin B_{12} that are needed for erythropoiesis. Options 2, 3, and 4 contain lesser amounts. **Cognitive Level:** Application **Client Need:** Health Promotion and Maintenance **Integrated Process:** Nursing Process: Implementation **Content Area:** Adult Health: Hematological **Strategy:** Which food list contains the best sources of needed nutrients? Although good sources are included in all the options, recognize that one option contains more protein, minerals, and needed vitamins than the others. **Reference:** LeMone, P., & Burke, K. (2008). *Medical-surgical nursing: Critical thinking in client care* (4th ed.). Upper Saddle River, NJ: Pearson/Prentice Hall, pp. 1103–1104.

6 **Answer: 2** Iron dextran can be given intravenously or as deep IM injection. A test dose for allergic response should be given before starting the therapy. The gluteal muscle is the best route for IM administration since the muscle is large and highly vascular. The Z-track method is preferable to prevent tattooing of the skin and tissue necrosis caused by infiltration into the subcutaneous tissue.
Cognitive Level: Application **Client Need:** Physiological Integrity: Pharmacological and Parenteral Therapies **Integrated Process:** Nursing Process: Implementation **Content Area:** Adult Health: Hematological **Strategy:** The core issue of the question is knowledge of the properties of injectable iron and how this impacts on administration. Review this medication if the question was difficult. **Reference:** Porth, C. M. (2005). *Pathophysiology: Concepts of altered health states* (7th ed.). Philadelphia, PA: Lippincott Williams & Wilkins, p. 309.

7 **Answer: 3** In hemostasis, after vascular spasm, platelet aggregation immediately forms a platelet plug at the site of bleeding (option 1), but fibrin reinforces the platelet plug in the next step. Pressure can be safely released once the fibrin clot is formed – usually in a few minutes. Clot retraction (option 2) and clot dissolution (option 4) occur in later phases of the process.
Cognitive Level: Application **Client Need:** Physiological Integrity: Physiological Adaptation **Integrated Process:** Nursing Process: Implementation **Content Area:** Adult Health: Hematological **Strategy:** Apply knowledge of the blood clotting process to clinical actions. **Reference:** Porth, C. M. (2005). *Pathophysiology: Concepts of altered health states* (7th ed.). Philadelphia, PA: Lippincott Williams & Wilkins, pp. 289–290.

8 **Answer: 4** Pernicious anemia is caused by the body's inability to absorb vitamin B_{12}. This is caused by a lack of intrinsic factor in the gastric juices or surgical removal of the terminal ileum where the vitamin is absorbed. The Shilling test, a 24-hour urine test for excretion of vitamin B_{12}, is seldom used today because detection of parietal cell and intrinsic factor antibodies (a blood test) is now possible for a definitive diagnosis of pernicious anemia.
Cognitive Level: Application **Client Need:** Physiological Integrity: Reduction of Risk Potential **Integrated Process:** Nursing Process: Planning **Content Area:** Adult Health: Hematological **Strategy:** Use nursing knowledge and the process of elimination to answer the question. Note the similarity between the words *parietal cell* and *intrinsic factor* in the correct option with the words *pernicious anemia* in the stem of the question. **Reference:** Porth, C. M. (2005). *Pathophysiology: Concepts of altered health*

states (7th ed.). Philadelphia, PA: Lippincott Williams & Wilkins, p. 310.

9 **Answers: 1, 2, 4, 5** In sickle cell anemia, if hypoxemia develops, the hemoglobin is deoxygenated and crystallizes into rod and chain shapes, deforming the erythrocyte into a crescent shape. Cells clump together, obstructing capillary blood flow. Conditions that predispose the client to hypoxemia, dehydration, or acidosis can trigger an episode. Options 1, 2, 4, and 5 are possible triggers.
Cognitive Level: Application **Client Need:** Physiological Integrity: Physiological Adaptation **Integrated Process:** Teaching/Learning **Content Area:** Adult Health: Hematological **Strategy:** Consider what conditions can predispose the client to problems. Notice that several options are similar and since the instructions are to select all that apply, choose the similar options if guessing. **Reference:** LeMone, P., & Burke, K. (2008). *Medical-surgical nursing: Critical thinking in client care* (4th ed.). Upper Saddle River, NJ: Pearson/Prentice Hall, p. 1108.

10 **Answer: 3** The client with neutropenia is unable to mount an inflammatory response. Fever is usually the first sign of infection. Options 1, 2, and 4 are all true statements, but they do not provide the clearest and most direct explanation about why the neutropenic client is at greater risk for infection.
Cognitive Level: Analysis **Client Need:** Physiological Integrity: Physiological Adaptation **Integrated Process:** Nursing Process: Analysis **Content Area:** Adult Health: Hematological **Strategy:** Relate the function of neutrophils to the inflammatory process. What is expected if the counts are low? **Reference:** LeMone, P., & Burke, K. (2008). *Medical-surgical nursing: Critical thinking in client care* (4th ed.). Upper Saddle River, NJ: Pearson/Prentice Hall, pp. 1138–1139.

Posttest

1 **Answers: 1, 4, 5** Cerebral tissue hypoxia is commonly associated with dizziness, faintness, and headache. Recognition of cerebral hypoxia is critical since the body will attempt to shunt oxygenated blood to vital organs and away from the skin. Dyspnea, fatigue, and sometimes angina are observed.
Cognitive Level: Application **Client Need:** Physiological Integrity: Physiological Adaptation **Integrated Process:** Nursing Process: Assessment **Content Area:** Adult Health: Hematological **Strategy:** Recall first how hemoglobin causes reduced oxygen to the tissues and symptoms of hypoxia. Look for options that describe findings caused by hypoxia. **Reference:** Porth, C. M. (2005). *Pathophysiology: Concepts of altered health states* (7th ed.). Philadelphia, PA: Lippincott Williams & Wilkins, pp. 304, 311.

2 **Answer: 3** Approximately 95% of clients with CML are Philadelphia chromosome-positive. This represents a translocation of the long arms of chromosomes 9 and 22. The other types of leukemia are not characterized by the Philadelphia chromosome.
Cognitive Level: Application **Client Need:** Physiological Integrity: Physiological Adaptation **Integrated Process:** Nursing Process: Analysis **Content Area:** Adult Health: Hematological **Strategy:** Specific knowledge is needed to answer this question. If you need to make an educated guess, consider that chromosome changes are most likely present in a chronic condition. **Reference:** Porth, C. M. (2005). *Pathophysiology: Concepts of altered health states* (7th ed.). Philadelphia, PA: Lippincott Williams & Wilkins, p. 332.

3 **Answer: 1** The risk for bleeding is of greatest risk since a large-bore needle is used to perform the biopsy and aspiration. Many of these clients often have an altered clotting capability. While the risk of infection is also a consideration, the procedure is performed under sterile conditions and is less of a concern than hemorrhage.
Cognitive Level: Application **Client Need:** Physiological Integrity: Physiological Adaptation **Integrated Process:** Nursing Process: Assessment **Content Area:** Adult Health: Hematological **Strategy:** Any biopsy carries similar risks. Consider the additional problems a client who needs a bone marrow study may experience. **Reference:** LeMone, P., & Burke, K. (2008). *Medical-surgical nursing: Critical thinking in client care* (4th ed.). Upper Saddle River, NJ: Pearson/Prentice Hall, p. 1126.

4 **Answer: 3** Organ meats like liver are a good source of iron as well as green, leafy vegetables and egg yolks. Whole-grain breads also contain iron; however, not in as high a quantity as organ meats.
Cognitive Level: Application **Client Need:** Health Promotion and Maintenance **Integrated Process:** Nursing Process: Implementation **Content Area:** Adult Health: Hematological **Strategy:** The critical word in the question is *iron.* Use knowledge of diet therapy to determine which foods have highest iron value. **Reference:** LeMone, P., & Burke, K. (2008). *Medical-surgical nursing: Critical thinking in client care* (4th ed.). Upper Saddle River, NJ: Pearson/Prentice Hall, p. 1110.

5 **Answer: 3** Options 1, 2, and 4 relate to the white blood cells, which are involved in protecting the client against infection. A platelet count lower than 20,000/mm^3 increases the client's risk for severe bleeding because of reduced platelets to assist in the clotting cascade to form a clot.
Cognitive Level: Analysis **Client Need:** Physiological Integrity: Reduction of Risk Potential **Integrated Process:** Nursing Process: Analysis **Content Area:** Adult Health:

Hematological **Strategy:** Recall the normal values of common laboratory tests. For this question, look for a result that relates to bleeding—a clue word in the question. **Reference:** Porth, C. M. (2005). *Pathophysiology: Concepts of altered health states* (7th ed.). Philadelphia, PA: Lippincott Williams & Wilkins, p. 293.

6 **Answer: 2** Leukemia is a result of erratic production of white blood cells by the bone marrow, which replace normal marrow components. It can arise from both a lymphatic and a myelocytic etiology. White blood cells are often immature and incapable of performing their expected function(s). Although the malignancies present with proliferation of different cells, they all arise from unregulated WBCs in the bone marrow.
Cognitive Level: Analysis **Client Need:** Physiological Integrity: Physiological Adaptation **Integrated Process:** Nursing Process: Analysis **Content Area:** Adult Health: Hematological **Strategy:** Select the option that relates to both acute and chronic leukemia. **Reference:** Porth, C. M. (2005). *Pathophysiology: Concepts of altered health states* (7th ed.). Philadelphia, PA: Lippincott Williams & Wilkins, pp. 328–332.

7 **Answer: 4** Sickle hemoglobin is transmitted by recessive inheritance. Sickle cell trait is generally a mild condition that produces few if any manifestations. These clients are considered carriers of the disease and require genetic counseling to determine presence of the hemoglobin S. Certain stressors result in a sickle cell crisis.
Cognitive Level: Application **Client Need:** Health Promotion and Maintenance **Integrated Process:** Nursing Process: Planning **Content Area:** Adult Health: Hematological **Strategy:** Do not confuse sickle cell trait with sickle cell anemia. **Reference:** Porth, C. M. (2005). *Pathophysiology: Concepts of altered health states* (7th ed.). Philadelphia, PA: Lippincott Williams & Wilkins, pp. 305–306.

8 **Answer: 1** All of the medications in the first option can affect platelet aggregation and should be avoided in a client with bleeding tendencies. A thorough review of all medications taken at home should be done whenever clients are issued new medications. Generally, the NSAIDs and aspirin-containing products interfere with platelet function while acetaminophen is safe.
Cognitive Level: Application **Client Need:** Physiological Integrity: Physiological Adaptation **Integrated Process:** Nursing Process: Implementation **Content Area:** Adult Health: Hematological **Strategy:** Recall that all parts of the option must be correct if it is the correct answer. Eliminate any option that contains one or more drugs that do not affect platelets. **Reference:** LeMone, P., & Burke, K. (2008). *Medical-surgical nursing: Critical thinking in client care* (4th ed.). Upper Saddle River, NJ: Pearson/Prentice Hall, p. 1126.

ANSWERS & RATIONALES

9 **Answer: 2** Hemophilia is a group of hereditary clotting factor disorders characterized by prolonged coagulation time that results in prolonged and sometime excessive bleeding. It is an X-linked recessive characteristic transmitted by female carriers, displayed almost exclusively in males, often resulting in spontaneous bleeding into the joints and resulting in hemoarthrosis with joint deformity and potential disability. Although he will have bleeding risks with dental work and surgery, there is not excess von Willebrand factor. Vitamins will not help.

Cognitive Level: Application **Client Need:** Physiological Integrity: Physiological Adaptation **Integrated Process:** Communication and Documentation **Content Area:** Adult Health: Hematological **Strategy:** An honest answer to prepare the client to manage the disease is the best response. **Reference:** Porth, C. M. (2005). *Pathophysiology: Concepts of altered health states* (7th ed.). Philadelphia, PA: Lippincott Williams & Wilkins, pp. 295–296.

10 **Answers: 1, 2, 4** The sore, beefy red tongue is very suspicious of pernicious anemia. The nurse should assess for other findings including altered sensations such as numbness or tingling in the extremities, and difficulty identifying one's position in space (proprioception), which may progress to difficulty with balance and spinal cord damage. Pallor and jaundice may be observed, but memory is not affected. The etiology is malabsorption rather than dietary deficiencies.

Cognitive Level: Application **Client Need:** Physiological Integrity: Physiological Adaptation **Integrated Process:** Nursing Process: Assessment **Content Area:** Adult Health: Hematological **Strategy:** Identify that the sore, beefy red tongue may indicate pernicious anemia. Next consider what other findings are expected, recalling also general symptoms common to all forms of anemia. **Reference:** LeMone, P., & Burke, K. (2008). *Medical-surgical nursing: Critical thinking in client care* (4th ed.). Upper Saddle River, NJ: Pearson/Prentice Hall, pp. 1110–1114.

References

Alexander, J. (2005). Nursing care of the client with lymphoma and multiple myeloma. In J. K. Itano & K. N. Taoka (Eds.), *Core curriculum for oncology nursing* (4th ed.). Philadelphia, PA: W. B. Saunders.

Bochmenkamp, S., & Wagner, K. D. (2006). Acute hematologic dysfunction. In P. S. Kidd, K. Johnson, & K. D. Wagner (Eds.), *High acuity nursing* (2nd ed.). Upper Saddle River, NJ: Prentice Hall.

Camp-Sorrell, D. (2005). Myelosuppression. In J. K. Itano & K. N. Taoka (Eds.), *Core curriculum for oncology nursing* (4th ed.). Philadelphia, PA: W. B. Saunders.

Fitzgerald, M. A. (2005). Hematologic disorders. In E. Q. Youngkin, K. J. Sawyer, J. F. Kissinger, & D. S. Israel (Eds.), *Pharmacotherapy: A primary care clinical guide.* (2nd ed.). Upper Saddle River, NJ: Prentice Hall.

LeMone, P., & Burke, K. M. (2008). *Medical-surgical nursing: Critical thinking in client care* (4th ed.). Upper Saddle River, NJ: Prentice Hall.

Moran, M. J., & Ezzone, S. A. (2005). Nursing care of the client with leukemia. In J. K. Itano & K. N. Taoka (Eds.), *Core curriculum for oncology nursing* (5th ed.). Philadelphia, PA: W. B. Saunders.

Olsen, S. J., Morrison, C. H., & Ashley, B. W. (2005). Prevention of cancer. In J. K. Itano & K. N. Taoka (Eds.), *Core curriculum for oncology nursing* (5th ed.). Philadelphia, PA: W. B. Saunders.

Porth, C. M. (2005). *Pathophysiology: Concepts of altered health states* (7th ed.). Philadelphia, PA: Lippincott Williams & Wilkins.

Wilkes, G. M., & Burke, M. B. (2005). *Oncology nursing drug handbook.* Boston, MA: Jones and Bartlett.

Wilkinson, J. M. (2006). *Nursing diagnosis handbook* (8th ed.). Upper Saddle River, NJ: Prentice Hall.

ANSWERS & RATIONALES

4 The parent of a child born with albinism type I asks the nurse how this happened. The nurse's best response is that the disorder is:

1. Autosomal dominant.
2. Autosomal recessive.
3. X-linked.
4. Multifactorial.

5 A priority nursing intervention for the infant with cleft lip is which of the following?

1. Monitoring for adequate nutritional intake
2. Teaching high-risk newborn care
3. Assessing for shallow respirations
4. Preventing injury

6 The nurse explains to a parent of a child with cystic fibrosis that the parent should administer the pancre-lipase (Pancrease) how often?

1. Three times daily
2. After each loose stool
3. Upon arising in the morning
4. With each meal and snack

7 A child is noted to have a very short stature, non-pitting lymphedema of the hands and feet, webbed neck, and low posterior hairline. The nurse will expect which of the following diagnoses?

1. Turner's syndrome
2. Down syndrome
3. Marfan's syndrome
4. Klinefelter's syndrome

8 A child with cleft palate begins pulling on his left ear, is irritable, and begins to run a temperature of 102° F. Based on these findings, the nurse would next assess the child for signs of which of the following?

1. Pneumonia
2. Urinary tract infection (UTI)
3. Otitis media
4. Cellulitis

9 The nurse concludes that a male child with a karyotype showing XXY is a candidate for which of the following?

1. Turner's syndrome
2. Klinefelter's syndrome
3. Down syndrome
4. Marfan's syndrome

10 The nurse explains to the mother of an infant born with phenylketonuria (PKU) that the infant requires a low phenylalanine diet to prevent which of the following complications?

1. Irreversible brain damage
2. Kidney failure
3. Blindness
4. Neutropenia

➤ *See pages 482–483 for Answers & Rationales.*

I. RISK FACTORS FOR GENETIC AND DEVELOPMENTAL HEALTH PROBLEMS

    A. Miscarriage: genetic defects cause 60% of spontaneous abortions (miscarriages)

    B. Maternal and paternal influences

        1. Familial: tends to run in certain families or ethnic groups

        2. With each subsequent offspring, the incidence may increase, although each pregnancy should be viewed as an independent event

            a. Endocrine: higher incidence of type 2 diabetes mellitus in Native American families

            b. Cardiac: ventral septal defect has increased reoccurrence among siblings

            c. Hematology: Mediterranean descent increases risk for glucose-6-phosphatase deficiency (G6PD), thalassemia

C. Age

1. Increased age of sperm, ova, or **gametes** (one or two cells created by meiosis)

   a. Parents over 35 years of age; both mother and father increase incidence of abnormal **zygote** (end product of parent cells joined during reproduction) such as trisomy (a condition in which there are three chromosome instead of two in a cell)

   b. **Autosomal** (all chromosomes other than the sex [XX or XY]): dominant disorders such as Marfan's syndrome

2. Adolescent: younger age of mother leads to increased risk

   a. Factors related to hormonal changes

   b. Dietary insufficiency of protein, iron

   c. Risk-taking behaviors: smoking, drugs

D. Nutrition

1. Malnutrition leads to poor cell formation

2. Folic acid deficiency is a known factor in spina bifida

3. Low protein increases risk of congenital heart disease

4. Iron-deficiency anemia and small for gestational age (SGA)

E. Environment

1. Teratogens: interfere with fetal development

   a. Drugs

      1) Tobacco increases incidence of congenital defects

      2) Alcohol exposure leads to fetal alcohol syndrome (FAS)

      3) Drugs, i.e., phenytoin (Dilantin) has a higher incidence of congenital malformation

   b. Radiation leads to increase risk of **nondisjunction** (an abnormal separation) during **meiosis** (two stages of separating to create two gametes)

   c. Infection

      1) Can interfere with fetal development

      2) Rubella leads to increased risk of microcephaly

      3) Cytomegalovirus (CMV) leads to increased risk of optic atrophy

2. Oxygen deprivation

   a. Smoking leads to increased possibility of prematurity

   b. Maternal hypertension can lead to birth complications and cerebral palsy

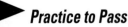

Practice to Pass

What is the rationale for developing a family tree (pedigree) as a part of family planning?

F. Multifactorial (combination of causes for a congenital defect)

1. Combination of all of the above: disruption in utero plus hereditary predisposition, such as cleft lip or palate

2. Genetic predisposition that leads to **malformation** (abnormal development process in utero leading to defect in organ or region of body)

   a. Approximately 5% to 10% of cancers have a **gene** (genetic material [DNA]) marker

   b. Positive human leukocyte antigen-B (HLA-B) allele in children with diabetes mellitus type 1

II. TRISOMY 21 (DOWN SYNDROME)

A. Overview

1. Defined as a chromosome disorder involving the 21st chromosome

2. **Syndrome** (a congenital defect associated with a characteristic set of anomalies) is a predisposition for:

   a. Congenital heart disease: atrial ventricular canal; 40% to 50% have improper development of separate atria and ventricles on left and right, which can cause congestive heart failure (CHF)

   b. Leukemia, 30 times higher incidence

   c. Hypothyroidism, 20 times higher incidence

   d. Hirschsprung's disease, higher incidence

B. Pathophysiology

1. Malformation involves 21st **chromosome** (23 pairs of protein structures consisting of DNA that map out the functions of cells within the body)

   a. **Trisomy**

      1) Nondisjunction: causes 92% to 95% of Down syndrome; zygote contains 3 chromosomes instead of normal pair at chromosome 21; increased incidence with paternal/maternal age

      2) **Mosaicism** (presence of cells from two different genetic materials in the same individual)—causes 1% to 3% of Down syndrome; trisomy occurs during **mitosis** (stages of separation to create a new daughter cell); leads to some normal and abnormal cell lines; milder form of the syndrome

   b. **Translocation** (after a chromosome breaks, a transfer of all or part of a chromosome to another chromosome leading to a severe or fatal defect)

      1) Causes 3–5% of Down syndrome

      2) Zygote has exchanged materials from break in chromosome 21

      3) No increased risk with age, but does have a 5–15% risk of reoccurrence

2. Signs and symptoms

   a. Physical characteristics

      1) Hypotonia: lack of general muscle tone

      2) Hyperflexibility: able to flex joints beyond 180 degrees

      3) Wide space between first and second toe

      4) Transverse palmar crease: (horizontal crease across palm) or plantar crease in foot is present in clients with Down syndrome (see Figure 16-1)

      5) Low-set ears: normal is along an imaginary line from eye to top of ear

      6) Epicanthal folds: folds of skin along external to internal edge of eye

      7) Depressed nasal bridge

      8) High, arched, narrow palate and protruding tongue

   b. Intellectual characteristics

      1) Moderate to severe mental retardation

      2) Emphasis is on concrete and individualized operations

   c. Sensory deficits

      1) Myopia

      2) Hyperopia

      3) Strabismus

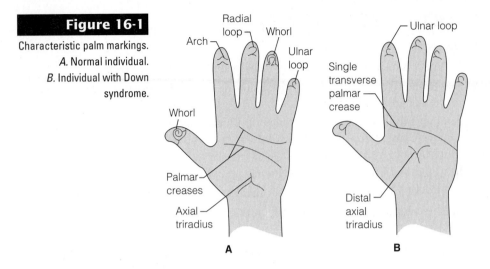

Figure 16-1

Characteristic palm markings.
A. Normal individual.
B. Individual with Down
syndrome.

C. **Nursing assessment**

1. Assessment

    a. Early detection (look for physical attributes in newborn nursery)

    b. Family assessment

       1) Use tool to measure family strengths Apgar, family profile

       2) Assess grieving process: denial, nonacceptance of diagnosis; depression; unable to care for self or others; withdrawal, not speaking with family; anger; being unreasonable with nursing staff

    c. Physical characteristics: muscle strength and flexibility, appearance and distinguishing features, growth and development, sensory status, respiratory and cardiac status for possible complications

2. Diagnostic tests include genetic screen to detect cause of abnormal chromosome 21

    a. Prenatal: amniocentesis to identify chromosome 21; chorionic villi sampling

    b. Postnatal: chromosome 21, detection of trisomy

D. **Nursing management**

1. Development

    a. Goal: promote optimal development; the infant may develop at a slower rate with smaller steps; involve family in setting goals for child

    b. Interventions should be planned according to developmental level

       1) Infant

          a) Cognition: Piaget's sensorimotor: Denver Developmental Screening Test (DDST) or comparable developmental screening tool to determine baseline level; monitor progression; enroll in infant stimulation program

          b) Social: Erickson's trust vs. mistrust: assessment of family, cultural, and feeding interaction to reinforce a positive family bond; refer to social services if suspect abuse/neglect

       2) Toddler

          a) Cognition: Piaget's sensorimotor, continue to promote sensory stimulation; reinforce realistic expectations/goals

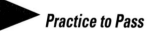

Practice to Pass

Why is it important to understand child development in the client with Down syndrome?

    b) Social: Erickson's autonomy vs. shame and doubt, unsuccessful toilet training can lead to child abuse; anticipatory guidance in relation to temper tantrums

  3) Preschool

    a) Cognition: Piaget's preoperational support; involvement in the child's early education program

    b) Social: Erickson's initiative vs. self-doubt, allow for successes within an integrated school program

  4) School-age

    a) Cognition: will usually remain in Piaget's concrete formations; give simple, visual cues for any teaching during hospitalizations

    b) Social: Erickson's industry vs. inferiority; inclusion programs are beneficial for schools and the child; after school activities

  5) Adolescence: social, Erickson's identity vs. role confusion; must involve in teen activities; information on reproduction and puberty at their level

  6) Adult: job placement; level of living independence; parent or guardianship and living will issues need to be resolved

2. Monitor for respiratory infections (especially in infant); because of large protruding tongue and hypotonia, child has an increased incidence of respiratory complications/compromise

  a. Vital signs: increased respiratory rate, fever

  b. Congestion

  c. Inability to tolerate feedings

  d. Prevent infection

    1) Liquify secretions with humidifier

    2) Use saline and bulb syringe to suction secretions

3. Cardiac defects: monitor for congestive heart failure

  a. Monitor for urine output, minimum 1 to 2 mL/kg/hr

  b. Monitor for edema

  c. Activity and feeding tolerance

  d. Note change in color, cyanosis

4. Postoperative care for the child with heart defect correction

5. Priority nursing diagnoses: Delayed development; Impaired parenting; Risk for ineffective airway clearance; Ineffective tissue perfusion; Decreased cardiac output

Practice to Pass

Why is it important to determine the cause of trisomy 21?

III. TURNER'S SYNDROME

A. Overview

1. Defined as a deletion or abnormal X on chromosome 45; there are a total of 45 chromosomes with 22 somatic pairs and only 1 sex chromosome (45, XO)

2. Syndrome predisposition for:

  a. Hypothyroidism

  b. Aortic coarctation

  c. Renal structure anomalies

  d. Behavior and learning disturbances

B. Pathophysiology

1. Female phenotype with incidence 1:2,500 female births
2. Not clear but thought to be nondisjunction or fragmented X
3. The only monosomy that is viable, yet 99% are spontaneously aborted
4. Signs and symptoms
   a. Newborn
      1) Low posterior hairline
      2) Lymphedema of feet and legs
      3) Webbed neck
   b. Child: short stature; growth slows after age 3; below 3% on growth chart
      1) No development of secondary sex characteristics during puberty
      2) Lack of or nonfunctioning ovaries
      3) Wide-spaced nipples
      4) Short 4th metacarpals
      5) "Shield-like" chest with underdeveloped breasts
      6) Normal intellectual development
      7) Frequent urinary tract infections (UTIs)

C. Nursing assessment

1. Assessment includes any signs or symptoms of renal, cardiac, or thyroid dysfunction
   a. Renal: note any UTIs
   b. Cardiac: aortic coarctation, decrease in lower extremity blood pressure
   c. Hypothyroidism: intolerance to cold, weight gain, lethargy, hair loss, enlarged thyroid gland
2. Early recognition: note physical characteristics in newborn nursery
3. Assessment of family and cultural characteristics, noting strengths of family
4. Additional assessment: growth charts (height and weight), observance of sex characteristics, physical characteristics
5. Diagnostic tests
   a. Labs: blood urea nitrogen (BUN), creatinine (CR) for kidney function
   b. Radiology: voiding cystourethrography (VCUP), cystoscopy
   c. Prenatal genetic testing before birth
   d. Genetic **karyotype** (pictorial analysis of the chromosomes of an individual after birth

D. Nursing management

1. Medications include (as appropriate)
   a. Estrogen prior to age 12 years
   b. Progesterone for secondary sexual characteristics
2. Monitor nonverbal and verbal suggestion of hopelessness
3. Encourage teen support group
4. Encourage verbalization
5. Early detection: note characteristics at birth in order to initiate genetic counseling for family

▶ *Practice to Pass*

How is it possible for the client with Turner's syndrome to not be diagnosed until adolescence?

6. Genetic counseling

   a. Educate on defect, sex-linked chromosome disorder

   b. Family planning; determine if possible the type of malformation

7. Nursing priority diagnoses: Disturbed body image; Ineffective sexuality patterns; Impaired family processes; Risk for imbalanced fluid volume

IV. KLINEFELTER'S SYNDROME

A. Overview

1. Defined as a polysomic **X-linked** (an inherited gene disorder located on X-chromosome) chromosome defect with one or more extra X-chromosomes in the **genotype** of the entire genetic make-up of individual male

2. Associated with increased parental age (maternal or paternal)

3. Incidence: 1:850 male births

B. Pathophysiology

1. During meiosis, nondisjunction of the X- and Y-chromosome causes the disorder

2. With an increase in Xs, there is an increase in mental retardation

3. Usually occurs as presence of extra chromosome 47; additional X and possibly Y chromosomes 47-XXY 48-XXYY, etc.

4. Signs and symptoms

   a. Tall, lean body with disproportionately long legs to trunk

   b. Small or undescended testicles

   c. Gynecomastia

   d. Sterility

   e. Sparse facial hair

   f. Voice does not change at puberty

   g. Normal intellectual development, may have delay in language

   h. Abnormalities

      1) Scoliosis

      2) Dental abnormalities

      3) Cardiac abnormalities

      4) Pulmonary disease

C. Nursing assessment

1. Assessment includes sexual characteristics, growth chart (height and weight), reproductive history

2. Early recognition of physical characteristics that may be delayed until puberty

3. Family and cultural assessment

D. Nursing management

1. Medication, including testosterone

2. Support child and family through diagnosis

   a. Verbalize positive attributes

   b. Demonstrate parenting

   c. Provide anticipatory developmental and safety guidance

   d. Support constructive discipline

   3. Early child development program
      a. Use face position and eye contact
      b. Stimulate cognitive development
      c. Monitor for achievement of physical, cognitive, and psychosocial milestones
   4. Genetic counseling
      a. Family planning
      b. Family support/referral
   5. Encourage teen support
      a. Identify effective ways to express anger/frustration
      b. Identify community resources
      c. Education on sterility
      d. Encourage peer support
   6. High priority nursing diagnoses: Disturbed body image, Impaired family processes, Risk for altered development

▶ *Practice to Pass*

Explain nondisjunction as the cause of Klinefelter's syndrome.

V. PHENYLKETONURIA (PKU)

A. Overview

1. Defined as a metabolic disorder defective in the enzyme phenylalanine hydroxylase that metabolizes phenylalanine, leading to accumulation of phenylalanine and other metabolites
2. Autosomal recessive disorder with **homozygous** presentation (malformation created with autosomal recessive presentation; both chromosomes must be present) (see Figure 16-2)
3. If untreated, will lead to severe mental retardation, seizures, and death
4. Incidence 1:15,000, carrier state can be detected; more common in Caucasians

Figure 16-2

Phenylketonuria: Autosomal Recessive Gene Pattern (Both Chromosomes Present)

A. Carrier father

		D	d
Carrier mother	D	DD	Dd
	d	dD	dd

B. Carrier father

		D	d
Disease mother	D	DD	Dd
	D	DD	Dd

C. Normal father

		d	d
Disease mother	D	Dd	Dd
	D	Dd	Dd

D. Normal father

		d	d
Carrier mother	D	Dd	Dd
	d	dd	dd

DD = Disease   D = disease gene
dD, Dd = Carrier   d = normal gene
dd = No risk

B. Pathophysiology

1. Enzyme phenylalanine hydroxylase is absent, which converts phenylalanine to tyrosine
2. Tyrosine is needed by the body for melanin pigment and for the hormones epinephrine and thyroxin
3. Phenylalanine is responsible for growth; the accumulation of serum phenylalanine leads to irreversible central nervous system damage and mental retardation
4. Increased metabolites in the blood (phenylpyruvic acid and phenylacetic acid) are excreted in urine, causing a musky odor and phenylketonuria (PKU)
5. Signs and symptoms
   a. Musky odor to urine
   b. Neuromuscular development delay
   c. Failure to thrive
   d. Mental retardation by age 6 months
   e. Acute episodes
      1) Possible seizures
      2) Vomiting
      3) Eczematous rashes

C. Nursing assessment

1. Assessment includes growth and development, urine, nutritional status, skin, signs of dehydration
2. Diagnostic tests (done after 24 hours of protein-containing fluids)
   a. Newborn screen: blood specimen taken after 48 hours but within 7 days of birth (if taken earlier, should be repeated at 1–2 weeks of age); phenylalanine levels over 10 to 15 mg/dL leads to brain damage
   b. Electroencephalography (EEG)

D. Nursing management

1. Newest recommendation is to maintain low phenylalanine diet for life
   a. Breastfeeding possible if phenylalanine levels are monitored
   b. Phenylalanine level must be maintained between 2 and 6 mg/dL
   c. Dietary products: Pro-Phree or Phenex-1 are examples of low phenylalanine products
   d. Avoid high-protein foods (especially meat and dairy products), which are highest in phenylalanine; as well as aspartame
   e. Older child can exchange some vegetables, but should maintain minimal meat consumption
   f. Adolescent females and child-bearing women should adhere to diet to prevent congenital anomalies (low birth weight, mental retardation, and microcephaly)
2. Monitor growth and development
   a. Must maintain adequate nutrition with an extremely limited diet
   b. Educate family on importance of maintaining routine primary health care visits for screening and growth assessment
3. Monitor phenylalanine levels
   a. Phenylalanine at dangerous levels if greater than 15 mg/dL

    b. Increased stress, illness, growth spurts will trigger increased phenylalanine levels

    c. Most common manifestation is vomiting leading to dehydration

    d. Maintain seizure precautions

4. Plan for genetic counseling with the family

    a. Genetic screening to assess offspring **carrier** (one affected and one unaffected autosome)

    b. Future pregnancy planning (see Table 16-1 again)

5. Female with PKU at puberty

    a. Counseling on secondary sexual developmental

    b. Counseling on family planning if mother has the disorder

      1) If partner is carrier, 2:4 chance of reoccurrence; if partner is not a carrier, all offspring will be carriers (see Table 16-1 again)

      2) Instruct on strict control of diet if planning pregnancy

6. Priority nursing diagnoses: Risk for injury related to seizure activity and increased phenylalanine levels; Deficient knowledge related to diet therapy; Risk for impaired development related to CNS damage

Practice to Pass

A client and her husband are carriers of the phenylketonuria (PKU) allele. She asks the nurse what the risk is that their children will present with the disease. How should the nurse respond?

VI. HUNTINGTON'S DISEASE

A. Overview

1. Defined as a rare, inherited disease caused by degeneration in the cerebral cortex and the basal ganglia; defect on chromosome 4

2. An autosomal dominant disease with **heterozygous** (only one abnormal autosomal has to be present) presentation (see Figure 16-3)

3. Usually evident between 25 and 55 years of age

4. 5/100,000 occurrence, occurs in all ethnic groups, life expectancy about 10 years

5. Also called Huntington's chorea

B. Pathophysiology

1. Degeneration in the cerebral cortex and basal ganglia causes a deficient inhibitory neurotransmitter system and neurotransmitters are lost; especially gamma-aminobutyric acid (GABA)

2. GABA is an inhibitory transmitter of the central nervous system (CNS) that inhibits specific target pathways to slow increased activity in these pathways

    a. A deficiency of GABA causes increased neural excitation

    b. Associated with epilepsy, anxiety disorders, depression

Figure 16-3

Huntington's Disease: Autosomal Dominant Gene Pattern (Only One Chromosome Present)

A. Normal father

		d	d
Disease	D	Dd	Dd
mother	d	dd	dd

B. Disease father

		D	d
Disease	D	DD	Dd
mother	d	dD	dd

DD, Dd, dD = Disease   D = disease gene
dd = No risk   d = normal gene

     c. Receptors are concentrated in two areas

       1) Limbic system, controlling emotional behaviors

       2) Locus cerulues, controlling arousal

3. An imbalance in basal ganglia occurs between dopamine and acetylcholine, and GABA

     a. Acetylcholine is decreased

     b. Dopamine not affected (unlike Parkinson's disease)

     c. **Choreiform** (rapid and jerky body motion that is involuntary) movements result from deficient neurotransmitter inhibition

4. Degeneration in cerebral cortex leads to progressive increase in labile emotions caused by decrease in GABA

     a. Violent behavior changes

     b. Dementia

5. Alleles inherited from the father results in onset later in life than if inherited from the mother

6. Other physiologic changes

     a. Lesions may occur in the putamen, corpus striatum, and thalamus

     b. Frontal lobes of brain atrophy, enlarge, and change the lateral ventricle structure

     c. Neurons in certain areas of the brain are reduced

7. Symptoms begin between the age of 25 to 55 years

8. Signs and symptoms

     a. Movement

       1) Choreiform movements

       2) Athetosis: slower movements than choreiform

     b. Intellect: progressive degeneration, impaired memory and judgment

     c. Severe dementia

       1) Impulsiveness

       2) Paranoia, delusions, and hallucinations

       3) Neurosis

       4) Verbal and emotional outbursts; irritability

       5) Suicidal tendency

       6) Personality changes

C. Nursing assessment

1. Assessment includes memory, ability to follow commands, ability to perform activities of daily living (ADLs) and degree of movement problems, mental status, history of recent changes in personality and level of consciousness, ability to stay on-task

2. Diagnostic tests

     a. Diagnosis made by clinical manifestations and family history

     b. No prognostic lab studies to treat or predict the disease

     c. Positive gene marker on DNA testing for conclusive diagnosis

     d. Magnetic resonance imagery (MRI) to assess brain involvement

D. Nursing management

1. Medications

    a. Antipsychotics such as phenothiazines and butyrophenones

    b. Antidepressants

2. Genetic counseling

    a. Autosomal dominance needs only one affected autosome (see Figure 16–3)

    1) 2:4 reoccurrence if one parent has Huntington's

    2) 3:4 reoccurrence if both parents have Huntington's

    b. Ethical considerations in testing gene presence

    1) The variance in age of presentation

    2) Currently no cure

    3) Family planning issues

3. Nutrition

    a. Establish baseline and monitor for weight loss; increase calories and protein to support increased activity level

    b. Maintain good oral hygiene

    c. Impaired swallowing could lead to aspiration

    1) Maintain in upright position during eating

    2) Give small amounts at one time

    3) Give thickened liquids

4. Long-term care

    a. Monitor family for issues related to behavior control

    b. Suicide precautions may be necessary

    c. Drug and alcohol abuse are common and should be monitored

    d. Institutionalization when home care no longer possible

5. Controversial therapies: fetal brain tissue transplants have been moderately successful, but ethical issues exist related to source of transplant

6. Future therapies

    a. Gene replacement therapy: replaces the abnormal gene on chromosome 4

    b. No medication available to cure the disease

7. Priority nursing diagnoses: Deficient knowledge, Imbalanced nutrition: less than body requirements, Risk for aspiration, Ineffective family coping

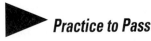

Practice to Pass

What are the ethical implications of early diagnosis by identifying gene marker 4 in offspring of the client with Huntington's chorea?

VII. MARFAN'S SYNDROME

A. Overview

1. Defined as a connective tissue disorder caused by atrophy of neurons in specific areas of brain; involves chromosome 15

2. An autosomal dominant disorder with heterozygous presentation; no carrier status

3. A **congenital** (present since birth) disorder with 25% spontaneous mutations

4. Incidence 1:10,000

B. Pathophysiology

1. A mutation occurs of frillin-1, a connective tissue protein that is found in body tissue

> **2.** Defect is in the elastic fibers of connective tissues causing long, thin extremities; hyperextendable joints; and spinal deformities

3. Associated defects

   a. Aortic aneurysm: most common cause of early death; weakness within the aorta leads to dilation and rupture

   b. Optic lens disorders: dislocated optic lens, retinal detachment, cataracts, glaucoma, and myopia

4. Signs and symptoms

   a. Tall, lean body with thin fingers (arachnodactyly) and winged scapula

   b. Vision disturbances

   c. Musculoskeletal deformities: pectus excavatum, curvature of thoracic spine, hyperextensibility of joints, scoliosis

5. Often associated with sports-related cardiac arrest

C. Nursing assessment

1. Assessment includes growth and development, proportioned body, visual examination, range of motion, scoliosis screening, auscultation of abdomen for pulse, blood pressure, cardiac status

2. Diagnostic tests: genetic screening, MRI if aneurysm suspected

D. Nursing management

1. Medications include beta blockers for cardiac problems

2. Community and school education

   a. Support automated external defibrillator (AED) implementation

   b. Health physical prior to participation in athletic events

   c. Scoliosis screening

3. Sensory: note any change in vision and encourage yearly eye exams

> **4.** Cardiac

   a. Monitor cardiac status: auscultation of abdomen, pulse, vital signs

   b. Aortic valve replacement may be indicated

   c. Maintain blood pressure within normal limits

5. Genetic counseling

   a. Discuss family planning and risk of recurrence

   b. Parent and child education on risks for associated anomalies

6. Priority nursing diagnoses: Risk for decreased cardiac output; Disturbed sensory perception: visual; Disturbed body image; and Deficient knowledge related to dysrhythmias

VIII. ALBINISM

A. Overview

1. Defined as a lack of skin pigmentation caused by the absence of tyrosinase, which is needed for melanin synthesis

2. An autosomal recessive chromosomal disorder with homozygous presentation

3. Incidence is 1:17,000 individuals

    4. Two types

        a. Type I: oculocutaneous

        b. Type II: less pigmented

B. Pathophysiology

    1. Autosomal recessive disorder; both parents are carriers

        a. 25% chance of mutation

        b. 25% chance not carrying gene

        c. 50% chance of having carrier status

        d. Risk is unchanged with each subsequent pregnancy

    2. Individuals are deficient in tyrosinase, an enzyme needed to synthesize melanin, but have a normal number of melanocytes

    3. Type I: *oculocutaneous*

        a. Defect in tyrosinase

            1) Unable to convert tyrosine to dopa

            2) Results in lack of melanin synthesis

        b. Associated visual problems

            1) Foveal hypoplasia can occur; abnormal retinal development because of lack of pigment

            2) Transillumination: the iris lacks sufficient pigment to screen light coming into eye

            3) Associated vision disturbances: nystagmus, strabismus, myopia, hyperopia, photophobia

    4. Type II: *less pigmented*

        a. May have slight pigmentation

        b. No ocular or integument variations

    5. Syndromes associated with albinism; Hermansky-Pudlak syndrome (HPS)

        a. Syndrome of albinism including bleeding tendencies

        b. Can include lung (pulmonary fibrosis) and bowel (inflammatory bowel disease)

        c. Bleeding problems result from malfunction of platelets and include nosebleeds, bruising or severe bleed during surgery or childbirth

        d. Client will have normal results in prothrombin time (PT), partial thromboplastin time (PTT); may lack Von Willebrand factor (less than 70% occurence, higher risk of bleed)

    6. Signs and symptoms

        a. Lack of pigment in skin, hair, eyes

            1) Skin (pale or pink)

            2) Hair (white or yellow)

            3) Eyes (light-colored or pink)

        b. Vision assessment

            1) Low vision 20/50

            2) Legally blind 20/200

            3) VEP: visually evoked potential for young infant

C. **Nursing assessment**

1. Nursing assessment includes visual exam and inspection of color in the skin, hair, eyes, ability to read because of nystagmus; any extraocular eye movement

2. Diagnostic test: none

D. **Nursing management**

1. Symptomatic care

   a. Screen vision

   b. Avoid sun exposure; use maximum sunscreen

   c. Wear sunglasses

   d. Frequent checks for potential melanoma

   e. Corrective visual wear/aids with dark lenses

2. Genetic counseling

   a. Teach parent/child potential for future children with albinism

   b. Genetic screening of family

3. Cultural competency

   a. Dispel myths related to mixed ethnicity or inbreeding as the cause

   b. Educate about genetics as the cause

4. Priority nursing diagnoses: Deficient knowledge; Risk for impaired skin integrity; Risk for impaired sensory perception

IX. CYSTIC FIBROSIS (CF)

A. **Overview**

1. Defined as an autosomal recessive chromosome disorder with exocrine gland dysfunction, which manifests in multiple body systems

2. Multisystem involvement: respiratory, pancreatic, liver, gastrointestinal (GI)

   a. Severity of symptoms varies on an individual basis

   b. Goal is to increase longevity

3. Incidence is 1:2,000; affects mostly Caucasians

B. **Pathophysiology**

1. Homozygous presentation: chromosome 7 defect affecting single gene on long arm of chromosome that encodes for the cystic fibrosis transmembrane regulator (CFTR)

2. Primary feature is lack of function of chloride channels: failure to open or absence of channels

3. Defective protein inhibits transport of sodium chloride, leading to an increased viscosity of secretions and an increase of sodium chloride (NaCl) in sweat

4. System pathophysiology

   a. Respiratory tract

      1) Decreased ciliary function and increased thickness of mucous secretions occurs

      2) Decreased function of alveoli and alveolar plugs leads to repeat infections and chronic obstructive pulmonary disease (COPD)

         a) COPD leads to cor pulmonale (right-sided heart failure caused by respiratory problems) and chronic hypoxemia

        b) *Pseudomonas aeruginosa* and *Staphylococcus aureus* are common organisms that resist antibiotics, leading to drug-resistant pneumonia

    3) Sinus tract disease with polyps and chronic thick mucus

  b. Gastrointestinal

    1) Thick secretions block the ducts leading from pancreas to duodenum

    2) Malabsorption occurs because digestive enzymes don't reach food

        a) Predominantly affects fats and fat-soluble vitamins A, D, K, E

        b) Leads to malnutrition if untreated

  c. Pancreas: damage to Islets of Langerhans causes an increased incidence of type 1 diabetes mellitus

  d. Liver: biliary obstruction leads to cirrhosis and gallbladder disease

5. Signs and symptoms

  a. Respiratory

    1) Frequent pneumonias (methicillin-resistant *staphylcoccus aureus* [MRSA] leads to high mortality rate)

    2) Productive cough with thick, foul-smelling secretions

    3) Clubbing of nails from chronic hypoxemia

    4) Persistent sinusitis for the adolescent

    5) COPD leads to chronic high CO_2 level

  b. Nutrition

    1) Large protruding abdomen

    2) Infant: failure to thrive

    3) Older child: osteomalacia (rickets), abnormal clotting times, and malnourishment

  c. Newborn: ilcus related to thick mucus from meconium

  d. Infant

    1) Rectal prolapse because of thick stools

    2) Steatorrhea (foul-smelling stool containing undigested fat)

  e. Older child

    1) Diabetes-related disorders if diabetic ketoacidosis unchecked

    2) Delayed secondary sexual characteristics

  f. Young adult

    1) Female: thick cervical secretions lead to decreased fertility

    2) Males: sterile or minimal sperm production related to blocked seminal ducts

C. Nursing assessment

  1. Nursing assessment includes: respiratory status, vital signs, auscultation of lung sounds, abdominal size, stool characteristics, sexual characteristics, reproductive history, analysis of sputum, daily weight, and growth chart

  2. Diagnostic tests

    a. Classic NaCl sweat test (2 to 5 times greater than normal)

    b. Newborn screen: decreased trypsin (pancreatic enzyme) level in stool indicates CF; normal is positive in small amounts (screen is required in most states)

    c. Prenatal and carrier status screening is available

    d. Arterial blood gases (ABGs) or pulse oximetry

      e. Chest x-ray (CXR)

      f. Pulmonary function studies (PFS)

D. Nursing management

  1. Medications

      a. Bronchodilators

      b. Antibiotics as needed

      c. Corticosteroids

      d. Dornase alfa (Pulmozyme) to reduce mucus viscosity (aerosol)

      e. Annual immunizations

      f. Pancrelipase (Pancrease) by mouth

  2. Nursing interventions

      a. Respiratory

        1) Administer oxygen (O_2) as needed: use caution with O_2 administration; chronically high CO_2 can alter respiratory drive

        2) Assess respiratory status

        3) Teach proper administration of inhalers and O_2: separate corticosteroids by 20 to 30 minutes from other inhalers; administer the corticosteroids last

        4) Monitor for side effects of medications, particularly tachycardia

        5) Increase fluids to liquefy secretions

        6) Chest physiotherapy: postural drainage and percussion/vibration to loosen and clear secretions; flutter device and huffing procedure used to assist in increasing expectoration; perform after bronchodilation

        7) Treat pulmonary infections; there is increased risk for antibiotic-resistant microorganisms; it is important to monitor therapeutic response

      b. Pancreas

        1) Pancreatic enzyme replacements such as pancrelipase (Pancrease) must be given before each meal or snack

        2) Note stool characteristics (steatorrhea) to determine absorption

        3) Assess growth while hospitalized; monitor daily weights at same time and using same scale

  3. Chronic degenerative disease

      a. Lung/heart transplant is current trend to treat irreversible lung/heart disease

      b. Developmental issues

        1) Support adolescents who struggle with sexuality and chronic illness

        2) Monitor parental characteristics of overprotection

        3) Discuss end-of-life issues as they arise

  4. Genetic counseling

      a. Provide anticipatory guidance to parents of a child with CF regarding future pregnancies

      b. Encourage genetic counseling for the client with CF

      c. Update client on therapies for gene replacement as they become available

  5. Priority nursing diagnoses: Failure to thrive r/t malabsorption; Impaired growth and development r/t chronic illness; Impaired gas exchange r/t increased mucus secretions; Risk for infection r/t decreased alveolar function; Impaired family processes r/t chronic disease; Deficient knowledge r/t care of child with CF

X. CLEFT LIP/PALATE

A. Overview

1. Cleft lip is defined as a vertical opening (cleft) in the upper lip
2. Cleft palate is defined as a fissure in the roof of the mouth creating a passageway between the mouth and nose
3. Is the most common craniofacial malformation
4. Cleft lip and palate can be:
   a. Together or separate
   b. Unilateral or bilateral
   c. Complete or incomplete
5. The cause is **multifactorial** and is associated with various syndromes (i.e., Pierre Robin's)

B. Pathophysiology

1. Interruption in development, leading to lack of fusion or rupture of palate or lip
   a. 6 to 8 weeks gestation for cleft lip (CL)
   b. 8 to 12 weeks gestation for cleft palate (CP)
2. Cleft lip may involve external nares, nasal cartilage, nasal septum, and alveolar process
3. Cleft palate may involve uvula and soft palate
4. Signs and symptoms include visual defect, crusting on cleft, swallowing air, vomiting, difficulty sucking, expulsion of formula through nose (cleft palate), aspiration, difficulty with speech, otitis media

C. Nursing assessment

1. Cleft lip apparent at birth: unilateral, bilateral, or complete
2. Cleft palate needs more thorough assessment in newborn
   a. Biuvula or split uvula is indicative of a cleft
   b. Note any feeding difficulties; is at high risk for aspiration
3. Overall assessment: nutritional status, abdominal distention, lung sounds (aspiration), signs of infection at site, weight, speech and dental (when older), hearing

D. Nursing management

1. Cleft lip: surgical repair recommended and can occur as a young infant (approximately 2 months)
2. Cleft palate
   a. Team approach with stages of repair occurring as young infant through adolescence
   b. Coordination of team
      1) Orthodontist: oral-pharyngeal development and dentition
      2) Speech and language therapist: develop sucking and treat altered speech
      3) Otolaryngologist: assesses and treats chronic otitis related to abnormal connection between Eustachian tube and posterior oropharynx
      4) Audiologist: chronic otitis leads to hearing loss
      5) Plastic surgeon: repairs craniofacial anomalies
      6) Social worker: monitors financial and emotional needs

3. Preoperative nursing interventions

   a. Nutrition

> **1)** Assess adequate intake

   2) Encourage parent to provide modified nipple or supplemental tube feeding

   3) Assess if child can adequately suck

> **4)** Monitor to prevent aspiration of formula or breast milk; feed in sitting position

   b. Oropharyngeal (CP)

   1) Understand and educate family on orthodontic hardware for the infant/child

   2) Monitor effectiveness of speech therapy for coordinating speech and adequate sucking

   c. Hearing

   1) Frequent monitoring for hearing loss

   2) Listen to family for reports of delayed or altered speech

4. Postoperative nursing interventions

   a. Prevent damage to surgical site

> **1)** Child with repair of cleft lip is not to be placed prone

> **2)** Keep objects away from mouth

> **3)** Elbow restraints: monitor for skin breakdown to area restrained

   4) Educate family to keep child's hands away from face if restraints off

   5) Cleanse area with prescribed solution, usually peroxide (H_2O_2) and sterile water (H_2O); follow current agency protocol

   6) Lubricate lip with antibiotic ointment

   7) Devices such as Logan bar or bow to relieve tension on incision site

   b. Monitor for adequate fluid/nutrition intake, weigh daily

   c. Monitor for incisional pain

5. Growth and development

> **a.** Monitor family for positive bonding with infant

   1) Important to bring child with cleft to parent soon after delivery

   2) Connect families early with support group and repair team

   b. Monitor child for positive self-image

   c. Genetic counseling for familial tendencies

6. Priority nursing diagnoses: Imbalanced nutrition: less than body requirements r/t poor sucking ability; Impaired parenting r/t child with a disability, Pain r/t surgical correction; Risk for aspiration r/t open communication within oropharyngeal cavity

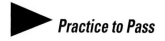

Practice to Pass

Why is it important to assess for a biuvula in the newborn?

Case Study

A 6-month-old male infant is admitted to the nursing unit with the diagnosis of recurrent pneumonia. On admission, the client has a respiratory rate of 50, heart rate of 170, and a temperature of 102°F. The client is retracting substernally with bilateral wheezes and rhonchi. The mother states that this is her son's third admission since birth for pneumonia. She also mentions that he hasn't been gaining weight like her older child had at 6 months of age.

1. How is this consistent with cystic fibrosis?
2. What tests could be ordered to confirm the diagnosis?
3. What nursing interventions could alleviate the respiratory distress?
4. What is the rationale behind the poor weight gain?
5. What teaching needs to be done with the family about the respiratory component of cystic fibrosis before the child goes home? What genetic counseling should occur for the family?

For suggested responses, see page 539.

POSTTEST

❶ A 16-year-old client comes to the pediatrician's office for a physical examination, which is required to join the high school basketball team. He is a tall, lean male with long, slender fingers. His mother states that the first game is next week, and she is concerned about his health because she has heard about high school athletes dying on the basketball court during games. The nurse interprets that which of the following is the congenital anomaly and associated life-threatening defect that the parent could be referring to?

1. Down syndrome and atrial-ventricular (AV) canal
2. Marfan's syndrome and aortic dilation
3. Phenylketonuria (PKU) and seizures
4. Turner's syndrome and hypothyroidism

❷ The nurse should plan to teach the parent of a client with albinism about which preventive health care measure?

1. Ulcerative colitis diet
2. Use of a high-SPF sunblock
3. Hair loss monitoring
4. Monitor for growth retardation

❸ A woman who has just been diagnosed with Huntington's disease asks the nurse if her children are likely to develop this disorder also. What is the best response by the nurse?

1. If the mother alone has the disease, they have a 50% chance of inheriting the same disorder
2. Both parents must have the disease for the offspring to inherit the same disorder
3. Disorder is a spontaneous disruption of the neurotransmitters with no inheritance principles
4. If the mother has the disease, they have a 1:4 chance of inheriting the same disorder

4 The symptoms in a client with cystic fibrosis have progressed rapidly over the past two years. Presently, the client is in the Emergency Department with significant respiratory distress. What physical characteristics should the nurse expect to see in the client? Select all that apply.

1. Low-set ears and long slender fingers
2. Increased anteroposterior chest diameter (barrel chest)
3. Clubbed fingernails
4. Bibasilar crackles on auscultation
5. Chronic cough

5 The nurse explains to parents of an infant with cystic fibrosis that the foul-smelling, frothy characteristic of the stool results from the presence of large amounts of which of the following?

1. Sodium and chloride
2. Undigested fat
3. Semidigested carbohydrates
4. Lipase, trypsin, and amylase

6 A client with cystic fibrosis (CF) is in obvious respiratory distress with circumoral cyanosis. What factor should the nurse consider when administering oxygen with a PRN order for this client?

1. Children with cystic fibrosis respond poorly to oxygen administration
2. Administration of oxygen could decrease respiratory drive
3. Higher the flow rate of oxygen, the better the child will breathe
4. Oxygen should only be administered via facemask

7 The parents of a baby with Down syndrome are seeking genetic counseling. The baby has been identified as having trisomy of chromosome 21. The nurse would include which information when counseling the clients about the risk of conceiving another child with trisomy 21?

1. Risk increases with maternal age
2. There is no risk of a second child with Down syndrome
3. Risk is 1 in 4 since there is already a child with Down syndrome
4. Age of the father is a bigger risk factor than the mother's age

8 Nursing care of an adolescent client with Klinefelter's syndrome focuses mainly on which of the following nursing diagnoses?

1. Alteration in fluid and electrolyte balance
2. Disturbed body image
3. High risk for complications
4. Impaired physical mobility

9 A 16-year-old girl comes to the clinic because she has not begun to menstruate like all of her friends. She is short and shows no signs of secondary sex characteristics. She reports swollen hands and feet, has skin folds in the neck and has a low hairline. She asks the nurse what to do about her concerns. What is the best response by the nurse?

1. "Don't worry. Many girls are late developing. Just wait a little longer."
2. "There must be something really wrong considering what you have told me. Let's see what the doctor says."
3. "We recommend that girls with problems like yours have chromosomal studies to find the reason and begin treatment."
4. "You have a severe chromosomal problem. There is no treatment but you could consider yourself lucky not to get periods."

10 The nurse would use which explanation in telling the mother of a child who is postoperative for cleft lip repair about the importance of keeping the elbow restraints in place?

1. "Your child could pull out his or her nasogastric tube."
2. "Your child might dislodge his or her intravenous catheter."
3. "Your child may aspirate formula."
4. "Your child may disrupt the lip suture line."

➤ *See pages 483–485 for Answers & Rationales.*

POSTTEST

ANSWERS & RATIONALES

Pretest

1 **Answer: 2** An individual with Huntington's develops chorea (rapid, jerky movements) and might have difficulty swallowing liquids, which could lead to the potential of aspiration of thin liquids. Death usually results from aspiration pneumonia or another infection. **Cognitive Level:** Application **Client Need:** Physiological Integrity: Physiological Adaptation **Integrated Process:** Teaching/Learning **Content Area:** Adult Health: Neurological **Strategy:** Eliminate the wrong options after identifying the risks reduced by thickening liquids. **Reference:** LeMone, P., & Burke, K. (2008). *Medical-surgical nursing: Critical thinking in client care* (4th ed.). Upper Saddle River, NJ: Pearson/Prentice Hall, pp. 1642–1643.

2 **Answer: 4** The child with Down syndrome will go through the same first developmental stage of trust vs. mistrust, only at a slower rate. Therefore, the nurse should concentrate on developing a bond between the primary caregiver and the child. **Cognitive Level:** Application **Client Need:** Health Promotion and Maintenance **Integrated Process:** Nursing Process: Assessment **Content Area:** Foundational Sciences: Growth and Development **Strategy:** Specific knowledge of the developmental stages is needed to answer the question. Note that the client is an infant to pick the first developmental stage, which sets the stage for how the infant will relate to the world after birth. **Reference:** Porth, C. M. (2005). *Pathophysiology: Concepts of altered health states* (7th ed.). Philadelphia, PA: Lippincott Williams & Wilkins, p. 142.

3 **Answer: 1** The connective tissue disorder of Marfan's syndrome can include aortic insufficiency, which can lead to aortic rupture or dissection, which is the primary cause of death for the disorder. Retinal detachment and hyperextensible joints are not life threatening. Seizure activity represents a neurological problem. **Cognitive Level:** Application **Client Need:** Physiological Integrity: Physiological Adaptation **Integrated Process:** Nursing Process: Assessment **Content Area:** Child Health **Strategy:** The critical words in the question are *potentially lethal*. Evaluate two options easily because they are not life threatening and then recall that Marfan's disease is a connective tissue disorder rather than a neurological disorder to choose between the remaining two. **Reference:** Porth, C. M. (2005). *Pathophysiology: Concepts of altered health states* (7th ed.). Philadelphia, PA: Lippincott Williams & Wilkins, p. 138.

4 **Answer: 2** Albinism type I is an autosomal recessive disorder. Both parents must be carriers for the child to inherit the congenital disorder. **Cognitive Level:** Application **Client Need:** Physiological Integrity: Physiological Adaptation **Integrated Process:** Teaching/Learning **Content Area:** Foundational Sciences: Growth and Development **Strategy:** Use general nursing knowledge to answer the question. Recall that when options are opposites, one of them must be incorrect. **Reference:** Porth, C. M. (2005). *Pathophysiology: Concepts of altered health states* (7th ed.). Philadelphia, PA: Lippincott Williams & Wilkins, p. 137.

5 **Answer: 1** The infant with cleft lip is unable to create an adequate seal for sucking. The child is at risk for inadequate nutritional intake as well as aspiration (not shallow respirations as in option 3). Although newborn care (option 2) and preventing injury (option 4) are general nursing interventions for all clients, the priority need is one that meets basic physiological needs. **Cognitive Level:** Application **Client Need:** Physiological Integrity: Physiological Adaptation **Integrated Process:** Nursing Process: Implementation **Content Area:** Foundational Sciences: Growth and Development **Strategy:** Consider Maslow's hierarchy when prioritizing. Recall that physiological needs are a priority before safety needs. **Reference:** Ball, J., & Bindler, R. (2006). *Child health nursing: Partnering with children & families*. Upper Saddle River, NJ: Pearson/Prentice Hall, p. 1095.

6 **Answer: 4** Pancrelipase should be given with each meal and snack so it is available before food enters the duodenum. Pancrelipase, a drug that is a pancreatic enzyme, allows a diet with normal amounts of fat and protein. The dose and product type are individualized for each client. The drug is not given to treat loose stools (option 2). It needs to be administered more than once per day (option 3). Option 1 is partially correct in that meals are eaten 3 times per day, but this option is nonspecific as to timing with food and does not account for intake of snacks. **Cognitive Level:** Application **Client Need:** Physiological Integrity: Pharmacological and Parenteral Therapies **Integrated Process:** Teaching/Learning **Content Area:** Child Health **Strategy:** Recall the role of the enzyme in aiding digestion to help focus on the option that is most accurate. **Reference:** Porth, C. M. (2005). *Pathophysiology: Concepts of altered health states* (7th ed.). Philadelphia, PA: Lippincott Williams & Wilkins, p. 708.

7 **Answer: 1** Short stature, nonpitting lymphedema of the hands and feet, webbed neck, and low posterior hairline are the key assessment features in Turner's syndrome. If the child is diagnosed early in age, proper treatment with growth hormone can be offered to the family. This description does not fit Down syndrome (option 2), Marfan's syndrome (option 3), or Klinefelter's syndrome (option 4).
Cognitive Level: Application **Client Need:** Physiological Integrity: Physiological Adaptation **Integrated Process:** Nursing Process: Assessment **Content Area:** Child Health **Strategy:** The question describes one of these genetic disorders. If guessing, eliminate the ones known to be incorrect. Otherwise, specific nursing knowledge is needed to answer the question. **Reference:** Porth, C. M. (2005). *Pathophysiology: Concepts of altered health states* (7th ed.). Philadelphia, PA: Lippincott Williams & Wilkins, p. 143.

8 **Answer: 3** The child with cleft palate has communication between the oropharnyx and the Eustachian tube. The child is at high risk for recurrent ear infections. The symptoms described are common with otitis media regardless of the congenital abnormality.
Cognitive Level: Analysis **Client Need:** Physiological Integrity: Physiological Adaptation **Integrated Process:** Nursing Process: Assessment **Content Area:** Child Health **Strategy:** Read the symptoms carefully. The phrase *pulling on his left ear* is a clue to the location of the infection. Recall also the pathophysiology of cleft palate in making a selection. **Reference:** Porth, C. M. (2005). *Pathophysiology: Concepts of altered health states* (7th ed.). Philadelphia, PA: Lippincott Williams & Wilkins, p. 1333.

9 **Answer: 2** The child with Klinefelter's has an extra X chromosome. The karyotype shows the pictorial analysis of the total chromosomes of a cell (or an individual).
Cognitive Level: Application **Client Need:** Physiological Integrity: Physiological Adaptation **Integrated Process:** Nursing Process: Analysis **Content Area:** Child Health **Strategy:** Recall that *karyo-* refers to the nucleus of a cell. In this question, if the word karyotype is unfamiliar, relate your answer to the extra X chromosome. **Reference:** Porth, C. M. (2005) *Pathophysiology: Concepts of altered health states* (7th ed.). Philadelphia, PA: Lippincott Williams & Wilkins, p. 144.

10 **Answer: 1** The child with PKU must maintain a strict low-phenylalanine diet to prevent central nervous system damage, seizures, and eventual death. The child lacks phenylalanine hydroxylase, an enzyme needed to metabolize phenylalanine.
Cognitive Level: Application **Client Need:** Physiological Integrity: Physiological Adaptation **Integrated Process:**

Teaching/Learning **Content Area:** Child Health **Strategy:** Recall that PKU tests are routinely done on all newborns and that damage is neurological. Otherwise specific nursing knowledge is needed to answer this question. **Reference:** Ball, J., & Bindler, R. (2008). *Pediatric nursing: Caring for children* (4th ed.). Upper Saddle River, NJ: Pearson/Prentice Hall, p. 1247.

Posttest

1 **Answer: 2** The physical characteristics of the client are consistent with Marfan's syndrome. This connective tissue disorder can involve the heart and specifically the aorta and can lead to a fatal aortic aneurysm. Clients with Down syndrome are typically not tall and lean; they tend to be shorter in height and of average build. Clients with PKU have an inborn error of metabolism and require a low phenylalanine diet. Turner's syndrome is a chromosomal anomaly with the absence of one X chromosome, and hypothyroidism is a disorder in which the thyroid gland has less than adequate function in producing T3 and T4 for bodily metabolism.
Cognitive Level: Analysis **Client Need:** Physiological Integrity: Physiological Adaptation **Integrated Process:** Nursing Process: Assessment **Content Area:** Child Health **Strategy:** Consider the physical characteristics given in the question. After you have identified the disorder, what is the life-threatening aspect? **Reference:** Porth, C. M. (2005). *Pathophysiology: Concepts of altered health states* (7th ed.). Philadelphia, PA: Lippincott Williams & Wilkins, pp. 137–138.

2 **Answer: 2** Without melanin production, the child with albinism is at risk for severe sunburns. Maximum sun protection should be taken, including use of hats, long sleeves, minimal time in the sun, and high-SPF sunblock, to prevent any problems. It is unnecessary to alter the diet because there is not an associated risk of ulcerative colitis (option 1); hair loss (option 3) and growth retardation (option 4) are not of concern.
Cognitive Level: Application **Client Need:** Safe, Effective Care Environment: Safety and Infection Control **Integrated Process:** Nursing Process: Planning **Content Area:** Child Health **Strategy:** This question asks about preventive health maintenance. Eliminate the options that do not apply to albinism. **Reference:** LeMone, P., & Burke, K. (2008). *Medical-surgical nursing: Critical thinking in client care* (4th ed.). Upper Saddle River, NJ: Pearson/Prentice Hall, pp. 426–427.

3 **Answer: 1** Huntington's is an autosomal dominant disorder needing only one chromosome to be present. The risk of transmission of the chromosome 4 defect is 2:4 incidences if one parent has the disease, meaning 2

children will have the disorder and 2 will be normal. If both parents have it, 3 of the 4 children will have the disease and 1 will be normal.
Cognitive Level: Analysis **Client Need:** Health Promotion and Maintenance **Integrated Process:** Nursing Process: Assessment **Content Area:** Child Health **Strategy:** The core issue of the question is the risk of developing a disease with an autosomal dominant disorder. Use principles of genetics and recall that this is an autosomal dominant disorder to make a selection. **Reference:** Porth, C. M. (2005). *Pathophysiology: Concepts of altered health states* (7th ed.). Philadelphia, PA: Lippincott Williams & Wilkins, p. 137.

4 **Answers: 2, 3, 4, 5** The child with cystic fibrosis is chronically hypoxic because of progression of chronic obstructive pulmonary disease (COPD). Clubbing of nail beds occurs after six months of inadequate oxygenation. The client will have a chronic cough, bibasilar crackles, barrel chest, and possibly signs of right-sided heart failure. Low-set ears are seen with Down syndrome, and long slender fingers with Marfan's syndrome.
Cognitive Level: Application **Client Need:** Physiological Integrity: Physiological Adaptation **Integrated Process:** Nursing Process: Assessment **Content Area:** Child Health **Strategy:** Look for respiratory system findings. Do not choose abnormalities for other syndromes. **Reference:** LeMone, P., & Burke, K. (2008). *Medical-surgical nursing: Critical thinking in client care* (4th ed.). Upper Saddle River, NJ: Pearson/Prentice Hall, p. 1340–1342.

5 **Answer: 2** The client with cystic fibrosis poorly absorbs fats because of the thick secretions blocking the pancreatic duct. The lack of natural pancreatic enzyme leads to poor absorption of predominantly fats in the duodenum. Foul-smelling frothy stool is termed steatorrhea.
Cognitive Level: Application **Client Need:** Physiological Integrity: Physiological Adaptation **Integrated Process:** Teaching/Learning **Content Area:** Child Health **Strategy:** Recall that in CF, the pancreatic insufficiency results in digestive problems, causing the stool described in the question. Consider the role of the exocrine pancreas in digestion. Do not be fooled by an option with pancreatic-sounding names. **Reference:** LeMone, P., & Burke, K. (2008). *Medical-surgical nursing: Critical thinking in client care* (4th ed.). Upper Saddle River, NJ: Pearson/Prentice Hall, pp. 1340–1342.

6 **Answer: 2** Clients with CF develop COPD and chronic carbon dioxide retention (hypercapnia), becoming dependent on hypoxia to drive the respiratory system. Too much oxygen will decrease the body's desire to breathe. Therefore, the nurse should monitor the respiratory status/rate of a client with cystic fibrosis for potential apnea.

Cognitive Level: Application **Client Need:** Physiological Integrity: Basic Care and Comfort **Integrated Process:** Nursing Process: Implementation **Content Area:** Child Health **Strategy:** Consider the chronic obstruction with CF and apply knowledge of safe oxygen administration. **Reference:** Porth, C. M. (2005). *Pathophysiology: Concepts of altered health states* (7th ed.). Philadelphia, PA: Lippincott Williams & Wilkins, p. 706.

7 **Answer: 1** The risk of Down syndrome increases with the age of the mother since the oocytes have been formed since birth. The risk is 1 in 1300 at 25 years and increases to 1 in 30 at 45 years. Since males produce sperm throughout their life, the paternal age is not thought to be a factor. If the child had translocation of the 21st chromosome, there would be no relation to maternal age but a high recurrence risk if the mother was a carrier. This information is important to disclose to the family in genetic counseling.
Cognitive Level: Application **Client Need:** Health Promotion and Maintenance **Integrated Process:** Nursing Process: Analysis **Content Area:** Child Health **Strategy:** Specific nursing knowledge is needed to answer this question. Apply knowledge of birth defects and risks. **Reference:** Porth, C. M. (2005). *Pathophysiology: Concepts of altered health states* (7th ed.). Philadelphia, PA: Lippincott Williams & Wilkins, p. 142.

8 **Answer: 2** The adolescent client with Klinefelter's syndrome is a tall, lean male with no secondary sex characteristics. Body image is the appropriate nursing diagnosis for the adolescent client after taking into account growth and developmental considerations. Fluid and electrolyte balance and impaired physical mobility are not of concern, and high risk for complications is too vague to be of use for this client.
Cognitive Level: Application **Client Need:** Psychosocial Integrity **Integrated Process:** Nursing Process: Analysis **Content Area:** Child Health **Strategy:** The core issue of this question is an understanding of the key growth and developmental concerns of an adolescent client with an inherited disorder that affects physical appearance. Use these concepts and the process of elimination to make a selection. **Reference:** Ball, J., & Bindler, R. (2008). *Pediatric nursing: Caring for children* (4th ed.). Upper Saddle River, NJ: Pearson/Prentice Hall, p. 1245–1246.

9 **Answer: 3** It is recommended that girls who have lymphedema, delayed puberty, and are below the fifth percentile in height have chromosomal studies. This client has the appearance of Turner's syndrome. It needs to be confirmed and treated. Options 1 and 4 are incorrect because they ignore the client's concerns. Option 2

would increase the client's fear although the statement about physician input is correct.
Cognitive Level: Application **Client Need:** Physiological Integrity: Physiological Adaptation **Integrated Process:** Communication and Documentation **Content Area:** Child Health **Strategy:** The problems of this client are greater than delayed puberty. Choose an option that gives true information. **Reference:** Porth, C. M. (2005). *Pathophysiology: Concepts of altered health states* (7th ed.). Philadelphia, PA: Lippincott Williams & Wilkins, pp. 143-144.

10 **Answer: 4** For optimal appearance and healing of the suture line for cleft lip repair, the child should not be allowed to touch the mouth.
Cognitive Level: Application **Client Need:** Safe, Effective Care Environment: Management of Care **Integrated Process:** Communication and Documentation **Content Area:** Child Health **Strategy:** Consider the need for postoperative healing, remembering that the principle of restraints is to use the least restraint for the shortest time. **Reference:** Porth, C. M. (2005). *Pathophysiology: Concepts of altered health states* (7th ed.). Philadelphia, PA: Lippincott Williams & Wilkins, pp. 399-401.

References

Ball, J., & Bindler, R. (2008). *Pediatric nursing: Caring for children* (4th ed.). Upper Saddle River, NJ: Pearson Education.

LeMone, P., & Burke, K. M. (2008). *Medical surgical nursing. Critical thinking in client care* (4th ed.). Upper Saddle River, NJ: Prentice Hall.

McCance, K., & Huether, S. (2006). *Pathophysiology: The biologic basis for disease in adults and children* (5th ed.). St. Louis, MO: Elsevier Science.

Porth, C. M. (2005). *Pathophysiology: Concepts of altered health states* (7th ed.). Philadelphia, PA: Lippincott Williams & Wilkins.

Venes, D., & Thomas, C. L. (Ed.). (2006). *Taber's cyclopedic medical dictionary* (20th ed.). Philadelphia: F. A. Davis.

Wilkinson, J. M. (2006). *Nursing diagnosis handbook with NIC interventions and NOC outcomes* (8th ed.). Upper Saddle River, NJ: Prentice Hall.

Wilson, B. A., Shannon, M. T., & Stang, C. L. (2006). *Nursing drug guide 2006.* Upper Saddle River, NJ: Prentice Hall.

ANSWERS & RATIONALES

17 Multisystem Health Problems

Chapter Outline _____

Risk Factors for Multisystem Health Problems

Shock

Trauma

Disseminated Intravascular Coagulopathy (DIC)

Acute Respiratory Distress Syndrome (ARDS)

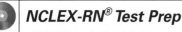

NCLEX-RN® Test Prep

Use the CD-ROM enclosed with this book
to access additional practice opportunities.

Objectives _____

➤ Define key terms associated with multisystem health problems.

➤ Identify risk factors associated with the development of multisystem health problems.

➤ Explain etiologies of multisystem health problems.

➤ Describe the pathophysiological processes associated with specific multisystem health problems.

➤ Distinguish between normal and abnormal multisystem findings obtained from nursing assessment.

➤ Prioritize nursing interventions associated with multisystem health problems.

Review at a Glance

acute respiratory distress syndrome (ARDS) a form of acute respiratory failure with respiratory insufficiency and inefficient gas exchange

anaphylactic shock shock resulting from an immune response to the presence of antigens; a form of distributive shock

antigen a foreign substance introduced into the body that triggers antibody production and can cause allergic reactions

bacteremia the presence of bacteria within the bloodstream

cardiac tamponade compression of the heart muscle by excess fluid or blood within the pericardial sac

cardiogenic shock shock caused by abnormal cardiac functioning or "pump failure"

contusion a bruising of tissue

disseminated intravascular coagulopathy (DIC) a disorder of coagulation in which the body alternately clots and hemorrhages in response to injury; the body's clotting substance reserves are overwhelmed resulting in massive hemorrhaging

fibrinolysis process in which thrombi (clots) are broken down

hypovolemic shock shock caused by a decrease in the circulating volume as a result of actual fluid or blood loss

laceration any tearing or slicing of the flesh and possibly underlying fleshy structures

metabolic acidosis a condition caused by the abnormal decrease in bicarbonate concentrations within the body; the body's pH becomes acidic

neurogenic shock shock that results from a decrease in sympathetic control of vasomotor responses, usually as a result of spinal injury; a form of distributive shock

obstructive shock shock in which the ventricles are not able to fill or empty appropriately because of a block in the flow of blood from the heart

pulse pressure the difference between systolic and diastolic pressure readings; normally about 30 to 40 mmHg

pulsus paradoxus a notable decrease in the pulse upon inspiration

shock the state of inadequate perfusion and oxygenation to vital organs and tissues throughout the body

septic shock shock that occurs in response to the release of endotoxins from bacteria, generally Gram-negative; a form of distributive shock

toxic shock syndrome a form of septic shock that occurs most commonly in women who utilize tampons while menstruating; Staphylococcus aureus is generally thought to be the bacteria involved

trauma a physical injury caused by outside forces

PRETEST

1 A client involved in a motor vehicle accident presents with a BP 120/62, pulse 100, respirations 28 to 32 and labored, and temperature 98.4° F orally. Examination of the anterior chest reveals obvious rib fractures, and breath sounds are absent in this area. The client's trachea is deviated to the left side of the neck. The nurse concludes that the client is probably experiencing which of the following?

1. Spontaneous pneumothorax
2. Tension pneumothorax
3. Iatrogenic pneumothorax
4. Open pneumothorax

2 A client presents after a near-drowning incident in which the client was submerged for an undetermined amount of time. The client has since regained consciousness and is alert and oriented, but anxious. Vital signs are BP 120/72, pulse 92, respirations 26, temperature 98.0°F orally. Pulse oximetry indicates an SaO_2 of 93% on 4 L/min of oxygen via nasal cannula. The nurse concludes that the client is at greatest risk to develop which of the following?

1. Cardiogenic shock
2. Spontaneous pneumothorax
3. Renal failure
4. Acute respiratory distress syndrome (ARDS)

3 A client was brought to the Emergency Department following a motorcycle accident. The client is alert and oriented with intermittent periods of confusion and reports moderate to severe thirst and left thigh pain. Vital signs are BP 100/60, pulse 112, respirations 28, and temperature 98.4°F orally. Capillary refill is three seconds and urinary output is 30 mL/hour. On examination there is an obvious pelvic deformity and the left thigh is distended. A diagnosis of hypovolemic shock is established. The nurse interprets by these findings that the client is in which phase of shock?

1. Initial phase
2. Compensatory phase
3. Progressive phase
4. Irreversible phase

4 A client reports difficulty breathing and generalized weakness after experiencing chest pain for approximately one hour the previous night. On exam, the client's skin is pale and diaphoretic, breath sounds are equal with crackles noted throughout all lung fields, capillary beds are dusky, and jugular venous distention is present. Vital signs are BP 98/50, pulse 118 and thready to palpation, respirations 26 and labored, temperature 98.6°F orally. The nurse will take action for which of the following suspected conditions?

1. Obstructive shock
2. Neurogenic shock
3. Hypovolemic shock
4. Cardiogenic shock

5 A client who has ingested the third dose of an antibiotic prescribed for a urinary tract infection arrives at the urgent care clinic. The client is weak, diaphoretic, reports difficulty breathing and itching, and appears flushed. The nurse ensures that epinephrine is at hand considering that the client is likely experiencing which form of shock?

1. Septic
2. Anaphylactic
3. Hypovolemic
4. Neurogenic

6 A client arrives in the Emergency Department after a fall from approximately 10 feet. The initial body point of contact was the upper-middle back, and the client reports sharp pain in this area with movement. The nurse suspects which type of injury?

1. Head injury
2. Spleen injury
3. Cervical spine injury
4. Liver injury

7 A client reports chest pain, rapid heart beat, and difficulty breathing. On exam, heart sounds are muffled. Which of the following assessment findings by the nurse would support a diagnosis of cardiac tamponade? Select all that apply.

1. Deviated trachea
2. Weak peripheral pulses
3. Absent breath sounds to the lower lobes
4. Diminished or absent carotid or femoral pulses during inspiration
5. Blood pressure 94/72 during inspiration, 10 mm Hg lower systolic than the blood pressure on expiration

8 A client who sustained a penetrating bowel injury has several concerns to be addressed regarding future care that require prioritizing. Which of the following conditions would receive priority by the nurse in developing the client's plan of nursing care?

1. Constipation
2. Peritonitis
3. Paralytic ileus
4. Intestinal adhesions

9 A client seeks treatment for a laceration to the forehead sustained in a fight. The client reports no loss of consciousness but is confused and has a strong alcohol odor on the breath. The Emergency Department nurse prepares the client for which of the following priority diagnostic assessments?

1. Skull x-ray and urine alcohol
2. MRI of the brain and blood alcohol
3. Blood alcohol and glucose
4. Electroencephalography (EEG) and blood alcohol

10 A client has a suspected femoral fracture from an injury sustained three hours ago. There is gross swelling to the left thigh, and the skin is tight and bruised. The client complains of numbness and tingling in the toes. What other assessments would the nurse expect to make if compartment syndrome exists? Select all that apply.

➤ *See pages 519–520 for Answers & Rationales.*

1. Toes cool and dusky
2. Bounding pulses distal to the fracture
3. Pain in the leg unrelieved by narcotics
4. Inability to move the ankle and toes in the affected leg
5. Changes in level of consciousness

I. RISK FACTORS FOR MULTISYSTEM HEALTH PROBLEMS

A. Shock

1. Hypovolemic shock

   a. Hemorrhagic: trauma (internal and external), aneurysm dissection, disseminated intravascular coagulopathy (DIC)

   b. Nonhemorrhagic: burns, vomiting, diarrhea, inadequate intake, excessive sweating, severe third-spacing of body fluids (such as edema, ascites)

2. Cardiogenic shock: myocardial infarction (MI; most common), cardiac dysrhythmias (heart block, supraventricular tachycardia [SVT], atrial fibrillation), electrolyte imbalances, cardiac tamponade, cardiomyopathy, cardiac valve disease, cardiac surgery, pericarditis, genetic anomalies

3. Obstructive shock: cardiac tamponade, pulmonary embolism, obstructive valve disease, tension pneumothorax, pulmonary hypertension

4. Distributive (*normovolemic*)

   a. Anaphylactic shock: antibiotic therapy, immunizations, food, animal or chemical exposure (sensitization must occur prior to event), allergies, new drug therapy, insect bites, venomous bites

   b. Septic shock: trauma, surgical procedures of the gastrointestinal (GI) and urinary tract, therapy involving invasive devices and procedures (IVs, urinary catheter, tracheal intubation), burns, immunosuppressed states (cancer, human immunodeficiency virus [HIV], acquired immunodeficiency syndrome [AIDS], steroid therapy), diabetes, tampon usage, elderly

B. Trauma

1. Factors predisposing an individual to traumatic injury are limitless

2. Certain lifestyle patterns, hobbies, and professions greatly increase the risk such as fire and police personnel, motorcycling, farmworkers, construction workers, electricians; high impact sports such as football, skiing, racing; and ingesting alcohol or controlled substances while operating equipment

3. Exposure to forces of acceleration, deceleration, or various forces of thrust and energy upon an inadequately protected individual because of neglect to utilize safety devices such as seat belts or harnesses or nonadherance to standard safety procedures

C. Disseminated intravascular coagulopathy (DIC): shock, complications of pregnancy, hemolytic reactions, trauma, metabolic acidosis

D. Acute respiratory distress syndrome (ARDS): shock, trauma, major insult to any organ system, characterized by reduced perfusion to major organs, massive infection

II. SHOCK

A. Overview

1. **Shock** is the state of inadequate perfusion and oxygenation to vital organs and tissues throughout the body; it cannot be defined as one specific disease

2. Manifests itself as a syndrome within many diseases or traumatic injuries that may be life-threatening

3. The body normally maintains perfusion to the cellular level by cooperation of:

   a. The pumping mechanism of the heart

   b. An intact vascular "highway" that facilitates blood flow

   c. An adequate amount of oxygenated blood that is exchanged at the capillary level with metabolic wastes

   d. An intact clotting cascade (intrinsic and extrinsic)

4. Any disruption of any component within this system results in an algorithmic attempt to compensate, which manifests itself in the classic signs and symptoms of shock

5. Types of shock

   a. Hypovolemic: hemorrhagic and nonhemorrhagic

   b. Cardiogenic

   c. Obstructive

   d. Distributive: anaphylactic and septic

6. Cause is usually related to a major insult to the body

7. Hemodynamic concepts that are the basic components of vascular homeostasis are important in identifying and treating shock states (see Figure 17-1)

   a. Stroke volume (SV): amount of blood that is ejected from the left ventricle into the aorta with each ventricular contraction

   b. Cardiac output (CO): amount of blood pumped from the left ventricle every minute; calculated by the equation *Stroke volume × Heart rate*

   c. Systemic vascular resistance (SVR): amount of resistance provided by the vascular bed against the flow of blood being ejected from the left ventricle; when the sympathetic nervous system (SNS) is stimulated in response to a threat, vasoconstriction occurs, increasing the SVR

   d. Mean arterial pressure (MAP): the average pressure maintained within the arterial system of the body; calculated by *Cardiac output × Systemic vascular resistance*

      1) When any component increases, MAP increases

      2) Conversely, with any decrease, there is a drop in MAP

      3) An increase or decrease in the intravascular volume effects MAP in a parallel manner

8. Whatever the cause of a shock state, the reactions and symptoms will generally follow the same course with a few notable signs defining the particular type of shock or the underlying cause

9. It is important to *first* identify that a state of shock is occurring rather than to identify the particular type

B. Pathophysiology

1. Shock is a syndrome that manifests itself as a result of the body's attempts to achieve homeostasis in direct response to a perfusion and oxygenation insult

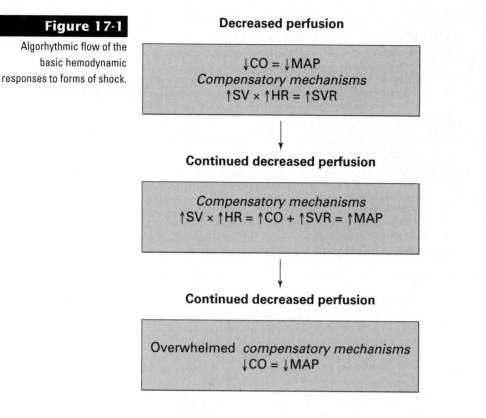

Figure 17-1

Algorhythmic flow of the
basic hemodynamic
responses to forms of shock.

Decreased perfusion

$\downarrow$CO = $\downarrow$MAP
Compensatory mechanisms
$\uparrow$SV $\times$ $\uparrow$HR = $\uparrow$SVR

Continued decreased perfusion

Compensatory mechanisms
$\uparrow$SV $\times$ $\uparrow$HR = $\uparrow$CO + $\uparrow$SVR = $\uparrow$MAP

Continued decreased perfusion

Overwhelmed *compensatory mechanisms*
$\downarrow$CO = $\downarrow$MAP

2. The origin of the insult may differ, but the compensatory mechanisms for all
types will be similar (see Box 17-1)

a. *Initial phase of shock* (mild)

1) A decline in circulating blood volume (500 mL or less) activates baroreceptors in the vascular system to note the decline in MAP; SNS activity is
activated; beta receptors are stimulated to increase oxygen (O_2) consumption of the cardiac muscle

2) Catecholamines (epinephrine and norepinephrine notably) are released,
creating vasoconstriction in areas that can more easily undergo periods of
ischemia, such as fat, bone, and skin; SVR is increased as a result

3) Bronchodilation and increased cardiac output occurs as a result of beta receptor stimulation

4) Few objective physical assessment findings are noted because vasoconstriction is minimal and little anaerobic activity occurs

b. *Compensatory phase of shock* (moderate shock)

1) With volume loss of 25% to 30%, more intense compensatory measures
are initiated; MAP continues to decline

2) Cardiac contractility, rate, and peripheral vasoconstriction increase

3) In an attempt to shunt blood flow to vital organs (heart, lungs, brain), there
is diminished blood flow to the kidneys, liver, GI tract, and extremities

4) Capillary pressure decreases allowing fluid shifts from interstitial spaces
into the vascular compartment in order to expand the circulating volume

Box 17-1

**Systemic Effects
and Compensatory
Response of Shock**

Neurologic

➤ Hypoxia with decreasing volume and systemic pressure

➤ Cerebral edema with severe, continuing hypoxia

➤ Circulatory collapse as sympathetic nervous system (SNS) stimulation is lost

Respiratory

➤ Bronchodilation and increase in respiratory rate in response to hypoxic status at cellular level

➤ Diminished respirations as a result of continued hypoxia to pulmonary tissue

Cardiac

➤ Increase in rate and contractility as a result of SNS stimulation in response to decreasing volume

➤ Decreasing blood pressure as shock progresses

➤ Diminished perfusion to the heart itself as a result of continued hypoxia

Gastrointestinal

➤ Ischemia as a result of the shunting of blood to the heart, lungs, and brain

➤ Ulcer and paralytic ileus may occur as a result of prolonged ischemia

Renal

➤ Ischemia as a result of compensatory shunting to heart, lungs, and brain

➤ Release of renin in response to decreased renal perfusion and decreased glomerular filtration, which results in decreased urine production in an effort to raise BP

➤ Tubular necrosis with prolonged renal hypoxia and renal failure

Integumentary

➤ Vasoconstriction with SNS stimulation

➤ Edema occurs in late shock as a result of fluid shifting to the interstitial spaces

    5) Decreased renal perfusion initiates the renin-angiotensin-aldosterone (RAA) system, causing thirst and an increased reabsorption of water and sodium

    6) Objective findings become apparent

  c. *Progressive phase of shock* (severe or decompensated)

    1) As shock continues to progress, compensatory mechanisms from the previous phase continue unchecked, worsening the status

    2) Volume loss of 35% to 50% occurs because of hemorrhage or fluid leakage

    3) Continued vasoconstriction worsens the already hypoxic state of cells and tissues

    4) As cells die because of hypoxia, they release destructive enzymes and proteins into the surrounding tissues, increasing the oncotic pressure in the interstitial space, and decreasing the circulating volume even further

    5) The body shifts from aerobic to anaerobic respiration at the cellular level and lactic acid is produced as a byproduct; **metabolic acidosis** (as acid-base

imbalance caused by an abnormal decrease in bicarbonate concentrations in the blood, shifting the pH of the body to an acidotic state)

    6) Dramatic physical changes in assessment parameters occur

  d. *Irreversible phase of shock*

    1) Despite restoration of circulating volume or the stabilization of vital signs, death will occur

    2) Microcirculation has been compromised beyond repair, resulting in widespread cellular death that eventually encompasses the tissues of vital organs

    3) Symptoms displayed during shock are part of the "survival" physiology the body initiates in response to a disease or injury

    4) Systemic changes are closely correlated with advancing SNS stimulation and the byproducts of that stimulation

3. The overall course of shock states is very similar; however, the underlying cause may vary the pathological processes

  a. Four types of shock: hypovolemic, cardiogenic, obstructive, and distributive (including anaphylactic, septic, and neurogenic)

  b. Anaphylactic, septic, and neurogenic shock are known as *distributive* forms of shock because there is an adequate intravascular volume; however, it is distributed in a manner within the body that does not sustain perfusion and oxygenation

  c. Hypovolemic shock

    1) **Hypovolemic shock** is caused by a decrease in circulating volume of more than 15%

    2) Loss of volume is from obvious hemorrhaging, extracellular fluid and/or plasma loss from burns, peritonitis, or ruptured aneurysms

    3) Fluids can also be lost from the GI tract because of severe vomiting, diarrhea, or gastric suctioning

    4) Inadequate intake, excessive sweating, diuretic usage, and interstitial shifting (third-spacing) associated with processes such as liver disease and severe protein wasting may cause this form of shock

    5) Loss of circulating volume causes an inadequate MAP, activating the SNS and initiating compensatory mechanisms

    6) Signs and symptoms (see Table 17-1)

  d. Cardiogenic shock

    1) **Cardiogenic shock** is caused by abnormal cardiac functioning or "pump failure"

    2) There is adequate volume within the intravascular space, however, perfusion and oxygenation at the cellular level is inadequate because of the inability of the heart to move blood throughout the body with acceptable force

    3) The most common and dangerous cause of cardiac failure is MI; cardiomyopathy, cardiac tamponade, valve disease, and dysrthymias are contributing factors

    4) A decrease in MAP stimulates the SNS; beta receptors within the heart are stimulated as a result, creating a dangerous scenario in that O_2 consumption is increased in the very organ that is compromised, thus placing greater stress on cardiac tissue

Table 17-1	Clinical Manifestations of Hypovolemic Shock			
	Initial	**Compensatory**	**Progressive**	**Irreversible**
Subjective	Reports pain and thirst; sensorium intact	Anxious; restless; reports greater thirst; episodes of confusion	Confused; restless; agitated	
Objective	Tachycardia; respirations baseline; normotensive; fleshtone or pallor of extremities; skin dry or slightly moist; capillary refill < 3 sec; normal or slightly decreased urine output; ABGs normal	Hypotension; tachycardia; tachypnea; skin cool, pale, and dry/diaphoretic; capillary refill < 4–6 sec, urine output less than 30 mL/hr; ABGs indicate trend toward metabolic acidosis	Profound hypotension; tachycardia with weak or nonpalpable peripheral pulses; cardiac dysrhythmias; tachypnea; skin pale, dusky, and/or mottled capillary beds without refill, blanching; ABGs—metabolic acidosis; diminished or absent urine output; no purposeful movement	Severe hypotension; tachypnea with shallow depth; diminishing air exchange with crackles; cardiac dysrhythmias; skin ABGs—profound metabolic acidosis; anuria; comatose

5) Distal vascular beds become congested with deoxygenated blood creating the hallmark nail bed cyanosis with this form of shock

6) Increased SVR occurs from the pooling that occurs in the periphery

7) Pressure is then exerted on the left ventricle, causing pulmonary congestion as fluid cannot exit the lungs to the left ventricle

8) Signs and symptoms (see Table 17-2)

e. Obstructive shock

1) **Obstructive shock** results from an inability of the cardiac ventricles to fill or empty appropriately because of an obstruction in the blood flow from the heart; cardiac preload is decreased and severely compromised; may be difficult to diagnose

2) There is an increased pressure on the right side of the heart and an inadequate blood return

3) This form of shock is differentiated from cardiogenic shock in that the heart itself can pump adequately and is not necessarily diseased; it is the

Table 17-2		Signs and Symptoms
Clinical Manifestations of Cardiogenic Shock	**Subjective**	Restless Agitated
	Objective	Hypotension Tachycardia with weak, thready pulse Cardiac dysrhythmias Decreased or narrowed pulse pressure Tachypnea with labored depth and crackles Jugular venous distention (JVD) Skin cool and moist Circumoral cyanosis Nail beds dusky

presence of some "obstruction" outside of the heart that compromises perfusion; trauma may create obstructions

4) Pulmonary embolism (PE) is the most common cause of obstructive shock; damage to the alveoli from the "explosion" of the embolus in the lung creates an increasing pressure on the right side of the heart because blood cannot enter easily into the lung from the right ventricle; in the presence of a suspected PE, signs and symptoms of shock should be correlated to obstruction

5) Signs and symptoms often correlate with right-sided heart failure: jugular venous distention, hepatomegaly, and edema (see Box 17-2)

f. Distributive shock

1) Anaphylactic shock

a) Anaphylactic shock results from an overwhelming immune response to an allergen or **antigen** (a foreign substance introduced into the body that causes the body to produce antibodies)

b) This form of shock is particularly catastrophic and requires aggressive and immediate intervention as circulatory collapse is rapid

c) Associated with the administration of antibiotics or exposure to a foreign protein; parenteral medication administration routes are more prone to cause true anaphylaxis than oral routes

d) On exposure to an antigen, the body's immune system produces an antibody specific to the allergen

e) With subsequent exposure, a reaction occurs wherein large amounts of histamines are released into the blood stream in response to the foreign body

f) Histamines cause marked dilation in the arterioles as well as increasing capillary permeability

g) There is a profound fluid shift into the interstitial spaces from the intravascular compartment, creating edema (third–spacing)

Box 17-2	**Signs and Symptoms**
Clinical Manifestations of Obstructive Shock	Anxiety
	Somnolence
	Hypotension
	Tachycardia
	Tachypnea with dyspnea
	Jugular venous distention (JVD)
	Pallor
	Pericardial friction rub
	Muffled heart sounds or gallop (S_3)
	Chest pain
	Decreased to absent urinary output
	Possible signs and symptoms of a pneumothorax
	Possible open chest wound or fractured ribs
	Possible diminished or absent breath sounds
	Possible whistling or rushing sounds with inspiration
	Possible tracheal deviation

Box 17-3	**Signs and Symptoms**
Clinical Manifestations of Anaphylactic Shock	Marked restlessness Anxiety Severe itching and difficulty swallowing Hypotension Tachycardia Tachypnea with wheezing and possible stridor Diminished breath sounds Hypersalivation and/or drooling Generalized urticaria Edema (focusing on orbital and facial components) Cardiac dysrhythmias Skin cool and moist Flushing Abdominal cramping Emesis

h) Overwhelming vasodilation and pooling of circulating blood in the periphery causes a precipitous drop in MAP; vasodilation produces the characteristic skin flushing and warmth

i) Laryngeal edema may occur, and bronchospasms further compromise pulmonary function and airway clearance

j) Signs and symptoms (see Box 17-3)

2) Septic shock

a) Septic shock is most often associated with release of endotoxins from Gram-negative bacteria into the bloodstream, although it may also be caused by some Gram-positive bacteria; massive vasodilation occurs in response to the pathogen's release of toxins into the bloodstream

b) An initial infection occurs and progresses to frank **bacteremia,** (presence of bacteria in the blood); sepsis follows in most instances

c) Some shock states may be present without obvious bacteremia if a localized infection is large enough to generate a sufficient toxic release

d) Toxic shock syndrome is a form of septic shock that occurs most commonly in menstruating women who use tampons and is often produced by *Staphylococcus aureus;* blood cultures may not always be positive with this form of septic shock

e) As pathogens release their poison into the blood stream, the inflammatory process with the help of the immune system responds to the destruction of blood cells and the presence of bacteria

f) Initial presentation is generally with a fever and flushing that is not seen in other forms of shock

g) Disseminated intravascular coagulopathy (DIC) is associated with this form of shock and will be reviewed later in this chapter

h) Signs and symptoms (see Table 17-3)

3) Neurogenic shock

a) Neurogenic shock occurs as a result of decreased SNS control of vasomotor responses; parasympathetic stimulation is unchecked, allowing peripheral vasodilation to occur, thereby decreasing MAP

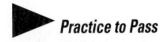

Practice to Pass

A 23-year-old woman who has suffered no apparent injury or recent illness is diagnosed as being in shock. What predisposing risk factor would be investigated and why?

Table 17-3	Early Shock	Late Shock
Clinical Manifestations of Septic Shock	Sensorium intact with restlessness and agitation Nausea Possible abdominal tenderness Normotensive Tachycardia Tachypnea Skin flushed Warm and moist Moderate to severe hyperthermia Shivering Emesis Exudate from wound sources	Hypotension Tachycardia Cardiac dysrhythmias Tachypnea with laboring and shallow depth Skin cool and pale Normothermic to hypothermic (indicates decreasing basal metabolic rate) Somnolence to coma Decreased to absent urinary output

   b) This form of shock is somewhat rare and generally associated with significant spinal trauma

   c) Because neurogenic shock is often associated with trauma, it is important to remember to rule out hypovolemic shock initially, even in the absence of obvious volume loss or bleeding

   d) Signs and symptoms (see Box 17-4)

  4. General signs and symptoms are common to all forms of shock (see Figure 17-2)

C. Nursing assessment

  1. Assessment criteria for each category

   a. *Hypovolemic shock*

    1) Assessment includes symptom analysis of pain and thirst, level of consciousness (LOC), vital signs (VS), skin color and temperature, capillary refill, urinary output, evidence of coping (or lack of), cardiac rhythm, heart and lung sounds, movement, peripheral pulses, and presence of risk factors

    2) Diagnostic tests

     a) Hemoglobin and hematocrit (H&H): baseline levels should be obtained and serial monitoring performed to reflect changes; H&H levels with whole blood loss will reflect a decrease; an increase of the H&H levels will occur when the majority of fluid lost is within the vascular system (such as occurs with dehydration and third-spacing)

     b) Urinalysis may indicate the presence of blood secondary to direct injury or indirect "shaking" of the kidney during the traumatic incident

Box 17-4	**Signs and Symptoms**
Clinical Manifestations of Neurogenic Shock	Level of consciousness varies according to the underlying cause Hypotension Bradycardia followed by tachycardia (especially in brain and spinal trauma) Skin flushed followed by pallor and coolness Possible hypothermia Decreased to absent urinary output Respiratory rate is dependent on cause of shock *Note:* Traumatic injuries and central nervous system depressants vary the objective findings accordingly.

Figure 17-2 Multisystem effects of shock.

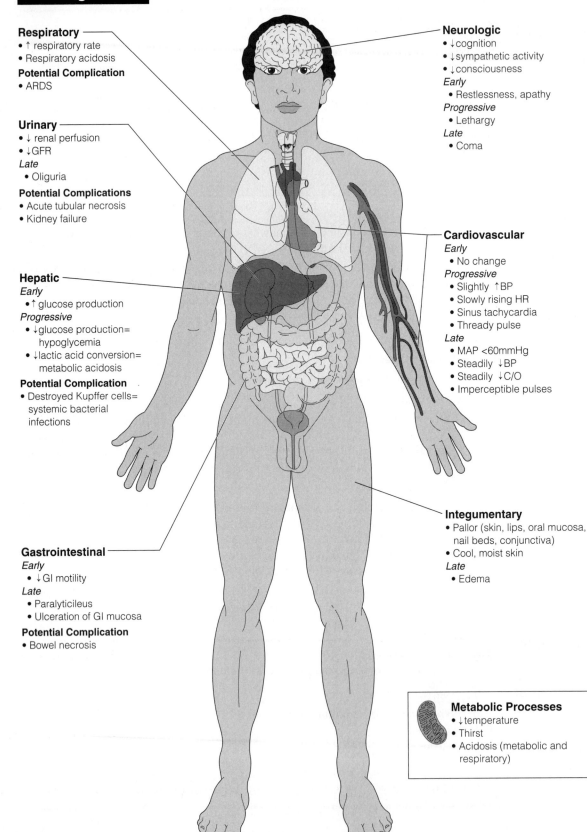

Respiratory
- ↑ respiratory rate
- Respiratory acidosis

Potential Complication
- ARDS

Urinary
- ↓ renal perfusion
- ↓GFR

Late
- Oliguria

Potential Complications
- Acute tubular necrosis
- Kidney failure

Hepatic
Early
- ↑ glucose production

Progressive
- ↓glucose production=
  hypoglycemia
- ↓lactic acid conversion=
  metabolic acidosis

Potential Complication
- Destroyed Kupffer cells=
  systemic bacterial
  infections

Gastrointestinal
Early
- ↓GI motility

Late
- Paralyticileus
- Ulceration of GI mucosa

Potential Complication
- Bowel necrosis

Neurologic
- ↓cognition
- ↓sympathetic activity
- ↓consciousness

Early
- Restlessness, apathy

Progressive
- Lethargy

Late
- Coma

Cardiovascular
Early
- No change

Progressive
- Slightly ↑BP
- Slowly rising HR
- Sinus tachycardia
- Thready pulse

Late
- MAP <60mmHg
- Steadily ↓BP
- Steadily ↓C/O
- Imperceptible pulses

Integumentary
- Pallor (skin, lips, oral mucosa,
  nail beds, conjunctiva)
- Cool, moist skin

Late
- Edema

Metabolic Processes
- ↓temperature
- Thirst
- Acidosis (metabolic and
  respiratory)

       c) Arterial blood gases (ABGs): normal to metabolic acidosis

       d) Type and cross match (TXM): in preparation for blood administration

       e) Coagulation studies such as partial thromboplastin time (PTT), prothrombin time (PT)

  b. *Cardiogenic shock*

    1) Assessment includes preexisting cardiac dysfunction such as MI or trauma and other risk factors; VS; heart rhythm; pulses; lung sounds; heart sounds; presence of edema; skin color and temperature; capillary refill and color of nailbeds; mentation; urinary output (note: damage from MI versus cardiac tamponade may be differentiated by noting signs and symptoms of tamponade such as jugular venous distention [JVD] without symptoms of pulmonary congestion and presence of a pericardial friction rub; this is an important distinction because treatment for tamponade must be instituted immediately)

    2) Diagnostic tests

       a) H&H levels may be decreased with a long medical history of heart disease from chronic renal hypoperfusion

       b) Cardiac enzymes, isoenzymes, and troponin may be elevated as a result of cardiac tissue damage

       c) Chest x-rays (CXR) may indicate cardiomegaly and pulmonary edema

       d) Electrocardiogram (EKG) 12-lead

       e) ABGs: metabolic acidosis

  c. *Obstructive shock*

    1) Assessment includes risk factors and predisposing diagnoses such as thrombophlebitis, deep vein thrombosis (DVT), and risk factors for DVT such as smoking and contraceptive use; VS; presence of edema; skin color and temperature; complaints of respiratory or cardiac problems; lung sounds; heart sounds; trachea midline

    2) Diagnostic tests

       a) Cardiac enzymes, isoenzymes, and troponin may be elevated secondary to myocardial tissue damage

       b) CXR may indicate pneumothorax

       c) Echocardiogram may indicate pericarditis or valve disease

       d) ABGs

       e) 12-lead EKG

  d. *Distributive shock*

    1) Anaphylactic shock

       a) Assessment includes preexisting exposure to medication, foods with high allergic potential (iodine-containing foods, coarse wheat products, various nuts), animals, insect bites and other risk factors; perform a thorough head-to-toe assessment to locate source of bite/sting after aggressive treatment has been initiated; assess for mentation; complaints of itching and difficulty swallowing; VS; lung sounds; heart sounds; presence of edema; GI complaints; respiratory status; in many instances anaphylactic shock progresses to circulatory collapse and coma within minutes

       b) Diagnostic tests: complete blood counts (CBC) may indicate an overall increase in white blood cells (WBC) in response to the inflammatory process; eosinophil counts may also be elevated in response to allergens; other laboratory or radiology tests are noncontributory for anaphylaxis; ABGs determine acid–base balance

2) *Septic shock*

a) Assessment includes preexisting signs or symptoms of infection even if current treatment for an infection is in progress; assess for other risk factors; VS; mentation; skin color and temperature; GI complaints; signs of infection/inflammation; urinary output; vaginal exam to check for retained tampon

b) Diagnostic tests: CBC shows elevated WBC count initially; as shock progresses, the body's immune response is overwhelmed and there is a decrease in the overall WBC count; monocytes may increase in response to macrophage activity against bacteria; blood and wound C&S identifies bacteria (spinal fluid may be cultured to diagnose neurological infections); radiology tests (ultrasound, magnetic resonance imaging [MRI], or computerized tomography [CT]; coagulation studies

3) *Neurogenic shock*

a) Assessment includes risk factors to include traumatic injury, central nervous system (CNS) depressants, and anesthesia; VS; skin color and temperature; urinary output; mentation

b) Diagnostic tests: laboratory testing is limited in diagnosing this form of shock; radiology studies may reveal spinal or cranial trauma

2. Primary diagnostic tests (common to most forms)

a. ABGs: reflect metabolic acidosis (lowering of pH) that develops as a result of increasing carbon dioxide levels in the blood secondary to hypoxia

b. Urinalysis: indicates an increasing specific gravity and osmolality as the urine becomes more concentrated

c. Blood urea nitrogen (BUN): increases in response to diminishing renal function

D. **Nursing management**

1. Organization

a. Prehospital: baseline history to include VS, mechanism of injury, machinery involved if traumatic situation, environmental factors surrounding an accident; if no preadmission report is available, obtain prehospital data simultaneously with physical assessments and interventions

b. Specialty personnel within the hospital should be organized prior to the arrival of a trauma victim in shock if possible, and include respiratory therapists, radiology personnel (to include CT), additional nursing support, surgeons, anesthesiologists, orthopedists, and radiologists

c. Ancillary units such as intensive care unit (ICU) and operating room (OR) need to be notified of a potential admission

d. In many facilities a trauma protocol (team approach) is initiated within the emergency department so that care is delivered in an organized manner; nurses may be assigned to an anatomical area or to a procedure, becoming the "IV nurse" or the "thoracic nurse"

2. General treatment measures

a. Maintain life support by instituting ABC (airway, breathing, circulation) guidelines

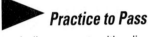

Practice to Pass

A client presents with a diagnosis of cardiogenic shock. What diagnostic value is the most accurate for gauging the severity of shock and why?

    b. Supine position with spinal alignment maintained (all head injuries are considered spinal injuries also until ruled out as negative)

    c. Airway should be secured, protected, and supplemental oxygen should be initiated using as appropriate delivery device according to the client's overall assessment

    d. Immediately initiate an appropriate IV access, usually an 18-gauge catheter for peripheral IV

    e. Initiate continuous cardiac and SaO_2 (pulse oximetry) monitoring and prepare for frequent VS assessments

    f. Maintain stabilization to all deformities and prevent hypothermia by covering the client

    g. All clients suspected of shock should have an indwelling urinary catheter inserted to accurately measure urine output; do not attempt to place in the presence of obvious pelvic deformity or active bleeding from the urethra

    h. Sympathomimetic medications may be ordered for their inotropic and vasoconstrictive effects, such as epinephrine (Adrenalin), dopamine (Intropin), isoproterenol (Isuprel), and amiodarone (Cordarone), as well as glucose to rule out hypoglycemia

        1) A positive inotropic effect provides for increased cardiac contractility

        2) Sympathomemetics stimulate beta–1 receptors, creating an increase in O_2 consumption by heart

        3) Sympathomimetics may not be given to those in cardiogenic shock or with serious heart disease secondary to the cardiac stress they create

3. *Hypovolemic shock*

    a. Medications include sympathomimetics, vasopressors, and medications to treat acid-base and electrolyte imbalances

    b. Place the client in a supine position with legs elevated (modified Trendelenberg or shock position) to increase cerebral blood flow; keep the neck and obvious deformities stabilized; avoid this position, however, if a head injury is suspected

    c. Prepare for the potential application of antishock trousers (inflatable pant-like devices that compress the lower half of the body to enhance circulation to the heart, lungs, and brain)

    d. Gain IV access by inserting at least two large-bore IV cannulas (18-gauge or larger)

        1) Insert lines on admission to enable rapid fluid resuscitation; avoid the jugular and subclavian veins if possible

        2) Intraosseous infusions may need to be initiated in cases of severe burns or in pediatric clients

    e. Initiate IV fluids

        1) Crystolloids (isotonic or balanced solutions such as normal saline [NS] and lactated Ringer's [LR]) may be initiated to treat mild shock

        2) Moderate to severe shock may require administration of colloidal solutions to expand plasma volume; however, beware that coagulation disorders may develop as well as hypersensitivity reactions

        3) Colloidal solutions also increase oncotic pressure in the intravascular space, which may predispose the client to circulatory overload, pulmonary edema, and allergic reactions

    f. Blood, a type of colloid, is also given with caution

        1) Infection, as well as hemolytic reactions are a concern

        2) Obtain a type and crossmatch lab specimen to identify blood type; however, universal O-negative blood should be requisitioned if time does not allow for specific matching and hospital protocol allows

        3) Monitor vs every 15 minutes, a febrile reaction (fever) usually indicates a reaction

    g. In severe, unremitting shock, autotransfusions may be administered, in which the client's own blood is collected using special equipment and is reinfused

4. *Cardiogenic shock*

    a. Medications include agents to correct acid-base and electrolyte imbalances, cardiac agents amiodarone (Cordarore) or positive inotropic agents may be used

    b. Typically, sympathomimetic agents that stimulate alpha and beta receptors indiscriminately are avoided due to the increased oxygen demand they place on cardiac tissue

    c. Place the client in a supine position or with slightles elevation if the systolic BP is low; this position is contraindicated in those clients experiencing respiratory distress associated with pleural effusion

    d. Obtain IV access, however, clients experiencing cardiogenic shock may have fluids restricted

5. *Obstructive shock*

    a. Medications include vasopressors such as norepinephrine bitartrate (Levophed)

    b. Prepare for the insertion of a thoracostomy tube to relieve a tension pneumothorax

    c. Prepare for pericardiocentesis to relieve cardiac tamponade

    d. Provide supportive treatment with fluids

6. *Distributive shock*

    a. Septic shock

        1) Medications include positive inotropics and broad spectrum antibiotics; empirical antibiotic therapy is often initiated before C & S resulted available; however, all cultures should be collected before starting antibiotic therapy

        2) Prepare to administer crystolloid fluids

    b. *Anaphylactic shock*

        1) Medications include crystolloids, sympathomimetics (specifically epinephrine) as well as antihistamines, vasopressors, and glucocorticoids; use sympathomimetics with great caution in clients with heart disease

        2) Aerosol treatments for bronchodilation may be given in the presence of bronchospasms

        3) Maintain the client in a supine position and do not overheat with excessive sheets and blankets

    c. *Neurogenic shock*

        1) Medications include IV fluids (crystalloids) and vasopressors; this type of shock may or may not respond well to fluid therapy

        2) Place the client in a supine position, maintaining skeletal alignment in the presence of suspected spinal trauma

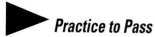

7. Reassessment

    a. Nursing management of all forms of shock includes continuous, accurate monitoring of the client's status to identify improvement or deterioration

    b. VS, urine output, and laboratory parameters are fundamental

    c. Clients experiencing shock are also at great risk to develop GI ulcers secondary to GI ischemia, and ARDS

    d. Various monitoring devices may include central venous pressure, pulmonary artery or capillary wedge pressure, or intracranial pressure

    e. Signs of resolution of a shock state include stable vs with signs of adequate perfusion, improved and/or adequate urine output, appropriate level of consciousness (LOC) with orientation and alertness, an H&H level within normal parameters or improving, and a pH within normal limits

▶ Practice to Pass

A client presents with a diagnosis of septic shock. When would antibiotics be initiated and what classification of therapy would be given?

III. TRAUMA

A. Overview

1. **Trauma** is defined as the physical injury to the body from external forces; there are many predisposing factors and all parts of the body are vulnerable

2. Trauma may range from simple to complex, depending on the organs and systems involved

3. Injury is generally a result of

    a. Accelerating forces: gunshot wound is an example

    b. Decelerating forces: impact from motor vehicle accident (MVA)

4. Injuries may be blunt, penetrating, or shearing in nature

5. Body organs and tissues may also experience traumatic injury as a result of medical procedures and treatment

6. It is impossible to predict with certainty the effects that one type of injury may have on an individual, so care must be approached in an algorithmic, organized, and rapid manner

B. Pathophysiology

1. *Skull/brain trauma*

    a. Trauma to the skull may take the form of soft tissue or bone injury and is often associated with acceleration and deceleration of great velocity

    b. The scalp and face have an extensive vascular system so that wounds may bleed in copious amounts; if this is combined with other areas of hemorrhage, a hypovolemic state may occur

    c. Intracranial hemorrhages may be classified according to their location in relation to the protective meningeal coverings of the brain; the dura (outer), the arachnoid (middle), and the pia mater (internal); hemorrhaging may also occur within any other area within the brain itself forming an intracerebral hematoma

    d. Subdural (below the brain's lining) or epidural (above the brain's lining) hematomas may develop; these may be acute in nature or develop over the course of hours

        1) Subdural hematomas are common and usually from venous tissue bleeding

        2) Epidural hematomas usually result from arterial bleeding (usually middle meningeal artery)

  e. The symptoms of brain injury closely relate to the amount and location of damage and may be diffuse or specific in nature

  f. *Closed* trauma to the head may occur with or without a fracture to the skull; there is no passage formed by the injury from the brain to the atmosphere

   1) Hemorrhaging within the brain creates pressure; as pressure elevates, more damage from the force created by the bleeding leads to more injury; hypoxemia increases cerebral blood flow in response to the elevating CO_2 levels, creating more swelling

   2) The brain injury itself may suppress vital functions such as ventilation, worsening the hypoxic state

   3) Depending on the location of the injury, sensory and motor function may be impaired, reflected in paresthesias, paralysis, and an altered sensorium (leaving the client open to further injury)

   4) Injuries that hemorrhage rapidly and profusely may cause a "shift" of the brain as pressure is exerted

  g. *Open* head injuries are those in which the integrity of the cranial cavity has been compromised, leaving a passage for material (such as bacteria) to move from the atmosphere to the brain; however, the swelling that occurs may be lessened with an open head injury

   1) This type of trauma may also result in brain tissue swelling and hemorrhage; many of the symptoms will be the same as those involved with a closed head injury (depending on its location) and extent

   2) Open head injuries tend to be more focal in nature rather than diffuse

  h. Injuries to the protective tissues of the brain pose a unique problem of infection in that bacteria may be introduced, resulting in the infectious process of meningitis

  i. Trauma to the ear, sinus, and eye may also provide potential routes for infection to the brain and must be investigated

  j. Facial bone injury may be isolated or complicate a skull injury

   1) Mandibular and maxillary fractures are generally a result of blunt or crushing forces to the facial area and pose a unique problem to airway management

   2) Trauma to facial nerves may also be present

  k. Orbital fractures, often seen with fractures of the zygomatic bones, may also involve damage to the eye sphere itself

  l. All fractures of the face, with or without the presence or hemorrhaging, should be viewed with suspicion, and cranial integrity should be verified

2. *Cervical/neck trauma*

  a. Cervical and neck trauma should automatically be suspected with head injuries, falls, or injuries to the chest and upper back

  b. May involve soft tissue and/or the cervical portion of the spinal column

  c. Great vessel injury to the carotid arteries or jugular veins is life-threatening in nature, and a hypovolemic state may be immediate and profound

  d. Damage to the trachea may occur simultaneously with great vessel injury and may result in either mechanical blocking of air, or diminished air exchange secondary to the presence of active hemorrhaging

  e. Cervical spinal injuries involve the vertebrae from C1 to C8; these injuries should be suspected in the presence of head injuries as well as injuries that

Figure 17-3 Spinal injury mechanisms. *A.* Compression of cord. *B.* Stretching of cord. *C.* Compression fracture.

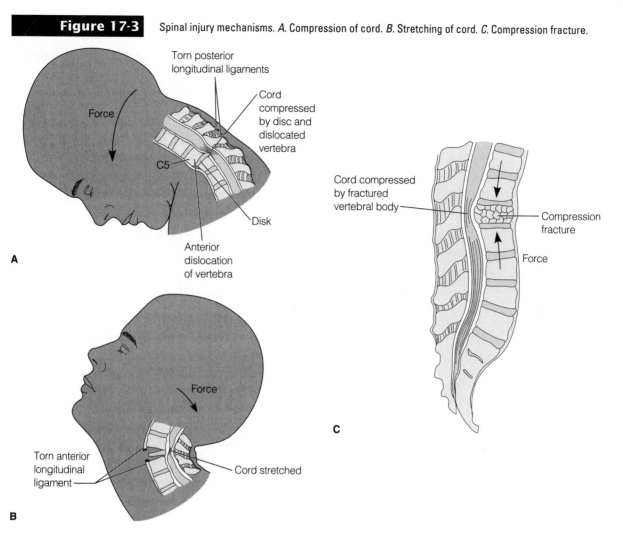

Torn posterior
longitudinal ligaments

Cord
compressed
by disc and
dislocated
vertebra

Force

C5

Disk

A

Anterior
dislocation
of vertebra

Cord compressed
by fractured
vertebral body

Compression
fracture

Force

C

Force

Torn anterior
longitudinal
ligament

Cord stretched

B

may result in hyperflexion (bending back) of the neck, such as car accidents that "whip" the head back

  f. Traumatic injuries that strike the top of the head and push the head down into the body (axial loading) should also be suspected of creating spinal injuries (see Figure 17-3)

  g. Depending on the specific location and whether the cord itself has been transected (complete severance), a variety of symptoms may occur as innervation of various organs and structures is disrupted

  h. Higher cord damage may result in the cessation of vital life functions such as respiration

  i. Lower cervical cord injury may also mimic higher lesions because of the paralysis of other functions; therefore, it is of higher priority to carry out emergency interventions than to try to diagnose the *specific* location of injury

 3. *Chest trauma*

  a. Injuries to the chest are most often the result of blunt or penetrating trauma

  b. Bone injury may occur to the surrounding protective cage of the chest, with or without trauma to the underlying tissues and organs; however, cardiac and pulmonary injury should always be ruled out when there is enough force to injure the bony structures encasing these organs

  c. With significant chest injuries, air exchange and tissue perfusion may be profoundly impaired; a hypovolemic state may be created as a result

  d. Great vessel injury is another potential complication of chest trauma and may result in the severance or tearing of these structures

  e. Significant heart problems

    1) Cardiac tamponade results when the heart is compressed by excess fluid or blood in the pericardial sac

      a) The ensuing decrease in output results in cardiogenic or obstructive shock

      b) This condition progresses rapidly and is a medical emergency

      c) A hallmark sign of cardiac tamponade is the finding of **pulsus paradoxus** or paradoxical pulses, a notable decrease in the pulse upon inspiration

      d) The **pulse pressure** (difference between systolic and diastolic pressure, about 30–40 mmHg) also begins to diminish in tamponade

    2) To differentiate a myocardial infarction from cardiac tamponade in initial assessment be aware that jugular venous distention will occur in tamponade without the concurrent pulmonary congestion that is seen with heart failure from myocardial infarction; a friction rub may also be auscultated in tamponade

    3) A **contusion,** or bruising of tissue, is assigned differently in that cardiac tissue itself is injured as opposed to the pericardial area; contusions should always be suspected with cardiac tamponade

    4) A preexisting cardiac condition may further complicate the scenario as a result of the diseased heart's inability to tolerate the additional stress

  f. Significant lung problems

    1) Pneumothorax: a pneumothorax is an emergent condition in which air leaks into the pleural space, either through the lung itself (closed) or from the outside atmosphere (open)

      a) The negative pressure within the pleural space becomes equal to the atmosphere, resulting in the collapse of the area of the lung involved

      b) A pneumothorax may be spontaneous in nature and not evolve from an injury, however, most occur as the result of blunt or penetrating trauma to the pleural space

    2) Tension pneumothorax: in the event that the pleural cavity becomes open to the outside atmosphere through penetrating trauma to the chest, a tension pneumothorax may result

      a) The wound itself becomes a valve, allowing air to enter the chest cavity and none to escape

      b) The increasing pressure may cause a shift of the mediastinum away from the side of the injured lung

      c) The trachea also deviates to the side of the unaffected lung, a hallmark sign of tension pneumothorax

      d) Increasing pressure on the unaffected lung compromises the already impaired gas exchange

    3) Hemothorax: a collection of blood in the pleural space caused by blunt or penetrating trauma; hemorrhaging into the pleural cavity impairs gas exchange as well as potentially causing a significant source of hypovolemia

4) Flail chest: results when two or more ribs are fractured in two areas, resulting in chest wall instability

a) With inspiration and expiration, this segment moves paradoxically with the rest of of the chest

b) On inspiration the involved area moves inward, while on expiration, the area may appear to bulge

c) This paradoxical movement mechanically impairs the normal expansion of the lungs and is often associated with underlying pulmonary injuries such as a contusion or pneumothorax

4. *Abdominal trauma*

a. Injury to the abdomen may cause many complications in the trauma client because of the numerous organs and major blood vessels located within the abdominal cavity

b. In the event that a specific determination of the organ involved cannot be made initially, basic life support and shock management should take precedence

c. After a specific diagnosis is made to the injured organ(s), the functional limitation of the organ(s) should be considered and included in the continuing plan of care

d. Any rupture of an abdominal organ should include focus on the spillage of organ contents into the abdominal cavity that may result in infectious or chemical peritonitis

1) Liver: injuries to this organ may result from blunt or penetrating trauma

a) The liver has a large reservoir of blood, so significant injury to this organ may cause a hypovolemic crisis

b) Contusions and hemorrhaging within this organ may be insidious in nature and signs and symptoms may not initially appear

c) Liver injury should be suspected in the presence of lower rib fractures, pulmonary trauma, and thoracic and abdominal injuries

2) Pancreas: injury to the pancreas from trauma carries a high risk of other associated injuries because of its location; hypovolemia may result as well as injury to the surrounding organs from released pancreatic fluids containing digestive enzymes

3) Spleen: injury to the spleen may result from blunt or penetrating forces and is a significant source of hemorrhaging

a) As a part of the lymph system, the spleen is not essential to maintenance of vital life functions and may be removed

b) Acute injury may result in hypovolemia

c) Injury in clients who have previously enlarged spleens, such as pregnant women and those suffering from mononucleosis, occurs with greater ease

4) Bowel: bowel injury may be specific to the small or large intestines

a) Both areas may be injured by blunt or penetrating sources, however, the large bowel, or colon, is more often associated with abdominal trauma

b) Trauma to the colon is frequently associated with peritonitis from intracolonic bacteria being released into the abdominal cavity

       5) Stomach: injury to the stomach is a rare finding in trauma, probably as a result of its location within the protective shell of the rib cage

          a) Penetrating injuries, such as gunshots, comprise the majority of gastric injuries associated with trauma

          b) Because of its anatomical location, injury to the spleen is very often associated with stomach trauma and can rapidly lead to death due to hemorrhage; assess for an enlarging abdomen

          c) Damage may cause the spillage of gastric juices and air into the surrounding cavities

5. *Genitourinary trauma* (closely associated with abdominal trauma)

    a. Renal trauma: the kidneys are well protected by the spinal column and ribs, however, traumatic injury may result from blunt or penetrating forces

       1) Because the kidneys are somewhat "free-floating" in nature they can be jostled, resulting in hematuria with minimal trauma

       2) The renal system is also prone to significant damage as a result of diminished blood flow secondary to shock

       3) In the presence of identified abdominal, thoracic, or pulmonary trauma, injury to the renal system should be highly suspected even when no hematuria is present

       4) Most renal injuries are minor in nature, but profound blood loss may occur with vessel tearing or rupture

       5) Injuries to the ureter are very rare and are usually penetrating in nature

    b. Bladder trauma: bladder trauma is most often associated with blunt trauma; however, penetrating injury may result from external forces as well as from fractures of the pelvis

       1) Bladder rupture occurs most often when the bladder is distended or full at the time of injury

       2) While the bladder is not viewed as a significant source of bleeding, bladder injury should be assessed in conjunction with pelvic injuries that may cause gross hemorrhaging; its location near the great pelvic vessels warrants high levels of attention in assessment

    c. Urethral trauma: trauma to the urethra is somewhat uncommon and is usually associated with blunt injury in males

       1) "Saddle"-type injuries may occur in both females and males wherein the pubis symphysis impacts an object while decelerating, such as a steering column or cross beam

       2) Pelvic fractures are often associated with urethral injury

6. *Fractures*

    a. A break in the continuity of any bone is considered a fracture

    b. Fractures result when the bone cannot withstand the exertion of mechanical forces being exerted upon it; the force may be direct or indirect in nature, such as spontaneous fractures that occur when body weight upon standing alone is enough to injure weakened bony matter

    c. When the integrity of the bone is broken, there is hemorrhaging within the site that begins the inflammatory process

    d. Swelling causes pain and reduces movement of surrounding muscles and tissues

    e. Severe fractures may impinge on neurological innervation and/or may compromise blood flow to the extremity involved

        1) Compartment syndrome can occur: any excess swelling or pressure that constricts blood flow to the muscles and nerves

        2) Hypoxemia and cellular death may result at the site and distal to the injury, creating a potential loss of limb

    f. Fractures near great vessels that tear or rupture as a result of the injury may also cause secondary hemorrhaging, creating a hypovolemic state

    g. Large bone fractures such as the pelvis or femur may create a hypovolemic state due to the blood loss from the bone itself

    h. *Spinal fractures*

        1) Fractures to the spinal column at the cervical level are generally the result of deceleration and acceleration, which flex, hyperextend, or rotate the neck

        2) Penetrating or crushing injuries are more common below the cervical spine

        3) Vertebral fractures may completely sever the spinal cord, resulting in paralysis below the fracture site

        4) Disruption of the blood supply to the cord may also cause permanent damage

        5) The extent and location of the fracture determines the degree of system impairment, which results from damage to the neural pathways from the spinal cord to the organs and tissues they control

        6) Injury to the spine may also be seen in post-traumatic states when ligaments and bones are unstable and subsequent maneuvering occurs

    i. *Pelvic fractures*

        1) Pelvic fractures occur most frequently in order adults from low-velocity falls; these are generally closed and non-displaced

        2) In younger, healthier individuals, high-velocity deceleration injuries to the pelvis are seen as a result of motor vehicle accidents and falls

        3) These fractures may be a significant source of hemorrhage and may signal additional trauma to other systems such as the abdominal and urinary organs

        4) Pelvic fractures and other long bone fractures are prone to the release of fat, potentially forming a life-threatening fat embolus

    j. *Acetabulum, hip, and proximal femur fractures*

        1) The proximal portion of the femur meets the pelvis at the acetabulum and forms the hip; this area of the body is prone to fracture within the geriatric population from falls or pathologic fractures, which occur as a result of porous bone density

        2) The femur is the largest bone in the body and contains a significant amount of blood stored in the shaft; a great amount of force is needed to break this bone, and as such, assessment for other pelvic and knee injuries should be done

        3) Because of their close location to the femoral vessels, injuries to these bones may also result in injury to arteries, veins, and nerves; hypovolemia may be of significant concern

        4) Peripheral blood flow and neurological function to the lower extremities may be severely compromised

▶ **Practice to Pass**

A client presents with a small caliber gunshot wound to the lower left lateral chest with signs and symptoms suggesting a pneumothorax and shock. No other injury is noted. What type of shock and pneumothorax is suspected and why?

k. *Soft tissue injuries*

1) Soft tissue injuries are those injuries resulting in damage to tissues and their underlying vasculature

2) These may be crushing in nature or as a result of a puncture or **laceration** (injuries to soft tissue that result in a tearing or slicing of the skin and possibly the underlying fleshy structures)

3) These injuries may also be seen within industrial settings where liquid or air is utilized under high pressure

   a) The substance is introduced to the tissues at great volumes and under tremendous pressure

   b) Tissues are crushed, altering circulation in the area

4) Bone or ligament and tendon involvement are usually not seen in the presence of a primary diagnosis of tissue injury

5) Hemorrhage into the surrounding tissue at the site of the injury results in diminished perfusion to the area that may cause tissue necrosis or delayed healing

C. Nursing assessment

1. Multisystem injury that threatens life or limb requires rapid and sequential assessment and intervention for a successful outcome

2. Each primary assessment phase will correspond with an immediate intervention if an injury is discovered

   a. Remember also that there are generally multiple members of a trauma team who assess and intervene almost simultaneously

   b. A secondary assessment occurs after life-threatening injuries are maintained and airway, breathing, and circulation (ABCs) are restored

3. Treatment for a "higher" level system, such as the airway, should never be postponed in order to complete the entire sequence

4. Many hospitals utilize rapid assessment forms that allow for a determination of the intensity or severity of a trauma client's condition; these tools provide great assistance in organizing the most common needs of clients at differing levels of acuity

5. Assessment

   a. Prearrival

      1) Vital signs

      2) Focused injury findings

      3) Neurological status (to include if victim has lost consciousness)

      4) Machinery involved (includes type and caliber of weapon)

      5) Current medications, medical history, allergies

      6) Safety belt usage

      7) Mechanism of injury, time of injury

      8) Environmental factors such as chemical spills

      9) Tetanus immunization status if wounds are present

   b. If no report is available prior to the client's arrival, gather pertinent information simultaneously while assessing the client's condition; *treatment should never be delayed because of an absent or incomplete history*

   c. Obtaining data about the circumstances of the injury is important to rule out secondary and delayed manifestations of an injury; however, life support is carried out in the same and consistent manner for all victims of trauma

    d. Upon arrival

       1) Assess airway and adequate ventilation through observation and auscultation; note abnormalities such as absence of breathing or inadequate ventilations and irregular depth or rate

       2) Assess for vomitus or debris in the mouth

       3) Assess for flail segments of the ribs, diminished or absent breath sounds, presence of a deviated trachea (trachea is "pushed" to one side rather than midline in the anterior neck), and the sounds of any air movement through a wound

       4) Assess cardiac activity through gentle palpation of the carotid pulse and/or auscultation

       5) Assess cardiac rhythms via a cardiac monitor, noting any dysrhythmias

       6) Assess for distant heart sounds, pericardial friction rub and the presence of distended jugular veins

       7) Assess for obvious sources of hemorrhage, to include the urethral meatus and the rectum

       8) Be sure to assess the client's back while maintaining spinal alignment

       9) Assess for signs and symptoms of shock, specifically hypovolemic or cardiogenic shock (give close attention to diminishing urinary output, as pulse and BP may not alter dramatically until late shock is reached)

      10) Assess neurological status including LOC, peripheral posturing, sensation, and mobility

      11) Assess pupillary size in millimeters and response to light

      12) Assess for paralysis and symmetry of movement

      13) Loss of rectal tone may be assessed in the presence of spinal cord injury

      14) Assess for fractures with special attention provided to the thoracic, pelvic, and femoral areas

      15) Assess for pain, shortening, and external rotation of the affected leg commonly found in hip fractures

      16) Assess peripheral pulses and extremity temperature and color

      17) Assess for fracture variations and locations, numbering sites in the event there are multiple injuries; crushing injuries may mask displaced bones, but may be threatening in and of themselves; areas of gross distention may produce a *compartment* or tourniquet effect at the site and distal to the injury, blocking blood flow and producing a limb-threatening emergency

6. Diagnostic tests

    a. H&H: hypovolemic shock is always a significant risk for the trauma client; decreasing levels and the rate of deterioration may indicate severe hemorrhaging

    b. WBC: may elevate with the inflammatory response to trauma or in response to blood in the abdominal cavity, indicating a source of hemorrhage

    c. ABGS: indicates respiratory failure and acid/base imbalances; used to direct supplemental oxygen therapy

       1) Respiratory failure is indicated by a $PO_2 < 50$ mmHg or a $PCO_2 > 50$ mmHg

       2) If the failure is acute in nature, the pH (normal 7.35 to 7.45) will fall as CO_2 is retained

    d. EKG: may reveal dysrhythmias requiring treatment or procedural interventions

    e. Cardiac enzymes: an elevation indicates cardiac tissue damage has occurred

Practice to Pass

A client presents with a cast on the lower left arm because of a fracture from falling. The upper-left arm is severely bruised and distended, and the client is complaining of severe "pressure" to this area. What emergent condition could be related to the client's injuries?

    f. Urinalysis: urine with microscopic hematuria may indicate minor to significant genitourinary trauma

     g. Blood alcohol and/or toxicology screen: traumatic injuries are often associated with alcohol ingestion or substance use

        1) Severe intoxication compromises airway clearance and respiratory effort

        2) The client is at more risk for injury; assess carefully to differentiate diminished mentation caused by injury from that brought on by intoxication or an abnormal glucose

    h. Glucose testing: hyperglycemia may be mistaken for alcohol intoxication because of the pungent, fruity smell of the breath and the confusion clients typically exhibit

D. Nursing management

   1. Prearrival

      a. Organize ancillary staff such as additional nursing support, respiratory and radiology personnel and any other medical consultants based upon the client's status

      b. Equipment: organize equipment to include resuscitative equipment (crash cart with airway management equipment and medications), IV access equipment and fluid, urinary catheterization equipment, bandaging supplies, sterile water and basins, lab specimen collectors and other supplies as needed for procedures such as cricothyrotomy, thoracostomy, thoracotomy, peritoneal lavage, and pericardiocentesis

   2. Standard interventions

       a. Assistance with ventilation using supplemental O_2

      b. Establishing intravenous (IV) access; two large-bore IV catheters (18 gauge or larger) are usually inserted

      c. Cardiac monitoring and continuous/intermittent VS monitoring to include pulse oximetry

      d. Maintaining alignment at all times in the supine position until an appropriate diagnosis is made; splint and support obvious deformities; slightly elevate the legs in the absence of head injury, cardiac decompensation or pulmonary edema/congestion

      e. Accurate observation of intake and output (I&O)

        1) A urinary catheter should be inserted when accurate measurements are required

        2) Do not insert a catheter when bleeding from the urethral meatus is noted or there is obvious hip and pelvic deformity until bladder injury is ruled out

      f. Document all assessments, interventions, and responses

      g. Maintain airway, circulation, and neurological assessment (see Table 17-4)

      h. Manage shock state

   3. Fractures

      a. Medications include analgesics and antibiotics, which may be given prophylactically for open wounds

      b. Support and split obvious fractures without manipulating or "reducing" (bending a fracture into alignment) the bone, utilizing pillows, folded linens, and tape

      c. Release any constricting garments or splints without manipulating the fractured area, frequently performing neurovascular checks distal to the site of injury

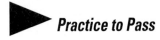

Practice to Pass

A pre-hospital report by emergency medical personnel indicates a near-drowning victim dove head first into shallow waters. What preparations, including department contacts, would be made prior to the client's arrival?

Table 17-4	Nursing Management of Trauma	
Airway	**Circulation**	**Neurological**
• Establish and maintain adequate airway • Use supplemental oxygen • Remove debris with tongue depressor and suction • Utilize airway supplements such as oropharyngeal or endotracheal tubes • Utilize nasal intubation if cervical injury suspected • Prepare for thoracostomy (chest tube) if needed	• Monitor for cardiac dysrhythmias • Prepare to administer medications and perform procedures specific to dysrhythmia, such as defibrillation • Prepare for a thoracotomy if necessary • Pericardiocentesis may be needed if cardiac tamponade is evident • Monitor vital signs every 5 to 15 minutes	• Assess neurological status every 15 minutes as needed • Medications include osmotic diuretics and steroids for cerebral edema; antibiotics for open head injury • Maintain immobile and aligned cervical spine while neurological assessment is unstable • Restrict fluids if level of consciousness is changing and shock is not evident • Use hyperventilation to lower cerebral edema • Control seizures

    d. Ice may be applied to cool the area, avoiding direct contact with the skin or injured area

    e. In the presence of an open or suspected open fracture, sterile, saline-soaked gauze should be applied until the area is thoroughly cleansed

  4. Hemorrhage

    a. Treat obvious sources of external hemorrhage by direct pressure applied through moist, sterile bandages

    b. A hemothorax may contain over one liter of blood and may constitute a significant source of volume loss; a thoracostomy tube may be inserted and an autotransfusion may be performed

    c. Bleeding from within the abdomen and retroperitoneum may occur with or without abdominal distention and rigidity until late into the shock sequence; peritoneal lavage may be performed to determine the presence of blood

    d. Fractures of the pelvis and femur are also capable of producing profound hypovolemic states; as with all states of hypovolemia, the intravascular volume is restored by infusing crystalloids or colloids (including blood) and by administering sympathomimetics

IV. DISSEMINATED INTRAVASCULAR COAGULOPATHY (DIC)

  A. Overview

    1. Disseminated intravascular coagulopathy (DIC) is a complex and abnormal response of the body's normal clotting mechanisms to an injury

    2. Clotting processes are accelerated and normal clothing substances become depleted, leaving the client open to massive hemorrhaging

    3. DIC may become a complicating side effect in some forms of shock, most commonly with septic shock; it also occurs secondary to other disorders but does not occur alone

    4. It is associated with a high mortality rate

    5. Causes of DIC include sepsis, shock, malignant neoplasms, liver disease, metabolic disorders, circulatory disorders, gynecological conditions, spinal or brain injuries, transfusion reactions, and immune disorders including venomous bites

B. Pathophysiology

1. In healthy individuals, homeostasis is maintained between vessel injury and bleeding when an appropriate size clot forms; clotting only becomes a problem when no injury has been sustained or when hemorrhaging depletes the client's reservoir of clotting factors

2. The intrinsic and/or extrinsic clotting pathways are activated in response to a traumatic injury

3. Thromboplastin is released from damaged cells and as a result, platelets begin to adhere to the damaged vessel or blood cell forming a "barrier" to prevent further hemorrhaging and injury

4. A plug of fibrinogen and fibrin is stabilized at the site of the injury through the processes of normal clot formation; the clot or plug is then removed through a process called **fibrinolysis** (process by which a clot is broken down)

5. Fibrinolysis may occur immediately or days after an injury and causes the release of fibrin degradation products (FDPs) and fibrin degradation fragments (FDFs); in healthy individuals or those suffering only minor injuries, the process is restricted to the area of injury

6. Clients suffering from massive tissue and cellular damage, such as traumatic or shock states, deplete the clotting factors as they are used up in an attempt to prevent further hemorrhaging

7. This cycle becomes self-defeating in that circulating fibrin clots become widespread throughout the body's intravascular volume, often causing widespread thrombosis (blood clots in the bloodstream)

8. Thrombi indicate to the body that further damage is occurring and the body responds by releasing more clotting factors that are also consumed until, finally, massive hemorrhaging occurs; circulating FDPs also have an anticoagulant affect, worsening the scenario

9. The client hemorrhages at a life-threatening level, while at the same time clotting extensively in an unrelenting cycle

10. Signs and symptoms

    a. Decreased blood pressure and peripheral pulses

    b. Purpura, ecchymosis, petechiae

    c. Cyanosis and bleeding that may range from mild oozing around catheter/IV sites and oral mucosa to profound volume loss noted by hematuria or occult blood in the stool or vomitus

    d. Intraabdominal bleeding may manifest itself with pain, distention, and rigidity

    e. Hypoxemia, dyspnea, and air hunger

    f. Neurologic symptoms: confusion, decreased LOC, seizures

    g. Renal symptoms: oliguria

    h. GI symptoms: nausea, vomiting

    i. Epistaxis

    j. Seizures

    k. Pain in chest, muscles, back, and abdomen

Practice to Pass

A client presents with frank hematuria, bleeding from the gums, and an elevated prothrombin time and partial thromboplastin time. What other diagnostic test may be ordered to support a diagnosis of disseminated intravascular coagulopathy (DIC) versus another coagulation abnormality and why?

C. Nursing Assessment

1. Assessment

   a. Risk: any client who presents with obvious signs and symptoms of frank hemorrhaging without obvious injury; or predisposing conditions such as shock, septicemia, or those transfusion of blood products

   b. Assessment includes VS, pulses, respiratory and cardiac status, assessment of all orifices and venipuncture sites, symptom analysis of pain, skin color, capillary refill, mentation, urinary output, and GI complaints

2. Diagnostic tests

   a. PT International normalized ratio (INR) or and PTT: elevated

   b. FDPs or FDFs: elevated

   c. D-dimer test will be elevated

      1) Serial testing is very important and assists in determining the diagnosis of DIC as opposed to other bleeding disorders

      2) A steady increase in these values indicates ongoing, massive clot breakdown rather than a lack of clotting factors

   d. CBC

   e. Electrolyte panel

   f. BUN, creatinine

D. Nursing management

1. Medications include heparin (in some clients) to neutralize the effects of circulating thrombin

   a. However, heparin should be administered with great care and only when extreme circumstances warrant its use

   b. Generally this anticoagulant is administered when DIC is not rapidly reversed through treatment of the underlying cause or in clients who are threatened by bleeding or massive thrombis formation

2. It is important to treat the underlying cause of DIC as quickly as possible and treat for a shock state that has precipitated the crisis

3. Fresh frozen plasma and cryoprecipitate are administered to replace clotting factors

4. Monitor coagulation tests not only for diagnosis, but for treatment

V. ACUTE RESPIRATORY DISTRESS SYNDROME

A. Overview

1. **Acute respiratory distress syndrome (ARDS)** is acute respiratory failure caused by many factors such as shock, trauma, burns, bacterial or viral pathogens, aspiration of fluids, and toxic injury

B. Pathophysiology

1. Alveolar walls are severely impaired; pulmonary capillaries are injured or there is damage to alveolar lining

2. The result is increased permeability of alveolar blood vessels, which allows fluid to accumulate in alveolar spaces and alveoli become airless; a tremendous strain is placed on the heart and cardiac complications are likely

3. Fluid in alveoli causes a decrease in surfactant and increased surface tension, leading to a loss of lung compliance, decreased ventilation, and hypoxia; lungs become stiff and noncompliant because of alveolar collapse

4. As alveoli are damaged, hypoxia ensues and eventually cell injury and death occurs
   a. Inflammatory reactions can occur as alveoli and capillaries are damaged
   b. The inflammation causes release of cytokines that leads to damage of capillaries and alveoli nearby
   c. Hyaline membranes form inside alveoli and further hinder exchange of oxygen and carbon dioxide

5. A spontaneous pneumothorax can occur

6. Supplemental oxygen does not improve the condition, a hall mark of diagnosing AROS

C. Nursing assessment

1. Assessment includes respiratory distress (tachypnea, use of accessory muscles, marked dyspnea), lung sounds (crackles or rhonchi), abnormal ABGs (hypoxia and/or hypercapnia), cyanosis, retractions, agitation, and confusion (late stage)

2. Diagnostic tests: CXR (large, diffuse infiltrates or "white outs" with normal heart size), ABGs ($PaO_2 < 50$ mmHg and respiratory alkalosis), PFS (decreased lung compliance; reduced vital capacity, minute volume, and functional vital capacity), and pulmonary artery pressure monitoring for diagnostic purposes (normal pressures will be evident in ARDS versus elevated pressures in pulmonary edema)

D. Nursing management

1. Medications
   a. Nitrous oxide for its analgesic effect or to dilate blood vessels and improve oxygenation
   b. Nonsteroidal anti-inflammatory drugs (NSAIDs), interleukin-1 receptor antagonists, neutrophil inhibitors, or corticosteroids to reduce inflammation
   c. Lung surfactants: beractant (Survanta), calfactant (Infasurf), and colfosceril (Exosurf Neonatal) to lower surface tension of alveoli and prevent alveolar collapse; this action restores pulmonary compliance and oxygenation
   d. Antibiotics if an infection is suspected as the cause
   e. Heparin to prevent complication of ARDS such as thrombophlebitis, pulmonary embolus, or disseminated intravascular coagulopathy (DIC)
   f. Sedative agents or skeletal muscle relaxants such as pancuronium bromide (Tubocurarine) to control the agitation associated with mechanical ventilation

2. Foremost therapy is to treat the cause

3. Main form of therapy is endotracheal intubation and mechanical ventilation
   a. Continuous positive airway pressure (CPAP) or positive-end expiratory pressure (PEEP) is often used to open airways and alveoli and to improve gas exchange
   b. PEEP has been associated with decreased cardiac output, lung injury caused by high mechanical pressure to lung tissue known as barotrauma; and decreased vital signs (VS), especially a drop in blood pressure (BP), monitor lung sounds

4. Maintaining a prone position may improve oxygen perfusion

5. Monitor pulmonary arterial pressure through use of a Swan-Ganz line

> ### ▶ Practice to Pass
>
> A client, who has suffered a large myocardial infarction (MI) and has had difficulty recuperating, suddenly goes into acute respiratory distress syndrome (ARDS). Why should treatment be aggressive in this situation?

6. Maintain adequate fluid and nutritional status

7. Monitor oxygen saturation and signs of a pneumothorax, which is a complication of ARDS

Case Study

A trauma victim presents to the Emergency Department after a motor vehicle accident in which the pre-hospital report indicates that the car's steering wheel was broken and no seat belt was worn. Vital signs are BP 100/58, pulse 116, respirations 26 and labored, temperature 97.2°F oral. The client is intermittently confused and is lethargic. There is a 6-inch laceration to the frontal scalp. Pupils are equal and reactive. Upon exam, there is a large ecchymotic area to the right anterior chest and paradoxical movement is noted. Breath sounds are absent to the right base, anteriorly and posteriorly. The right leg is externally rotated and shortened.

1. What fundamental interventions would be initiated immediately upon arrival based on this information?

2. What procedures would potentially be performed?

3. What phase and type of shock is suspected on presentation? What diagnostic values would contribute to determining the phase and type?

4. What are the potential injuries that are most highly suspected of contributing to the shock state?

5. What physical finding would cause concern when determining whether to place a urinary catheter for accurate output monitoring?

For suggested responses, see page 539.

POSTTEST

1 A client presents with suspected chest and spinal injuries after a motor vehicle accident. On receipt of the client from ambulance personnel, the Emergency Department nurse determines that which of the following is a priority intervention?

1. Preparing spinal traction to align head and spinal cord
2. Checking interior of the mouth for broken teeth or other injuries
3. Applying pressure to areas of gross hemorrhaging
4. Auscultating and inspecting chest for the presence of pneumothorax or tamponade

2 A trauma client has been admitted to the Emergency Department. The nurse analyzes the hemoglobin and hematocrit levels to monitor for which of the following shock states?

1. Hypovolemic
2. Cardiogenic
3. Anaphylactic
4. Distributive

3 A 57-year-old man who suffered a large myocardial infarction develops acute respiratory distress syndrome (ARDS) as a complication. The client is intubated and placed on positive end expiratory pressure (PEEP). The nurse becomes most concerned about which of the following findings while the client is on PEEP?

1. Sinus tachycardia of 125 beats per minute
2. Anxiety
3. Blood pressure of 88/52
4. Temperature of 100.5°F

POSTTEST

4 A client has developed hypovolemic shock. The nurse would use which of the following indicators when prioritizing the ongoing plan of care?

1. Urinary output
2. Skin turgor
3. Range of mobility
4. Temperature

5 A client involved in a motor vehicle accident is brought by ambulance to the trauma unit. She was thrown against the right side of an older car that has standard hand cranks for the window. Her abdomen is distended and painful to touch, hematocrit and hemoglobin (H&H) are low, and BP is 80/50. Which of the following would be the nurse's major concern?

1. Head injury
2. Spontaneous pneumothorax
3. Ruptured liver or spleen
4. Ruptured kidney

6 A client who sustained a head injury from a blow to the head 10 hours ago is brought to the Emergency Department in a lethargic state with one pupil larger and sluggish in responding to light. The computed tomography (CT) scan shows a venous bleed and subdural hematoma. The nurse would look to what changes or assessments as an indication of worsening status? Select all that apply.

1. Further loss of consciousness
2. Lowering of systolic blood pressure
3. Bradycardia
4. Projectile vomiting occurring without warning
5. Papilledema on fundoscopic examination

7 A client presents to the Emergency Department with a gunshot wound to the upper anterior left chest. Which assessment would the nurse perform next after completing the primary survey?

1. Patency of the airway
2. Secondary injuries such as extremity fractures
3. Chest excursion and gas exchange
4. Constipation and smoking history

8 When evaluating the status of a client who is recovering from hypovolemic shock following administration of blood products and other colloids, which indicators would the nurse use to determine whether the client has had the best outcome?

1. Vital signs, hematocrit and hemoglobin (H&H), and coagulation tests within normal limits
2. Vital signs and a hematocrit and hemoglobin (H&H) level within normal limits and a urinalysis without hematuria
3. Vital signs and a hematocrit and hemoglobin (H&H) level within normal limits and a negative C-spine x-ray
4. Vital signs and neurological exam within normal limits

9 The nurse assesses a client who sustained a fracture of the femur 16 hours ago for which complication for which the client is at greatest risk?

1. Disuse syndrome
2. Fat embolism syndrome
3. Reflex sympathetic dystrophy
4. Infection

10 The nurse determines that successful outcome measurements for a client who experienced open trauma to the head includes the:

1. Recall of the actual event of injury.
2. Loss of consciousness of no greater than 24 hours.
3. Absence of signs of meningitis.
4. Absence of pain.

➤ *See pages 520–522 for Answers & Rationales.*

ANSWERS & RATIONALES

Pretest

1 **Answer: 2** All forms of pneumothorax may progress to the extent that tension develops within the affected lung space and exerts pressure on the unaffected lung. A deviated trachea is a classic sign of tension pneumothorax. **Cognitive Level:** Application **Client Need:** Physiological Integrity: Physiological Adaptation **Integrated Process:** Nursing Process: Analysis **Content Area:** Adult Health: Respiratory **Strategy:** Look for the abnormal manifestations and reflect on the mechanism of injury to determine the problem. **Reference:** Porth, C. M. (2005). *Pathophysiology: Concepts of altered health states* (7th ed.). Philadelphia, PA: Lippincott Williams & Wilkins, pp. 691–692.

2 **Answer: 4** Aspiration of any liquid into the lungs places the client at risk for development of ARDS. Assessments to evaluate the onset of this syndrome should focus on the respiratory system and diminishing oxygen saturation despite increasing supplemental oxygen. **Cognitive Level:** Analysis **Client Need:** Physiological Integrity: Physiological Adaptation **Integrated Process:** Nursing Process: Assessment **Content Area:** Adult Health: Respiratory **Strategy:** The clues are the near-drowning situation and the poor respiratory status. Recall that with drowning, there is aspiration of water into the lungs. **Reference:** Porth, C. M. (2005). *Pathophysiology: Concepts of altered health states* (7th ed.). Philadelphia, PA: Lippincott Williams & Wilkins, pp. 715–716.

3 **Answer: 2** During the compensatory phase of shock, the body attempts to correct the progression of a decrease in intravascular volume through an increase in pulse and respiration and the subjective sensation of thirst. Shunting of blood begins to occur from organs not vital for immediate survival. Renal blood flow is diminished, and urinary output falls. Blood pressure is decreasing but adequate for current homeostasis. Thirst is a response to decreased blood volume. **Cognitive Level:** Analysis **Client Need:** Physiological Integrity: Physiological Adaptation **Integrated Process:** Nursing Process: Analysis **Content Area:** Adult Health: Cardiovascular **Strategy:** Consider that tissue perfusion is still being maintained although the heart rate, blood pressure, and oliguria indicate moderate severity of shock. **Reference:** Porth, C. M. (2005). *Pathophysiology: Concepts of altered health states* (7th ed.). Philadelphia, PA: Lippincott Williams & Wilkins, pp. 619–620.

4 **Answer: 4** The presenting signs and symptoms are associated with the compensatory phase of shock. Myocardial infarction is the most common cause of cardiac damage resulting in cardiac insufficiency or "pump failure" leading to cardiogenic shock. Jugular venous distention and pulmonary congestion are consistent with heart failure. **Cognitive Level:** Analysis **Client Need:** Physiological Integrity: Physiological Adaptation **Integrated Process:** Nursing Process: Analysis **Content Area:** Adult Health: Cardiovascular **Strategy:** All the options are for a type of shock. Determine the origin from the situation. **Reference:** Porth, C. M. (2005). *Pathophysiology: Concepts of altered health states* (7th ed.). Philadelphia, PA: Lippincott Williams & Wilkins, pp. 614–615.

5 **Answer: 2** The client is exhibiting the standard immunological reaction to the administration of an antibiotic. Sensitizing dosages have already occurred as reported by the client. Anaphylactic shock is a form of distributive shock. More information would be needed to determine whether this client is developing septicemia or septic shock. There is no supporting evidence in the client's situation for hypovolemic or neurogenic shock. **Cognitive Level:** Application **Client Need:** Physiological Integrity: Physiological Adaptation **Integrated Process:** Nursing Process: Analysis **Content Area:** Adult Health: Immunological **Strategy:** Read the client situation of receiving a few doses of an antibiotic and then developing symptoms of a problem. **Reference:** Porth, C. M. (2005). *Pathophysiology: Concepts of altered health states* (7th ed.). Philadelphia, PA: Lippincott Williams & Wilkins, p. 622.

6 **Answer: 3** Cervical and thoracic spinal injuries are often associated with trauma to the head, chest, and upper back, as well as falls and deceleration incidents. **Cognitive Level:** Analysis **Client Need:** Physiological Integrity: Physiological Adaptation **Integrated Process:** Nursing Process: Analysis **Content Area:** Adult Health: Neurological **Strategy:** Consider the history of fall and the impact to the upper-middle back. Use knowledge of anatomy and pathophysiology when eliminating the incorrect options. **Reference:** Porth, C. M. (2005). *Pathophysiology: Concepts of altered health states* (7th ed.). Philadelphia, PA: Lippincott Williams & Wilkins, pp. 1216–1217.

7 **Answers: 2, 4, 5** Paradoxical pulses, or pulsus paradoxus, is a hallmark symptom of cardiac tamponade. As pressure is exerted on the left ventricle from fluid, the natural increase in pressure from the right ventricle during inspiration creates even more pressure, diminishing cardiac output. Narrowed pulse pressure, hypotension, and weak pulses are also manifestations of cardiac tamponade. A deviated trachea is a sign of a tension pneumothorax, and atelectasis is not associated with tamponade. **Cognitive Level:** Analysis **Client Need:** Physiological Integrity: Physiological Adaptation **Integrated Process:** Nursing Process: Assessment **Content Area:** Adult Health: Cardiovascular **Strategy:** Recall that in cardiac tamponade, there is rising intracardiac pressure resulting in decreased diastolic filling and decreased cardiac output. Consider what manifestations will be observed because of these events. **Reference:** Lemone, P., & Burke, K. (2008). *Medical-surgical nursing: Critical thinking in client care* (4th ed.). Upper Saddle River, NJ: Pearson/Prentice Hall, pp. 1050–1051.

8 Answer: 2 Penetrating injury to the bowel releases intracolonic material into the peritoneal cavity, predisposing the individual to a serious infection that may progress to septicemia. While a paralytic ileus is of concern any time the abdominal cavity has been accessed through surgery or injury or with the administration of certain medications, it is not of the life-threatening nature that is found with the diagnosis of peritonitis. Peritonitis may cause the occurrence of a paralytic ileus. **Cognitive Level:** Application **Client Need:** Safe, Effective Care Environment: Management of Care **Integrated Process:** Nursing Process: Planning **Content Area:** Adult Health: Gastrointestinal **Strategy:** Consider which option poses a potential for life-threatening complications. When narrowing the options to two, determine which one needs the most immediate intervention. **Reference:** Lemone, P., & Burke, K. (2008). *Medical-surgical nursing: Critical thinking in client care* (4th ed.). Upper Saddle River, NJ: Pearson/Prentice Hall, p. 259.

9 Answer: 3 Many traumatic injuries occur as a result of the slowed responses and judgment associated with alcohol intoxication. Hyperglycemia may exhibit similar signs and symptoms to intoxication so it is necessary to assess both values. Skull x-rays are noncontributory for brain injuries unless there is an obvious or highly suspected fracture. The client reports no loss of consciousness but a CT scan may be done if head injury in addition to the laceration is suspected. An MRI is not appropriate at this time. An EEG measures the electrical brain waves to determine brain death or some type of seizure and abnormal cerebral activity. **Cognitive Level:** Analysis **Client Need:** Physiological Integrity: Reduction of Risk Potential **Integrated Process:** Nursing Process: Assessment **Content Area:** Adult Health: Neurological **Strategy:** Note that blood alcohol levels ap-

pear in many options. Both tests in the option must be appropriate for the option to be correct. Consider what etiology besides alcohol intoxication may cause this client's symptoms. **Reference:** Lemone, P., & Burke, K. (2008). *Medical-surgical nursing: Critical thinking in client care* (4th ed.). Upper Saddle River, NJ: Pearson/Prentice Hall, p. 261.

10 Answers: 1, 3, 4 Compartment syndrome is a result of swelling or pressure that constricts blood flow to musculature and nerves. Hemorrhaging and loss of intravascular fluid to the interstitial spaces creates a tourniquet effect, compromising the circulation at the site of injury and distally. Unrelieved pain, signs of compromised arterial circulation, sensory loss, and motor weakness are important symptoms. Nerve symptoms develop within 30 minutes of ischemia and muscle weakness in two to four hours—the time frame for this client. **Cognitive Level:** Application **Client Need:** Physiological Integrity: Physiological Adaptation **Integrated Process:** Nursing Process: Assessment **Content Area:** Adult Health: Musculoskeletal **Strategy:** Consider that when circulatory changes occur with musculoskeletal trauma, there is an increased likelihood of compartment syndrome. Read each option carefully and use the process of elimination to make a selection. **Reference:** Porth, C. M. (2005) *Pathophysiology: Concepts of altered health states* (7th ed.). Philadelphia, PA: Lippincott Williams & Wilkins, pp. 499–500.

Posttest

1 Answer: 2 The client's airway is priority in all phases of life support. Remember ABCs for life support. A trauma team usually consists of many people and others can be assessing less critical areas. Spinal traction is not the same as immobilizing the cervical spine, which is another priority of care. **Cognitive Level:** Analysis **Client Need:** Safe, Effective Care Environment: Management of Care **Integrated Process:** Nursing Process: Implementation **Content Area:** Adult Health: Respiratory **Strategy:** Remember ABCs of life support to prioritize your answer. **Reference:** Lemone, P., & Burke, K. (2008). *Medical-surgical nursing: Critical thinking in client care* (4th ed.). Upper Saddle River, NJ: Pearson/Prentice Hall, pp. 265–266.

2 Answer: 1 Hematocrit and hemoglobin (H&H) levels will continue to decrease with ongoing hemorrhaging, indicating the aggressiveness of interventions to replace intravascular volume in hypovolemic shock. Cardiogenic shock would not be characterized by a drop in H&H, nor would anaphylactic shock or distributive shock. **Cognitive Level:** Application **Client Need:** Physiological Integrity: Physiological Adaptation **Integrated Process:**

Nursing Process: Analysis **Content Area:** Adult Health: Cardiovascular **Strategy:** Identify what mechanism causes the hemoglobin and hematocrit to steadily fall. Recall what happens to the blood volume and blood pressure if this occurs to make a selection. **Reference:** Porth, C. M. (2005). *Pathophysiology: Concepts of altered health states* (7th ed.). Philadelphia, PA: Lippincott Williams & Wilkins, pp. 617–619.

3 Answer: 3 Barotrauma (decreased cardiac output and damage to lung tissue) is a complication of PEEP. A drop in blood pressure is associated with a decrease in cardiac output. The sinus tachycardia may be a compensatory mechanism to raise the BP or a response to the ARDS. Anxiety is expected with intubation and the small temperature elevation may or may not indicate a serious problem.
Cognitive Level: Analysis **Integrated Process:** Nursing Process: Analysis **Client Need:** Physiological Integrity: Physiological Adaptation **Content Area:** Adult Health: Respiratory **Strategy:** The clue is to select an option that is of concern with the PEEP. The other options are related to the client's status but not necessarily to the PEEP. **Reference:** Porth, C. M. (2005). *Pathophysiology: Concepts of altered health states* (7th ed.). Philadelphia, PA: Lippincott Williams & Wilkins, pp. 1161, 1163.

4 Answer: 1 All forms of shock diminish perfusion to the renal system. A decreasing output is indicative that the kidneys may be losing function as a result of significant tubular necrosis. Skin turgor (option 2) will generally reflect circulating volume, but is not a precise indicator. Range of mobility (option 3) is irrelevant to circulating volume. Temperature (option 4) could elevate with fluid volume loss but is again an imprecise indicator.
Cognitive Level: Application **Integrated Process:** Nursing Process: Planning **Client Need:** Physiological Integrity: Physiological Adaptation **Content Area:** Adult Health: Cardiovascular **Strategy:** Consider which assessment will give the best information related to blood volume and circulation. **Reference:** Lemone, P., & Burke, K. (2008). *Medical-surgical nursing: Critical thinking in client care* (4th ed.). Upper Saddle River, NJ: Pearson/Prentice Hall, p. 269.

5 Answer: 3 A distended, painful abdomen with signs of hypovolemic shock and a low H&H should trigger the nurse to consider a ruptured liver or spleen. Although a ruptured kidney could also occur, the major concern would be the liver because of its vascular nature. A head injury or pneumothorax should be assessed next.
Cognitive Level: Analysis **Client Need:** Physiological Integrity: Physiological Adaptation **Integrated Process:** Nursing Process: Assessment **Content Area:** Adult Health: Gastrointestinal **Strategy:** The manifestations and history

suggest trauma and hemorrhage. What body area is most likely injured? **Reference:** Lemone, P., & Burke, K. (2008). *Medical-surgical nursing: Critical thinking in client care* (4th ed.). Upper Saddle River, NJ: Pearson/Prentice Hall, p. 259.

6 Answers: 1, 3, 4, 5 Subdural hematomas are formed most often from venous tissue bleeding and are more common than other forms of brain injury. They have a high mortality because of secondary brain injury due to edema and increased intracranial pressure (ICP). Signs of increased ICP include projectile vomiting, deteriorating level of consciousness, papilledema (swelling of the optic disk) or, in late stages, the Cushing's triad (increased mean arterial pressure, widening pulse pressure, and bradycardia).
Cognitive Level: Application **Client Need:** Physiological Integrity: Physiological Adaptation **Integrated Process:** Nursing Process: Assessment **Content Area:** Adult Health: Neurological **Strategy:** Recall the signs of increased ICP after considering that the ICP would rise because of accumulating blood in the subdural space. **Reference:** Porth, C. M. (2005). *Pathophysiology: Concepts of altered health states* (7th ed.). Philadelphia, PA: Lippincott Williams & Wilkins, pp. 1235–1239.

7 Answer: 2 A secondary assessment or survey occurs once the airway, breathing, and circulation (primary survey) are assessed and interventions begun. Life-threatening injuries located during the primary assessment must be stabilized prior to reviewing for additional injuries or wounds. Airway and breathing assessments have already been done. Assessing for constipation and smoking is not a priority at this time.
Cognitive Level: Application **Client Need:** Physiological Integrity: Physiological Adaptation **Integrated Process:** Nursing Process: Assessment **Content Area:** Adult Health: Musculoskeletal **Strategy:** Remember ABCs. Utilize principles of conducting a secondary survey to recall what step comes after the client is stabilized from the life-threatening injury. **Reference:** Lemone, P., & Burke, K. (2008). *Medical-surgical nursing: Critical thinking in client care* (4th ed.). Upper Saddle River, NJ: Pearson/Prentice Hall, pp. 260, 266–267.

8 Answer: 1 Administering colloidal solutions may diminish the blood's ability to coagulate by reducing platelet adhesion while expanding the intravascular volume needed in severe shock states. Vital signs within established parameters indicate support of vital functions. Acceptable hematocrit and hemoglobin levels substantiate and support perfusion at a cellular level as well as resolution of volume loss. The presence or lack of hematuria is not a viable indicator of the level of shock states or their resolution.

Cognitive Level: Analysis **Client Need:** Physiological Integrity: Physiological Adaptation **Integrated Process:** Nursing Process: Evaluation **Content Area:** Adult Health: Cardiovascular **Strategy:** Differentiate between the physiological effects of intravenous crystalloids and colloids. What is the desired client response? **Reference:** Lemone, P., & Burke, K. (2008). *Medical-surgical nursing: Critical thinking in client care* (4th ed.). Upper Saddle River, NJ: Pearson/Prentice Hall, pp. 277–279.

9 **Answer: 2** Fat is more easily expressed from the larger bones such as the hip and femur when they are fractured. Other answers are not associated with a specific bone group.

Cognitive Level: Application **Client Need:** Physiological Integrity: Physiological Adaptation **Integrated Process:** Nursing Process: Analysis **Content Area:** Adult Health: Musculoskeletal **Strategy:** The critical word in the question is *femur*. Consider what serious complication may

follow a fracture of a long bone such as the femur. **Reference:** Lemone, P., & Burke, K. (2008). *Medical-surgical nursing: Critical thinking in client care* (4th ed.). Upper Saddle River, NJ: Pearson/Prentice Hall, p. 266.

10 **Answer: 3** An injury to the protective tissues of the brain poses a risk for infection in that bacterium can be introduced, especially with an open injury. Meningitis would be the manifestation exhibited.

Cognitive Level: Analysis **Client Need:** Physiological Integrity: Physiological Adaptation **Integrated Process:** Nursing Process: Evaluation **Content Area:** Adult Health: Neurological **Strategy:** The critical words *open trauma* relate to the body's protective barriers being breeched in the trauma. Consider what can enter the body to select an answer. **Reference:** Lemone, P., & Burke, K. (2008). *Medical-surgical nursing: Critical thinking in client care* (4th ed.). Upper Saddle River, NJ: Pearson/Prentice Hall, pp. 266–267.

References

Copstead-Kirkhorn, L., & Banasik, J. (2005). *Pathophysiology* (3rd ed.). Philadelphia, PA: Saunders.

Kee, J. L. (2005). *Laboratory and diagnostic tests* with nursing implications (7th ed.). Upper Saddle River, NJ: Pearson Education.

Lemone, P., & Burke, K. (2008). *Medical-surgical nursing: Critical thinking in client care* (2nd ed.). Upper Saddle River, NJ: Prentice Hall.

McCance, K., & Huether, S. (2006). *Pathophysiology: The biologic basis for disease in adults and children* (5th ed.). St. Louis, MO: Elsevier Science.

Porth, C. (2005). *Pathophysiology: Concepts of altered health states* (7th ed.). Philadelphia, PA: Lippincott, Williams & Wilkins.

Venes, O. & Thomas, C. (Eds). (2006). *Taber's cyclopedic medical dictionary* (19th ed.). Philadelphia, PA: F.A. Davis Co.

Wagner, K., Johnson, K., & Kidd, P. (2006). *High acuity nursing* (4th ed.). Upper Saddle River, NJ: Pearson Education.

Appendix

➤ Practice to Pass Suggested Answers

Chapter 1

Page 11: *Suggested Answer*—Beclomethasone (Vanceril) is a steroid; a common as well as concerning side effect in children is growth retardation. A child's asthma may require a medication on a daily basis as strong as the steroids. A decline in height and weight has been documented while children are on continuous doses of steroid therapy, and these should be monitored monthly.

Page 11: *Suggested Answer*—Steroids such as prednisone are often used for exacerbations of COPD with effective results. A side effect of steroids, however, is fluid retention, which could easily occur in a cardiac client with a history of CHF. Careful monitoring of intake and output, weight, presence of edema, and lung sounds should be implemented in order to identify early signs of CHF should they occur.

Page 16: *Suggested Answer*—Either the antibiotic is not the correct treatment for the type of organism causing the pneumonia or the pneumonia is viral in nature. A culture and sensitivity should be obtained to identify the organism causing the problem and to ensure sensitivity of the antibiotic to the organism. If the problem is viral pneumonia, antibiotics will not usually help anyway. Any time fever persists after an individual has been on an antibiotic for at least 72 hours, additional considerations should be made.

Page 18: *Suggested Answer*—Remember that two groups at risk for tuberculosis are the disadvantaged and HIV-positive individuals. This client carries those risk factors and could be HIV-positive without knowing at this time. Also, females with sexually transmitted infections (STIs) often test positive for resistant strains of TB.

Chapter 2

Page 43: *Suggested Answer*—The fact that she has CAD does not mean she has had damage (injury) to the heart muscle itself. CAD indicates blockage in the arteries that bring blood to the heart and supply the needed oxygen. She can live with coronary artery disease and never have a heart attack if she modifies her lifestyle and corrects the behaviors that lead to CAD. The symptoms of a heart attack need to be explained (nausea, vomiting, crushing chest pain, shortness of breath, diaphoresis) as well as the difference between angina and a myocardial infarction.

Page 45: *Suggested Answer*—The nurse should explain to the client that having stable angina does not mean that the client will have a heart attack. As long as the causes of the pain are known and it stops with rest or responds to nitroglycerin, it should not cause permanent injury to the heart. However, if the pain changes in duration or intensity, or if the number of attacks increases, a health care provider should be seen as soon as possible. During an angina attack, if the pain stays longer, is more intense, or does not respond to rest or nitroglycerin, call for emergency help.

Page 48: *Suggested Answer*—An example of an acceptable response might be: "I know you feel that way, but now that you are here we can help you. Try to take deep, even breaths. We will give you some medication to help with the pain." Explain the procedures that are being ordered and what appears to be happening. Also explain that the feeling is normal when someone is having chest discomfort and shortness of breath. Do not offer false reassurance that everything will be all right when it may not.

Page 56: *Suggested Answer*—The nurse should explain to the client that he has been very ill and it will take some time for his body to return to normal. The doctor should talk to him about follow-up care. It is important that he follow the directions and rehabilitation schedule and not try to return to work too soon or further problems or complications may develop. An appropriate explanation and comparison for clients with heart problems is to compare it to a broken leg. The broken bone cannot always be seen, but it's still there and takes time to heal. The crutches are often the only reminder of the problem. The heart needs time to heal also and the signs and symptoms experienced are the only reminders of the problem. The client should check with the physician as to when the proper time is to return to work.

Page 67: *Suggested Answer*—The nurse should go immediately to the room and assess the client. If he is unresponsive and pulseless, call a code and call for the crash cart and defibrillator. If the client is awake, alert, and talking, check the monitor leads for proper connection. Chaotic activity could be caused by ventricular fibrillation, interference, a disconnected lead wire, a loose monitor pad, or activity such as bathing or respiratory percussion. Regardless, the client should always be assessed first.

Page 72: *Suggested Answer*—Inform the client that close follow-up care is needed. The disease progression must be monitored, as well as how well the client tolerates the progression. The client will have many tests done to determine the progression. If signs of congestive heart failure begin, the client will be treated with medication to help the heart beat more effectively. If angina occurs, clients often respond to beta blockers and nitroglycerin. Sometimes it is necessary to have a valve replaced. That is a decision that the client and the doctor must make together. The client must know that prior to any invasive procedure (including dental procedures), prophylactic antibiotics must be taken to prevent infection from getting to the valve and causing further problems or complications.

Chapter 3

Page 88: *Suggested Answer*—Discuss with the client what the client means by forgetting medicines and making up the dose at the next medication time. It would be very helpful to determine which medications the client is taking in this manner—prescription drugs, an over-the-counter medicine, or some alternative medicine. The nurse should review the medication schedule with the client. The primary outcome is to have the client's blood pressure reading be less than 140/90. Ask the client and family members if the medication schedule is convenient. Also, the purpose of each medication should be reviewed with the client and family members. The nurse should determine if the client is experiencing any side effects. If so, the nurse should ask which medications are involved, how long these problems have been present, and whether the client has notified the health care provider. Writing medication schedules on a card or pre-pouring the medicines for the client on a weekly basis might take the confusion out of the schedule. Determine if the client can adequately read and see the medication labels in order to read the dosage and times. If the client cannot read, pictures or a video describing what is to be done and how should be provided. If the client cannot see to read the names of the medications, specific directions could be developed by the nurse and big numbers used to indicate the time of day the medicine is to be taken. In addition, a referral to a home health agency for supervisory visits focused on medication compliance might be helpful. Time for client questions should be provided.

Page 91: *Suggested Answer*—The focus of the plan of care is to assist the client in the prevention and reduction of risk factors. This may be accomplished by:

- Avoiding sitting or standing in one place for prolonged periods of time. Frequently, support hose will help manage venous congestion.
- Avoiding the use of round garters and the wearing of tight abdominal garments, which constrict blood flow.
- Elevating the legs while sitting if venous congestion is a problem.
- Encouraging the client to begin walking and gradually increase distance up to 1 mile per day.
- Weight loss, if the client is obese. A referral to a weight reduction program within the community.
- Suggesting the adding of bulk to the diet to eliminate constipation to prevent straining and following a healthy-heart diet low in sodium, cholesterol, and fat.
- Discussing the cessation of smoking and limiting caffeine if these are present factors. Explain that cardiac disease such as congestive heart failure, myocardial infarction, and cardiomyopathy are risk factors for PVD and that PVD can lead to a thrombus or emboli.
- Educating the client on maintaining a normal blood pressure and having it monitored frequently if hypertension exists.

Page 93: *Suggested Answer*—The family should be commended on their concern and the nurse should identify that their concern is very important. Explain that surgery to repair an aneurysm is a serious operation and should not be considered lightly. The major complications are hemorrhage, stroke, and possibly death. Explain that an aneurysm that is not growing larger or leaking is often better left alone. The client should be compliant in having the MRIs every 6 months and keeping weight and blood pressure under control. Surgery is usually recommended when the aneurysm is at 5 cm (or greater) or shows signs of rapid growth or hemorrhage. Stress that the surgery will be a major operation for a 70-year-old individual; therefore, careful consideration should be made when the time is appropriate. The family should be instructed to seek medical advice if the back pain worsens or continues.

Page 98: *Suggested Answer*—Smoking is a primary cause of Buerger's disease, whereas genetics or unknown etiology is associated with Raynaud's disease. Raynaud's disease affects women more than men, while Buerger's affects mostly men. Raynaud's is usually triggered by stress or cold temperatures, while smoking triggers Buerger's disease. Raynaud's involves the digits mostly and more commonly the hands, while Buerger's usually affects the lower extremities. The blue-white-red color changes in the hands are classic for Raynaud's. Intermittent claudication is associated with Buerger's disease. Clients with either disease should stop smoking to limit the events and protect the extremities from cold injury during an event.

Chapter 4

Page 120: *Suggested Answer*—Encourage discussion of concerns and major goals of rehabilitation based on the client goals. These may include improved mobility, maintenance of range-of-motion, self-care, bladder and bowel control, improved communication, optimal family functioning, and prevention of complications and repeated stroke. Stress that the goal of rehabilitation is to allow the client to learn his or her strengths and limitations and hopefully improve on the latter. The family should be encouraged to support the health care professionals and not to offer to "do things" for their loved one. Explain that an acute care setting usually offers a lot of assistance during the acute phase versus a rehabilitation facility that encourages clients to perform their own ADLs under supervision.

Page 129: *Suggested Answer*—Consult and follow the Infection Control Policies and Procedures recommended by the facility. Isolation is no longer recommended in most cases. Careful "standard precautions" are always important to protect the client and nurse with the exception of meningicoccal meningitis. Good handwashing, use of gloves, and proper disposal of waste products should be initiated. Small infants and pregnant women should always avoid any potential risk.

Page 133: *Suggested Answer*—Review the procedure with the client to assess understanding and emphasize that there is no pain involved; provide open-ended questions to encourage discussion; recommend washing hair to decrease oil and avoid gels or hairspray; no sedatives or hypnotics should be administered beforehand, except as part of the EEG study; do not allow client to fast before study or to use stimulants like caffinated drinks or coffee; clarify with physician if any routine medications are to be held; explain what the placement of the electrodes means.

Page 135: *Suggested Answer*—

- Ineffective airway clearance, ineffective breathing pattern, impaired gas exchange
- Impaired physical mobility
- Self-care deficit
- Imbalanced nutrition: less than body requirements
- Constipation, diarrhea, urinary retention
- Risk for infection
- Risk for impaired skin integrity
- Impaired verbal communication (if tracheostomy)
- Pain
- Anxiety
- Powerlessness

Page 140: *Suggested Answer*—Assess the nature of the swallowing difficulty. Is the client having difficulty swallowing liquids and/or solids or chewing his food?

- Sit the client upright to eat and at least 30 to 45 minutes after eating.
- Observe the client swallow a sip of water; note coughing during and after eating.
- Observe as the client projects the tongue and moves it back and forth; refer to speech therapist for thorough evaluation; assist client to erect sitting position.
- Stay with the client while eating; cut food in small bites.
- Teach the client to think through the act of swallowing: close lips with teeth together, move the tongue up to the roof of the mouth with food on it; swallow with head bent forward.
- Try soft foods and thickened liquids.
- Massage client's face and neck muscles before eating.

Chapter 5

Page 162: *Suggested Answer*—The most effective way to increase joint mobility and maintain joint function is to participate in a regular exercise program and implement measures that decrease joint stress. The regular exercise program should be developed in collaboration with a physical therapist and include isometric exercises, PROM, and AROM. Some examples of measures that will decrease joint stress include pacing activities, performing activities when sitting if possible, using a splint for hands and wrists, and relaxation techniques. Water aerobics are significantly helpful, especially to elderly clients.

Page 163: *Suggested Answer*—To determine the appropriate pharmacological therapy in the client diagnosed with gouty arthritis it is important to know if elevated levels of uric acid are related to an increase in the production of uric acid or a decrease in the excretion of uric acid. A 24-hour urine specimen is collected to determine if the client is excreting normal levels of uric acid, 200 to 750 cc/24 hrs. A level that exceeds 750 cc/24 hrs indicates that the production of uric acid is increased, levels below 200 cc/24 hrs indicate that the excretion of uric acid is impaired.

Page 166: *Suggested Answer*—Bone deformities occur in Paget's disease as a result of excessive bone remodeling. Normal bone marrow is replaced with vasclar, fibrous connective tissue and bones eventually enlarge. Often one of the first symptoms of Paget's disease is increased head size.

Page 171: *Suggested Answer*—The following factors differentiate these bone tumors; growth rate, age of onset, tissue origin, and location. All three bone tumors are classified as primary bone tumors: chondrosarcomas are characterized by slow growth; Ewing's sarcomas and osteosarcomas are characterized by rapid growth; Ewing's sarcomas metastasize to the lung tissue. Chondrosarcomas occur more frequently in adult males, the other two primary bone tumors occur more frequently in young males during periods of optimal growth, 10 to 25 years of age. The tissue of origin for osteosarcomas is the metaphysis of long bones and they are usually found in the distal femur, proximal tibia, and proximal humerus following an injury. The tissue of origin for chondrosarcomas is cartilage located in the pelvis, femur, and humerus. Ewing's sarcomas originate in the nerve tissue within the bone marrow, located in the pelvis, humerus, ribs, and femur.

Page 176: *Suggested Answer*—

Nursing diagnosis: Deficient knowledge related to cast care

Goal: Client and significant other will care for cast correctly and report problems to health care provider for early intervention.

Interventions: Instruct client and caregiver on the following:

- Report increase in pain, decrease in movement, changes in color, coolness of fingers, loss of sensation, and/ or increased swelling.
- Apply ice directly over fracture for first 24 hours.
- Elevate the cast on pillows and expose to air while drying.
- Check areas of skin at cast edges for skin breakdown, provide padding as needed.
- Do not place any objects in the cast; use a blowdryer on cool setting for itching.
- Report drainage or odor from cast.
- Wear a sling to support the arm.
- Keep cast dry; cover with a plastic bag during bathing.

Chapter 6

Page 191: *Suggested Answer*—Explain to the client that open-angle glaucoma is a treatable condition and that blindness is not an inevitable result. Careful physician monitoring of intraocular pressure along with strict compliance to the medical regimen (i.e., use of prescribed beta adrenergic eye drops, miotics, and/or carbonic anhydrase inhibitors) will preserve sight.

Page 192: *Suggested Answer*—Postoperative instructions should include the importance of strict compliance with the administration of prescribed eye drops, the need to leave the eye covered between administration of eye drops, the need to avoid bending over, and the importance of sleeping on the nonoperative side.

Page 196: *Suggested Answer*—The macula is an area in the center of the retina that receives light from the center of the visual field. It is the center of greatest visual acuity. Degeneration of the macula occurs when the outer layer of the retina deteriorates or "fails" and waste products build up. These waste products cause death of retinal cells and loss of vision.

Page 197: *Suggested Answer*—Retinal detachment occurs when the retina (the inner layer of the eye) pulls away from the choroid (the middle layer of the eye). The retina is the sensory part of the eye that is essential for sight. When it separates, damage and/or death occurs to the nerve cells and loss of vision occurs. Retinal detachment is a medical emergency and requires surgical correction. However, surgical procedures like scleral buckling along with photocoagulation can reattach the retina and preserve sight.

Page 202: *Suggested Answer*—The nurse should urge the mother to avoid allowing the child to lie down while drinking from a bottle since this position increases the risk of acute otitis media. In addition, the mother should be advised that exposure to tobacco smoke in the home poses risks for otitis media.

Page 209: *Suggested Answer*—The nurse should discuss with the client the availability of various types of speech generators as well as the possibility of learning esophageal speech. Surgical procedures to restore speech such as tracheoesophageal puncture (TEP) in conjunction with a prosthesis are also available.

Chapter 7

Page 220: *Suggested Answer*—Although the indigestion of GERD and that associated with a heart attack can feel very similar, angina usually feels like a tightness or heaviness, associated with shortness of breath, sweating, lightheadedness, and sometimes nausea. The discomfort of GERD will be centered more around mealtime with stress and other factors increasing the acidity in the stomach. Instruct the client not to let indigestion unrelieved by medicine continue without seeking medical attention.

Page 222: *Suggested Answer*—Prevention of a peptic ulcer includes caution in the use of nonsteroidal anti-inflammatory drugs (NSAIDs), including acetylsalicylic acid (aspirin); avoiding excessive physiologic and psychologic stress; and avoiding cigarettes and too much caffeine. Additional risk factors are a positive family history for ulcers as well as type O blood. Clients should always know the side effects of any over-the-counter (OTC) and prescription medications, which could cause ulcers also. Consumption of spicy, hot foods in excess along with high stress levels add to the risk.

Page 225: *Suggested Answer*—Assessment criteria used for any client with possible dehydration are appropriate, including checking for skin turgor and sunken eyeballs, as well as observation for dryness of skin; dry mucous membranes; dark, amber urine with decreased output; and complaints of thirst. Lab data would include a high hematocrit level, increased blood urea nitrogen (BUN), increased specific gravity of urine, hypernatremia, and hypokalemia.

Page 228: *Suggested Answer*—An unrelieved obstruction that is accompanied by such significant symptoms needs immediate attention. The condition could worsen with increased distention, change in level of consciousness, electrolyte imbalances, and increased pain, especially if the bowel ruptures or peritonitis occurs.

Page 229: *Suggested Answer*—The lack of fever and normal WBC would help in determining a diagnosis of appendicitis. Rebound tenderness should be checked and an IV started. Without any further symptoms and no rebound tenderness, the condition may be only a stomach virus and the IV fluids will cause improvement in the pain within 24 hours. Remember, however, if appendicitis is an appropriate diagnosis, sudden cessation of the pain could mean the appendix ruptured.

Chapter 8

Page 245: *Suggested Answer*—Determination of ascites can be made through objective observation of the size and contour of the abdomen, weight gain, firmness to the abdomen, taunt skin over the abdomen, distant, low-pitched bowel sounds, intake greater than output, and daily increase in the measurement of the abdominal girth. Subjectively, the client may complain of fullness or back pain. Lab data should include: serum albumin, protein, electrolytes, and tests specific to the cause such as liver function tests for cirrhosis or hepatitis.

Page 245: *Suggested Answer*—In alcoholic (Laënnec's) cirrhosis, scarring of the liver occurs such as in biliary cirrhosis but there is also fat accumulation. Both of these (scarring and fat accumulation) cause a decrease in the function of the liver. The alcohol is transformed to acetaldehyde, which begins the process of altering hepatic function. The acetaldehyde inhibits the removal of proteins from the liver and alters metabolism of vitamins and minerals. Ammonia is unable to be metabolized, therefore a serum level is high in an alcoholic (hence the odor). Failure of the liver to work properly can lead to a GI bleed. An alcoholic often forfeits good meals for drinking either because of lack of appetite, lack of money (money spent on alcohol instead of food), or remaining in a stuporous state and failing to eat. Blood pressure (BP) elevates in the client because of portal hypertension and can often reach stroke range.

Page 248: *Suggested Answer*—Hepatitis A and E can be prevented by avoiding contaminated food and water, by avoiding situations in which one might come in contact with food handlers who do not use the necessary precautions. The client also should avoid contact with possibly contaminated shellfish. Hepatitis B, C, and D may be avoided by preventing contact with contaminated blood and body fluids. This includes needles, syringes, pooled blood, and unprotected sexual activity. A vaccine for hepatitis A and B is available for prophylaxis. Immunoglobulin may be given after exposure to hepatitis A, B, and D.

Page 250: *Suggested Answer*—Nursing diagnoses would include Pain, Imbalanced nutrition: less than body requirements, and Risk for fluid volume deficit. If cholecystitis occurs and surgery is necessary, additional diagnoses would be: Risk for infection; Impaired skin integrity; and Risk for impaired gas exchange. Nursing interventions would include keeping the client NPO, administering pain medication as needed, administering oral bile acids or dissolvers, monitoring lab work, assessing for pain, stool characteristics, GI complaints, and nutritional status. Teaching should be instituted when appropriate about eating less fat-containing foods and losing weight.

Page 254: *Suggested Answer*—Because these three diagnoses have similar elevated lab work, the nurse should be able to differentiate specific symptoms and lab work related to each.

Cholecystitis: A classic symptom is pain radiating to the back or right shoulder, intolerance to fat-containing foods, and fever. Remember, *-itis* signifies inflammation, and fever is usu-

ally present. Lab work specific for cholecystitis is elevated direct bilirubin and alkaline phosphatase with a normal serum amylase.

Pancreatitis: A classic symptom is pain that radiates to the back and is relieved by sitting up, leaning forward, flexing the left leg, or by walking, and fever. Classic lab work is an elevated amylase and lipase level.

Cirrhosis: Pain is usually not present, but ascites are characteristic as are spider angiomas, palmar erythema, and hepatomegaly. Specific lab work indicating cirrhosis are elevated liver function tests (alanine aminotransferase [ALT], aspartate aminotransferase [AST], alkaline phosphatase, gamma-glutamyl transpeptidase [GGT]).

The symptoms of jaundice and clay-colored stools can be present in all three as well as an elevated bilirubin level.

Chapter 9

Page 273: *Suggested Answer*—Essential information to provide the client newly diagnosed with hypothyroidism includes the following:

- Take thyroid medications as prescribed; do not abruptly discontinue.
- Take medications 1 hour before or 2 hours after meals for optimal absorption.
- Monitor weight and report changes as instructed.
- Do not use iodized salt or drugs containing iodine.
- Avoid excessive intake of foods such as cabbage, turnips, spinach, and carrots because these foods inhibit the thyroid hormone (TH) utilization.
- Consume adequate fluids, at least 2000 mL, or as prescribed.
- Consume a high-fiber diet to avoid constipation.
- Obtain adequate rest.
- Maintain skin integrity by proper care of dry skin.

Page 274: *Suggested Answer*—Because there is a high risk of damage to the parathyroid glands during a thyroidectomy, the client should be monitored for hypoparathyroidism. Manifestations are attributed to hypocalcemia and include tetany, muscle spasms, positive Chvostek's sign, positive Trousseau's sign, a decreased serum calcium level, and increased serum phosphorus level.

Page 278: *Suggested Answer*—Fluid volume excess is a complication of Cushing's syndrome as a result of excess cortisol which leads to sodium and water reabsorption. Interventions would include the following actions:

- Weigh client daily at the same time, using the same scale.
- Measure and record intake and output every 8 hours; compare with previous 72 hour totals to identify trends.
- Monitor heart rate, blood pressure, respirations, lung sounds.
- Assess for jugular vein distention and peripheral edema.
- Educate client about fluid restriction as prescribed.

Page 279: *Suggested Answer*—In Addison's disease, an insufficient amount of glucocorticoids and mineralocorticoids leads to fluid volume deficit, hyperkalemia, and hyponatremia. Instructions on nutritional management of Addison's disease would include the following:

- Consume a diet high in sodium and low in potassium; high-potassium foods to avoid include fruits, vegetables, chicken, liver, tuna, turkey.
- Consume at least 3000 mL of fluid daily, or as prescribed.
- Do not skip meals.
- Weigh self daily and report changes as instructed.

Page 284: *Suggested Answer*—Chronic diabetes insipidus will require lifelong replacement of antidiuretic hormone (ADH). Failure to replace the water loss can result in severe hypovolemia and hypernatremia. Instructions would include the following information:

- Treatment is lifelong.
- Take antidiuretic hormone as prescribed.
- Consume fluids as prescribed.
- Wear Medic-Alert bracelet.
- Signs and symptoms of diabetes insipidus.

Chapter 10

Page 299: *Suggested Answer*—Obtain history of present illness: duration of symptoms, history of kidney stones, previous UTI, kidney or bladder disease; past history of diabetes, hypertension, allergies, pregnancy; last menstrual period, use of birth control methods, date of last sexual contact, history of new sex partner; assess recent medication use including antibiotics; family history of kidney disorders; inquire about diet: caffeine or carbonated drinks and water intake. Instructions should include the following: take medication as prescribed; explain indications of medications and side effects; increase water intake to at least 8 glasses of water per day; avoid food or beverages that contribute to urine acidity, which may promote bacterial growth; explain the importance of follow up urinalysis to assure resolution of infection; and teach women hygiene measures to prevent contamination or irritation.

Page 301: *Suggested Answer*—Teach the client what factors increase the risk of stone formation (male, Caucasian race, prior or family history, medications such as vitamins A, C, and D, antacids with calcium, gout) and what they can do to minimize this risk; emphasize increasing fluid intake and dietary restrictions (such as limiting foods high in vitamin D, calcium, purines, oxalate, acidic and alkaline foods) to prevent further stone formation; teach the client regarding signs and symptoms of urinary tract infection; demonstrate how to strain all urine and save any stones for further analysis.

Page 302: *Suggested Answer*—Polycystic kidney disease is a hereditary disease and causes cysts to form in the kidney thereby causing the kidney to enlarge; these cysts may form a blockage of the kidney causing destruction of the kidney tissue; common symptoms include flank pain, blood in the urine, infection, and stones.

Page 304: *Suggested Answer*—Glomerular filtration rate is the amount of fluid filtered from the blood into the capsule per minute; this rate is influenced by three factors: total surface area available for filtration, permeability of the filtration membrane and the net filtration pressure; the normal GFR in both kidneys is 120 to 125 mL/min in adults; one advantage of a high GFR is that it allows the kidneys to rapidly filter waste products from the body and it allows the body fluid to be filtered and processed by the kidney many times a day; glomerulonephritis causes a decreased GFR which leads to azotemia and activation of the RAA system; this in turn causes sodium and water retention and edema.

Page 310: *Suggested Answer*—Fluids are usually limited in CRF, especially if dialysis is being done; the more fluid consumed, the sooner dialysis will be needed and edema will be evident; the client should be educated on the amount of fluid allowed in a 24-hour period and plan with the client how this will be distributed, accounting for medicine administration; provide an explanation that fluids are usually offered based on total allowance rather than randomly with each meal; explain that research has indicated that lowering protein in CRF slows the progression of the disease and decreases common signs of uremia such as anorexia, nausea, and vomiting.

Chapter 11

Page 322: *Suggested Answer*—There is a familial tendency to develop hypospadias, but no gene has yet been identified. Therefore, the client's sons may, but the risk is less than 50 percent. Assurance should be given to the parents that if the son does have the condition, surgery can be performed to correct the situation.

Page 324: *Suggested Answer*—Nonsteroidal anti-inflammatory drugs (NSAIDs) should have been discontinued 10 days preoperatively. Additionally, clients with BPH should avoid taking OTC allergy medications, as they can induce urinary retention from spasm of the bladder sphincter.

Page 327: *Suggested Answer*—Testicles are comprised of tiny tube-like structures (seminal vesicles and vas deferens). If a lumpectomy were performed, any cancer present would escape into the tube systems and begin growing there, thus spreading the cancer. The inguinal route of surgery allows the testicle to be removed intact and prevent cancer seeding into the tissues surrounding the tumor.

Page 332: *Suggested Answer*—Primary dysmenorrhea is the condition where menses are painful from menarche. This condition is caused by an excessive production of prostaglandins. Although fairly common, not every woman has this condition. Familial tendencies exist, therefore asking the client whether her mother and sisters have always had painful periods would be a better predictor.

Page 334: *Suggested Answer*—The first mammogram should be performed between the ages of 35 and 40, with yearly mammograms beginning at 40 according to the American Cancer Society's recommendations. She should have a mammogram now and yearly from this point on.

Page 336: *Suggested Answer*—Doxycycline is a tetracycline and therefore contraindicated during pregnancy (Pregnancy Category D drug). Tetracycline is known to cause discoloration of tooth enamel. A pregnancy test must be performed. If the client is pregnant, withhold the doxycycline and notify the provider of the client's pregnancy. Expect the provider to order a different medication such as azithromycin (Zithromax).

Chapter 12

Page 356: *Suggested Answer*—The nurse should know that allergies to dust, mold, grasses, pollens, and spores trigger a type I hypersensitivity response that is localized rather than systemic. Systemic type I hypersensitivity would lead to anaphylaxis. In a localized type I hypersensitivity, cell-bound IgE in the bronchial tree, nasal mucosa, and conjunctival tissues come in contact with the allergen and releases histamine and chemical mediators that produce the symptoms of asthma, rhinitis, and conjunctivitis. A good explanation for the mother is to inform her that small doses of the agent the child is allergic to will be given in order to help the body develop antibodies. These antibodies will then build the immune system so that her child will react less or perhaps not at all when the allergen is introduced. Calm her fears about a severe reaction by explaining that the dose is usually diluted and will be slowly increased in strength to prevent major complications. Also inform her that the child will be monitored during the time immediately after receiving the injection for any complications.

Page 357: *Suggested Answer*—An autoimmune disease is when the body no longer recognizes self as self, but instead identifies and targets self as non-self. The basis of the immune system is that it has the ability to recognize self vs. non-self in order to target any foreign cell or particle. In essence, the body turns on itself in an autoimmune disease. In rejection of an organ tissue, the body recognizes the tissue as foreign and the immune system responds as it should to any foreign particle, rejecting its presence in the body. Although the desired outcome is for the body not to reject the tissue, the immune system is working correctly in this situation. Immunosuppressant drugs are given to stop the body from rejecting the donor organ tissue.

Page 357: *Suggested Answer*—The presence of antihistamines would prevent the test from producing true positive or negative results. When an allergen comes in contact with the individual, the response is for the immune system to release histamine and other chemicals (inflammatory symptoms). If an antihistamine is on board, the release of histamine will be blocked and a reaction may not occur.

Page 359: *Suggested Answer*—The mildest and most common symptoms would be dry, itchy, red rash on the back of the hands and fingers. Blistering and weeping may occur along with swelling. These symptoms constitute an irritant contact dermatitis. A true type I immediate hypersensitivity reaction would occur within 5 to 30 minutes and stop when the gloves were removed. Immediate itching and swelling of the fingers or hand occurs. The gloves should not be snapped because the latex can adhere to the particles of starch powder inside the gloves and the inhalation of the powder aerosol may provoke symptoms also.

Page 360: *Suggested Answer*—Individuals exhibiting a true anaphylaxis are usually highly sensitive individuals and the reactions, which may be mild or severe, develop in minutes, are almost instantaneous. Second, anaphylactic shock is always a potential concern for anyone exhibiting anaphylactic symptoms. The effects may involve the respiratory or cardiac system along with vasodilation and fluid loss from the vascular system.

Page 364: *Suggested Answer*—In a client who has been exposed to HIV, antibodies may not be produced for 6 weeks to 6 months after the initial infection (known as seroconversion). The ELISA test identifies HIV antibodies. Therefore, depending on the timing of infection and antibody production, an ELISA may return negative initially but return positive later on. Hence, a second ELISA is often conducted to confirm a suspicion of positive HIV results. To actually confirm the diagnosis of positive HIV, a Western blot antibody test, which is more reliable than ELISA, is conducted once a positive ELISA has been obtained.

Chapter 13

Page 376: *Suggested Answer*—Clients with immune deficiency disorders, clients receiving chemotherapy, or clients receiving long-term corticosteroid therapy are often those who contract opportunistic infections. In all of these states, the immune system, which normally defends against pathogens, is suppressed and unable to perform normally.

Page 382: *Suggested Answer*—Some viruses enter the host cell and insert their genome into the chromosome of the host, remaining in a latent, nonreplicative state for long periods of time. A virus can remain communicable during recurrence. Stress increases the recurrence of latent or recurrent viruses. The lack of symptoms may be problematic in that the client is contagious and does not know it. Also, a virus can recur and be more virulent than the first time, without a cure.

Page 383: *Suggested Answer*—Bacteria may be described as cocci (spherical), bacilli (rod-shaped), clavate (club-shaped), or spirochetal (corkscrew-shaped). Staining characteristics include Gram-positive or Gram-negative characteristics. Typically, Gram-negative organisms are more virulent. Bacteria may also be classified as aerobic (requiring oxygen) or anerobic (not needing oxygen).

Page 389: *Suggested Answer*—Corticosteroids are immunosuppressant and therefore enhance the growth of fungal skin infections. A fungal infection as well as tuberculosis will be exaccerbated if a corticosteroid is used.

Page 395: *Suggested Answer*—Intestinal obstruction can occur with helminth infestation and can be a life-threatening event. The organisms may also affect other organs: cestodes (brain), nematodes (alveoli), trematodes (blood vessels, intestines, liver, or lungs).

Chapter 14

Page 409: *Suggested Answer*—Sunburn is a minor burn injury of the superficial layer of the skin. Sporadic, intense sunburns are more damaging to the skin than everyday exposure with use of a sunscreen. Use of sunscreens and limiting sun exposure to the less hazardous hours of the day (before 10:00 A.M. and after 3:00 P.M.) can prevent sunburn. Recurrent sunburn can lead to other skin disorders such as early skin aging, seborrheic keratosis, basal and squamous cell carcinoma, and malignant melanoma.

Page 412: *Suggested Answer*—Instruct the client to wash the skin with a mild soap and water at least twice a day to remove accumulated oils. Eat a regular, well-balanced diet. Exposing the skin to sun may help but sunburns should be avoided; get regular exercise and sleep. Do not squeeze the pimple; this causes the material to go deeper into the skin and usually the pimple gets larger and infected. The client should be instructed to be patient because treatment for acne can take months for a noticeable difference.

Page 414: *Suggested Answer*—Stress the importance of good nutrition and cleanliness through good handwashing and proper disposal of dressings. Teach the client never to squeeze or try to open the infected area. Teach the client signs and symptoms that should be reported to a health care provider such as fever, swelling, redness, pain, and drainage. Teach the importance of taking the full course of medication that has been prescribed.

Page 419: *Suggested Answer*—HSV 2 is a herpes simplex virus that usually involves the genitalia and skin below the waist in sexually active individuals. Explain the natural history of the disease with emphasis on recurrent episodes, asymptomatic viral shedding, and sexual transmission. Antiviral therapy can be used on an episodic basis or as suppressive therapy. Stress the importance of use of condoms during sexual intercourse, but the need to abstain from all sexual activity when lesions or prodromal symptoms are present.

Page 419: *Suggested Answer*—Do not share linens; use a clean towel and washcloth daily. Carefully dry between the toes. Do not wear the same pair of shoes every day, and avoid wearing rubber or plastic-soled shoes. Wear cotton socks that are changed frequently. Educate on the use of talcum powder and that over-the-counter fungal powder/spray should be used twice daily or prescribed medication for at least 2 weeks even though the symptoms have disappeared. Inquire if others in the family have the same symptoms. Educate on cleaning bathing surfaces after each bath/shower.

Chapter 15

Page 438: *Suggested Answer*—Since the client is in his nadir period, he is experiencing pancytopenia with all of his blood counts being affected. He is at high risk for infection and will require education on a neutropenic diet, limiting exposure to others, taking his temperature orally every four hours, and the importance of hand-washing, especially after toileting. The client is also at risk for hemorrhage, secondary to a low platelet count. The client should be educated to avoid aspirin and aspirin-containing products, avoid straining to have a bowel movement, and use electric razors while shaving. He can expect frequent lab work, transfusions with red cells and platelets, as well as possible antibiotic and antifungal administration.

Page 442: *Suggested Answer*—Both Hodgkin's and non-Hodgkin's arise from the lymph nodes and then disseminate throughout the body. Hodgkin's disease usually affects younger people, while non-Hodgkin's lymphoma occurs in the middle to later years. The causative etiology for both is unknown; however, chemical exposure may be a causative agent. Hodgkin's disease is classified by the presence of Reed-Sternberg cells, which don't occur in non-Hodgkin's lymphoma. Both clients are diagnosed by lymph node biopsy. Depending on bone marrow invasion, both clients are at risk for infection and bleeding. Depending on the stage of the disease, the client may need surgery only, surgery and radiation, therapy, or surgery, radiation, and chemotherapy. The chemotherapeutic protocols are unique for each of the diagnoses.

Page 443: *Suggested Answer*—With bone involvement the client is at risk for developing hypercalcemia. The family needs to be educated on the importance of maintaining mobility and to ensure the client ambulates with assistance due to her increased risk for falling. The role of hydration also needs to be emphasized, and the family needs to be educated on the importance of an intake and output record. The family should understand the signs and symptoms of hypercalcemia, and the importance of reporting these to the client's physician. Finally, the family should be educated on the administration of long-acting morphine and the importance of administering it on a specific schedule to avoid breakthrough pain.

Page 446: *Suggested Answer*—Both platelets and factor VIII play an important role in clot formation; therefore, the client with a decreased platelet count is just as susceptible to hemorrhage as the client with a factor VIII deficiency. The client with thrombocytopenia is at greater risk for spontaneous hemorrhage, and the problem is usually treated with platelet transfusions, except in idiopathic thrombocytopenia papura (ITP), when the treatment of choice is steroid therapy. The client with factor VIII deficiency usually receives scheduled factor VIII infusions and is at greater risk of bleeding into the joints. Both clients need to be educated on bleeding and safety precautions.

Page 449: *Suggested Answer*—Both pernicious anemia and folic acid deficiency are macrocytic (megaloblastic) anemia. Pernicious anemia is caused by a deficiency in vitamin B_{12}, usually caused by a lack of intrinsic factor, while folic acid deficiency is caused by a deficiency of folic acid. Both present with a smooth, sore, beefy, red tongue, while pernicious anemia presents with paresthesias and prioception, which delineates it from folic acid deficiency.

Page 451: *Suggested Answer*—The nurse should educate the client and his parents about the importance of adequate hydration during their vacation since dehydration will increase intravenous viscosity, triggering a crisis. The client should also be encouraged to take rest breaks while at any water or amusement parks, since extreme body heat and excessive exercise can trigger an event. Since high altitude can trigger a sickling episode, the nurse should discuss the feasibility of using ground transportation to get to the vacation destination.

Chapter 16

Page 462: *Suggested Answer*—The pedigree can demonstrate the risk for congenital defects in future offspring. The pedigree can also establish patterns of inheritance and what diseases the family is prone to develop.

Page 465: *Suggested Answer*—The child with Down syndrome is following the same pattern of development as peers of a similar age, but at a slower pace. The family needs anticipatory guidance as the child nears each phase of development. Erickson's stages of development can still be identified and need the same attention. Helping the client deal with social concerns as well as sexual questions should consist of fair treatment.

Page 465: *Suggested Answer*—There are three known types of chromosome 21 abnormalities; nondisjunction, translocation, and mosaicism. Translocation has a 5 to 15% chance of reoccurrence and should be considered in future family planning. Prevention of another child with trisomy 21 may be an option.

Page 466: *Suggested Answer*—The adolescent with Turner syndrome has no development of secondary sex characteristics and growth is below standard level. Because these clinical manifestations don't occur until adolescence, the diagnosis and treatment may be delayed.

Page 468: *Suggested Answer*—Nondisjunction is an abnormal separation during meiosis. This can lead to interference with fetal development. In nondisjunction, one zygote receives too many alleles and the other too few. Examples are trisomy 21, monosomy in Turner's syndrome, and Klinefelter's syndrome (which can be trisomy or multiple additions of X and possibly Y). In particular, Klinefelter's syndrome is an X-linked de-

fect with one or more extra X chromosomes in a genotype; e.g., XXY, XXXY.

Page 470: *Suggested Answer*—Refer to Figure 16-2 (p. 468) for autosomal recessive patterns. The risk of having children with PKU is 1:4, 2:4 risk of being carriers, and 1:4 risk being normal.

Page 472: *Suggested Answer*—At present there is no cure for Huntington's and no predictor of when symptoms will begin. If a client knows he or she has a disease, but no control over when and how it will develop, it can be an overwhelming piece of information. Yet a client has the right in family planning to know what might potentially be passed along to his or her children.

Page 479: *Suggested Answer*—The newborn with biuvula has a cleft palate that could possibly go undetected. The child with a cleft needs to be referred for treatment and prevent complications such as otitis media, aspiration, and speech impairment. Sometimes the biuvula is the only obvious physical characteristic.

Chapter 17

Page 496: *Suggested Answer*—In the absence of illness or injury, a woman in the childbearing years would have the predisposing risk factor of utilizing tampons for menstruation. A thorough assessment of recent menstruation and sanitary product utilization would be indicated. The concern for toxic shock syndrome is high in light of her age.

Page 500: *Suggested Answer*—Arterial blood gases (ABGs) are the most accurate measure of progressing shock. All forms of shock are a syndrome that result in inadequate perfusion and oxygenation of tissues. As shock progresses, anaerobic respiration replaces aerobic. Lactic acid production builds, causing metabolic acidosis. ABGs measure the pH of the blood. Other tests that may be ordered are creatinine phospholinase (CPK) and isoenzymes and troponin level, but these determine heart damage, not shock.

Page 503: *Suggested Answer or CHF*—A broad-spectrum antibiotic is usually begun initially as soon as the diagnosis is made. A narrow-spectrum antibiotic cannot be initiated until the culture and sensitivity returns, which then confirms the actual diagnosis. It is imperative to collect all cultures prior to the start of any antibiotic. Failure to collect all specimens can and most likely will result in improper treatment or incorrect diagnosis.

Page 510: *Suggested Answer*—An open hemothorax is suspected. A bullet wound provides an opening to the outside atmosphere so the development of a tension pneumothorax is possible. A tension pneumothorax is a life-threatening medical emergency. Bleeding within the pleural space could provide a significant source of hemorrhage so the shock state is hypovolemic in nature.

Page 511: *Suggested Answer*—Swelling from edema and bleeding may create a tourniquet-like effect, creating compartment syndrome. The nurse should assess circulation to the lower arm: pulses, capillary refill, color of extremities, and have client rank his or her pain. The physician should be notified immediately so that the casts can be removed or the client may need surgery.

Page 512: *Suggested Answer*—Necessary staff should be summoned including additional nursing support, as well as respiratory and radiology personnel. In a smaller institution or one that has on-call personnel, a representative from neurology and perhaps radiology should be made available. Resuscitative equipment should be ready including airway management equipment; an intravenous line should be primed and ready to infuse; cardiac monitor readied; suction available; a catheterization tray on hand; and typical wound care supplies available. Although most trauma rooms will be stocked with these supplies, a quick survey decreases time once the client arrives.

Page 514: *Suggested Answer*—A D-dimer test is indicated for a differential diagnosis. This test measures fragments, which elevate in response to clot breakdown. A steady increase in these values indicates ongoing clot breakdown rather than a lack of clotting factors.

Page 516: *Suggested Answer*—ARDS often occurs suddenly and is extremely fatiguing for the client. A client already stressed because of an acute MI doesn't need the additional respiratory stress, nor can the body tolerate extreme respiratory difficulty for long periods. Insufficient oxygenation coupled with a heart that has impaired circulation could be fatal. Treatment should be quick in order to prevent further complications.

▶ Case Study Suggested Answers

Chapter 1

1. The mother should be given an explanation as to what each drug does and any specific side effects. The montelukast (Singulair) carries few side effects, headaches being the most common. Stress to the mother that this medication should be taken every day regardless of the event of an asthma attack. Explain the difference between the maintenance inhaler nedocromil (Tilade) and the rescue inhaler albuterol (Ventolin). Be sure the mother understands that the maintenance drug is given every day and the albuterol is given only if an attack occurs and should be used immediately. If the attack does not stop within 30 to 60 minutes, the albuterol drops plus saline can be used via nebulization. Specific instructions on using a nebulizer and mixing the saline with albuterol should be given to the mother before discharge. The rescue inhaler as well as the nebulizer can cause extreme nervousness in clients. An explanation should be given on how to use the inhaler (complete exhalation; administering the correct number of puffs while inhaling to the count of 10), correctly cleaning the mouthpiece, and checking for fullness of the canister (if empty, the canister will float; if half full, it will sink halfway; if full, it will sink completely).

2. Explain to the mother that asthma is an inflammation of the airways that leads to constriction (or closing) of the bronchi, but this constriction is reversible with medications. The closing of the bronchi causes clients to feel like they cannot get enough air, which can be very frightening. The wheezing that can be heard when these clients breathe is also due to the closing of the bronchi; the air is trying to pass through a smaller opening than usual.

3. Usually the physician will give specific instructions on when to seek medical attention. However, standard protocol is to seek treatment when first the rescue inhaler and then the nebulizer have been used without any results. If the physician allows more than one nebulizer treatment, encourage the mother to give the allowed number of treatments before seeking immediate attention; explain that some attacks may take longer to stop than others. However, any time the child is having more frequent or more severe attacks, a physician should examine the child. Also, if attacks are occurring right after another or an attack is prolonged (status asthmaticus), immediate attention is necessary.

4. The child should be given a brief explanation of what asthma is in terms he or she can understand. If the child is extremely anxious during an attack, assurance should be given that he or she will always be able to breathe, but may not be able to get a good, deep breath. Address the child's fears and allow the child to voice his or her concerns. Explain that the higher the anxiety level, the more difficult it is to breathe.

5. Triggers are stimuli that produce the initial inflammatory response that proceeds to the asthma attack, causing mucosal edema, mucous secretion, and inflammation of the airways. Triggers cause the bronchospasm and can be specific allergies (mold, dust, pollen, etc.) or such things as cold air, strong odors, high altitude, intense exercise, and emotional stress. An individual may also find other unusual triggers that are not common to all people with asthma.

Chapter 2

1. Begin by assessing the ABCs—airway, breathing, and circulation. He has an open airway and is breathing adequately. Assess his circulation by checking his pulse (apical and radial) and blood pressure and placing him on the monitor to assess his heart rhythm. Assess the level of pain on a pain scale of 1 to 10, with 10 being the worst pain. Assess the duration and location of the pain (does it radiate?) and have the client describe the pain in his own words. Listen to his heart sounds; note any abnormal sounds such as murmur, friction rub, or S_3 or S_4 gallops. Assess his skin color and temperature; note capillary re-

fill (should be less than 3 seconds). Listen to his lung fields anteriorly and posteriorly for crackle, rhonchi, or wheezes. Note any labored respirations or use of accessory muscles and ask whether he feels short of breath. Assess his abdomen and extremities for signs of swelling. Assess distal pulses.

2. The nurse would ask if he has had prior history of cardiac disease or episodes of angina, any previous heart attack, or history of coronary artery disease. Does he have a history of hypertension, hypercholesterolemia, or hyperlipidemia? The nurse needs to assess if he has a strong family history of cardiac problems. Is he diabetic? Has he ever had previous ECGs done and where? Who is his family doctor and does he have a cardiologist?

3. Laboratory data would include troponin, CK-MB, CBC with differential, complete chemistries (electrolytes, glucose, BUN/Cr, liver functions), PT and PTT, as well as a chest x-ray and 12-lead ECG at bedside. If necessary, ABGs or continuous pulse oxymetry may be ordered.

4. Possible medications ordered include nitroglycerin (Nitrostat, NTG) sublingual 0.4 mg or nitroglycerin IV drip, titrated to pain and/or systolic blood pressure of 100 mmHg; nitrol paste (Nitro-Dur) 1 or 2 inches to chest wall; acetylsalicylic acid (aspirin) as an antiplatelet drug to prevent clots; and morphine sulfate 2 to 5 mg IV push if nitroglycerin is not effective in relieving chest pain or if BP is too low. After the initial chest pains are relieved, a beta blocker, nitrate, and/or calcium channel blocker would probably be ordered.

5. The nurse should look for inverted T waves and depressed S-T segments as a sign of ischemia; elevated S-T segments as a sign of injury; Q waves in two contiguous leads as a sign of infarct of undetermined age; tachycardia that may be present because of the effects of pain and anxiety; any abnormal rhythm or ectopic beats such as PVCs as a sign of irritability.

Chapter 3

1. Since the client has had several colds, the health care provider should assess what medications, both prescription and over-the-counter (OTC), the client took during these periods of illness and whether they are still being taken. Many OTC products can cause an increase in blood pressure. Second, data should be collected on whether the client has ever had a sudden increase in BP before; if so, what was the reason (if known), and what was done about it? It is always suggested to verify that the client is indeed compliant with medicine administration and diet. It would be helpful to know if a family member has been visiting the health care provider with the client in order to relay accurate information. Last, verify that the instructions about correct dose and time of administration are being followed by the client.

2. The family and client should be counseled on what is meant by a high blood pressure value and the possible complications (stroke, death, etc.). If medications are not being taken correctly, educate on each medication—what it is for, how much should be taken, and setting up a dosing schedule that meets the needs of the client. Explain what side effects can occur and the consequences of skipping a dose. If diet is a concern, educate the client on low-sodium foods and the relationship of sodium to blood pressure. Using the readings from the Council on Aging, establish a normal range of blood pressure that is safe for the client. Be sure the family knows how to monitor the BP as well as when to report to a healthcare professional.

3. Essential information includes drug name, dosage, and time for administration, need to assess pulse and/or blood pressure prior to taking the medication, reason for taking the medication, and side effects that need to be reported to the health care provider. Report any chest pain or problems with respirations. Some medications require the client to move slowly when changing positions to avoid lightheadedness. Emphasis should be placed on not "making up" a missed medication; rather wait until the next time the medicine is due to take the dose prescribed unless instructed otherwise. Parameters for low pulse and blood pressure reading should be provided as well.

4. Priority of care is decreasing the blood pressure to a range acceptable for the client. Once this is established, priorities include:
   - Teaching the client and family about the medication regime.
   - Awareness of the possibility of compliance issues.
   - Assisting the client in maintaining compliance through clear instructions; make accommodations for clients with poor eyesight and those who are unable to read or speak English.
   - Implementing the plan to form a partnership with the client, the significant others, and the health team for support, information, and care.

5. Essential hypertension is usually from an unknown cause and is also termed primary hypertension. It occurs in a majority of hypertensive clients (about 95 percent). Secondary hypertension, on the other hand, is usually related to a disease process. Secondary hypertension is often easier to control because control of the disease will often regulate the blood pressure (BP). It is important to understand that in essential hypertension the left ventricle (the power chamber of the heart) must work harder to overcome the resistance it encounters when blood is pumped out. When the ventricle must continuously work hard, the muscle will hypertrophy (or stiffen); this can cause heart problems later on. When the heart is unable to adjust to the hypertension, the kidneys become involved in an effort to regulate the pressure. One of the serious concerns is that there are rarely obvious symptoms, and often there are no symptoms at all. A headache or nosebleed may occur when the pressure rises extremely high.

Chapter 4

1. Anticipated signs and symptoms of Parkinson's include resting tremors, stooped posture, masklike face, soft monotone voice, drooling, poor balance, shuffling propulsive gait, rigidity, insomnia, weight loss, constipation, depression, and dementia. In addition, the client might be withdrawn, uncooperative, and noncompliant because of his reluctance to be at the facility.

2. A priority nursing diagnosis for the client is Impaired physical mobility, as well as Risk for injury. The client with Parkinson's disease has difficulty initiating ambulation, is unsteady, and often has difficulty stopping and righting himself if he begins to fall. Safety should be a primary goal in the care of this client. Other diagnoses would include Self-care deficit; Imbalanced nutrition: less than body requirements; Risk for constipation; Noncompliance; Interrupted thought processes; Hopelessness; and Powerlessness.

3. It would be best to schedule his physical therapy to coincide with peak drug action. Planned rest periods should be a part of his daily routine to allow him to prevent fatigue and frustration during physical therapy. An explanation should be given to the client as to the importance of the physical therapy.

4. A good approach to handling the client with Parkinson's disease who has become upset would be to:
   - Acknowledge to him that you recognize he is frustrated and upset.
   - State that you are sorry if it seemed you were trying to rush him.
   - Encourage and praise him for his efforts to maintain independence. Stress that you recognize it is important for him.
   - Allow him as much time as he needs to dress.

5. Some specific instructions to assist with mobility problems are:
   - Daily exercise to maintain function: walking, swimming, stretching.
   - Stretching and posture exercises as suggested by physical therapy.
   - Take big steps and lift legs.
   - Think about stepping over an object for episodes of "freezing."

Chapter 5

1. Emergency nursing care for the client with a fracture includes:
   - Immobilizing the fracture: Anything sturdy can be used to immobilize the fractured area; belts can be used to secure the fracture to the hard surface. The extremity or limb should be placed in the same position on the area where it is to be immobilized.
   - Controlling any bleeding: Pressure should be held to control bleeding. If clean linens are available, these can be applied to the area. Firm pressure should be held constantly if an artery has been severed.
   - Cleaning the wound if there is an open fracture: Open fractures should be cleaned if possible and a moist, clean towel applied to keep the bone from drying.

2. The nurse should assess the 5 Ps: pain, paresthesia, pulses, pallor, and paralysis; elevate the extremity and apply ice during the first 24 hours; keep the cast open to air and supported on pillow to allow for drying; assess for signs and symptoms of compartment syndrome during the first 48 hours.

3. Provide instructions to client and caregivers regarding cast care and complications to report.
   - Report increase in pain, decrease in movement, changes in color, coolness of fingers, loss of sensation, and/ or increased swelling.
   - Apply ice directly over fracture for first 24 hours.
   - Elevate the cast on pillows and expose to air while drying.
   - Check areas of skin at cast edges for skin breakdown, provide padding as needed.
   - Do not place any objects in the cast; use a blow dryer on cool setting for itching.
   - Report drainage or odor from cast.
   - Wear a sling to support the arm.
   - Keep cast dry; cover with a plastic bag during bathing.
   - Instruct the client to expect pain, especially during the first 24 to 48 hours. The client should also be instructed to use pain medicine at the first sign of pain and avoid waiting since this makes pain control more difficult.

4. Compartment syndrome is usually the reason for excruciating pain after 48 hours. Even with a crushing fracture, pain will begin to decrease within 48 hours if a cast has been applied and the area is immobilized. Swelling and pressure account for the excruciating pain and should be relieved immediately.

5. Notify the physician immediately. The cast will need to be removed to assess the limb. Then elevate the extremity and apply ice to relieve the edema. Next, assist with bivalving the cast or prepare client for fasciotomy as indicated. Usually, the relief of the edema and pressure relieves the pain. If not, analgesics should be administered. Remember to obtain a surgical permit before medication is administered in the event of surgery. An explanation of the problem should be given to the client and family, especially if pain medicine is being held.

Chapter 6

1. Assessment findings in acute Ménière's disease include the symptoms outlined in the case study as well as hypotension, diaphoresis, and nystagmus. The vertigo may be so severe that the client becomes immobilized and may even fall to the floor.

2. Medical interventions for acute attacks may include the use of anticholinergics (i.e., scopolamine [Isopto

Hyoscine], atropine [Isopto Atropine]), antiemetics (i.e., prochlorperazine [Compazine], meclizine [Antivert]), and central nervous system (CNS) depressants (i.e., diazepam [Valium]) to control the nausea, vomiting, and symptoms of motion sickness. Bedrest should be initiated as well as fluid and electrolyte replacement if necessary.

3. Diagnostic tests include audiometry, x-rays, and computed tomography (CT) scans of the vestible, and an electronystagmography (ENG) test battery including caloric ice water testing. In addition, an auditory dehydration test that uses glycerine or fast-acting diuretics to dehydrate the inner ear is often used. Acute, temporary improvement in symptoms following this test is considered diagnostic of Ménière's disease.

4. Ménière's disease is a chronic disorder of the inner ear that presents with three major symptoms: dizziness (vertigo), ringing in the ears (tinnitus), and hearing loss. The cause of the disorder is unknown and usually affects only one ear. The symptoms appear to be caused by the accumulation of fluid in a part of the inner ear known as the membranous labyrinth. Factors that cause acute symptoms include increased sodium intake, stress, allergies, and premenstrual fluid retention.

5. Discharge instructions for clients with Ménière's disease should include:
   - The signs of impending attacks (i.e., feeling of fullness in the ear, increasing tinnitus, dizziness, nausea, and/or vomiting).
   - Avoidance of attack triggers (i.e., stress, fatigue, blinking lights, loud noises, and/or quick or jerky body movements).
   - The need for adequate rest and sleep as well as relaxation techniques.
   - Safety measures to utilize if attacks occur while driving.
   - Sodium-restricted diets.
   - The avoidance of substances causing vasoconstriction (i.e., tobacco, alcohol, and caffeine).

Chapter 7

1. Questions would include the following:
   - What caused you to come to the health facility?
   - Have you been vomiting? What other symptoms have you had? When did these start?
   - How many bowel movements do you usually have a day?
   - Have you had this problem before?
   - What are your usual dietary habits?
   - How much weight have you lost? Over what period of time?
   - Are you able to care for yourself?
   - Have you noticed blood or mucus in your bowel movements?
2. Objective data should include observation of color, consistency, and character of stools; level of pain; relationship between diarrhea and mealtime; abdominal palpation to determine areas of tenderness; check for rebound tenderness as an indication of peritonitis or appendicitis; monitor hemoglobin, hematocrit, WBC, serum Na, K, and Cl.

3. Social history information that would assist in her plan of care would be identification of job or family stress; use of cigarettes or alcohol; and presence of family or support systems. Stress factors have been known to aggravate the exacerbation of symptoms. Cigarettes and alcohol also are aggravating symptoms. The client will need to depend on family and/or social support systems as a part of her adjustment to home care.

4. Nursing measures would include administering antidiarrheal medications as ordered, teaching good skin care, monitoring and encouraging fluid intake, being sure the client has easy access to the bedpan or bathroom, supplying room deodorizers as necessary, and weighing the client daily.

5. Other nursing measures include administering corticosteroid or immunosuppressive drugs as ordered, implementing a low-fiber diet, promoting rest, using antianxiety measures (planned rest periods, decreasing excess stimuli if pain medicine is administered, allowing privacy if diarrhea occurs), and preparing for surgery if indicated. In addition, client education should be given on what the illness is, complications that can occur and prevention techniques, type of medications used and possible side effects, and how to lower stress.

Chapter 8

1. The risk factors present for pancreatic cancer in this client are age and cigarette smoking. Other risk factors include industrial chemicals, environmental toxin exposure, high-fat diet, pancreatitis, and diabetes mellitus.
2. The likely location of the pancreatic tumor based upon the symptoms of pain when supine, jaundice, and weight loss, is the body of the pancreas. The jaundice could be significant of cancer of the head of the pancreas, but the pain when supine does not correlate. There are usually no symptoms if the cancer is in the tail of the pancreas.
3. The primary preoperative nursing interventions are:
   - Evaluate physical and psychological status. Create a collaborative care plan, which includes physical, psychological, and spiritual interventions.
   - Determine client's acuity level.
   - Provide a teaching plan for client and family for postoperative care.
   - Explain that client may be cared for in the intensive care unit for a period of time.
   - Provide comfort measures through proper positioning and administration of pain medication as needed.
   - Monitor and maintain nausea and vomiting.
   - Assess lab work as ordered.
4. The primary postoperative nursing interventions are:
   - Monitor respiratory status.

- Monitor renal output.
- Monitor cardiac status.
- Prevent wound infections.
- Maintain patency of the gastric suction.
- Administer pain medications at regular intervals.
- Monitor blood chemistries.
- Watch for complications of hemorrhage, hypovolemic shock, and hepatorenal failure.

5. The prognosis for this client is poor—nearly all pancreatic cancer is fatal within the first year. 85 percent of cases are not diagnosed until too late because the symptoms are not specific and the onset is slow. Although this type of cancer is rare (3 to 4% of the cancers in United States), it is more likely to occur in adults between 50 and 70 years of age.

Chapter 9

1. Diabetes mellitus at a young age occurs when beta cells in the pancreas fail to work properly and do not control glucose (sugar) correctly. The glucose builds up in the bloodstream; this is called hyperglycemia. Normally, a certain amount of glucose is produced by the beta cells, then the body uses what glucose it needs and gets rid of what it doesn't need. With diabetes, the increased level of glucose spills into the urine. Glucose acts to draw fluid with it, resulting in increased urination and thirst. A third problem is hunger. The body needs insulin to use the carbohydrates, which our body needs for energy. The body finds other things for energy, like protein and fat and often any other stored nutrients, which causes the hungry feeling and results weight loss.

2. The most important symptoms are the 3 Ps (polyphagia, polyuria, polydipsia), the signs of hypoglycemia (nervousness, weakness, faint feeling, and possible coma), and the signs and symptoms of diabetic ketoacidosis (fruity breath, a change in respirations, extreme fatigue, nausea, and vomiting).

3. Although DM is often familial, it is considered an autoimmune disease and may occur without any family history. Explain what an autoimmune disease is and that diabetes at age 16 may be from genetics, environmental, or immunological factors. Calm the mother by including her in the teaching sessions and allowing her to ask questions and share concerns.

4. Explain what peak time means and what the time is for each type of insulin. Explain that the most likely time for a hypoglycemic reaction is 2 to 4 hours after taking regular insulin and 6 to 8 hours after taking NPH insulin. Be sure she understands that she has to consider both peak times if the medications are mixed in the morning.

5. The client will most likely experience symptoms of hyperglycemia. The goal of maintaining her glucose values within a normal range should be emphasized, especially since teenagers do not always eat healthy foods. Without scaring her, stress the long-term consequences of DM. At the same time, factors that affect her glucose level, such as exercise, over- or undereating, and stress, could cause her glucose to drop and therefore she should know the symptoms of hypoglycemia. Instructions should be given to her about taking candy, fruit, or a regular cola if her glucose level does drop, especially during school hours.

Chapter 10

1. L. J. is experiencing metabolic acidosis, which is common in ARF. Hydrogen ions, which are high in acidosis, are unable to be eliminated along with other metabolic wastes. Remember, if the pH is low, H^+ ions are high. The pH and bicarbonate are both low and the carbon dioxide is normal, which indicates metabolic acidosis.

2. The hyperkalemia could cause cardiac arrhythmias. The normal potassium level is 3.5 to 5.0 mEq/L and the heart does not tolerate values too low or too high.

3. L. J. is in the maintenance phase of ARF. Most of the signs and symptoms presented by L. J. are typical of this phase. The initial phase has very few manifestations and hopefully the recovery phase shows renal improvement. This phase should last from 1 to 2 weeks.

4. L. J. could possibly experience CHF or pulmonary edema. The edema, rales, and low urinary output are suggestive of these disorders. The strain placed on the heart by the ARF episode could also trigger a cardiovascular event.

5. The diet should not be high in sodium because of the retention of fluid being experienced by the client. The low sodium is of least concern in his present state. Sodium supplements may be used to exchange potassium, thereby increasing sodium and lowering potassium levels. The main dietary restriction is protein and high carbohydrates should be given to accommodate for the low proteins.

Chapter 11

1. General anesthesia is usually used. A low abdominal incision is made. The prostate is resected and lymph nodes are also obtained. If it appears that the prostate capsule has been invaded with cancer, additional tissue around the prostate may be removed. Postoperative pain medication is provided. An indwelling urinary catheter will be in place.

2. The pathology report of the tissue removed (the prostate gland, surrounding tissue if taken, and lymph nodes) reveals the extent of the disease. Additional scans may also be utilized to stage the disease.

3. Prostate cancer in the elderly is a very slow-growing cancer, and conservative treatment is utilized because of the expectation that the client's eventual demise will result from a cause other than the prostate cancer. The younger the client is at diagnosis, the more likely it is that the cancer is an aggressive form that will require more aggressive treatment. Another factor in determining what type

of anesthesia to use is based on the surgical procedure and the age of the client.

4. Radiation therapy and chemotherapy will most likely be required after the surgery.

5. Stage 3 prostate cancer indicates that the cancer is outside the capsule of the prostate and may also be in the seminal vesicles. It has not spread to the lymph nodes or other organs.

Chapter 12

1. Immediate assessment should focus on airway patency (respiratory rate, depth, lung sounds, any dyspnea or stridor). The client is exhibiting initial signs of possible anaphylaxis (type I hypersensitivity reaction). Although his blood pressure (BP) is within normal limits (WNL), it is on the lower side and with tachycardia, the nurse should be proactive at this time. The welts definitely indicate a localized reaction, and his anxiety may or may not be related to anaphylaxis. If the airway is not patent, oxygen should be administered and an oropharyngeal of nasopharyngeal airway instituted immediately.

2. The nurse should first determine what the client's normal BP range is and then identify how he reacted to bee stings in the past for comparison. If the client runs a much higher BP than this, the nurse may be concerned that hypotension is developing. Individuals allergic to a specific insect often react similarly when bitten or stung by other insects. This reaction may be typical for this client when venom is injected. If this response is exaggerated, the nurse should again be proactive and monitor the client closely. The reaction may be caused by the multiple stings of the hornets.

3. Drug therapy would involve topical and oral antihistamines and possibly corticosteroids. Epinephrine should be on hand for administration if airway management or severe edema presents.

4. The wife should be informed that her husband apparently has a type I hypersensitivity reaction to insect bites and stings (if he has presented with similar symptoms to bees) and that he probably always will respond in this fashion. Explain that each subsequent episode may be more exaggerated because the body has become sensitized to the allergen. Emphasize that the massive amount of welts is probably caused by the number of hornet stings, as hornets swarm and attack in large numbers. Calm the wife by explaining that the antihistamines will help with his symptoms and that he may be sleepy because of the antihistamines.

5. This client needs to be instructed on the following:
   • Have a "bee sting kit" available at all times, which includes a prefilled syringe of epinephrine (Epi-pen). The wife should be taught how to administer the Epi-pen. If the kit contains an inhaler, teach her on the use of the inhaler also.
   • Have antihistamine lotion and tablets available.

   • Have corticosteroid lotion available.
   • Teach her the symptoms of a true anaphylactic reaction and when to bring the client in by ambulance versus trying to drive him.
   • Discuss strategies to avoid allergens as much as possible.
   • Purchase a Medic-alert bracelet that should be worn at all times.
   • Encourage the wife to have an alternate plan if a local ambulance service is not available where she lives.
   • Demonstrate and have her return demonstrate steps to take when an anaphylactic reaction occurs: open the airway, place the client in high Fowler's position, count the respirations, calm the victim.

Chapter 13

1. This is classified as a nosocomial infection, hospital-acquired, and is probably related to the surgical procedure. Good handwashing and use of aseptic technique in changing the dressing are the best interventions.

2. A culture and sensitivity of the wound is the diagnostic test. If this is positive, an antibiotic showing sensitivity will be ordered. If this is negative, other tests will be ordered. Complete blood count (CBC), blood culture, and sensitivity, chest x-ray (CXR) to rule-out sepsis or pneumonia are recommended.

3. A white blood count (WBC) and differential should be analyzed. If an infection as described here is present, bacteria are the most likely cause. The WBC will probably be elevated with elevated neutrophils (since the onset is new).

4. Vancomycin (Vancocin) is the recommended treatment because it has bactericidal and bacteriostatic action. It interferes with cell membrane synthesis in multiplying organisms. It is active against both Gram-positive and Gram-negative organisms.

5. Neurotoxicity, ototoxicity, nephrotoxicity, fever, and chills are adverse effects. "Red neck syndrome" can be reduced by slowing the infusion.

6. Quinupristin and dalfopristin (Synercid); linezolid (Zyvox), or the synergistic effect of vancomycin (Vancocin) and gentamycin (Garamycin) are effective against vancomycin-resistant *Staphylococcus aureus* (VRSA). Daptomycin (Cubicin) is also effective with MRSA.

Chapter 14

1. The nurse should inquire as to when the eruption began, the appearance, and where the rash is located. Questions should be asked about any pain, itching, or burning around the area before the blisters appeared. The nurse should inquire about a history of chickenpox and any other medical diagnoses that may have compromised her immune status. A thorough review of all medications she is currently taking would be indicated, as some drugs also depress the immune system.

2. The nurse should thoroughly examine the skin for characteristic lesions and distribution. A determination should be made as to whether the involvement is dermatomal or unilateral and whether there is opthalmic involvement. If the eyes are involved, emergency treatment and referral is indicated. Assessment for pain management is also essential as this can be very painful, especially for an elderly client.

3. Herpes zoster is caused by a reactivation of the varicella virus (chickenpox) that remained dormant in the basal ganglia after an episode of chickenpox. It is a viral infection usually involving the skin of a single dermatome and usually resolves within about 2 weeks. An antiviral medication will be necessary to shorten the duration of the disease, help lessen the itching, and control the pain.

4. The goal of therapy is suppression of pain, inflammation, and infection. Use of over-the-counter nonsteroidal antiinflammatory drugs (NSAIDs) is recommended for pain and fever. Oral antiviral medications are available: valacyclovir HCL (Valtrex) 1 gm, 3 times a day for 7 days; famiciclovir (Famvir) 500 mg, three times a day for 7 days; and aysyekloever (Acyclovir) 800 mg, 5 times a day for 7 days. Antipruritic medications such as corticosteroids or antihistamines will decrease itching and scratching.

5. Wet compresses using Burow's solution or cool tap water can be used for a soothing effect. Avoid scratching the area to prevent secondary infection. Stress keeping follow-up appointments in 3 days and again a week later to monitor the disease. Fever, chills, increased pain, or drainage should be reported promptly. The client needs to isolate herself from neonates, pregnant women, and immunosuppressed persons. Explain that she is contagious to those persons who have never had chickenpox. The disease usually resolves, but there may be scarring at the site of the lesions.

Chapter 15

1. Nursing diagnoses should be prioritized as follows:
   - Risk for infection related to decreased circulating granulocytes secondary to acute lymphocytic leukemia and decreased ability to heal properly secondary to diabetes mellitus.
   - Risk for injury: bleeding related to decreased circulating platelets secondary to acute lymphocytic leukemia.
   - Ineffective airway clearance related to increased phlegm, decreased secondary defenses, prolonged bed rest, and age.
   - Altered nutrition: less than body requirements related to increased metabolism secondary to acute lymphocytic leukemia.
   - Altered oral mucous membranes related to the effect of chemotherapeutic medications and neutropenia.
   - Altered role performance related to recent cancer diagnosis.
   - Anticipatory grieving related to fear of impending death secondary to recent cancer diagnosis.

Since infection is the number one cause of death in these clients and the client's circulating granulocytes are decreased (Absolute granulocyte count [AGC] = 990), the risk for infection is more life threatening than the other diagnoses and therefore is listed first. Since she is already experiencing petechiae and her platelet count is decreased (12,000/mm^3), bleeding becomes the second most life-threatening complication and should be considered second. Her weight loss of 10 pounds makes Altered nutrition an important diagnosis.

2. The client's absolute granulocytes/neutrophil count (AGC or ANC) is extremely low. The AGC is calculated by taking the WBC (% bands + % segs) and normally should be greater than 1,000. In this case: 9,000 (0.01 + 0.10) = 990, makes the client extremely susceptible to opportunistic infection. When the client's granulocytes are decreased, the client will lose first line of defense against infection. Neutrophils are the first cells to arrive at a site of infection; they engulf the invading organism and trigger the inflammation response. These clients are highly susceptible to life-threatening infections and often don't produce the normal response to infection. Fever may be the only sign of infection in these clients.

3. Monitor for manifestations of infection, which include elevated temperature, chills, throat pain, chest pain, cough, burning on urination, rectal or vaginal itching or irritation. Monitor vital signs and oxygenation every four hours. Assess for temperature spikes with chills, tachypnea, tachycardia, restlessness, change in PaO$_2$, and hypotension. Although the body temperature is usually elevated in infection, clients with leukemia may have an altered response and sepsis may be present before abnormal vital signs occur. Hypotension is usually a late symptom of sepsis. The presence of yellow-colored sputum and redness to the Hickman catheter are concerning since these are significant signs of infection.

4. Part of the client's treatment protocol includes prednisone. Steroid therapy will cause an increase release of glycogen from the liver thereby increasing the glucose level in the blood. As a result, the client will require frequent glucose monitoring and sliding scale insulin to regulate her diabetes. This will create an increase in the number of invasive procedures, since both capillary blood glucose monitoring and insulin injects will require a needle stick. Because of the underlying leukemia diagnosis, the client is more susceptible to infection, and with her diabetes diagnosis, she is susceptible to delayed healing. The nurse should use meticulous skin preparation for this client, and keep capillary blood glucose testing to a minimum. The nurse may consider discussing accessing a blood sample from the Hickman, but due to the small sample required, the risk may outweigh the benefit.

5. Primary caregiver support and place of discharge needs to be determined early in the hospital stay. Many clients are discharged at the completion of their chemotherapy induction to nadir at home. Because this client's children are dispersed all over the country and her spouse travels a good deal with his job, the nurse should discuss how

the family plans to assist the client after discharge. The nurse also needs to begin teaching the primary caregiver about Hickman catheter maintenance as well as preparation of the home to decrease infection exposure. Subcutaneous injection technique also needs to be assessed since the client will be discharged on insulin as well as other medications such as filgrastim (Neupogen), epoetin alfa (Procrit), and daunorubicin (Cerubidine).

Chapter 16

1. Cystic fibrosis is a multisystem disease. Respiratory compromise, recurrent pneumonia, and failure to thrive (FTT) are all symptoms of cystic fibrosis. The client with cystic fibrosis has thick, increased viscosity of secretions, decreased ciliary function, decreased alveolar function and alveolar plugs that lead to repeat infections and long-term chronic obstructive pulmonary disease (COPD). *Pseudomonas* and *Staphylococcus* are the most common organisims and are often resistant to antibiotics. The gastrointestinal tract is also involved and malabsorption occurs due to blockage of the ducts leading from the pancreas to the duodenum. Fats and fat-soluble vitamins are not absorbed and malnutrition can occur. In an infant, this is manifested as failure to thrive.
2. The test most commonly performed to confirm cystic fibrosis is the sweat chloride test revealing an elevated sodium chloride level. The defective protein inhibits transport of sodium chloride and these electrolytes are excreated in the sweat. The nurse could also refer to pulmonary function tests to determine the level of respiratory compromise. Hypoxia is chronic because of the COPD and can lead to Cor pulmonale (right-sided congestive heart failure from a respiratory cause). Arterial blood gases (ABGs) or pulse oximetry are usually also conducted. In the newborn screen, a decreased trypsin in the stool indicates pancreatic insufficiency or cystic fibrosis.
3. Medications the nurse may administer would be bronchodilators such as albuterol (Ventolin), beclomethasone (Vanceril), and dornase alfa (Dnase). The Ventolin and Vanceril should aid in opening the lungs and improving respirations. The Dnase alters the mucous viscosity, which should allow greater ease in expectorating any secretions. Antibiotics may also be ordered. Other interventions include administering low dose oxygen, chest physiotherapy (CPT), and suctioning as needed.
4. The client with cystic fibrosis has plugging of the pancreatic duct, which leads to decrease in absorption of fats, carbohydrates, and protein. The malabsorption leads to failure to thrive.
5. The family needs to be able to perform CPT, respiratory aerosol treatments, and know the potential side effects of those treatments. The family also must be able to recognize the signs and symptoms of infection and respiratory distress. Teaching the client concerning signs of hypoxia and use of a pulse oximetry is useful to avoid frequent visits to a health care provider. The nurse should also stress the need to keep the child current on immunizations in order to avoid other diseases that may be exaggerated in cystic fibrosis. The nurse can review with the family what an autosomal recessive pattern is and if both parents are carriers what is the chance of reoccurrence. The family can also have the disease diagnosed in the prenatal and perinatal period.

Chapter 17

1. Fundamental interventions would include maintaining spinal alignment, providing supplemental oxygen and maintaining the airway. Initiation of two large bore cannulas, control of scalp hemorrhage, and laboratory/radiology testing to include arterial blood gases, complete blood count, chemistry panel (glucose), urinalysis, blood alcohol, type and crossmatch for donor specific blood and cervical spine, chest, hip, and pelvic x-rays. Further assessment of the client would include heart sounds, respiratory status, cardiac monitoring, peripheral pulses, complaints voiced by the client, especially chest or leg pain. A thorough head-to-toe assessment would then need to be made.
2. A thoracostomy (chest tube) may be inserted for the diagnosis of pneumothorax. A CT scan or MRI may be performed for possible brain injuries. A urinary catheter would also need to be inserted unless contraindicated.
3. The client is in the compensatory phase of hypovolemic shock. The rise in pulse and respiration, along with the change in level of consciousness are indications. ABGs indicate the level of cellular perfusion and acid-base balance that is affected by respiration at the cellular level. Hematocrit and hemoglobin levels are also useful in determining active blood loss for hypovolemic shock.
4. While the scalp is very vascular and will bleed profusely depending on the size of the laceration, the potential for pelvic and hip fractures constitute the greatest threat of hemorrhage from both the bone itself and the possible injury to great vessels in the femoral area. With a diagnosis of flail chest, the potential for a pneumothorax or hemothorax could contribute to the overall volume loss. The client could also suffer a cardiac contusion or a hematoma.
5. It is vitally important to maintain an accurate output recording, however, in the presence of pelvic or hip injury there may also be penetrating damage to the bladder. Bleeding from the meatus would indicate bladder trauma or actual urethral damage that would contraindicate the insertion of a urinary catheter.

Index

Pages numbers followed by b indicate box; those followed by f indicate figure; those followed by t indicate table.